.e Fro

SPORTS MEDICINE CONSULT

A Problem-Based Approach to Sports Medicine for the Primary Care Physician

SPORTS MEDICINE CONSULT

A Problem-Based Approach to Sports Medicine for the Primary Care Physician

BRIAN D. BUSCONI, MD

Associate Professor
Orthopedics and Physical Rehabilitation
Pediatrics, and Family Medicine and Community Health
University of Massachusetts Medical School
Worcester, Massachusetts
and
Chief, Sports Medicine and Arthroscopy
University of Massachusetts Memorial Medical Center
Director, Sports Medicine Center
University of Massachusetts Memorial Medical Center
Worcester, Massachusetts

J. HERBERT STEVENSON, MD

Director Sports Medicine Fellowship
Department of Family and Community Medicine
University of Massachusetts Medical School
Worcester, Massachusetts
and
Director Sports Medicine
Family and Community Medicine
University of Massachusetts Health Center
Worcester, Massachusetts

Wolters Kluwer | Lippincott Williams & Wilkins
Health

Philadelphia • Baltimore • New York • London
Buenos Aires • Hong Kong • Sydney • Tokyo

Acquisitions Editor: Robert Hurley
Managing Editor: Elise M. Paxson
Marketing Manager: Lisa Lawrence
Production Manager: Alicia Jackson
Designer: Stephen Druding
Compositor: Macmillan Publishing Solutions

© 2009 by LIPPINCOTT WILLIAMS & WILKINS, a WOLTERS KLUWER business

530 Walnut Street
Philadelphia, PA 19106 USA
LWW.com

Printed in China

13 digit ISBN: 978-0-7817-8720-8
10 digit ISBN: 0-7817-8720-3

Library of Congress Cataloging-in-Publication Data

Sports medicine consult : a problem-based approach to sports medicine for the primary care physician / [edited by] Brian D. Busconi, J. Herbert Stevenson.
    p. ; cm.
Includes bibliographical references and index.
ISBN 978-0-7817-8720-8 (alk. paper)
 1. Sports medicine—Handbooks, manuals, etc. 2. Primary care (Medicine)—Handbooks, manuals, etc.
 3. Medical consultation—Handbooks, manuals, etc. I. Busconi, Brian D. II. Stevenson, J. Herbert.

  [DNLM: 1. Athletic Injuries—diagnosis—Handbooks. 2. Athletic Injuries—therapy—Handbooks.
 3. Primary Health Care—Handbooks. 4. Sports Medicine—Handbooks. QT 29 S76395 2009]

    RC1211.S663 2009
    617.1'027—dc22

                                                                                    2009025937

DISCLAIMER

Care has been taken to confirm the accuracy of the information presented and to describe generally accepted practices. However, the authors, editors, and publisher are not responsible for errors or omissions or for any consequences from application of the information in this book and make no warranty, expressed or implied, with respect to the currency, completeness, or accuracy of the contents of the publication. Application of the information in a particular situation remains the professional responsibility of the practitioner.

   The authors, editors, and publisher have exerted every effort to ensure that drug selection and dosage set forth in this text are in accordance with current recommendations and practice at the time of publication. However, in view of ongoing research, changes in government regulations, and the constant flow of information relating to drug therapy and drug reactions, the reader is urged to check the package insert for each drug for any change in indications and dosage and for added warnings and precautions. This is particularly important when the recommended agent is a new or infrequently employed drug.

   Some drugs and medical devices presented in the publication have Food and Drug Administration (FDA) clearance for limited use in restricted research settings. It is the responsibility of the health care provider to ascertain the FDA status of each drug or device planned for use in their clinical practice.

To purchase additional copies of this book, call our customer service department at **(800) 638-3030** or fax orders to **(301) 223-2320**. International customers should call **(301) 223-2300**.

Visit Lippincott Williams & Wilkins on the Internet: at LWW.com. Lippincott Williams & Wilkins customer service representatives are available from 8:30 am to 6 pm, EST.

10 9 8 7 6 5 4 3 2 1

CCS1009

We would like to dedicate this book to our wonderful and loving families, parents, and children. Most of all we would like to dedicate the book to our patient and loving wives Meridith and Karolyn along with our children Hannah, Amelia, and Carter; Liam and Aidan, who are always there for us despite the many long days and lost weekends. We also dedicate the book to our teachers and mentors who have led the way before us and continue in their support.

J. Herbert Stevenson
Brian D. Busconi

CONTRIBUTORS

AMY E. ABBOT, MD
Assistant Professor of Orthopedics and Physical Rehabilitation
University of Massachusetts Medical School
Worcester, Massachusetts

JOSEPH BERNARD, DO
Family Practitioner
Family Medicine and Sports Medicine
Exeter Hospital
Exeter, New Hampshire

MICHAEL A. BROWN, MD
Assistant Professor of Orthopedics and Physical Rehabilitation
University of Massachusetts Medical School
Worcester, Massachusetts

KELTON M. BURBANK, MD
Orthopedic Surgeon
Department of Orthopedic Surgery
University of Massachusetts Memorial Health Care-Health Alliance Campus
Leominster, Massachusetts

VASILIOS CHRISOSTOMIDIS, DO
Assistant Professor
Department of Family and Community Medicine
University of Massachusetts Medical School
Worcester, Massachusetts

GREGORY CZARNECKI, DO
Program Director
Internal Medicine Osteopathic Residency Program
University of Connecticut Health Center
Department of Medicine
Hartford Hospital
Hartford, Connecticut

NICOLA A. DEANGELIS, MD
Assistant Professor
Department of Orthopedics
University of Massachusetts Medical School
Worcester, Massachusetts

JONATHAN M. FALLON, DO, MS
Sports Medicine Fellow
Department of Orthopedic Surgery
University of Massachusetts Medical Center
Worcester, Massachusetts

ZACHARY A. GEIDEL, MD
Sports Medicine Fellow
Primary Care Sports Medicine
University of Massachusetts
Fitchburg, Massachusetts

PATRICK GUERRERO, DO
Orthopedics and Sports Medicine Surgeon
Orthopedics
Central Cal Orthopedic
Turlock, California

ETHAN M. HEALY, MD
Orthopedic Resident
Orthopedics
University of Massachusetts Medical Center
Worcester, Massachusetts

PETER L. HOTH, MD
Vice Chairman
Department of Family Medicine
Exempla Lutheran Medical Center
West Ridge, Colorado

XINNING LI, MD
Orthopedic Surgery Resident
Department of Orthopedic Surgery
University of Massachusetts Medical Center
Worcester, Massachusetts

CHRISTOPHER J. LUTRZYKOWSKI, MD
Associate Residency Director
Maine Dartmouth Family Medicine Residency Program
Augusta, Maine

LEE A. MANCINI, MD, CSCS, CSN
Assistant Professor
University of Massachusetts Sports Medicine Fellowship
Department of Family Medicine and Community Health
University of Massachusetts Medical Center
Worcester, Massachusetts

T. MICHELLE MARIANI, MD
Attending Surgeon
Department of Orthopedic Surgery
Waterbury Hospital/St. Mary's Hospital
Waterbury, Connecticut

ROBERT M. MASELLA, MD
Sports Medicine Fellow
Orthopaedic Surgery
University of Massachusetts Medical Center
Worcester, Massachusetts

JEREMY J. MCCORMICK, MD
Chief Resident
Department of Orthopedics and Physical Rehabilitation
University of Massachusetts Medical Center
Worcester, Massachusetts

ROBERT J. NASCIMENTO
Orthopedic Resident
Department of Orthopedic Surgery
University of Massachusetts Medical Center
Worcester, Massachusetts

DANIEL B. OSUCH, MD
Resident Physician
Department of Orthopedics and Physical Rehabilitation
University of Massachusetts Medical Center
Worcester, Massachusetts

JESSICA L. PELOW, MD
Resident
Orthopaedic Surgery
University of Massachusetts Medical Center
Worcester, Massachusetts

KATHERINE M. RIGGERT, DO
Assistant Professor of Family Medicine and Community Health
University of Massachusetts Medical School
Worcester, Massachusetts

PIERRE ROUZIER, MD
Head Team Physician
University Health Services
University of Massachusetts Amherst
Amherst, Massachusetts

CAROLYN M. SALUTI, DO
Associate Staff Member
Pediatrics
Jordan Hospital
Plymouth, Massachusetts

AGAM SHAH, MD
Department of Orthopedics
Newton-Wellesley Hospital
Newton, Massachusetts

BENJAMIN M.J. THOMPSON, MD
Resident
Department of Orthopedic Surgery
University of Massachusetts Medical Center
Worcester, Massachusetts

JAKE D. VEIGEL, MD
Sports Medicine Fellow
Primary Care Sports Medicine
University of Massachusetts
Fitchburg, Massachusetts

FAREN WILLIAMS, MD
Professor
Clinical Orthopedics and Physical Rehabilitation
University of Massachusetts Medical School
Chief, Physical Medicine and Rehabilitation
UMass Memorial Medical Center
Worcester, Massachusetts

CONTENTS

PREFACE

T he genesis of *Sports Medicine Consult: Problem-Based Approach to Sports Medicine for the Primary Care Physician* came from the realization that there were no adequate or up-to-date resources that could be used at the point of care to help the busy clinician bridge the transition from a chief complaint to an accurate diagnosis and, finally, to a functional sports-specific treatment plan. The reason why this text is unique is it not only addresses the specific diagnosis and treatment but also helps one develop a rational differential diagnosis and, ultimately, an accurate diagnosis.

The goal of *Sports Medicine Consult* is to be a reference at the point of care. Bulleted sections, icons, and a uniform layout allow the reader to quickly find key information to make a diagnosis, order a test, initiate treatment, recognize indications for referral, and identify red flags. Evidence-based references and many exam maneuvers are incorporated where possible to help assess the evidence to support a diagnostic test or efficacy of a treatment.

A final goal of *Sports Medicine Consult* is to address the breadth and depth of the issues faced in the treatment of the athlete. The contributing authors include experts in sports medicine, orthopaedics, physical medicine and rehabilitation, nutrition, and strength and conditioning. The lead authors bring over 25 years of experience teaching sports medicine to medical students, residents, fellows, and practicing physicians as well as medical providers. It is that experience that has helped *Sports Medicine Consult* maintain a focus on key complaints and conditions for which athletes commonly present. Nonsurgical treatments and ways to expedite safe return to play are highlighted. We believe *Sports Medicine Consult: A Problem-Based Approach to Sports Medicine for the Primary Care Physician* will be an indispensable resource for the primary care physician, nurse practitioner, physician assistant, resident physician, physical therapist, and athletic trainer.

We thank the many contributing authors who gave their expertise and time to the development of this book. We also thank our editors for their guidance and tireless assistance in the editing process.

INTRODUCTION

Sports Medicine Consult: Problem-Based Approach to Sports Medicine for the Primary Care Physician is a problem-focused, evidence-based approach to sports medicine for the primary care provider, primary care resident, orthopaedic resident, physical therapist, and athletic trainer. The book is intended to assist medical providers treating athletes at the point of care with concise, practical keys to the evaluation and functional treatment of their sports medicine patients. The goal is to be a practical reference for the diagnosis and management of common sports medicine conditions found in athletes and active patients.

The book is organized to allow quick and easy access to the key information needed in the treatment of athletes. It is organized in three main sections: Approach to Athletes with Medical Conditions, Approach to Athletes with Musculoskeletal Disorders, and Approach to Athletes with Special Conditions or Special Athlete Populations.

The individual chapters have a uniform structure to further assist in quick access to specific information. The chapters have two main sections, with the first being an approach to a specific presenting complaint, e.g., Athlete with Knee Pain. The subsections within the first half of the chapters are: Introduction, Pathophysiology/Functional Anatomy, Epidemiology, Narrowing the Differential Diagnosis, History, Evidence-based Physical Exam, and Diagnostic Testing. The first half of the chapter is intended to help the medical provider develop a rational, organized approach to a presenting complaint along with an appropriate differential. Key pearls on how a thorough history and physical exam will affect the differential diagnosis are highlighted along with the sensitivity and specificity of exam maneuvers when available. Finally, the reader will have the understanding of what tests to order if the diagnosis remains unclear.

The second half of each chapter focuses on the specific conditions that can result in a common complaint. Each diagnosis is reviewed in an organized fashion that is thorough but concise. Bulleted sections allow quick review of treatment and return-to-play information. Each diagnosis has subsections on History and Physical Exam, Diagnostic Testing, Treatment, Prognosis/Return to Play, and Complications/Indications for Referral. Finally, each chapter has a Key Points section that summarizes the most important information for each problem. Icons are used throughout for quick reference to indicate complications/indications for referral and return to play/prognosis for the athlete.

The three appendices cover Injection Techniques, Interval Throwing Program, and Interval Running Program. All three subjects are extremely helpful in expanding nonsurgical treatment options and assisting in the safe and progressive return to play for the running or throwing athlete.

Sports Medicine Consult: Problem-Based Approach to Sports Medicine for the Primary Care Physician is a problem-focused approach intended to be an efficient, but thorough, resource for the busy medical provider. It allows rapid access to the key information needed to assist in the evaluation and treatment of athletes and active patients.

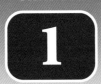

Preparticipation Physical Examination

Vasilios Chrisostomidis

INTRODUCTION

The preparticipation physical examination (PPE) was designed with the safety and health of the athlete in mind. Its goal is to detect the athlete's injuries, illnesses, or factors that may put him or her or other athletes at risk. The history is the single most important factor in determining whether an athlete has a medical or orthopaedic condition. An effective screening examination should have a high level of sensitivity and specificity. In addition it should be cost-effective and practical. Currently, data supporting the PPE meeting these attributes are lacking. Despite this the PPE is required at most high schools and colleges prior to participation.[1] The PPE denies clearance to only 0.3% to 1.3% of all athletes.[2] Additionally, 1.9% to 3.2% require further evaluation prior to participation.[3]

Role of PPE

The primary objective of the PPE is to screen for life-threatening problems as well as conditions that may predispose an athlete to injury or illness. There is no empirical evidence that the PPE is able to screen for silent but deadly illness; however, the consensus panel does recommend it be performed.[4]

Secondary objectives include that the PPE often meets administrative requirements of a school, college, or governing body. Currently, most states as well as the National Collegiate Athletic Association (NCAA) require some form of a preparticipation examination prior to sports participation. There may be annual or biannual requirements or an entrance physical followed by yearly interval history updates. Frequency, appropriate documentation, as well as who is able to perform the examination vary from state to state and also from high school to college athletics. Referencing appropriate requirements is essential to perform a proper PPE for the individual athlete. In most settings/states, a physician, nurse practitioner (NP), or physician assistant (PA) is generally acceptable for performing the PPE.

In addition the PPE may serve as an access point for health care and allow for the discussion of health care maintenance topics as well as general health. This may be the only entry for an athlete into the health care delivery system prior to an acute issue. It should be stressed, however, in the absence of the athlete's primary care provider performing the examination, the standard PPE should not supplement a well child or annual physical examination.

Timing and Setting

The PPE should ideally be performed 6 weeks prior to the start of the athletic season. This allows adequate time to evaluate and treat any conditions requiring further evaluation, testing, or treatment. Unfortunately, most athletes do not present for a PPE until just prior to the commencement of the season. One way to address this is to screen all returning athletes to a team/school who will need a PPE in the spring prior to return to school.

The setting of the preparticipation examination should ideally be in the athlete's primary care provider's office. This allows for confidentiality and continuity of care as well as the ability to address nonsports-related medical issues if the athlete is otherwise healthy to participate in sports. The main limitation is the time utilized and cost.

In order to reduce costs and improve efficiency, some schools and teams opt for a mass PPE session utilizing multiple health care providers. When the PPE is performed by a group of physicians, it is often split up into stations. Often one person will review the medical questionnaire, while another performs the physical examination and finally another provides clearance. An advantage of this format is that a multispecialty team is often created (i.e., primary care, orthopaedic, dentist, etc.), which may decrease the need for referral and avoid delay in clearing athletes for participation. It is important to have separate areas for male and female athletes as well as privacy for the examination portion of the physical. Confidentiality should be maintained at all times.

An alternative format for the mass PPE is the "locker-room" format where the entire examination is performed by one physician, but there are simultaneous examinations performed at the same time in separate examination rooms. This format requires a large number of physicians capable of performing the entire examination but can be an efficient and cost-effective format as well.

Standard Preparticipation Examination

The medical history is the most important part of the PPE. It will identify roughly 75% to 90% of all problems affecting the athlete. There are roughly 4 million competitive athletes in high school alone and 30 million athletes under the age of 18 who play organized sports in the United States.[4] It is important to remember that the PPE screens for conditions that result in unacceptable risk but does not reach a zero-risk circumstance. An excellent resource for the clinician providing preparticipation physicals is the most recent joint consensus monograph *Preparticipation Physical Evaluation*, 3rd Edition (American Academy of Family Physicians, American Academy of Pediatrics, American Medical Society for Sports Medicine, American Orthopaedic Society for Sports Medicine, American Osteopathic Academy of Sports Medicine). The form is composed of standardized history, physical examination, and clearance sections, which allows for efficient and thorough evaluation of the athlete. A copy of this form is shown in Figure 1.1.

HISTORY

Key components to the history that warrant further evaluation are highlighted below. For a complete detailed description of each component, please refer to the most recent PPE joint consensus monograph.[4]

Medical Problems

- Previous disqualification or surgeries
- Recent injuries/illness
- Ever spent a night in a hospital
- May indicate serious condition not highlighted by other questions

Medication/Supplements

- Prescription/nonprescription (over-the-counter)/herbal medications
- May clue the physician about medical conditions an athlete may have forgotten to mention

Allergy/Anaphylaxis

- Food or insect stings
- Necessity of medications on the sidelines is ultimately the responsibility of the athlete, though the trainer or medical provider covering an event or practice may as well choose to carry them

Cardiovascular

- Syncope, chest pain, shortness of breath (SOB) with activity, murmur, or positive family history (sudden death/ myocardial infarction [MI]) should prompt a work-up for cardiac conditions. Do not forget to ask about illicit drug (cocaine) or steroid abuse as a causative factor
- Family history of sudden cardiac death under the age of 50 (particularly first-degree relative)
- History of any cardiac testing (ECG [electrocardiogram], ECHO, stress test, etc.)
- It is difficult to diagnose life-threatening cardiac conditions—only 20% are diagnosed prior to sudden cardiac death[5,6]
- The most common cause of cardiac death in athletes under the age of 35 is hypertrophic cardiomyopathy (HCM), while coronary artery disease (CAD) is the most common cause over 35 years[5,6]

Pulmonary

- Prior history of asthma or exercise-induced asthma (EIA)
- SOB, wheezing, or coughing with exercise
- Family history of asthma
- Prior use of an inhaler or asthma medication

Viral Illness

- Recent viral illness with special attention paid to recent mononucleosis

Paired Organs

- Presence of any unpaired organs (kidney, eye, testicle)
- Ramifications of absence of one may affect clearance or require appropriate risk stratification. Please refer to "Clearance" section for details

Dermatologic Conditions

- Presence of any rashes, sores, or skin lesions
- Herpes, tinea, methicillin-resistant *Staphylococcus aureus* (MRSA) important in contact sports, particularly if active

Neurologic

- History of concussion, burners/stingers, seizures
- History of repetitive concussion or burners/stingers should prompt further inquiry and possibly a work-up

Heat Illness

- Often recurrent so detailed history may help to prevent recurrence
- Consider pre-exercise and postexercise weights as well as proper acclimatization

Musculoskeletal Injury

- Acute or overuse injuries including but not limited to fractures, sprains, strains, contusions, as well as overuse injuries

Preparticipation Physical Evaluation

DATE OF EXAM_____

Name_____ Sex_____ Age_____ Date of birth_____

Grade____ School_____ Sport(s)_____

Address_____ Phone_____

Personal physician_____

In case of emergency, contact

Name_____ Relationship_____ Phone (H)_____ (W)_____

Explain "Yes" answers below.
Circle questions you don't know the answers to.

	Yes	No
1. Has a doctor ever denied or restricted your participation in sports for any reason?	□	□
2. Do you have an ongoing medical condition (like diabetes or asthma)?	□	□
3. Are you currently taking any prescription or nonprescription (over-the-counter) medicines or pills?	□	□
4. Do you have allergies to medicines, pollens, foods, or stinging insects?	□	□
5. Have you ever passed out or nearly passed out DURING exercise?	□	□
6. Have you ever passed out or nearly passed out AFTER exercise?	□	□
7. Have you ever had discomfort, pain, or pressure in your chest during exercise?	□	□
8. Does your heart race or skip beats during exercise?	□	□

9. Has a doctor ever told you that you have (check all that apply):
   □ High blood pressure   □ A heart murmur
   □ High cholesterol   □ A heart infection

	Yes	No
10. Has a doctor ever ordered a test for your heart? (for example, ECG, echocardiogram)	□	□
11. Has anyone in your family died for no apparent reason?	□	□
12. Does anyone in your family have a heart problem?	□	□
13. Has any family member or relative died of heart problems or of sudden death before age 50?	□	□
14. Does anyone in your family have Marfan syndrome?	□	□
15. Have you ever spent the night in a hospital?	□	□
16. Have you ever had surgery?	□	□
17. Have you ever had an injury, like a sprain, muscle or ligament tear or tendinitis, that caused you to miss a practice or game? If yes, circle affected area below:	□	□
18. Have you had any broken or fractured bones, or dislocated joints? If yes, circle below:	□	□
19. Have you had a bone or joint injury that required x-rays, MRI, CT, surgery, injections, rehabilitation, physical therapy, a brace, a cast, or crutches? If yes, circle below:	□	□

Head	Neck	Shoulder	Upper arm	Elbow	Forearm	Hand/ fingers	Chest
Upper back	Lower back	Hip	Thigh	Knee	Calf/shin	Ankle	Foot/toes

	Yes	No
20. Have you ever had a stress fracture?	□	□
21. Have you been told that you have or have you had an x-ray for atlantoaxial (neck) instability?	□	□
22. Do you regularly use a brace or assistive device?	□	□
23. Has a doctor ever told you that you have asthma or allergies?	□	□

	Yes	No
24. Do you cough, wheeze, or have difficulty breathing during or after exercise?	□	□
25. Is there anyone in your family who has asthma?	□	□
26. Have you ever used an inhaler or taken asthma medicine?	□	□
27. Were you born without or are you missing a kidney, an eye, a testicle, or any other organ?	□	□
28. Have you had infectious mononucleosis (mono) within the last month?	□	□
29. Do you have any rashes, pressure sores, or other skin problems?	□	□
30. Have you had a herpes skin infection?	□	□
31. Have you ever had a head injury or concussion?	□	□
32. Have you been hit in the head and been confused or lost your memory?	□	□
33. Have you ever had a seizure?	□	□
34. Do you have headaches with exercise?	□	□
35. Have you ever had numbness, tingling, or weakness in your arms or legs after being hit or falling?	□	□
36. Have you ever been unable to move your arms or legs after being hit or falling?	□	□
37. When exercising in the heat, do you have severe muscle cramps or become ill?	□	□
38. Has a doctor told you that you or someone in your family has sickle cell trait or sickle cell disease?	□	□
39. Have you had any problems with your eyes or vision?	□	□
40. Do you wear glasses or contact lenses?	□	□
41. Do you wear protective eyewear, such as goggles or a face shield?	□	□
42. Are you happy with your weight?	□	□
43. Are you trying to gain or lose weight?	□	□
44. Has anyone recommended you change your weight or eating habits?	□	□
45. Do you limit or carefully control what you eat?	□	□
46. Do you have any concerns that you would like to discuss with a doctor?	□	□

FEMALES ONLY

	Yes	No
47. Have you ever had a menstrual period?	□	□

48. How old were you when you had your first menstrual period? _____

49. How many periods have you had in the last year? _____

Explain "Yes" answers here: _____
_____
_____
_____
_____
_____
_____
_____

I hereby state that, to the best of my knowledge, my answers to the above questions are complete and correct.

Signature of athlete_____ Signature of parent/guardian_____ Date_____

FIG. 1.1. Standardized PPE form. Adapted from American Academy of Family Physicians, American Academy of Pediatrics, American College of Sports Medicine, American Medical Society for Sports Medicine, American Orthopaedic Society for Sports Medicine, and American Osteopathic Academy of Sports Medicine.

Preparticipation Physical Evaluation

PHYSICAL EXAMINATION FORM

Name _____ Date of birth _____

Height _____ Weight _____ % Body fat (optional) _____ Pulse _____ BP___/____ (___/___ , ___/___)

Vision R 20/ _____ L 20/ _____   Corrected: Y N   Pupils: Equal _____ Unequal _____

Follow-Up Questions on More Sensitive Issues	Yes	No
1. Do you feel stressed out or under a lot of pressure?	☐	☐
2. Do you ever feel so sad or hopeless that you stop doing some of your usual activities for more than a few days?	☐	☐
3. Do you feel safe?	☐	☐
4. Have you ever tried cigarette smoking, even 1 or 2 puffs? Do you currently smoke?	☐	☐
5. During the past 30 days, did you use chewing tobacco, snuff, or dip?	☐	☐
6. During the past 30 days, have you had at least 1 drink of alcohol?	☐	☐
7. Have you ever taken steroid pills or shots without a doctor's prescription?	☐	☐
8. Have you ever taken any supplements to help you gain or lose weight or improve your performance?	☐	☐
9. Questions from the Youth Risk Behavior Survey (http://www.cdc.gov/HealthyYouth/yrbs/index.htm) on guns, seatbelts, unprotected sex, domestic violence, drugs, etc.	☐	☐

Notes: _____
_____
_____

	NORMAL	ABNORMAL FINDINGS	INITIALS*
MEDICAL			
Appearance			
Eyes/ears/nose/throat			
Hearing			
Lymph nodes			
Heart			
Murmurs			
Pulses			
Lungs			
Abdomen			
Genitourinary†			
Skin			
MUSCULOSKELETAL			
Neck			
Back			
Shoulder/arm			
Elbow/forearm			
Wrist/hand/fingers			
Hip/thigh			
Knee			
Leg/ankle			
Foot/toes			

*Multiple-examiner set-up only.
†Having a third party present is recommended for the genitourinary examination.

Notes: _____
_____

Name of physician (print/type)_____ Date _____

Address _____ Phone _____

Signature of physician _____ , MD or DO

FIG. 1.1. (Continued).

- Previous treatments including physical therapy (PT)/surgery/braces
- Assess the adequacy of evaluation and treatment as the athlete may need new work-up or treatment

Gastrointestinal (GI)

- Active or recent vomiting/diarrhea predisposes to dehydration as well as heat illness

Genitourinary (GU)

- Testicular masses, hernias, pain
- Female menstrual history including absence of menses, age of menarche, and frequency may indicate underlying risk for female athletic triad and energy imbalance

Eyes/Vision

- Best corrected acuity
- Greater than 20/40 considered abnormal
- If "functionally one eyed," may require mandatory eye protection[7]

Nutrition

- Eating disorders, disordered eating
- History of stress fractures, female triad

Psychosocial Concerns

- Drug use/illicit substances
- Tobacco/smokeless tobacco
- Performance-enhancing drugs
- Nutritional supplements
- Depression/anxiety screening
- Safety screening

Immunizations

- Make sure up to date

PHYSICAL EXAMINATION[4]

Vital Signs/Body Mass Index (BMI)

- Brachial artery blood pressure (BP) in the seated position (preferably bilateral)
- Make sure to refer age-appropriate normative values for BP
- If BP elevated, record bilateral BP and readings should be performed on at least two separate occasions
- It is important to use the appropriate-sized BP cuff as a small cuff may cause an elevated reading in a large individual

Visual Acuity

- Minimum 20/40 corrected vision in each eye

Head, Eyes, Ears, Nose, and Throat (HEENT)

- Evaluate for anisocoria so that there is a baseline in case of head injury/concussion

Cardiovascular

- Femoral artery pulses should be checked. If decreased then BP measurements should be taken from the lower extremity as well as bilateral upper extremity due to possible coarctation of the aorta.
- Cardiac auscultation should be performed in the supine and standing positions (or with Valsalva maneuver) specifically to identify murmurs of dynamic left ventricular outflow tract obstruction.
- The examiner should be listening for murmurs, irregular heartbeats, or extra heart sounds (S3/S4).
- Special attention should be paid to the murmur of HCM. Systolic murmurs 3/6 or greater, all diastolic murmurs, and any murmur that increases in intensity with Valsalva should be evaluated further prior to clearance.
- Examination should be performed for physical stigmata for Marfan's due to increased risk for cardiovascular complications.

Pulmonary

- This examination should focus on listening for good air movement with clear lung fields. Findings such as rhonchi, rales, or wheezes may require further work-up.

Abdomen

- Athlete should be supine and relaxed. Abdominal masses or organomegaly may require further work-up prior to clearance.

Genitalia

- A testicular examination as well as a hernia examination should be performed in males. This is an opportunity to discuss the self-testicular examination with the male athlete.
- The GU examination is deferred in females. Routine papanicolau tests should be encouraged.

Skin

- Examine for any signs of contagious infection including herpes, carbuncles, fungal infections, impetigo, and scabies.

Musculoskeletal System

- The goal is to determine if there are any injuries (acute or chronic) that affect safe participation by the athlete.
- Key factors include identifying any strength deficits, atrophy, or instability that may require rehabilitation or further treatment prior to participation.

- The physician may perform one of two types of examinations: "general musculoskeletal screening" or "joint specific."
- A general musculoskeletal screening may be performed followed by joint-specific examination for those joints failing the screening or having an acute or chronic injury requiring further assessment.

General Musculoskeletal Screening Examination

1. Inspect for any gross deformities or abnormalities
2. Check active neck range of motion (flexion/extension/side bending and rotation)
3. Have athlete shrug shoulders against resistance to assess trapezius strength
4. Abduct shoulders against resistance
5. Range of motion of shoulders in internal rotation and external rotation with elbows flexed
6. Flex and extend elbows
7. Pronate and supinate the wrist
8. Clench the fist and spread the fingers
9. Inspect lumbar spine for asymmetry or scoliosis
10. Check lumbar extension for pain or lack of range of motion
11. Check lumbar flexion for pain or lack of range of motion as well as scoliosis
12. Assess lower extremities for alignment and asymmetry
13. Perform the "duck walk" which assesses the function of the hips, knees, ankles, and feet simultaneously
14. Perform toe walk as well as heel walk to assess strength and stability

Note that any abnormalities should prompt the joint-specific examination.

Joint-specific Examination

- This examination includes inspection and range of motion testing of the spine, neck, shoulders, elbows, wrists, hands, hips, knees, ankles, and feet.
- Appearance and symmetry should be noted. The examination should be performed in a stepwise fashion in the same order each time so that no part of the examination is omitted.
- The specific joint examinations/maneuvers, along with their respective sensitivities and specificities, are illustrated throughout the other chapters of this text and as such will not be reviewed here at this time.

DIAGNOSTIC TESTING

Laboratory

- The routine use of blood or urine tests has not been substantiated and is not currently recommended as part of the PPE.[8]
- Some institutions screen for sickle cell trait and anemia given relatively high prevalence in some groups, but there is no evidence to support this action at this time.[8]

ECG

- The routine use of ECG to determine HCM, congenital anomalies, or significant cardiac arrhythmias has not been substantiated and is not currently recommended as part of the PPE by the American Heart Association.[6]

Echocardiogram

- While this tool may be effective in determining if an athlete has HCM, it is not recommended as a routine part of the PPE. It is considered cost-prohibitive and is not easily accessible at this time.[6,9]

CLEARANCE

Clearance is the determination of whether the athlete may safely participate in sports to the best judgment of the medical provider (physician, NP, PA). Some providers prefer to consider it a risk assessment rather than clearance. The athlete and family need to be involved when dealing with a minor. Fortunately, the need to deny clearance is rare, occurring in only 0.3% to 1.3% of all athletes.[2] A larger percentage (1.9% to 3.2%), however, may require further evaluation or treatment prior to participation.[3]

There can be different levels of clearance as shown in the PPE clearance form (Fig. 1.2). The medical provider may decide that no athletic participation is allowed, that the athlete may participate after certain conditions are met, or that the athlete may participate in athletics.

The last category may be further broken down into participation in events based on classification by contact or strenuousness of the activity as noted in Tables 1.1 and 1.2.

Regardless of the type of evaluation done, it is important that coaches and trainers understand restrictions in participation or further work-up in the athlete. It is also important to keep the lines of communication open with the athlete to avoid misunderstandings.

KEY POINTS
• The PPE is designed to detect the athlete's injuries, illnesses, or factors that may put him or her or other athletes at risk.
• The PPE does not replace the annual physical examination.
• The history is the key component of the PPE.
• History and physical examination findings should guide and work up as well as a clearance decision.
• Currently, the recommendation is not to use routine labs, ECG, or ECHO for PPE screening.

Preparticipation Physical Evaluation

| CLEARANCE FORM |

Name_____ Sex _____ Age _____ Date of birth_____

❑ Cleared without restriction

❑ Cleared, with recommendations for further evaluation or treatment for: _____

_____

_____

_____

❑ Not cleared for ❑ All sports ❑ Certain sports: _____ Reason: _____

Recommendations: _____

_____

EMERGENCY INFORMATION

Allergies _____

Other Information _____

IMMUNIZATIONS (eg, tetanus/diphtheria; measles, mumps, rubella; hepatitis A, B; influenza; poliomyelitis; pneumococcal; meningococcal; varicella)

❑ Up to date (see attached documentation) ❑ Not up to date Specify_____

Name of physician (print/type) _____ Date _____

Address _____ Phone_____

Signature of physician _____ , MD or DO

© 2004 American Academy of Family Physicians, American Academy of Pediatrics, American Medical Society for Sports Medicine, American Orthopaedic Society for Sports Medicine, and American Osteopathic Academy of Sports Medicine.

Preparticipation Physical Evaluation

| CLEARANCE FORM |

Name_____ Sex _____ Age _____ Date of birth_____

❑ Cleared without restriction

❑ Cleared, with recommendations for further evaluation or treatment for: _____

_____

_____

_____

❑ Not cleared for ❑ All sports ❑ Certain sports: _____ Reason: _____

Recommendations: _____

_____

EMERGENCY INFORMATION

Allergies _____

Other Information _____

IMMUNIZATIONS (eg, tetanus/diphtheria; measles, mumps, rubella; hepatitis A, B; influenza; poliomyelitis; pneumococcal; meningococcal; varicella)

❑ Up to date (see attached documentation) ❑ Not up to date Specify_____

Name of physician (print/type) _____ Date _____

Address _____ Phone_____

Signature of physician _____ , MD or DO

© 2004 American Academy of Family Physicians, American Academy of Pediatrics, American Medical Society for Sports Medicine, American Orthopaedic Society for Sports Medicine, and American Osteopathic Academy of Sports Medicine.

FIG. 1.2. Clearance form. Adapted from American Academy of Family Physicians, American Academy of Pediatrics, American College of Sports Medicine, American Medical Society for Sports Medicine, American Orthopaedic Society for Sports Medicine, and American Osteopathic Academy of Sports Medicine.

TABLE 1.1 **Classification of Sports by Contact**

Contact/Collision	Limited Contact	Noncontact
• Basketball • Boxing • Diving • Field hockey • Football (tackle, flag) • Ice hockey • Lacrosse • Martial arts • Rodeo • Rugby • Ski jumping • Soccer • Team handball • Water polo • Wrestling	• Baseball • Bicycling • Cheerleading • Canoeing/kayaking (white water) • Fencing • Field events (high jump, pole vault) • Floor hockey • Gymnastics • Handball • Horseback riding • Racquetball • Skating (ice, inline, roller) • Skiing (cross-country, downhill, water) • Softball • Squash • Ultimate Frisbee • Volleyball • Windsurfing/surfing	• Archery • Badminton • Bodybuilding • Bowling • Canoeing/kayaking (flat water) • Crew/rowing • Curling • Dancing • Field events (discus, javelin, shot put) • Golf • Orienteering • Power lifting • Race walking • Riflery • Rope jumping • Sailing • Scuba diving • Strength training • Swimming • Table tennis • Tennis • Track • Weight lifting

Adapted from Schepsis AA, Busconi BD. *Sports Medicine.* Philadelphia: Lippincott Williams & Wilkins; 2006:20.

TABLE 1.2 **Classification of Sports by Strenuousness**

High to Moderate Dynamic and Static Demands	High to Moderate Dynamic and Low Static Demands	Low Dynamic and High to Moderate Static Demands	Low Dynamic and Static Demands
• Boxing • Crew/rowing • Cross-country skiing • Cycling • Downhill skiing • Fencing • Football • Ice hockey • Rugby • Running (sprinting) • Speed skating • Water polo • Wrestling	• Badminton • Baseball • Basketball • Field hockey • Lacrosse • Orienteering • Table tennis • Race walking • Racquetball • Soccer • Squash • Swimming • Tennis • Volleyball	• Archery • Auto racing • Diving • Equestrian events • Field events (jumping, throwing) • Gymnastics • Karate or judo • Motorcycling • Rodeo • Sailing • Ski jumping • Water skiing • Weight lifting	• Bowling • Cricket • Curling • Golf • Riflery

Adapted from Schepsis AA, Busconi BD. *Sports Medicine.* Philadelphia: Lippincott Williams & Wilkins; 2006:20.

REFERENCES

1. DiFiori JP. Overuse injuries in children and adolescents. *Phys Sportsmed.* 1999;27(1).
2. Linder CW, DuRant RH, Seklecki RM, et al. Preparticipation health screening of young athletes: results of 1268 examinations. *Am J Sports Med.* 1981;9(3):187–193.
3. McKeag DB. Preseason physical examination for the prevention of sports injuries. *Sports Med.* 1985;2(6):413–431.
4. Matheson GO, et al. *Preparticipation Physical Evaluation.* 3rd ed. American Academy of Family Physicians, American Academy of Pediatrics, American Medical Society for Sports Medicine, American Orthopaedic Society for Sports Medicine, American Osteopathic Academy of Sports Medicine; 2005.
5. Van Camp SP. Sudden death in athletes. In: Grana WA, Lombardo JA, eds. *Advances in Sports Medicine and Fitness.* Chicago: Year Book Medical Publishers; 1988:121–142.
6. Maron BJ, Thompson PD, Ackerman MJ, et al. American Heart Association Council on Nutrition, Physical Activity, and Metabolism. Recommendations and considerations related to preparticipation screening for cardiovascular abnormalities in competitive athletes: 2007 update: a scientific statement from the American Heart Association Council on Nutrition, Physical Activity, and Metabolism: endorsed by the American College of Cardiology Foundation. *Circulation.* 2007;115(12):1643–455.
7. American Academy of Pediatrics, American Academy of Ophthalmology. Protective eyewear for young athletes. *Pediatrics.* 1996;98(2):311–313.
8. Taylor WC III, Lombardo JA. Preparticipation screening of college athletes: value of the complete blood cell count. *Phys Sportsmed.* 1990;18(6):106–118.
9. Feinstein RA, Colvin E, Oh MK. Echocardiographic screening as part of a preparticipation examination. *Clin J Sport Med.* 1993;3(3):149–152.

CHAPTER

2

Athlete with a Head or Facial Injury

Peter Hoth and Zachary A. Geidel

INTRODUCTION

Head and facial injuries in athletes often create anxiety in the provider caring for the athlete, as these injuries can be a source of significant morbidity, disability, disfigurement, or even death. Types of head injury encountered during sports activities include concussion, also known as mild traumatic brain injury (MTBI), second-impact syndrome, postconcussion syndrome, and intracranial hemorrhage. Facial injuries include dental injury, facial fractures, nasal fractures, epistaxis, and ocular injuries.

Concussion is the most common head injury encountered in sport, with as many as 300,000 concussions occurring annually in the United States due to sports participation.[1] Approximately 90% or more of concussions do not involve loss of consciousness.[2,3] Thankfully, the rates of head and facial injuries are decreasing in sport due to the implementation of helmets and facial protectors. Levy et al. (2004) showed a 74% decrease in fatalities and an 86% decrease in serious head injury since 1976 due to the implementation of the National Operating Committee on Standards for Athletic Equipment (NOCSAE) helmet standards as well as the implementation of new tackling laws to prevent spearing in football.[4]

PATHOPHYSIOLOGY

The mechanism of concussion can be a direct blow to the head, indirect trauma suffered during a fall, or a whiplash-type injury (Fig. 2.4). The underlying pathophysiology is an area of active research, with current data drawn largely from animal models and more severe forms of brain trauma in humans. The current theory proposes that a concussion results in a neurometabolic cascade that creates an increased glucose demand to restore normal cell membrane ionic homeostasis with a concomitant decrease in cerebral perfusion at the cellular level.[5] This can lead to axonal injury and potential cell death. While the acute onset of ionic changes occurs over hours, late onset effects can take days to weeks to resolve with normalization of brain function.[5]

Other etiologies of altered cognition due to a head injury other than concussion or intracranial bleed include second-impact syndrome and postconcussion syndrome. Second-impact syndrome is defined as a repeat head insult that occurs prior to the complete resolution of initial concussion, which may not have been recognized or evaluated. There is currently much debate regarding the prevalence and etiology of second-impact syndrome, but the most widely held position is that the brain loses its autoregulatory ability due to the first concussion, and with onset of the second injury, there is rapid onset of cerebral edema, often leading to significant morbidity and mortality, despite aggressive and rapid treatment.[3] Although second-impact syndrome is not seen in all athletes that return to play with ongoing concussive symptoms, the severe and devastating nature of this condition is one of the reasons why it is critical that athletes are asymptomatic prior to returning to play.

FUNCTIONAL ANATOMY

Given that concussion is the most common traumatic head injury, it is important to understand the anatomy of the brain (Fig. 2.2). The brain is a soft tissue structure floating in and surrounded by cerebrospinal fluid inside a thick, bony skull. If there is a direct or an indirect injury to the skull, the brain will move within the skull, colliding with the inner lining of the skull and causing a soft tissue injury or a concussion. If there is a severe impact to the skull, often in the temporoparietal region, with sheer forces that transect the middle meningeal artery, there can be an epidural hematoma, which can be a life-threatening emergency (Fig. 2.3).

The facial bones are anatomically situated to support the functions of vision, breathing, eating, and smell. Any damage to the facial structures therefore, by definition, can result in loss of functionality and impairment of these sensory modalities. Most notably, the inferior bony wall of the ocular cavity is extremely thin, and direct ocular trauma can result in a "blow out" fracture (Fig. 2.4). This is actually a protective mechanism that can spare the actual globe and helps to prevent blindness. An important anatomic factor regarding the mandible is that it is a U-shaped structure. Given this anatomy, any injuries to the mandible often result in fractures in more than one location.

Primary injury

Contusions, lacerations, shearing injuries, hemorrhage, and swelling can occur at the time of impact and cannot be reversed by treatment.

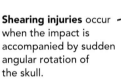

Contusions typically occur over the frontal and temporal poles of the brain regardless of the cranial impact site.

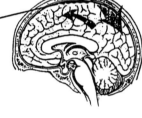

Lacerations, with or without associated fractures, are usually located near the midline, adjacent to the floor of the anterior or middle cranial fossa, and often involve the corpus callosum or pontomedullary junction.

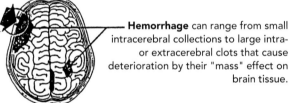

Shearing injuries occur when the impact is accompanied by sudden angular rotation of the skull.

Hemorrhage can range from small intracerebral collections to large intra- or extracerebral clots that cause deterioration by their "mass" effect on brain tissue.

FIG. 2.1. Mechanisms of concussions. Reprinted with permission from McKeag DB, Moller JL. *ACSM's Primary Care Sports Medicine.* 2nd ed. Philadelphia: Lippincott Williams & Wilkins; 2007.

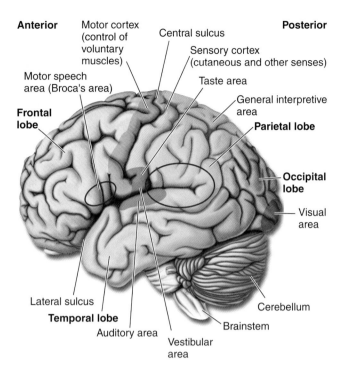

FIG. 2.2. Neuroanatomy and functional anatomy. Reprinted with permission from Bear M, Conner B, Paradiso M. *Neuroscience: Exploring the Brain.* 2nd ed. Baltimore: Lippincott Williams & Wilkins; 2000.

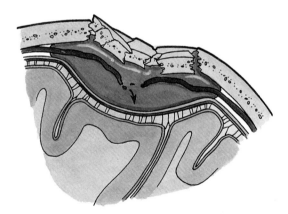

FIG. 2.3. Middle meningeal artery injury with epidural hematoma. Reprinted with permission from Moore KL, Agur A. *Essential Clinical Anatomy.* 2nd ed. Philadelphia: Lippincott Williams & Wilkins; 2002.

One important consideration regarding nasal anatomy is that the nasal septum is covered by a vascular web, Kiesselbach's plexus. Any fractures to the nasal septum can cause disruption of the vascular anatomy and a septal hematoma, which is an urgent condition requiring intervention to avoid nasal septal perforation.

The functional anatomy regarding sports-related ocular trauma is that the eye is a fluid-filled globe sitting in a thin-walled, bony socket. The medial border of the orbital socket is the lacrimal bone and the orbital plate of the ethmoid bone. Superiorly lies the orbital surface of the frontal bone. Laterally is the orbital surface of the zygomatic arch, and inferiorly is the orbital surface of the maxilla as well as a portion of the zygomatic arch. The main structure of this bony architecture is the orbital surface of the maxilla, which is the

thinnest of all the surrounding osseous structures and is most likely to fracture during an episode of blunt trauma to the globe. This anatomy is protective in that it allows for a blow-out fracture rather than resulting in globe rupture, which could cause blindness.

The most relevant ocular structures are the eyelids and the cornea. The lids are protective structures, which also have a role in tear production and tear removal through the lacrimal ducts. The lacrimal ducts exit the eye through

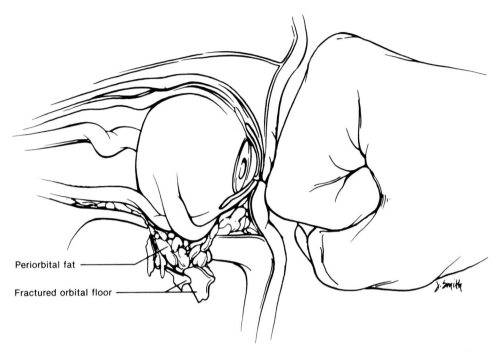

Periorbital fat

Fractured orbital floor

FIG. 2.4. Blow-out fracture. Reprinted with permission from Harwood-Nuss A, Wolfson AB, Christopher H, et al. *The Clinical Practice of Emergency Medicine.* 3rd ed. Philadelphia: Lippincott Williams & Wilkins; 2001.

the medial portion of both upper and lower eyelids; thus, any resulting injury or laceration to the region of the medial canthus should be thoroughly evaluated to ensure that lacrimal duct injury has not occurred. Injury to the lacrimal ducts that is not properly and promptly repaired by ophthalmology could result in a tear duct problem, eye watering, or dry eyes.

The cornea is the clear covering over the pupil and iris. It is an important structure in sport as it is commonly injured, usually due to a scratch or an abrasion. It usually heals well, but often needs a protective patch. The deeper structures include the anterior chamber, between the cornea and the lens; the posterior chamber, between the lens and the retina; and the retina itself. The remainder of the structures are all necessary for adequate visual acuity.

EPIDEMIOLOGY

Concussions are most often seen in the 12- to 24-year age range and are more frequently seen in male rather than female athletes. Current incidence data shows that there are 0.14 to 3.66 concussive injuries per 100 player-seasons versus athlete-seasons at the high school level. At the collegiate level, there are 0.5 to 3.0 injuries per 1,000 athlete exposures.[6] Approximately 90% or more of concussions do not involve loss of consciousness.[2,3]

Eye injuries related to sports or recreational activities account for 40,000 to 100,000 injuries annually in the United States, most of which may be preventable.[7,8] The highest risk of ocular injuries occurs in sports with sticks, balls, or racquets. In relation to ball sports, smaller balls (e.g., racquetball and handball) present higher risk of ocular injuries. Nonracquet sports that have a higher incidence of ocular trauma include boxing, basketball, and wrestling.

NARROWING THE DIFFERENTIAL DIAGNOSIS

On-field Assessment

The first rule for a head injury is that any athlete who is unconscious after an injury is assumed to have a cervical spine injury, and cervical spine precautions need to be taken with all further evaluation of the athlete until the cervical spine has been evaluated and cleared.

Once an athlete has been determined to be stable, they should be serially evaluated by a trained provider every 10 to 15 minutes. Use of a concussion scale such as the Sideline Assessment of Concussion (SAC) can assist with monitoring subtle changes, either improving or declining performance on any of the cognitive measures (Fig. 2.5).

The safest rule in caring for concussed athletes is that they should not be allowed to return to game play or practice until their symptoms have completely resolved. Additionally, the younger the athlete, the more restrictive the supervising provider should be in allowing them to return to play. Even if symptoms have resolved, it is recommended that athletes at the high school level or younger not return to participation on the day of injury. This recommendation is meant to protect the still-developing brain from further injury or insult.[9] If an

1) ORIENTATION:

Month: _____ 0   1
Date: _____ 0   1
Day of week: _____ 0   1
Year: _____ 0   1
Time (within 1 hr.): _____ 0   1

Orientation Total Score _____ / 5

2) IMMEDIATE MEMORY: (all 3 trials are completed regardless of score on trial 1 & 2; total score equals sum across all 3 trials)

List	Trial 1	Trial 2	Trial 3
Word 1	0 1	0 1	0 1
Word 2	0 1	0 1	0 1
Word 3	0 1	0 1	0 1
Word 4	0 1	0 1	0 1
Word 5	0 1	0 1	0 1
Total			

Immediate Memory Total Score _____ / 15

(Note: Subject is not informed of Delayed Recall testing of memory)

NEUROLOGICAL SCREENING:

Loss of Consciousness: (occurrence, duration)

Retrograde & Posttraumatic Amnesia:
(recall of events pre- and post-injury)

Strength:

Sensation:

Coordination:

3) CONCENTRATION:

Digits Backward (If correct, go to next string length. If incorrect, read trial 2. Stop after incorrect on both trials)

4-9-3	6-2-9 _____	0 1
3-8-1-4	3-2-7-9 _____	0 1
6-2-9-7-1	1-5-2-8-6 _____	0 1
7-1-8-4-6-2	5-3-9-1-4-8 _____	0 1

Months in reverse order: (entire sequence correct for 1 point)
Dec-Nov-Oct-Sep-Aug-Jul
Jun-May-Apr-Mar-Feb-Jan _____ 0   1

Concentration Total Score _____ / 5

EXERTIONAL MANEUVERS
(when appropriate):

5 jumping jacks   5 push-ups
5 sit-ups   5 knee-bends

4) DELAYED RECALL:

Word 1   0   1
Word 2   0   1
Word 3   0   1
Word 4   0   1
Word 5   0   1

Delayed Recall Total Score _____ / 5

SUMMARY OF TOTAL SCORES:

Orientation _____ / 5
Immediate Memory _____ / 15
Concentration _____ / 5
Delayed Recall _____ / 5

Overall Total Score _____ / 30

FIG. 2.5. Sideline Assessment of Concussion (SAC). Reprinted with permission from McCrea M. Standardized mental status assessment of sports concussion. *Clin J Sports Med.* 2001;11: 176–181.

athlete's condition is deteriorating rather than improving, especially if their level of consciousness is decreasing or they are starting to have localized neurologic deficits, such as abnormal papillary response, they need to be transported to an emergency medical facility immediately for further evaluation and treatment as they may have an intracranial hemorrhage, specifically an epidural hematoma that would require immediate surgical intervention to avoid increased intracranial pressure, brain stem herniation, and possible death.

Office-based Assessment

Concussed athletes presenting to the office may not realize they sustained a concussion. They may think they just had their "bell rung" or present with headache, dizziness, memory disturbances, or mood changes and not correlate it with head trauma. Furthermore, some symptoms can be delayed in onset and/or worsen as time progresses. The important point is to assess whether these were related to head trauma, and if so, a concussion must be assumed till ruled out. A thorough history of mechanism, symptoms, change in symptoms, as well as any evaluation or treatment done to date is essential. A thorough neurovascular examination with special focus on cognition, memory, and cerebella function is important in the concussed athlete. Any focal neurologic deficit or rapidly progressing symptoms imply potential cranial bleed, and transport to emergency medical facility should occur.

Facial trauma typically presents to the emergency department, but patients may present with minor complaints of double vision (potential orbital blow-out fracture) or tooth malocclusion (occult mandibular fracture) that may indicate more significant facial injuries.

Diagnostic Testing

Laboratory

Appropriate laboratory evaluation depends on the underlying condition but is typically not required with simple concussions or facial injuries.

Imaging

Appropriate imaging can be essential, depending on the suspected underlying condition. Most simple concussions do not require imaging, but complex concussions, presence of focal neurologic deficits, or progression of symptoms may warrant imaging studies. In the emergency department or when there is an acute deterioration of the athlete, emergent computed tomography (CT) is generally the imaging of choice. For postconcussion syndrome, chronic symptoms, or when CT is inconclusive but clinical suspicion remains, a magnetic resonance imaging (MRI) will provide the most accurate imaging of the brain structure for bleeds and cerebral hematomas. An MRI angiogram may be considered if ruling out vascular malformation. Functional MRIs (fMRIs) and positron emission tomography (PET) scans are

largely used for research at this time but may prove to be valuable with future research and validation.

X-rays are the initial imaging modality for facial injuries, with CT scan utilized for better visualization when clinically indicated. The extent of many facial fractures may not be evident until CT imaging is performed.

Other Testing

Neuropsychologic testing (traditional or computer based) has been advocated by some for the evaluation of the concussed athlete. Unfortunately, at this time, due to lack of independent validation, expense, and no outcome studies showing improved management of concussions, its use should largely be reserved for complex cases and research. This is the conclusion reached by the most recent 2nd International Conference on Concussion in Sport. Its future role may increase with better independent and outcome-based research, but currently, inappropriate use of neuropsychologic testing has the potential to give a false sense of security to athletes, parents, and medical providers. The gold standard remains management of concussed athletes by a trained physician.

APPROACH TO THE ATHLETE WITH CONCUSSION

The most frequent head injury encountered within athletics is a concussion or MTBI. There have been multiple definitions of concussion, but overall, a concussion is a complex pathophysiologic *process* affecting the brain and induced by traumatic biomechanical forces.[9] As previously discussed, the mechanism of concussion can be due to direct or indirect trauma, or from a whiplash-type injury (Fig. 2.1).

Concussion severity can be categorized as either simple or complex *only* in retrospect, once all of the concussive sequelae have resolved. Simple concussions constitute the majority of concussions and are those with progressive resolution of symptoms over 7 to 10 days.[9] Complex concussion "encompasses cases where athletes suffer persistent symptoms (including persistent symptom recurrence with exertion), specific sequelae (such as concussive convulsions), prolonged loss of consciousness (more than one minute), or prolonged cognitive impairment after the injury. This group may also include athletes who suffer multiple concussions over time or where repeated concussions occur with progressively less impact force."[9]

HISTORY AND PHYSICAL EXAMINATION

Key components of the history around concussion include evaluation of cognitive symptoms, somatic symptoms, and affective symptoms, as seen in Table 2.1.

TABLE 2.1 Categories of Concussive Symptoms		
Cognitive	Somatic	Affective
Confusion	Headache	Emotional
Posttraumatic amnesia (PTA)	Fatigue	Irritable
Retrograde amnesia (RGA)	Disequilibrium, dizziness	
Loss of consciousness (LOC)	Visual disturbances	
Disorientation	Phonophobia	
Feeling "in a fog," "zoned out"		
Inability to focus		
Delayed verbal and motor responses		
Slurred/incoherent speech		
Excessive drowsiness		

It is important to note that concussion symptoms can fluctuate, with some initial symptoms resolving quickly over minutes to hours (i.e., confusion, amnesia, ataxia) while others may take days to weeks to resolve (i.e., headache, memory disturbances, mood lability).

DIAGNOSTIC TESTING

Further evaluation of the concussed athlete may include structural neuroimaging such as MRI or CT. However, both of these modalities are usually normal in the setting of concussion and are not needed unless there is concern for intracranial hemorrhage or osseous damage, which may be indicated with prolonged loss of consciousness, focal neurologic deficit, or overall worsening symptoms in the setting of complex concussion. The role of fMRI is largely experimental and unvalidated at this time, but it may play a role in the future with complex cases.

Neuropsychologic testing (formal or computer based) may be needed for management of complex concussions but is *not* currently regarded as important for the management of *simple concussions.*[9] The most recent consensus statement does note that it may form a cornerstone role for management of complex concussions.[9] When computer-based testing is used, it is recommended that all data received from computerized testing be reviewed in the overall context of the concussion, and the final decisions regarding return to play should be made by a supervising physician with adequate experience in caring for concussed athletes.

TREATMENT

General Measures

The current recommendations for care of a concussed athlete include physical and cognitive rest until all of the physical, cognitive, and somatic symptoms have resolved. Beyond rest from sporting activity, rest from academic work as well as video games may facilitate more rapid recovery. It is important to note that while there is extensive variability in the duration and severity of concussions, the typical/simple concussion requires 7 to 10 days to resolve. Furthermore, neuropsychologic deficits can persist even after resolution of symptoms; therefore, a cautious rather than aggressive approach is recommended.

Once an athlete has become asymptomatic at rest, they should go through a progressive exercise challenge test prior to being returned to game play where they are at risk for sustaining another injury.[9] The exercise challenge progression includes light aerobic exercise, such as riding on a stationary bicycle, sport-specific exercise, noncontact training drills, full-contact training, and game play. If postconcussive symptoms occur, most commonly exertional headache, visual disturbance, or disequilibrium, decrease level of activity and try to progress again in 24 hours.[9] It is generally recommended that there be a 24-hour period in between each progression in activity level; however, the rapidity of progression and the final determination should be made by the supervising physician. Knowing, however, that the average recovery from concussion requires 7 to 10 days makes return to play prior to that time period potentially risky. In one study, 91% of repeat concussions occurred within 10 days and 75% within 7 days of the initial concussion.[11]

Pharmacologic Treatment

The role of pharmacologic treatment for concussions is an area of research with little evidence to support recommendations. Treatment of acute symptoms is largely for headaches, with over-the-counter Tylenol most commonly recommended. Non-steroidal anti-inflammatory drugs (NSAIDs) should be avoided unless underlying cerebral hematoma, bleed, or bleeding disorder has been ruled out.

In athletes with postconcussive symptoms, pharmacologic treatment may focus on controlling persistent symptoms including cognition deficits, mood disorders, and mood lability. There is little data in the area as well, but one may consider drawing data from consensus statements on the pharmacologic treatment of traumatic brain injury.[12]

Prognosis/Return to Play

Overall prognosis for a simple concussion is very good when it is properly treated. Risks for prolonged recovery or long-term sequelae include repeat or multiple concussions, prolonged loss of consciousness, and retrograde amnesia.[13] Whether genetic predisposition is a risk factor is an area of active research. Some are looking at a potential association between the apolipoprotein E allele and chronic traumatic brain injury.[14]

Return to play is based on asymptomatic graduated return to play as noted previously for an initial concussion. The general recommendation is that when an athlete suffers three concussions during a given season that they should be restricted from play for the remainder of the season. If there have been more severe concussions or head injuries, this may be decreased to two concussions within a given season.

Currently, the best way to prevent concussion is the use of adequate, properly fitting protective equipment and helmets. Additionally, the use and teaching of proper tackling and blocking techniques in football can help to minimize head injury.[15] Some authors have suggested use of mouth guards as a possible mechanism of concussion prevention. However, the current evidence regarding mouth guards and concussion prevention is inconclusive.[16]

Complications/Indications for Referral

Focal symptoms or rapidly progressive symptoms are indications for immediate emergent referral to a medical center with appropriate neurosurgical as well as emergent CT or MRI capabilities. Atypical symptoms or prolonged symptoms are indications for referral to a neurologist, neurosurgeon, or sports medicine physician with experience managing complex concussions. Neuropsychologists trained in assessing concussed athletes may be indicated at the discretion of the supervising physician.

APPROACH TO THE ATHLETE WITH EYE INJURIES

Eye traumas constitute common injuries in sports, particularly with ball and stick sports. Eye injuries range from eyelid lacerations, corneal abrasion, corneal/conjunctival lacerations, and subconjunctival hemorrhage to more severe injuries including hyphema induced by blunt trauma, traumatic iritis, retinal detachment, ruptured globe, and penetrating injuries or orbital wall fractures (Fig. 2.6).

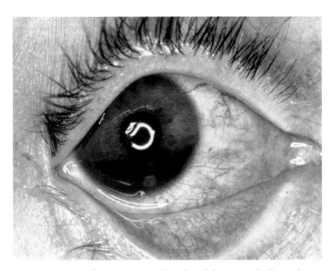

FIG. 2.6. Hyphema. Reprinted with permission from Harwood-Nuss A, Wolfson AB, et al. *The Clinical Practice of Emergency Medicine*. 3rd ed. Philadelphia: Lippincott Williams & Wilkins; 2001.

HISTORY AND PHYSICAL EXAMINATION

Approach to the patient with ocular injury includes obtaining a history of previous eye injury or decreased visual acuity. The history should include the use of eyeglass or contact lens or prior history of refractive eye surgery, such as LASIK. Athletes who have undergone eye surgery, such as corneal replacement or LASIK surgery, should be aware that there may be a risk for reinjury or LASIK flap displacement or corneal disruption following blunt trauma, thus increasing the risk of open globe injuries and indicating the need for athletes at risk for blunt ocular trauma to wear protective eyewear during athletic participation.[17,18] Mechanism of injury is important in determining possible injuries.

The preparticipation physical examination is used to identify athletes with monocular vision or significant decreases in visual acuity that would have long-lasting effects if the athlete suffered ocular trauma resulting in permanent vision impairment or disability. The visual examination should include a screening examination for equality of pupils, presence of amblyopia or lazy eye, or decreased visual acuity. Some people naturally have a degree of anisocoria, or unequal pupils. It is important to document this fact prior to injury. If anisocoria is first noticed on examination of a head injury, it can be indicative of increased intracranial pressure or possibly a cerebral hemorrhage.

The acute evaluation of the athlete with eye injury includes gross inspection for deformities, palpation for associated periorbital fracture, as well as proper inspection of pupils, sclera and cornea. Proper and equal pupil reflex should be noted as well as normal funduscopic examination.

DIAGNOSTIC TESTING

Plain radiographs or preferably CT of facial bones may be necessary if there is concern for fracture or hemorrhage.

TREATMENT

General Measures

The most important intervention for eye injuries is primary prevention. This is best done by the use of properly fitting protective eyewear for all practices and game play. The eyewear should be made of polycarbonate lenses and meet the ASTM (American Society for Testing and Materials) standards. Rest, cold compresses, and analgesics should be used for general blunt trauma if no fractures are suspected.

Pharmacologic Treatment

If a corneal abrasion or superficial corneal foreign body is present, appropriate antibiotics may be necessary.

Prognosis/Return to Play

The athlete needs to return to full baseline vision prior to being allowed to participate in athletic practice or game play. It is also imperative that there is no evidence of postconcussion syndrome prior to return.

Complications/Red Flags/Indications for Referral

Once an athlete has an eye injury, the more severe eye injuries such as hyphema, traumatic iritis, retinal detachment, decreased visual acuity, and new onset diplopia indicating possible orbital wall fracture or any possibility of an open globe injury require immediate referral to an ophthalmologist.

APPROACH TO THE ATHLETE WITH NASAL INJURIES

The two main nasal injuries encountered in athletics are nasal fracture and epistaxis, or nasal bleeding. Approximately 90% of nasal bleeding occurs in the anterior nasal passages. Kiesselbach's plexus is located in the anterior nasal passages, and it is a web of capillaries that is firmly adhered to the nasal septal cartilage. Given this anatomy, any damage to the septal cartilage can result in damage to the vascular plexus, resulting in epistaxis or possibly a septal hematoma.

HISTORY AND PHYSICAL EXAMINATION

The examination of the nose includes the nasal bone, the septum, and the cartilage. Discerning pre-existing deformities from acute injuries is important. Deviation of the nasal dorsum, epistaxis, and edema should prompt the examiner to look for septal dislocation and septal hematoma. Failure to identify a septal hematoma may result in necrosis of the septal cartilage and subsequent perforation and collapse. The main considerations necessary regarding nasal fractures are that if there is significant displacement of the fracture site, attempts at reduction may be focused at improving alignment and patency of the nasal airways as well as patient comfort. If done immediately after injury, reduction can be attempted without analgesia or sedation.

DIAGNOSTIC TESTING

Often radiologic studies are not necessary, but plain radiographs or facial bone CT may be obtained to rule out displaced fractures or hemorrhage.

TREATMENT

General Measures

If epistaxis is present, pressure is the key to treatment. Given that 90% of all nasal bleeds are in the anterior portion of the nose, the best initial treatment is constant, firm pressure while the athlete is leaning forward. This prevents significant amount of blood from passing into the posterior pharynx and either into the respiratory or into the gastrointestinal tract. If simple pressure is inadequate therapy, the nose can be packed with a simple gauze, nasal packing, or tampon.

Pharmacologic Treatment

The nasal packing can also be soaked with epinephrine to induce local vasoconstriction in an attempt to stop the bleeding.

Prognosis/Return to Play

The athlete should not be returned to play immediately after a nasal fracture. In general, nasal bones heal within 4 to 8 weeks; however, if the athlete returns sooner, a protective facial device is strongly recommended. It is also imperative that there is no evidence of postconcussion syndrome prior to return.

One key with acute nasal fractures is to inspect for a septal hematoma. If a hematoma is present, it needs to be drained with a large gauge needle and the nares subsequently need to be packed to avoid recurrence. Untreated nasal septal hematomas can put pressure on the septal cartilage, causing necrosis and possible septal perforation.

APPROACH TO THE ATHLETE WITH DENTAL INJURIES

Dental and mouth injuries are very common in contact sports, such as basketball, hockey, football, and lacrosse. Cohenca (2007) showed that basketball was the sport that had the highest rate of dental injuries at one collegiate institution, with 10.6 injuries per 100 athlete-seasons among men and 5.0 injuries per 100 athlete-seasons among women.[19] The American Dental Association recommends wearing custom mouth guards for the following sports: acrobatics, basketball, boxing, field hockey, football, gymnastics, handball, ice hockey, lacrosse, martial arts, racquetball, roller hockey, rugby, shot putting, skateboarding, skiing, skydiving, soccer, squash, surfing, volleyball, water polo, weight lifting, and wrestling. Mouth guards have been worn in sport to prevent maxillofacial injury since they were first worn by boxers in the 1920s and were mandated to be worn by high school football players since 1962. Knapik et al., in a 2007 meta-analysis, showed that the risk of orofacial sports injury was 1.6 to 1.9 times higher when a mouth guard was not used.[16] There are multiple types of dental injuries, including fracture, luxation, impaction, extrusion, and avulsion. Almost all of these injuries are true dental emergencies if they occur to permanent teeth. True tooth avulsion is one of the areas of dental injury where a trained provider acting quickly can help to provide a good outcome for the patient. The viability of the avulsed tooth depends on the viability of the periodontal ligament as well as the length of time the tooth has been avulsed. If the avulsed tooth is reimplanted within 5 minutes, there is an 85% to 97% chance of survival of the tooth, whereas the survival rate approaches 0% if the tooth is not reimplanted until one hour after injury.[20]

HISTORY AND PHYSICAL EXAMINATION

The anatomy of the tooth is important to understand for the appropriate treatment of dental injuries. Each tooth has an external crown and one or more internal roots. The crown is essentially made of a hard, protective layer of enamel, which protects the inner dentin and pulp. The pulp is the vascular chamber that provides nutrients to the tooth, as well as providing sensation. The root of each tooth is connected to the

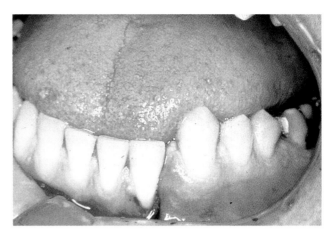

FIG. 2.7. Malocclusion/mandibular fracture. Reprinted with permission from Harries M, Williams C, Stanish W, et al. *Oxford Textbook of Sports Medicine*. New York: Oxford University Press; 1998.

socket via the periodontal ligament. Any major injury to the periodontal ligament increases the likelihood that an avulsed or broken tooth will not remain viable.[21]

One of the most important historical aspects of dental injury is the time, both the time of injury as well as time interval between injury and treatment, as they affect treatment and prognosis. The presence of primary versus secondary tooth injury also provides important information for diagnostic and treatment options. Other important aspects of the history that may indicate a more severe injury requiring immediate evaluation include spontaneous onset tooth pain or temperature sensitivity, which may indicate exposed dental pulp; pain with palpation or pressure, possibly indicative of a periodontal ligament injury; or malocclusion, which may indicate a mandibular or facial fracture[21] (Fig. 2.7).

DIAGNOSTIC TESTING

Any athlete with suspected dental or mandibular fracture or possible tooth displacement should undergo radiographs of the affected areas to rule out the possibility of bony or dental fracture.

TREATMENT

General Measures

There are a variety of dental fractures, all of which should undergo immediate evaluation by a maxillofacial surgeon to determine if urgent treatment is needed to prevent further morbidity or possibly to save the injured tooth. Basic initial management of dental or mandibular fractures involves stabilization of the jaw in the case of a mandibular fracture or stabilization of the portions of the tooth that are displaced.

If an avulsed tooth is found, it should be handled by the crown to avoid contact, and therefore destruction, of the periodontal ligament. If there is visible debris on the tooth, it may be rinsed with saline or water. The periodontal ligament should not be scrubbed as this may lead to damage and inability of the tooth to heal, even if it is rapidly reimplanted. If the tooth cannot be replanted within 5 minutes, it can be placed in a variety of solutions. The list of preferred solutions according to the American Academy of Pediatric Dentistry is Viaspan, Hanks' balanced salt solution, cold milk, saliva, physiologic saline, or water. The tooth should not be transported in the mouth due to risk of further tooth damage or aspiration or ingestion of the tooth. The tooth should then be held in place or a splint applied until urgent dental referral can be made.[22]

Pharmacologic Treatment

Appropriate antibiotic coverage is necessary if an avulsion or fracture is present to cover normal oral flora. The patient's tetanus status should be updated as well if either of these is present.

Prognosis/Return to Play

Athletes may return to play once cleared by a dental/maxillofacial surgeon. Follow-up is necessary within 24 hours of dental fractures. A dental mouth guard is highly recommended and effective for preventing further dental injuries.

Complications/Red Flags/Indications for Referral

Luxation injuries of teeth are another important aspect of dental injuries and were well described by Bernius and Perlin (2006).[21] When these injuries are encountered, prompt and proper management may allow for the ongoing viability of the injured tooth. The mildest form of luxation injury is a subluxation in which the tooth is injured and abnormally loosened but not displaced. In the majority of cases the tooth survives, but evaluation by a dentist is important to help stabilize and splint the tooth to prevent further injury and also to evaluate for more severe injury. Lateral luxation occurs when a tooth is displaced laterally. There may be associated root fracture or surrounding alveolar fracture or contusion. When these injuries occur in permanent teeth, they also require immediate dental referral for splinting and possible relocation. Other types of dental luxation injuries include intrusion, where the tooth is driven apically into the bony alveoli, extraction where the tooth is partially pulled from the socket, or avulsion injuries where the tooth is completely removed from the socket. The latter two injuries are

serious as urgent reposition and stabilization are critical to the survival of the tooth as previously described by Andreasen (1995).[20]

APPROACH TO THE ATHLETE WITH EAR TRAUMA

Ear problems are usually due to direct trauma or infection. Problems include ear lacerations, auricular hematoma, and tympanic membrane rupture. Infectious problems include otitis externa. Ear lacerations can be due to direct ear trauma such as an elbow to the ear while playing basketball or a stick injury to the helmeted head such as in hockey or lacrosse.

HISTORY AND PHYSICAL EXAMINATION

Inspection of the entire outer and inner ear is necessary after blunt trauma. Inspect the tympanic membrane for hemotympanum and the external canal for CNS leak. If an ear laceration is present, evaluation of the underlying auricular cartilage needs to be assessed to determine whether there is a cartilaginous tear present. Careful evaluation of the facial nerve is also necessary to rule out injury or palsy.

DIAGNOSTIC TESTING

Plain radiographs or CT of the head may be helpful if there is concern for associated skull fracture and subsequent hemorrhage.

TREATMENT

General Measures

All lacerations need to be irrigated and immediately repaired; however, if lacerations are complex, often these will be referred to a plastic surgeon. Hemostasis must be achieved to prevent subsequent hematoma formation.

Pharmacologic Treatment

If a cartilaginous injury is present, prophylactic antibiotics should be given to prevent chondritis. The main pathogens involved with otitis externa are *Pseudomonas* spp., *Proteus* spp., or *Escherichia coli*; therefore, appropriate antibiotic coverage would include coverage for these pathogens, with ciprofloxacin being a good choice if the athlete is not allergic.

Prognosis/Return to Play

In cases of minor trauma with appropriate treatment and a compression dressing, the athlete can be returned to play the same day of the injury with appropriate protective equipment, such as a headgear or a helmet. However, in cases of severe trauma that requires surgical repair, the athlete may need to be out for 6 to 8 weeks. It is also imperative that there is no evidence of postconcussion syndrome prior to return.

Complications/Indications for Referral

Auricular hematomas are due to pressure and sheer forces applied to the ear and represent a blood collection between the cartilage and the overlying skin. These lesions can be painful, and prompt treatment is necessary with drainage with an 18- to 20-gauge needle and a pressure dressing. If left untreated, an auricular hematoma can become calcified and disfiguring. This condition is known as "cauliflower ear." Overlying skin avulsion larger than 5 mm, severe crush injuries, complete or nearly complete avulsions or amputations, auricular hematoma, cartilage defects larger than 5 mm, wounds that require the removal of more than 5 mm of tissue, involvement of the auditory canal, obvious devitalization, and total ear avulsion all require referral to a plastic surgeon.

KEY POINTS

- Concussions are the most common head injury encountered in sports.

- On the field and office assessment are to include evaluation of cognitive, somatic, afferent and neurological deficits.

- CT scan and MRI are the imaging modalities of choice but most often are negative in the concussed athlete. Neuropsychological testing may also play a key role in evaluation of complex concussions.

- Treatment of concussion consists of physical and cognitive rest; most often, resolution occurs within 7–10 days.

- Return to play with gradual increase in exertion/sport with 24-hour asymptomatic periods in between.

- Eye, ear, nose, and dental injuries can be common and at times severe and may need specialist referral.

REFERENCES

1. Thurman DJ, Branche CM, Sniezek JE. The epidemiology of sports-related traumatic brain injuries in the United States: recent developments. *J Head Trauma Rehabil.* 1998;13:1–8.
2. McAlindon RJ. On field evaluation and management of head and neck injured athletes. *Clin Sports Med.* 2002;21(1):1–14.
3. Harmon KG. Assessment and management of concussion in sports. *Am Fam Physician.* 1999;60(3):887–892.
4. Levy ML, Ozgur BM, Berry C, et al. Birth and evolution of the football helmet. *Neurosurgery.* 2004;55:656–662.
5. Giza CC, Hovda DA. The neurometabolic cascade of concussion. *J Athl Train.* 2001;36(3):228–235.
6. Herring SA, et al. Concussion (mild traumatic brain injury) and the team physician: a consensus statement. *Med Sci Sports Exerc.* 2005 Nov;37(11):2012–2016.
7. American Academy of Pediatrics Committee on Sports Medicine and Fitness. Protective eyewear for young athletes. *Pediatrics.* 2004;113:619–622.
8. Classe JG. Sports related ocular trauma: a preventable epidemic. *J Am Optom Assoc.* 1996;67:66–67.
9. McCrory P, Johnston K, Meeuwisse W, et al. Summary and agreement statement of the 2nd International Conference on Concussion in Sport, Prague 2004. *Br J Sports Med.* 2005;39:196–204.
10. Herring SA, et al. Concussion (mild traumatic brain injury) and the team physician: a consensus statement. *Med Sci Sports Exerc.* 2006 Feb;38(2):395–399.
11. Guskiewicz KM, McCrea M, Marshall SW. Cumulative effects associated with recurrent concussion in collegiate football players: the NCAA Concussion Study. *JAMA.* 2003;290:2549–2555.
12. Warden D, Gordon B, McAllister TW, et al. Guidelines for the pharmacologic treatment of neurobehavioral sequelae of traumatic brain injury. *J Neurotrauma.* 2006;23(10):1468–1501.
13. Guskiewicz KM, Marshall SW, Bailes J, et al. Association between recurrent concussion and late-life cognitive impairment in retired professional football players. *Neurosurgery.* 2005;57(4):719–726; discussion 719–726.
14. Jordan BD, Relkin NR, Ravdin LD, et al. Apolipoprotein E epsilon4 associated with chronic traumatic brain injury in boxing. *JAMA.* 1997;278:136–140.
15. Levy ML, Ozgur BM, Berry C, et al. Analysis and evolution of head injury in football. *Neurosurgery.* 2004;55:649–655.
16. Knapik JJ, Marshall SW, Lee RB, et al. Mouthguards in sport activities: history, physical properties and injury prevention effectiveness. *Sports Med.* 2007;37(2):117–144.
17. Booth MA, Koch DD. Late laser in situ keratomileusis flap dislocation caused by a thrown football. *J Cataract Refract Surg.* 2003;29(10):2032–2033.
18. Oh-i K, Mori H, Kubo M, et al. LASIK flap dislocation by blunt trauma seven weeks after surgery. *J Refract Surg.* 2005;21(1):93–94.
19. Cohenca N, Roges RA, Roges R. The incidence and severity of dental trauma in intercollegiate athletes. *J Am Dent Assoc.* 2007;138(8):1121–1126.
20. Andreasen JO, Borum MK, Jacobsen HL, et al. Replantation of 400 avulsed permanent incisors. 1. Diagnosis of healing complications. *Endod Dent Traumatol.* 1995;11:51–58.
21. Bernius M, Perlin D. Pediatric ear, nose, and throat emergencies. *Pediatr Clin N Am.* 2006;53:195–214.
22. American Academy of Pediatric Dentistry (AAPD). Clinical guideline on management of acute dental trauma. *Pediatr Dent.* 2004;26(7):120–127.

CHAPTER

3

Athlete with Syncope

Christopher Lutrzykowski

INTRODUCTION

Syncope is defined as the temporary loss of consciousness and posture. Near syncope is defined as a prodromal symptom of fainting or near faint. These events can occur before, during, or after an athletic event and warrant an investigation. A cause for syncope can be found in up to 50% of patients.[1] A good patient history may be the single best determinant in guiding the clinician to the correct diagnosis.[1–3] The history is often obtained by interviewing the athlete, but it is paramount to include those who witnessed the event. This group includes parents, coaches, and trainers who can be of incalculable value in narrowing the differential diagnosis. Using the appropriate screening questions in a preparticipation examination may also be of benefit, as shown in Table 3.1.[2,3]

The athlete with syncope presents a diagnostic challenge due to the large list of potential etiologies ranging from the benign to the catastrophic. An excellent resource for the clinician caring for athletes is the 36th Bethesda Conference report: Eligibility Recommendations for Competitive Athletes with Cardiovascular Abnormalities.

There continues to be a highly visible and defined group of athletes who suffer a sudden cardiac death (SCD) event. This chapter includes guidelines for caring for the athlete with a variety of cardiac conditions including hypertension, arrhythmia, and syncope.

PATHOPHYSIOLOGY

Syncope occurs secondary to a sudden loss of blood pressure (BP) to the brain. Etiologies in athletes include both cardiac and noncardiac types. Hypertrophic cardiomyopathy (HCM) is a relatively common inherited medical condition, with the incidence estimated at 1:500 in the general population, and is inherited in an autosomal dominant fashion.[5] It is caused by mutations in any one of 10 genes that encode proteins of the cardiac sarcomere.[6] Initially thought to be a disease of white males, recent studies indicate a proportionate incidence among many ethnic groups.[6,7] Indeed it is estimated to be underdiagnosed in these populations as well as among

women.[7,8] Sudden death related to HCM also crosses ethnic lines with similar prevalence rates on autopsy of athletes after SCD.[8]

Postexertional syncope, also known as exercise-associated collapse, is a benign condition caused by venous pooling upon the completion of exercise. The cessation of normal muscular contraction of the lower extremity results in transient decreased venous return and subsequent cerebral hypoperfusion. Arrhythmias can occur for a variety of etiologies, with ischemia being the leading cause in the athlete over the age of 35. A full description of arrhythmias is listed later in the chapter.

EPIDEMIOLOGY

The rate of syncope among athletes is not known, but cardiac causes appear more defined. A recent study of 7,500 athletes revealed a syncopal history in 6% of athletes over a 5-year period.[9] This same study also noted that only 1% of those athletes had exertion-related syncope and no postexercise or nonexercise syncopal event was associated with structural heart disease.[9] The incidence of SCD has been estimated to be 1 per 200,000 athletes yearly in the United States, but true incidence may be higher.[10,11] The rate among young adults is less than 1% than that of SCDs among adults with the total number of cardiac-caused events reaching 10 to 13 per year.[1,12] Most causes of syncope are benign but deserve a workup due to both the potential for SCD as well as the disruptive nature of the event.[13] The majority of SCDs occur during sports activity or the immediate period thereafter. However, 20% of SCDs may occur in the ensuing 24-hour period post exercise, further complicating the correct identification of the true incidence rate.[14,15] Syncope can be recurrent; noncardiac syncope has a recurrence rate approaching 43% at 5 years.[16] The most common cause of nonexertional syncope among young competitive athletes appears to be vasovagal or "situational" (88% and 12%, respectively). Postexertional syncope (exercise-associated collapse) is most commonly associated with postural hypotension. Exertional syncope is most commonly associated with exertional-induced neurally mediated

TABLE 3.1 **AHA Consensus Panel Recommendations for Preparticipation Athletic Screening[4]**

Family History	Personal History	Physical Examination
Premature sudden cardiac death Heart disease in surviving relatives younger than 50 years old	Heart murmur Systemic hypertension Fatigue Syncope/near syncope Excessive/unexplained exertional dyspnea Exertional chest pain	Heart murmur (supine/standing[a]) Femoral arterial pulses (to exclude coarctation of aorta) Stigmata of Marfan syndrome Brachial blood pressure measurement (sitting)

[a]In particular, to identify heart murmur consistent with dynamic obstruction to left ventricular outflow. Modified from Maron BJ, Thompson PD, Puffer JC, et al. Cardiovascular preparticipation screening of competitive athletes. A statement for health professionals from the Sudden Death Committee (clinical cardiology) and Congenital Cardiac Defects Committee (cardiovascular disease in the young), American Heart Association. *Circulation.* 1996;94:850–856.

TABLE 3.2 **Causes of Sudden Death in 387 Young Athletes**

Cause	No. of Athletes	Percent
Hypertrophic cardiomyopathy (HCM)	102	26.4
Commotio cordis	77	19.9
Coronary artery anomalies	53	13.7
Left ventricular hypertrophy of indeterminate causation[a]	29	7.5
Myocarditis	20	5.2
Ruptured aortic aneurysm (Marfan syndrome)	12	3.1
Arrhythmogenic right ventricular	11	2.8
Tunneled (bridged) coronary artery[b]	11	2.8
Aortic valve stenosis	10	2.6
Atherosclerotic coronary artery disease	10	2.6
Dilated cardiomyopathy	9	2.3
Myxomatous mitral valve degeneration	9	2.3
Asthma (or other pulmonary condition)	8	2.1
Heat stroke	6	1.6
Drug abuse	4	1.0
Other cardiovascular cause	4	1.0
Long QT syndrome[c]	3	0.8
Cardiac sarcoidosis	3	0.8
Trauma causing structural cardiac injury	3	0.8
Ruptured cerebral artery	3	0.8

[a]Findings at autopsy were suggestive of HCM but were insufficient to be diagnostic.
[b]Tunneled coronary artery was deemed the cause of death in the absence of any other cardiac abnormality.
[c]The long QT syndrome was documented on clinical evaluation. Modified from Maron BJ. Sudden death in young athletes. *N Engl J Med.* 2003;349:1064–1075.
Adapted from data from the registry of the Minneapolis Heart Institute Foundation.[14]

syncope (66%). Cardiac anomalies appear to account for the rest.[9] Sudden death due to cardiac causes is most often attributed to HCM; as much as 50% of cardiovascular SCDs may be attributable to HCM.[15,17] HCM is followed by coronary artery anomalies, left ventricular hypertrophy (LVH), myocarditis, Marfan syndrome, and arrhythmogenic right ventricular cardiomyopathy in order of prevalence.[4,6,17] Latent coronary artery disease (CAD) dominates the incidence of SCD after the age of 35 with vast majority of causes

(80%).[17] Table 3.2 lists the causes of SCD based on order of frequency.

The Athlete's Heart

The athlete's heart undergoes physiologic changes with exercise, which impact diagnostic and therapeutic considerations. Cardiac remodeling and increased ventricular mass occur as a normal adaptation to prolonged exercise. In addition,

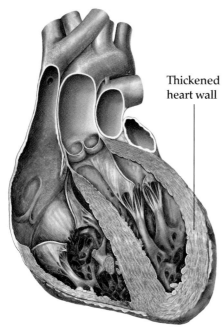

Thickened
heart wall

Cardiomyopathy

FIG. 3.1. Left ventricular hypertrophy. Modified from Opie LH. *Heart Physiology: From Cell to Circulation*. Philadelphia: Lippincott Williams & Wilkins; 2004. © LH Opie, 2004.

atrial and ventricular cavity size enlargement, without systolic or diastolic dysfunction, is also present because of increased blood volume. This is defined as the *athlete's heart*. These changes may occur within weeks of beginning a training program, are probably proportional to the intensity and duration of training, and resolve with decreasing exercise loads.[18] Electrocardiogram (ECG) findings in athletes can mimic cardiac injury patterns and may lead to unnecessary exclusion from participation.[4] Conversely, adolescent athletes rarely exhibit deep T-wave inversions;[19] 2% of athletes exhibit increased left ventricular (LV) wall thickness of 13 to 15 mm, thus overlapping the diagnostic criteria for HCM; and 15% of athletes have LV chamber size greater than 60 mm, which can raise concern for cardiomyopathy despite normal LV function.[20] Referral for further diagnostic testing is warranted, including echocardiogram (ECHO) (Fig. 3.1). Careful consideration should be given to athletes in this gray zone, as the risk for SCD is considerable, yet overly strict guidelines may exclude many athletes not otherwise at risk. ECG findings in athletes may return to normal, but ECHO findings continue to display HCM in those athletes with the disease.[21] Adolescent athletes rarely exhibit chamber size greater than 12 mm; LV wall thickness greater than 12 mm should prompt further evaluation for HCM.[22] Athletes with LV wall thickness greater than 15 mm on ECHO should be referred to a cardiologist.

NARROWING THE DIFFERENTIAL DIAGNOSIS
History

An adequate history of the event must be obtained from the athlete, coaches, parents, and trainers. It is a necessary but often time-consuming process. The history will often lead to the diagnosis and guide further workup and should include specific details of the event. The timing of the syncopal event should be noted; did the event occur before, during, or after the competition? How long after the event? Any prodromal symptoms such as palpitations or chest pain should be noted. Prior history and family history should be noted, including family history of sudden death. A dietary history should be obtained, including intrarace nutrition. Any medications, supplements, or ergogenic aids should be discussed and explored. The overall duration of the event and specific interventions should also be noted. Any physical stigmata of note, such as seizure activity, should also be recorded. A collapse "mid stride" is ominous as the majority of SCDs in athletes occur during or just after athletic participation.[6,21]

Evidence-based Physical Examination

The physical examination of the athlete will be guided by the history but should include measurement of bilateral BP, orthostatic BP, upper and lower extremity pulse, and dynamic cardiac examination.[23] Cardiac examination should include inspection of the chest wall for ventricular heave as well as palpation of the point of maximal impulse. Auscultation is facilitated by a quiet room and should include a dynamic examination with supine, squat, and standing maneuvers.[23] Respiratory and gastrointestinal examination as well as appropriate neurologic examinations would complete the evaluation.

Diagnostic Testing
Laboratory

Appropriate laboratory studies should be considered based upon clinical presentation and suspected etiology. Common tests to consider include complete blood count (CBC), renal function tests, and liver enzymes and thyroid studies. If infectious etiology considered monospot or Epstein–Barr virus (EBV) serology may be indicated.

Imaging

Diagnostic imaging may be considered when clinically indicated.

Other Testing

Additional workup in the office should include an ECG. Further testing will be guided by the history and physical and may include exercise tolerance test (ETT), and ECHO.

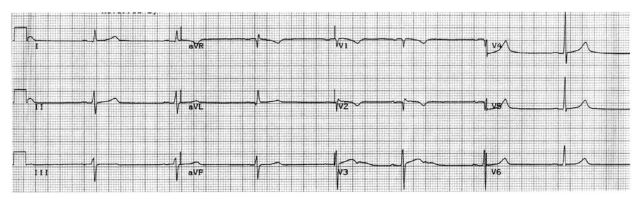

FIG. 3.2. ECG of left ventricular hypertrophy with long QT syndrome. Reprinted with permission from Topol EJ, Califf RM, Prystowsky EN, et al. *Textbook of Cardiovascular Medicine.* 3rd ed. Philadelphia: Lippincott Williams & Wilkins; 2006.

Ambulatory Holter/event monitoring, tilt-table testing, Electrophysiologic study (EPS) testing, and more invasive cardiac testings such as cardiac magnetic resonance imaging may be considered based on clinical presentation.[4]

APPROACH TO THE ATHLETE WITH HCM

As with other causes of syncope, HCM represents a diagnostic dilemma to the health care provider. Syncope and/or SCD are oftentimes the first-presenting finding for HCM. Up to 50% of cardiovascular SCDs may be attributable to HCM,[15,17] and the athlete with HCM may be asymptomatic until outflow obstruction occurs.

HISTORY AND PHYSICAL EXAMINATION

Symptoms can range from exertional chest pain, palpitations, and dyspnea on exertion to fatigue, syncope, or near syncope.[24] Physical examination findings can range from a normal physical examination to a clearly abnormal cardiac examination.

The murmur of HCM with outflow obstruction has been classically characterized as a harsh midsystolic murmur heard best over the aortic region, which increases with Valsalva maneuver and decreases with standing. Physiologically, Valsalva maneuver and squat to stand decrease venous return, which in turn creates turbulent blood flow in the outflow tract. Mitral valve prolapse may also be accentuated under these circumstances.[23] Physical examination findings may also include a reversal of the normal physiologic split S2 (a narrowing of the S2 on inspiration).[23]

Diagnostic Testing

ECG should be obtained and is frequently abnormal. ECG findings include evidence of LVH as well as Q waves in the inferior leads and deep T-wave inversions across the precordium. However, ECG findings overlap with normal findings of a normal athlete's heart. Additionally, the ECG may be normal in the early stages of the disease (Fig. 3.2).[25]

HCM is diagnosed on ECHO by end-diastolic asymmetric wall thickening of 15 mm or more in an adult patient. Genetic testing is available, and HCM has a heterogeneous presentation. This can lead to a normal ECHO in an individual with known risk for HCM.[7] It is generally accepted that the diagnosis of HCM in children is made with the same asymmetric wall thickening as in adults; that is 2 standard deviations above the mean for that age group in the presence of asymmetric wall thickening.[7] A recent study among highly trained adolescents helps further define this, as the vast majority of athletes aged 14 to 18 had LV wall thickness less than 12 mm in boys and 11 mm in girls.[19]

Treatment

General Measures

- Athletes suspected of HCM based on clinical examination are excluded from athletic participation until evaluated by an experienced cardiologist.[7]
- A period of deconditioning may help the cardiologist differentiate HCM from the athletic heart.[26]

Pharmacologic Treatment

- β-Blockers are the most commonly used medication in HCM. Verapamil may also be useful as a second-line agent.
- Disopyramide is a useful adjunct in select patients in conjunction with β-blockers.[27]

Prognosis/Return To Play

- If an athlete is suspected of having HCM based on physical examination findings, symptom complex, family history, or ECG findings, referral to cardiology and ECHO is mandatory.

- HCM presents a challenge to the sports provider and cardiologist, given its heterogeneous presentation and inability to accurately identify risk factors for disease progression and risk for SCD.
- The 36th Bethesda Conference guidelines recognize this, but at the present time, given that athletic activity may be a risk factor for fatal arrhythmia in HCM, the guidelines are broadly applied to all athletes with the diagnosis.[7]
- The 36th Bethesda Conference guidelines are as follows:
  - Athletes with a probable or unequivocal clinical diagnosis of HCM should be excluded from most competitive sports, with the possible exception of those of low intensity (class IA).
  - This recommendation is independent of age, gender, and phenotypic appearance, and does not differ for those athletes who are with or without symptoms, with LV outflow obstruction, or have had prior treatment with drugs or major interventions with surgery, alcohol septal ablation, pacemaker, or implantable defibrillator.
  - Although the clinical significance and natural history of genotype-positive–phenotype-negative individuals remain unresolved, no compelling data are available at present with which to preclude these patients from competitive sports, particularly in the absence of cardiac symptoms or a family history of sudden death.
- The guidelines are also clear on participation in athletics with implantable cardiac defibrillators (ICDs).
- Athletic participation in any sport other than class IA athletics is not recommended at this time, as ICD discharge may pose a risk to both the athlete and other participants.
- ICDs have not been fully tested under all athletic conditions and thus preclude participation.[7]
- The presence of an automated external defibrillator (AED) also does not warrant participation.
- While AEDs may be effective in aborting ventricular arrhythmias, they are not a reliable treatment intervention for an athlete with HCM.

Complications/Indications for Referral

All athletes suspected of having HCM should be excluded from participation and referred to an experienced cardiologist with knowledge of various stages of the disease.

APPROACH TO THE ATHLETE WITH ARRHYTHMIA

Arrhythmia may present in athletes with a constellation of symptoms including palpitations, unexplained dyspnea, or as syncope. The true incidence of arrhythmia as a cause of SCD in the absence of cardiac structural anomalies is not known. Arrhythmia as a cause of syncope is problematic in that it is usually fleeting and may not affect performance.

The arrhythmia may not exist every time an athlete takes the field and may not cause symptoms when present. However, it is important to recognize common arrhythmias among athletes and guide an appropriate workup to exclude those disease entities that may predispose athletes to SCD. Additionally, ECG findings in athletes may exhibit a number of findings that appear abnormal but in fact are common among highly trained athletes. These findings include but are not limited to sinus bradycardia, sinus arrhythmia, first-degree heart block, second-degree heart block type I, occasional uniform premature ventricular complexes (PVCs), and wandering atrial pacemaker.[1,28] Arrhythmias of atrial origin include sinus tachycardia, supraventricular tachycardia, atrial fibrillation, atrial flutter, and sinus arrhythmia. Sinus tachycardia is common, and indeed, the goal of exercise is to elevate the heart rate above resting values. Sinus arrhythmia is also common and considered normal among athletes. Sinus node–generated arrhythmias generally do not need additional workup unless they are symptomatic in the athlete and impair performance.[1] Atrial flutter is a rare cause of arrhythmia and syncope in athletes. Atrial fibrillation is more common and increases with advancing age in athletes. Master's athletes, in particular endurance athletes, may be at an increased risk of atrial fibrillation.[29]

Supraventricular tachycardia and AV nodal reentrant tachycardia (AVNRT) (retrograde conduction) can cause syncope and occasionally require more invasive testing and intervention. Wolff–Parkinson–White syndrome (WPW) is a concerning arrhythmogenic cause of syncope as it may lead in rare instances to SCD.[1] Premature ventricular contractions are common among athletes. Along with premature atrial contractions, this is the most common symptomatic presentation of arrhythmia in athletics.[13]

HISTORY AND PHYSICAL EXAMINATION

In addition to syncope, arrhythmia may present in a variety of different ways. The history includes fatigue, shortness of breath, dyspnea, reduced exercise performance, palpitations, and chest pain. The physical examination may be normal, reflecting the fleeting and often paroxysmal nature of most arrhythmias but may also exhibit irregularities in heart rate and rhythm. Atrial fibrillation is classically described as an irregularly irregular rhythm. PVCs may present with infrequent irregular beats and may be symptomatic.

DIAGNOSTIC TESTING

In addition to the ECG, ECHO is useful to evaluate structural anomalies. Risk factors for CAD should be thoroughly reviewed and consideration given to ETT in master's athletes.[1,11] Sport-specific participation with a loop recorder, when possible, can also help elucidate intermittent atrial arrhythmias. EPS may also be necessary. Angiography may be necessary in the master's level athlete with arrhythmia-induced syncope.

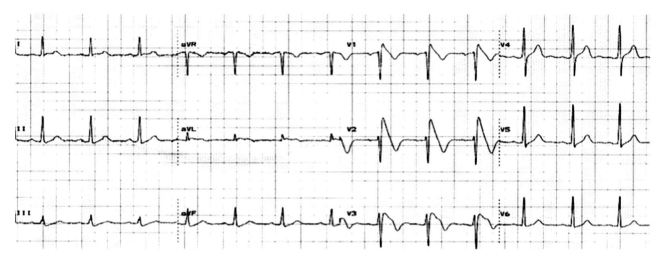

FIG. 3.3. ECG findings of Brugada syndrome. Reprinted with permission from Topol EJ, Califf RM, Prystowsky EN, et al. *Textbook of Cardiovascular Medicine.* 3rd ed. Philadelphia: Lippincott Williams & Wilkins; 2006.

Lab testing including thyroid function studies may be guided by the history and physical examination.

The athlete with ECG evidence of WPW requires a mandatory workup, including ECHO and exercise treadmill test. Additional studies such as 24-hour Holter monitoring during athletic activity and EPS may be necessary to adequately evaluate the patient.[1] Because of the rare but real risk of SCD in athletes with WPW, cardiac consultation including EPS and possible catheter ablation may be necessary.[1] Two recognizable ECG patterns of the athlete at risk for SCD include long QT syndrome and Brugada syndrome (see Figs. 3.2 and 3.3).

Short QT syndrome is identified by a corrected QT that is less than 300 milliseconds. The ECG in patients with Brugada syndrome displays an accentuated J wave in precordial leads 1 to 3 with ST segment elevation. Additionally, these abnormalities may also be followed by a negative T wave and an R prime. Athletes with these abnormalities are excluded from all sports participation except for class IA.[1]

TREATMENT

Atrial Flutter[1]

- Athletes with atrial flutter in the absence of structural heart disease who maintain a ventricular rate that increases and slows appropriately comparable to that of a normal sinus response in relation to the level of activity, while receiving no therapy or therapy with AV nodal-blocking drugs, can participate in class IA competitive sports with the warning that rapid 1:1 conduction still may occur. However, full participation in all competitive sports should not be allowed unless the athlete has been without atrial flutter for 2 to 3 months with or without drug treatment. Note that the use of β-blockers is prohibited in some competitive sports.

- Athletes with structural heart disease who have atrial flutter can participate in class IA competitive sports only after 2 to 4 weeks have elapsed without an episode of atrial flutter.

- Athletes without structural heart disease who have elimination of the atrial flutter by an ablation technique or surgery can participate in all competitive sports after 2 to 4 weeks without a recurrence, or in several days after an EPS showing noninducibility of the atrial flutter in the presence of bidirectional isthmus block.

- Athletes in whom anticoagulation is deemed necessary cannot participate in competitive sports where the danger of bodily collision is present.

Atrial Fibrillation[1]

- Athletes with asymptomatic atrial fibrillation in the absence of structural heart disease who maintain a ventricular rate that increases and slows appropriately and is comparable to that of a normal sinus response in relation to the level of activity, while receiving no therapy or therapy with AV nodal-blocking drugs, can participate in all competitive sports. Note that the use of β-blockers is prohibited in some competitive sports.

- Athletes with atrial fibrillation in the presence of structural heart disease who maintain a ventricular rate comparable to that of an appropriate sinus tachycardia during physical activity, while receiving no therapy or therapy with AV nodal-blocking drugs, can participate in sports consistent with the limitations of the structural heart disease.

- Athletes who require anticoagulation should not participate in sports with danger of bodily collision.

- Athletes without structural heart disease who have elimination of atrial fibrillation by an ablation technique, including surgery, may participate in all competitive sports after 4 to 6 weeks without a recurrence or after an EPS has confirmed noninducibility.

Supraventricular Tachycardia[1]

- Athletes without structural heart disease who are asymptomatic and have reproducible exercise-induced supraventricular tachycardia prevented by therapy and verified by appropriate testing can participate in all competitive sports.
- Athletes who do not have exercise-induced supraventricular tachycardia but experience sporadic recurrences should be treated.
- Because of the unpredictable nature of the tachycardia, end points for adequate therapy may be difficult to achieve.
- Once established, these athletes can participate in all activities consistent with their cardiac status.
- Asymptomatic athletes who have episodes of supraventricular tachycardia of 5 to 15 seconds that do not increase in duration during exercise can participate in all sports consistent with their cardiac status.
- Athletes with syncope, near syncope, or significant symptoms secondary to arrhythmia or who have significant structural heart disease in addition to the arrhythmia should not participate in any competitive sports until they have been adequately treated and have no recurrence for 2 to 4 weeks.
- At that time they can participate in class IA competitive sports.
- For those athletes with no structural heart disease who have had successful catheter or surgical ablation, are asymptomatic, and have no inducible arrhythmia on follow-up electrophysiologic testing, all competitive sports are permitted in several days. If no electrophysiologic testing is done, full participation is permitted on condition that there is no spontaneous recurrence of tachycardia for 2 to 4 weeks after ablation.

Ventricular Pre-excitation (WPW Syndrome)[1]

- Athletes without structural heart disease, without a history of palpitations, or without tachycardia (particularly those of ages 20 to 25 years or more) can participate in all competitive sports. However, in younger age groups, a more in-depth evaluation including an EPS may be recommended before allowing participation in moderate- to high-intensity competitive sports.
- Athletes with episodes of AV-reciprocating tachycardia should be treated as previously recommended (see section "Supraventricular Tachycardia"). However, it should be appreciated that they can develop atrial fibrillation with rapid ventricular rates. Electrical induction of atrial fibrillation to determine the shortest QRS interval between two complexes conducted over the accessory pathway during isoproterenol administration or exercise is recommended. Athletes in whom the shortest cycle length is less than 250 milliseconds should undergo ablation of the accessory pathway.
- Athletes with episodes of atrial flutter/fibrillation and syncope or near syncope whose maximal ventricular rate at rest (without therapy) as a result of conduction over the accessory pathway exceeds 240 beats/min should be considered for catheter ablation therapy of the accessory pathway prior to continuing competition. Those whose ventricular rate during isoproterenol administration is less than 240 beats/min and who have no episodes of syncope or near syncope appear to be at low risk for SCD.
- Athletes with no structural heart disease who have had successful catheter or surgical ablation of the accessory pathway, are asymptomatic, and have normal AV conduction and no inducible arrhythmia by follow-up EPS can participate in all competitive sports in several days. Those without an EPS and no spontaneous recurrence of tachycardia for 2 to 4 weeks after ablation can participate in all competitive sports.

Premature Ventricular Complexes[1]

- Athletes *without* structural heart disease who have premature ventricular complexes at rest and during exercise and exercise testing (comparable to the sport in which they compete) can participate in all competitive sports. Should the premature ventricular complexes increase in frequency during exercise or exercise testing to the extent that they produce symptoms of impaired consciousness, significant fatigue, or dyspnea, the athlete can participate in class IA competitive sports only.
- Athletes *with* structural heart disease who are in high-risk groups and have premature ventricular complexes (with or without treatment) can participate in class IA competitive sports only. Such athletes with premature ventricular complexes that are suppressed by drug therapy (as assessed by ambulatory ECG recordings) during participation in the sport can compete in only class IA competitive sports.

Prognosis/Return to Play

- Athletes without structural heart disease, palpitations, and supraventricular tachycardia and with age over 25 may participate without further workup.
- Further disposition of athletes who do not fall into this category should be based upon the 36th Bethesda Conference guidelines (Task Force 7: arrhythmia).
- Ventricular tachycardia and syncope caused by ventricular fibrillation and flutter always require additional workup and cessation of all activity.
- Further workup will be defined by underlying risk factors including CAD, congenital heart disease, and structural anomalies.

- Further athletic participation will be guided by the ability to permanently ablate the underlying cause for ventricular tachycardia or fibrillation.
- At the time of publication of this chapter, ICDs are an automatic disqualification for sports participation.[1]

Complications/Indications for Referral

Referral is indicated in the rare instance of sinus node disturbances leading to syncope, all AVNRT, atrial fibrillation/flutter, WPW, and significant ventricular arrhythmias.[1]

APPROACH TO THE ATHLETE WITH HYPERTENSION

A hypertensive athlete represents a therapeutic challenge to the clinician. Three recent guideline updates are essential to the clinician caring for athletes with hypertension. The Joint National Committee (JNC) VII update in 2003 simplified the diagnosis and treatment of hypertension in the general population. The 36th Bethesda Conference guidelines delineated specific criteria for treatment for athletes with hypertension. Finally, the fourth report on the diagnosis, evaluation, and treatment of high BP in children and adolescents from the National High Blood Pressure Education Program Working Group on High Blood Pressure in Children and Adolescents helps clarify the diagnosis and treatment of hypertension in young athletes. These guidelines are, as much as possible, evidence based and simplified from earlier renditions. Pediatric BPs are now based on age, height, and weight.[30,31]

Adult and pediatric hypertension classifications are similarly named: prehypertension and stage I and stage II hypertension that represent the current classification scheme.[30,32,33] Highlights of each of these recommendations are delineated in Table 3.3.

HISTORY AND PHYSICAL EXAMINATION

BP should be measured with the athlete in the seated position with feet on the floor and with an appropriately sized cuff. The athlete ideally should be resting comfortably for 5 minutes prior to the reading. This poses considerable delay with station-based screening of large populations of athletes. Ideally, no nicotine or caffeinated products should be consumed prior to the measurement. A second measurement within a reasonable time period should be obtained if the reading is elevated. A thigh BP measurement should be obtained in pediatric patients with elevated arm pressures;[33] bilateral and upper and lower extremity readings should be obtained to evaluate for possible coarctation of the aorta. An adequate history and physical must be obtained looking for end-organ damage and secondary causes of hypertension. Careful questioning may uncover use of anabolic steroids and ergogenic aids.

Diagnostic Testing

It is recommended that all athletes younger than 18 undergo a workup to exclude secondary causes of hypertension. The workup may include laboratory analysis and ECHO in particular for those athletes diagnosed with stage 2 hypertension. Adults with stage 1 hypertension should undergo limited laboratory analysis with further workup guided by a detailed physical examination. Adult athletes with stage 2 hypertension may also need further testing including ECHO to evaluate for LVH.[33]

Treatment

- Initial management of hypertension includes lifestyle modifications and avoidance of medications/supplements that elevate BP.
- Nonsteroidal anti-inflammatory drugs (NSAIDs) and nicotine can elevate BP, and athletes need to be counseled about the use of these agents. Weight reduction may prove beneficial. When medication is warranted, angiotensin-converting enzyme (ACE) inhibitors are often the first line of therapy in the athlete. ACE inhibitors are generally well tolerated with a low side effect profile and are effective in lowering BP.
- Angiotensin receptor blockers (ARBs) act similarly and may prove as effective.[34] There is a paucity of evidence from clinical trials, but general consensus supports usage of these agents as first-line therapy in athletes.
- Calcium channel blockers, in particular the nondihydropiridine class, are also generally well tolerated and do not have a negative performance effect.[34]

TABLE 3.3 **Stages of Hypertension**

Stages of Hypertension	Blood Pressure Guidelines	Blood Pressure Range
Prehypertension	Systolic or diastolic BP reading from the 90th to 95th percentile or if the reading exceeds 120/80 mm Hg even if the reading is below the 90th percentile	121–139/81–89[31,32]
Stage 1	BP reading from the 95th percentile to the 99th percentile plus 5 mm Hg	140–159/90–99[31,32]
Stage 2	Any BP higher than the 99th percentile plus 5 mm Hg	>160/100[31,32]

Prognosis/Return To Play

- All athletes with stage II hypertension are restricted from participation until BP is adequately controlled.
- Athletes with stage I hypertension may participate if no target organ damage is present including LVH.
- Athletes with evidence of LVH beyond the normal "athlete's heart" must be restricted from participating in most sports until BP is controlled,[33] recognizing the "gray zone" between LVH and athlete's heart.[31]
- Athletes may participate with prehypertension.
- The athlete should be followed every 3 months with repeat BP monitoring until BP is adequately controlled.[34]

Complications/Indications for Referral

Concern is raised regarding female athletes of childbearing age, as ACE inhibitors are prohibited in pregnancy. β-Blockers and diuretics, while the mainstay of initial therapy in the general population, are not recommended as initial therapy among athletes. β-Blockers negatively affect performance and are banned from some sports. Diuretics may pose a risk to athletes from depletion of certain electrolytes and reduced plasma volume. Diuretics are also banned in certain sporting events due to their capacity to mask anabolic agents.[31,34] Signs and symptoms of end-organ damage, recalcitrant hypertension, and significant secondary causes of hypertension should prompt exclusion from participation and referral to appropriate specialties until controlled.

KEY POINTS

- The athlete with syncope must be excluded from participation until a reasonable workup excludes potential causes of SCD.
- Athletes with HCM must be excluded from participation in all sports except class IA.
- Athletes with stage 2 hypertension must be excluded from participation in sports until BP is adequately controlled.
- ACE-I and ARBs are good first-line antihypertensive medications in athletes.

REFERENCES

1. Zipes DP, Ackerman MJ, Estes NA III, et al. Task Force 7: arrhythmias. *J Am Coll Cardiol.* 2005;45(8):1354–1363.
2. Beckerman J, Wang P, Hlatky M. Cardiovascular screening of athletes. *Clin J Sport Med.* 2004;14:127–133.
3. Joy EA, Paisley TS, Price R Jr, et al. Optimizing the collegiate preparticipation physical evaluation. *Clin J Sport Med.* 2004;14:183–187.
4. Maron BJ, Thompson PD, Puffer JC, et al. Cardiovascular preparticipation screening of competitive athletes. A statement for health professionals from the Sudden Death Committee (clinical cardiology) and Congenital Cardiac Defects Committee (cardiovascular disease in the young), American Heart Association. *Circulation.* 1996;94:850–856.
5. Maron BJ, Ackerman MJ, Nishimura RA, et al. Task Force 4: HCM and other cardiomyopathies, mitral valve prolapse, myocarditis, and Marfan syndrome. *J Am Coll Cardiol.* 2005;45(8):1340–1345.
6. Maron BJ. Hypertrophic cardiomyopathy in childhood. *Pediatr Clin North Am.* 2004;51:1305–1346.
7. Maron BJ, Spirito P, Roman MJ, et al. Prevalence of hypertrophic cardiomyopathy in a population-based sample of American Indians aged 51 to 77 years (the Strong Heart Study). *Am J Cardiol.* 2004;93:1510–1514.
8. Maron BJ, Carney KP, Lever HM, et al. Relationship of race to sudden cardiac death in competitive athletes with hypertrophic cardiomyopathy. *J Am Coll Cardiol.* 2003;41:974–980.
9. Colivicchi F, Ammirati F, Santini M. Epidemiology and prognostic implications of syncope in young competing athletes. *Eur Heart J.* 2004;25:1749–1753.
10. Maron BJ, Shirani J, Pliac LC, et al. Sudden death in young competitive athletes, clinical, demographic, and pathological profiles. *JAMA.* 1996;276:199–204.
11. Seto CK. Preparticipation cardiovascular screening. *Clin Sports Med.* 2003;22:23–35.
12. Van Camp SP, Bloor CM, Mueller FO, et al. Nontraumatic sports death in high school and college athletes. *Med Sci Sports Exerc.* 1995;27:641–647.
13. Mounsey JP, Ferguson JD. The assessment and management of arrhythmias and syncope in the athlete. *Clin Sports Med.* 2003;22:67–79.
14. Maron BJ. Sudden death in young athletes. *N Engl J Med.* 2003;349:1064–1075.
15. Firoozi S, Sharma S, McKenna WJ. Risk of competitive sport in young athletes with heart disease. *Heart.* 2003;89:710–714.
16. Colivicci F, Ammirati F, Biffi A, et al. Exercise-related syncope in young competitive athletes without evidence of structural heart disease. Clinical presentation and long-term outcome. *Eur Heart J.* 2002;23:1125–1130.
17. Pigozzi F, Spataro A, Alabiso A, et al. Role of exercise stress test in master athletes. *Br J Sports Med.* 2005;39:527–531.
18. Venckunas T, Stasiulis A, Raugaliene R. Concentric myocardial hypertrophy after one year of increased training volume in experienced distance runners. *Br J Sports Med.* 2006;40:706–709.
19. Sharma S, Whyte G, Elliott P, et al. Electrocardiographic changes in 1000 highly trained junior elite athletes. *Br J Sports Med.* 1999;33:319–324.
20. Maron BJ, Douglas PS, Graham TP, et al. Task Force 1: preparticipation screening and diagnosis of cardiovascular disease in athletes. *J Am Coll Cardiol.* 2005;45:1322–1326.
21. Sarto P, Merlo L, Noventa D, et al. Electrocardiographic changes associated with training and discontinuation of training in an athlete with hypertrophic cardiomyopathy. *Am J Cardiol.* 2004;93:518–519.
22. Sharma S, Maron BJ, Whyte G, et al. Physiologic limits of left ventricular hypertrophy in elite junior athletes: relevance to differential diagnosis of athlete's heart and hypertrophic cardiomyopathy. *J Am Coll Cardiol.* 2002;40:1431–1436.
23. Giese EA, O'Connor FG, Brennan FH, et al. The athletic preparticipation evaluation: cardiovascular assessment. *Am Fam Physician.* 2007;75(7):1008–1014.
24. Adabag AS, Kuskowski MA, Maron BJ. Determinants for clinical diagnosis of hypertrophic cardiomyopathy. *Am J Cardiol.* 2006;98:1507–1511.
25. Chee CE, Anastassiades CP, Antonopoulos AG, et al. Cardiac hypertrophy and how it may break an athlete's heart—the Cypriot case. *Eur J Echocardiogr.* 2005;6:301–307.
26. Basavarajaiah S, Wilson M, Junagde S, et al. Physiological left ventricular hypertrophy or hypertrophic cardiomyopathy in an elite adolescent athlete: role of detraining in resolving the clinical dilemma. *Br J Sports Med.* 2006;40:727–729.
27. Maron BJ, McKenna WJ, Danielson GK, et al. American College of Cardiology/European Society of Cardiology Clinical Expert Consensus Document on Hypertrophic Cardiomyopathy. A report of the American College of Cardiology Foundation Task Force on Clinical Expert Consensus Documents and the European Society of Cardiology Committee for Practice Guidelines. *Eur Heart J.* 2003;24: 1965–1991.

28. Wu J, Stork TL, Perron AD, et al. The athlete's electrocardiogram. *Am J Emerg Med.* 2006;24:77–86.
29. Farrar MW, Bogart DB, Chapman SS, et al. Atrial fibrillations in athletes. *MO Med.* 2006;103(3):297–301.
30. National High Blood Pressure Education Program Working Group on High Blood Pressure in Children and Adolescents. The fourth report on the diagnosis, evaluation, and treatment of high blood pressure in children and adolescents. *Pediatrics.* 2004;114(suppl):555–576.
31. O'Connor FG, Meyering CD, Patel R, et al. Hypertension, athletes, and the sports physician: implications of JNC VII, the Fourth Report, and the 36th Bethesda Conference Guidelines. *Curr Sports Med Rep.* 2007;6: 80–84.
32. Chobanian AV, Bakris GL, Black HR, et al. The seventh report of the Joint National Committee on Prevention, Detection, Evaluation, and Treatment of High Blood Pressure: the JNC 7 report. *JAMA.* 2003;289: 2560–2572.
33. Kaplan NM, Gidding SS, Pickering TG, et al. 36th Bethesda Conference: recommendations for determining eligibility for competition in athletes with cardiovascular abnormalities: Task Force 5: systemic hypertension. *J Am Coll Cardiol.* 2005;45:1346–1348.
34. Sachtleben T, Fields KB. Hypertension in the athlete. *Curr Sports Med Rep.* 2003;2:79–83.

4

Athlete with Shortness of Breath

Joseph J. Bernard and Zachary A. Geidel

INTRODUCTION

Shortness of breath is a common complaint in athletes and is a frequent reason for the athlete to seek medical attention. The potential etiologies range from benign deconditioning to serious cardiac or pulmonary disorders. Cardiac conditions that can cause shortness of breath in the athlete are covered in Chapter 3. The focus of this chapter will be on two common and similar pulmonary conditions: exercise-induced asthma (EIA) and exercise-associated bronchospasm (EAB). In addition, overtraining syndrome and anemia will be reviewed as causes for shortness of breath in the athlete.

PATHOPHYSIOLOGY

Asthma is a reversible condition of the tracheobronchial tree commonly encountered in children and young adults. The key clinical features include hyperresponsiveness that results in reversible narrowing of the airways. In 1995, the National Heart, Lung, and Blood Institute's "Global Initiative for Asthma" developed the following definition for asthma (Fig. 4.1):

"Asthma is a chronic inflammatory disorder of the airways in which many cells and cellular elements play a role, in particular, mast cells, eosinophils, T lymphocytes, macrophages, neutrophils, and epithelial cells. In susceptible individuals, this inflammation causes recurrent episodes of wheezing, breathlessness, chest tightness, and coughing, particularly at night or in the early morning. These episodes are usually associated with widespread but variable airflow obstruction that is often reversible either spontaneously or with treatment. The inflammation also causes an associated increase in the existing bronchial hyperresponsiveness to a variety of stimuli."[1]

Asthma is an inflammatory disorder of the airways involving several different inflammatory cells and mediators (Fig. 4.2). The inflammatory response causes characteristic structural changes in the airway, including an increase in airway smooth muscle. Subsequent airway narrowing results in the symptoms associated with asthma.

EIA is the transient narrowing of the airway in an athlete *with* chronic asthma following exercise or physical activity. EAB refers to bronchospasm in the athlete *without* the underlying findings of asthma. A key differentiation with asthma is the lack of significant inflammation as the underlying etiology seen in EAB.

There are two current theories on the underlying pathophysiology of EAB. The first is the *airway rewarming theory*, which postulates that hyperventilation in exercise leads to cooling of the airways. Upon cessation of exercise, small bronchiolar vessels dilate and become congested with the rewarming of the airways. This results in leakage into the submucosa of the airway walls stimulating bronchoconstriction.[2,3]

The second mechanism, the *hyperosmolarity theory*, proposes that during hyperventilation with exercise, there is water loss from the airway surface leading to hypertonicity and hyperosmolarity within the airway cells. Subsequently, mediators are released causing bronchoconstriction.[2,4] There is also some evidence that inflammation of the airway may be involved, similar to chronic asthma.[2]

A key component of normal lung function is the proper gas exchange at the alveolar level. Conditions that affect this process limit oxygenated blood from reaching the muscles and end organs. The affect on the gas exchange can result in clinical manifestations of performance decline, fatigue, and shortness of breath.

Key to the role of gas exchange is the hemoglobin molecule. In humans, the hemoglobin molecule is an assembly of four globular protein subunits. Each subunit is composed of a protein chain tightly associated with a nonprotein heme group. The heme group consists of an iron (Fe) atom held in a heterocyclic ring. The iron atom is the site of oxygen binding. Hemoglobin serves as the iron-containing oxygen transport system in red blood cells (RBCs). It transports oxygen from the lungs to the rest of the body, such as to the muscles, where it releases the oxygen load. Therefore, low levels of hemoglobin may hinder athletic performance.

Anemia refers to lower levels of hemoglobin than what is expected, resulting in a drop in one's hematocrit. Normal values for hemoglobin levels are as follows:

- Women: 12.1 to 15.1 g/dL
- Men: 13.8 to 17.2 g/dL
- Children: 11 to 16 g/dL

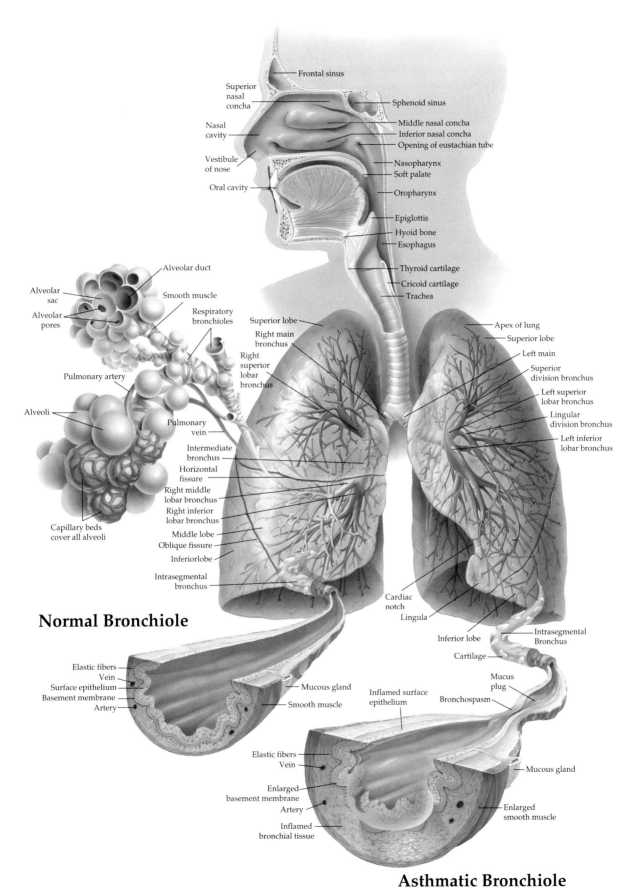

Normal Bronchiole

Asthmatic Bronchiole

FIG. 4.1. Respiratory system and asthma. Asset provided by Anatomical Chart Co.

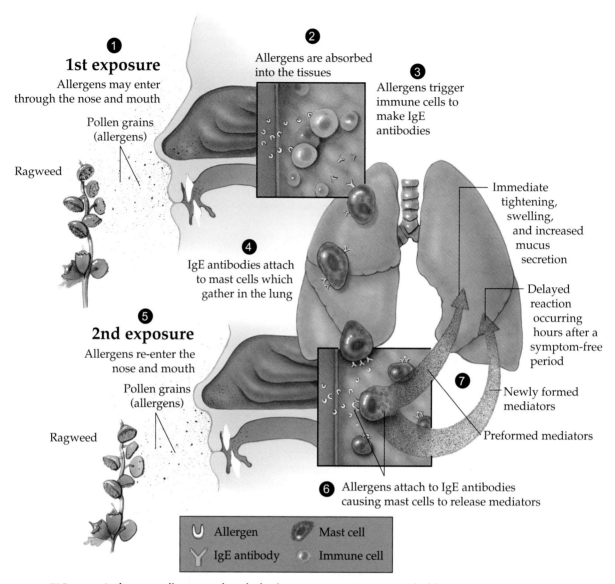

1 **1st exposure**
Allergens may enter through the nose and mouth

Pollen grains (allergens)

Ragweed

2 Allergens are absorbed into the tissues

3 Allergens trigger immune cells to make IgE antibodies

Immediate tightening, swelling, and increased mucus secretion

Delayed reaction occurring hours after a symptom-free period

4 IgE antibodies attach to mast cells which gather in the lung

5 **2nd exposure**
Allergens re-enter the nose and mouth

Pollen grains (allergens)

Ragweed

7 Newly formed mediators

Preformed mediators

6 Allergens attach to IgE antibodies causing mast cells to release mediators

∪ Allergen   Mast cell
Y IgE antibody   Immune cell

FIG. 4.2. Asthma mediators and pathologic responses. Asset provided by Anatomical Chart Co.

The term "sports anemia" or "athlete's anemia" is often used to refer to the lower levels of hemoglobin seen in the athletic population, especially in elite athletes. This is not a true anemia but a normal physiologic adaptation to exercise that results in increased plasma expansion.

In addition to dilutional anemia, other potential causes in athletes may include (1) excess destruction (i.e., foot strike anemia), (2) blood loss from gastrointestinal or genitourinary tract, and (3) decreased production (i.e., iron deficiency).

Other hematologic conditions that need to be considered in athletes include sickle cell disease/trait, in which abnormal hemoglobin is produced, or thalassemia, where there is a decrease in the production of normal hemoglobin chains.

The etiology of *overtraining syndrome* is controversial and an area of active research. Proposed pathophysiology includes the theory that an overactive pituitary gland is primarily responsible for physiologic responses to overtraining. This in turn results in elevated cortisol levels and added stress to the body's natural response to intense work. There is also an increase in serum creatine kinase levels and it is proposed that the body is in a state of catabolism, breaking down protein and muscle for energy. Overtraining has also been associated with overuse injuries, most commonly posterior tibialis syndrome, lower limb stress fractures, and tendonitis. It is unclear if this is due to excessive high training loads or inability of the body to recover and repair damage from training. The body's immune system is also compromised, possibly from decrease in C-reactive protein levels after intense exercise. Also it has been proposed that an acute phase response may occur in the overtrained athlete with leukocytosis, fever, decrease in copper and zinc levels, and increase in erythrocyte sedimentation rate (ESR). This in turn leads to an increase in colds, allergic reactions, and other infections. Psychologic factors are also manifested in overtrained athletes but much more difficult to detect at times.[5]

EPIDEMIOLOGY

EIA is seen in 80% to 90% of individuals with underlying asthma; however, many athletes only have bronchospasm associated with exercise without underlying chronic asthma.[6]

There is a variable reported incidence of EIA or EAB in the literature with range of 7% to 20% in the general population.[7,8] The variability appears to be related to the overall low quality of the studies, small numbers, and limited patient populations. Many studies have been done in certain subgroups, such as children, and in certain sports, such as figure skating and ice hockey. It is difficult to sort out which of these athletes only have bronchospasm associated with exercise and which have underlying chronic asthma. It does appear that certain sports are at higher risk for EIA or exercise-induced bronchospasm (EIB), including Nordic skiing, track and field, soccer, hockey, football, water polo, cycling, etc.

The incidence of anemia in the general public has been reported as 4% in males and 8% in females in the United States. The incidence of iron deficiency in premenopausal women has been found to be 4% to 8% in the United States. Regular nonprofessional sport activity does not cause an increased rate of anemia or of iron deficiency in fertile women. However, physical exercise has an impact on iron status, as it reduces serum iron and transferrin saturation and elevates soluble transferrin receptor. Nearly one-fifth of recreational athletes have anemia and one-third have iron deficit; these conditions can decrease their physical performance.[9] Sickle cell disease in the United States is estimated to be around 1 in 625 persons at birth; however, in black Americans the sickle gene is present in approximately 8% of the population. This reaches upward of 30% in Africa.

NARROWING THE DIFFERENTIAL DIAGNOSIS

While an exhaustive differential of conditions that might result in an athlete with exercise-associated shortness of breath are beyond the scope of this chapter, common conditions to consider include the following:

- EIA
- EAB (without underlying chronic asthma)
- Vocal cord dysfunction
- Chronic obstructive pulmonary disease
- Restrictive lung disease
- Cardiovascular disorder
- Upper/lower respiratory infection
- Deconditioning
- Anemia
- Overtraining
- Pneumothorax (spontaneous)
- Pulmonary embolism

History

When evaluating an athlete with shortness of breath, a thorough history should be obtained regarding the length of symptoms, precipitating and alleviating factors, and other associated symptoms. A past medical history of asthma would certainly make the diagnosis of EIA more likely. If there have been other associated infectious symptoms such as fever, sinus congestion, or productive cough, a respiratory infection may be likely.

Evidence-based Physical Examination

A thorough examination should be performed with special focus on the cardiovascular and pulmonary examinations. Key components of the cardiovascular examination should include bilateral blood pressure testing, cardiac auscultation, and peripheral pulse palpation. Key components of the pulmonary examination should include auscultation for expiratory wheezing and prolonged expiratory phase as well as inspiratory stridor in addition to any audible rales or rhonchi.

Diagnostic Testing

Laboratory

If clinically indicated, a complete blood count could help rule out anemia. Further iron and hemoglobin studies may be considered based on complete blood count (CBC) result and clinical scenario, including an athlete with a microcytic anemia and particularly in females and those of Mediterranean decent. This would include serum iron, ferritin, transferrin, total iron binding capacity, reticulocyte count, and possibly hemoglobin electrophoresis.

Thyroid studies, LFTs, and renal function tests may be considered. Blood tests to consider in the athlete with overtraining include CBC, cortisol level, luteinizing hormone level, testosterone level, creatine kinase level, C-reactive protein, and ESR.

Imaging

If a lower respiratory infection or spontaneous pneumothorax is suspected, a chest radiograph may be considered. Appropriate imaging studies would be indicated for suspected pulmonary embolism.

Other Testing

If clinical scenario and examination suggest cardiac findings ECG, echocardiogram, and exercise stress tests may be considered. Appropriate indications for cardiac testing are reviewed in the Chapter 3.

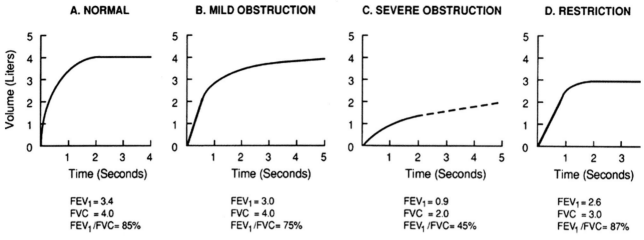

FIG. 4.3. Spirometry curves in respiratory disorders.

Pulmonary function tests (PFTs) are useful when looking for obstructive or restrictive lung disease. A full description of PFTs and spirometry are outlined in the following sections.

APPROACH TO THE ATHLETE WITH EXERCISE-INDUCED ASTHMA

HISTORY AND PHYSICAL EXAMINATION

Shortness of breath associated with exercise is usually the first complaint and will often prompt a workup for asthma. Athletes and coaches may have the misperception that the athlete is "just out of shape." There is often a decrease in exercise endurance as well. Questions regarding chest tightness, coughing, or wheezing associated with sports participation should be asked. Any athlete with shortness of breath should be questioned with regard to a history of asthma or bronchodilator use.

The symptoms of EIA may develop shortly after the onset of exercise, then improve after 15 to 30 minutes of exercise (refractory period), with recurrence after the termination of exercise. EIA will usually spontaneously resolve 30 to 60 minutes after cessation of exercise. Symptoms that begin early in exercise should be evaluated for other causes such as poorly controlled chronic asthma or vocal cord dysfunction.

A thorough physical examination should be done after obtaining a history suggestive of EIA. ENT examination should include looking for evidence of sinusitis or nasal allergies. A cardiac examination should be done to assess for murmurs or arrhythmias. Pulmonary examination should look for wheezing, rhonchi, rales, or stridor.

DIAGNOSTIC TESTING

Diagnosis of chronic asthma can be made by spirometry or PFT. Sport-specific challenge testing is the best way to

diagnose EIA, but this is often difficult, as spirometry is usually not available in the exercise setting that triggers the athlete's symptoms.

In the office or training room setting, baseline spirometry testing should be done before exercise, followed by having the athlete exercise on a treadmill or cycle ergometer (or maybe the stairs in an office). Postexercise testing can be done every 10 to 15 minutes after exercise for up to 30 to 60 minutes following exercise. A fall of 10% in the FEV1 is usually considered diagnostic for EIA[10] (Fig. 4.3). If other factors such as cold air are triggers, then the setting of the testing may need to be modified to accurately diagnose EIA.[10] The sensitivity and specificity of spirometry has been estimated to be around 61 and 60, respectively.[11]

An alternative mode of testing is to use peak expiratory flow (PEF) measurements. A fall of at least 10% of PEF is diagnostic for EIA.[12] The sensitivity and specificity for this form of testing is around 43 and 75, respectively.[11] Alternative methods of testing to evaluate and diagnose asthma also include the methacholine challenge and sputum eosinophil count, both of which are more sensitive and specific, with methalcholine challenge being 90 and 91 with respect to sensitivity and specificity and sputum eosinophil count being 72 and 80.[11]

TREATMENT

General Measures

- The mainstay of treatment of EIA is prevention and/or modifying the severity. This includes many nonpharmacologic and pharmacologic treatments.[13]
- Avoidance of any known triggers is the first-line nonpharmacologic treatment.
- Avoidance of cold, dry air by exercising in warmer and more humid conditions, or by wearing a mask if exercising in a cold environment, may improve symptoms.

Pharmacologic Treatment[14]

- Pharmacologic therapy consists of a variety of medications, but usually is initially treated with an inhaled β-agonist prior to exercise.
- These short-acting bronchodilators can be used 5 to 30 minutes prior to exercise for prophylactic use, as well as during exercise for any symptomatic relief if needed.
- Other pharmacologic therapies include inhaled corticosteroids, cromolyn compounds, and leukotriene inhibitors.
- Inhaled corticosteroids are the most consistently effective long-term control medication at all steps of care for persistent asthma.
- Cromolyn sodium may be used as alternative, but not preferred, medication for patients requiring step 2 care (for mild persistent asthma). They also can be used as preventive treatment before exercise or unavoidable exposure to known allergens.
- Leukotriene inhibitors are alternative, but not preferred, therapy for the treatment of patients who require step 2 care (for mild persistent asthma).
- Long-acting β_2-agonists are used in combination with inhaled corticosteroids for long-term control and prevention of symptoms in moderate or severe persistent asthma (step 3 care or higher in children 5 years of age and adults and step 4 care or higher in children 0 to 4 years of age, although few data are available for children 0 to 4 years of age).
- A long-acting β_2-agonist may be used before exercise to prevent EIB, but duration of action does not exceed 5 hours with chronic, regular use. Frequent or chronic use before exercise is discouraged, because this may disguise poorly controlled persistent asthma.

Prognosis/Return to Play

- Return of the athlete to sports participation can be done safely once the symptoms have been adequately treated.
- Albuterol metered dose inhaler (MDI) should be available for the athlete, with EIA at practice and at games.

Complications/Indications for Referral

If the athletes do not improve with standard treatment, they may need further workup for other underlying pulmonary conditions. Generally, athletes do well with medication therapy. It is important to know the rules of the governing body that dictates banned substances for the athlete, so as not to prescribe those medications.

APPROACH TO THE ATHLETE WITH EXERCISE-ASSOCIATED BRONCHOSPASM

Initial approach in the workup and treatment of EAB should include trying to differentiate whether there is underlying chronic asthma, or if the bronchospasm is only associated with exercise.

HISTORY AND PHYSICAL EXAMINATION

Shortness of breath associated with exercise, similar to an athlete with EIA, is the first complaint that often prompts a workup. Unlike chronic asthmatics, the athlete will not have symptoms at times other than with exercise-related activities. A decrease in exercise endurance, chest tightness, coughing, or wheezing associated with sports participation should be asked. It is also important to determine whether there is a history of asthma, so as to differentiate from EIA.

The symptoms of EAB, similar to EIA, may develop shortly after the onset of exercise, but more often will not be present until shortly after exercise has been terminated. It will usually spontaneously resolve 30 to 60 minutes after cessation of exercise. Symptoms that begin early in exercise should be evaluated for other causes such as poorly controlled chronic asthma or vocal cord dysfunction.

Physical examination findings of wheezing will not be present at times other than with exercise or physical activity. A thorough examination should be done to rule out transient causes of shortness of breath, such as upper or lower respiratory infections. A cardiac examination should be done to rule out cardiovascular causes. If you have the benefit of examining the athletes while they are exercising and experiencing symptoms, you may hear wheezing on auscultation.

DIAGNOSTIC TESTING

EAB is usually difficult to accurately diagnose due to lack of availability of testing equipment on the field or sidelines of most sporting facilities. Because there is not any underlying asthma, testing without the exercise trigger will be normal. Diagnostic testing is essentially the same as for EIA but to exclude an underlying asthmatic pathology. Exercise challenge testing can be performed as noted earlier in the EIA section.

TREATMENT

General Measures

- The mainstay of treatment of EAB is similar to EIA.
- This includes prevention and/or modifying the severity of the symptoms in addition to any nonpharmacologic and pharmacologic treatments.[13]
- Avoidance of any known triggers, such as cold, dry air, is a nonpharmacologic treatment that can be done by exercising in warmer and more humid conditions or by wearing a mask if exercising in a cold environment.
- Warming up prior to exercise may also reduce the symptoms of EAB.

- The athlete should try to warm up at 80% to 90% of their maximum workload for about 10 minutes before they compete.[15]

  This allows the athlete to compete during the "refractory period," where there is less bronchospasm. This phenomenon may last up to 2 hours, but is varied widely among individual athletes.

Pharmacologic Treatment

- Pharmacologic therapy consists of a variety of medications, but usually is initially treated with an inhaled β-agonist prior to exercise.
- A short-acting bronchodilator can be used 5 to 30 minutes prior to exercise for prophylactic use, as well as during exercise for any symptomatic relief if needed.
- Other pharmacologic therapies include inhaled corticosteroids, cromolyn compounds, and leukotriene inhibitors.

Prognosis/Return to Play

- Return of the athlete to sports participation can be done safely once the symptoms have been adequately treated.
- Albuterol MDI should be available for the athlete with EIA at practice and at games.

Complications/Indications for Referral

If the athletes do not improve with standard treatment, they may need further workup for other underlying pulmonary conditions. Generally, athletes do well with medication therapy. It is important to know the rules of the governing body that dictates banned substances for the athlete, so as not to prescribe those medications.

APPROACH TO THE ATHLETE WITH ANEMIA

There are numerous causes of anemia in athletes. Every anemia is caused by at least one of three problems: (1) decreased RBC production, (2) loss of RBCs by hemorrhage, or (3) early death (destruction) of RBCs (Fig. 4.4). Specific conditions are outlined.

HISTORY AND PHYSICAL EXAMINATION

Athletes who complain of shortness of breath or fatigue, or have a drop off in performance, should be evaluated for anemia as part of a comprehensive workup. Acute blood loss should be evaluated by questioning about melena or heavy menstrual bleeding. Questions about diet may point to

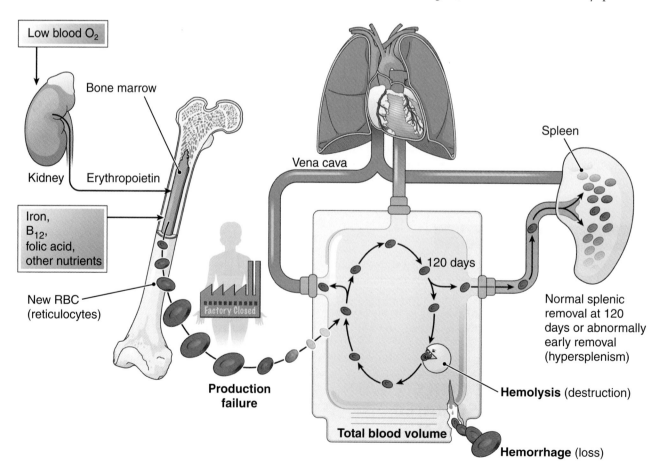

FIG. 4.4. Causes of anemia.

concerns about iron deficiency. Heavy and intense exercise may increase the likelihood of hemolysis.

As part of a comprehensive physical examination, the athlete should be evaluated for paleness of the skin or conjunctiva, epigastric discomfort that may be seen with gastritis associated with large amount of non-steroidal anti-inflammatory drugs use, and a rectal examination for fecal occult blood. Pulmonary and cardiac causes should also be evaluated as part of the complete examination. In addition to the physical examination, laboratory studies may be warranted.

DIAGNOSTIC TESTING

Basic laboratory studies should include a complete blood count, iron studies (iron, ferritin, transferrin saturation, and total iron binding capacity), and urinalysis.

APPROACH TO THE ATHLETE WITH DILUTIONAL PSEUDOANEMIA

Dilutional pseudoanemia is a temporary condition that occurs as a result of plasma volume expansion with exercise.

HISTORY AND PHYSICAL EXAMINATION

The plasma volume expansion with exercise does not occur immediately after exercise. It typically occurs well after exercise is complete and returns to baseline within a few hours.[16] When the plasma volume expands, the hemoglobin concentration reduces and results in the appearance of an anemia. There are no irregular physical findings or underlying medical causes associated with dilutional pseudoanemia.

DIAGNOSTIC TESTING

The hemoglobin will be transiently low, but other lab work for anemia, such as ferritin, mean corpuscular volume, hemoglobinuria, or haptoglobin should be normal.[16]

TREATMENT

No treatment is indicated for this benign process.

Prognosis/Return to Play

- There is no adverse effect on physical activity, and the athlete does not need to be kept out of participation.

Complications/Indications for Referral

Once the diagnosis is confirmed, there is no need for referral and the condition is self-limiting.

APPROACH TO THE ATHLETE WITH IRON DEFICIENCY ANEMIA

Iron deficiency is a common nutritional deficiency seen in the general population, as well as with athletes. Occasionally, there is also an associated anemia.

HISTORY AND PHYSICAL EXAMINATION

An athlete with shortness of breath or fatigue may need to be tested for anemia, and questions about dietary habits, menstrual periods, and gastrointestinal bleeding should be asked. If there is concern for gastrointestinal bleeding, a rectal examination should be done to include a test for fecal occult blood. Paleness of the skin or conjunctiva may also be noted.

DIAGNOSTIC TESTING

In stage I iron deficiency, there is an isolated decrease in the serum ferritin level, but hemoglobin levels will still be normal. In stage II, the iron level decreases, the transferrin saturation decreases, and the iron-binding capacity increases. There will be a mild normocytic anemia. In stage III, there is further depletion of the iron stores and development of a microcytic, hypochromic, iron-deficient anemia.[16]

TREATMENT

- If an athlete is determined to have an iron deficiency anemia and if he or she is not able to improve it with dietary modifications, he or she should be treated with oral iron replacement.
- Most commonly this is done with ferrous sulfate, but sometimes other choices such as ferrous gluconate may be used to minimize gastrointestinal side effects.
- Treatment may take several weeks before there is a noticeable improvement in the hemoglobin levels.
- Most show that 40 mg of elemental iron once daily is just as effective as three times daily dosing.[17]

Prognosis/Return to Play

- Athletes without any evidence of active bleeding can continue to participate without interruption.
- They may continue to exhibit symptoms of fatigue until they have been adequately treated.

Complications/Indications for Referral

If there is no improvement with oral replacement, the athlete has not been able to tolerate the iron supplements, or the etiology is unclear, a hematology consult may be needed.

If there is an associated menstrual or gastrointestinal bleeding issue, an appropriate referral for further workup may also be indicated.

APPROACH TO THE ATHLETE WITH INTRAVASCULAR HEMOLYSIS (EXERTION HEMOLYSIS)

Intravascular hemolysis can occur as a result of vigorous exercise. Originally it was thought that hemolysis was caused by the "foot strike mechanism" in which it was proposed that compression of capillaries was causing rupture of the RBCs, leading to hemolysis. However, this was also being seen in athletes such as swimmers and rowers and not specifically impact sports. It is now thought to be due to intravascular turbulence, acidosis, and increased temperature within the muscle tissue. Typically the amount of hemolysis is not significant enough to alter the CBC/RBC indices, and treatment is generally not necessary.[18]

HISTORY AND PHYSICAL EXAMINATION

Intravascular hemolysis is seen most commonly in endurance sports, such as long distance running.

DIAGNOSTIC TESTING

Testing should be done shortly after the completion of the workout. Findings include decreased serum haptoglobin and hemoglobinuria.

TREATMENT

- Alteration in training patterns or decrease in the intensity of training is the main treatment for intravascular hemolysis.
- Hemolysis will no longer be seen after a few days away from the exertion.

Prognosis/Return to Play

Intravascular hemolysis will not typically produce a significant enough anemia to cause the athlete to be removed from participation.

Complications/Indications for Referral

Intravascular hemolysis is generally a diagnosis of exclusion, and other more concerning causes of anemia should be ruled out first.

APPROACH TO THE ATHLETE WITH SICKLE CELL TRAIT/DISEASE

Some individuals produce not only the normal hemoglobin A but also an inherited hemoglobin S, which under physiologic stress can lead to sickling and destruction of the RBCs (Fig. 4.5). Athletes with sickle cell disease (SS) are not able to participate in intense physical activity due to the risk of developing a painful crisis, but those with sickle cell trait (AS) do participate in sports with certain precautions (Fig. 4.6).

HISTORY AND PHYSICAL EXAMINATION

Sickle cell trait is generally a rare trait, but is much more common in African-Americans. It is estimated that approximately 8% of African-Americans carry the sickle cell trait.[16,19] There have been reported deaths in young athletes with sickle cell trait due to rhabdomyolosysis, exertional heat stroke, and sudden cardiac arrhythmia.[16,20]

DIAGNOSTIC TESTING

Testing for the presence of hemoglobin S should be considered in high-risk populations.

TREATMENT

- Treatment in an athlete with a sickle cell trait is aimed at minimizing the risk of sudden death.

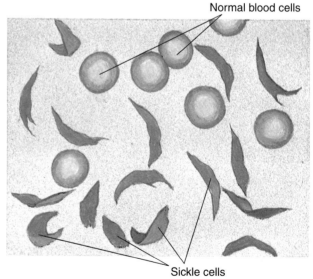

FIG. 4.5. Sickling of red blood cells. Reprinted with permission from Cohen BJ, Wood DL. *Memmler's The Human Body in Health and Disease.* 9th ed. Philadelphia: Lippincott Williams & Wilkins; 2000.

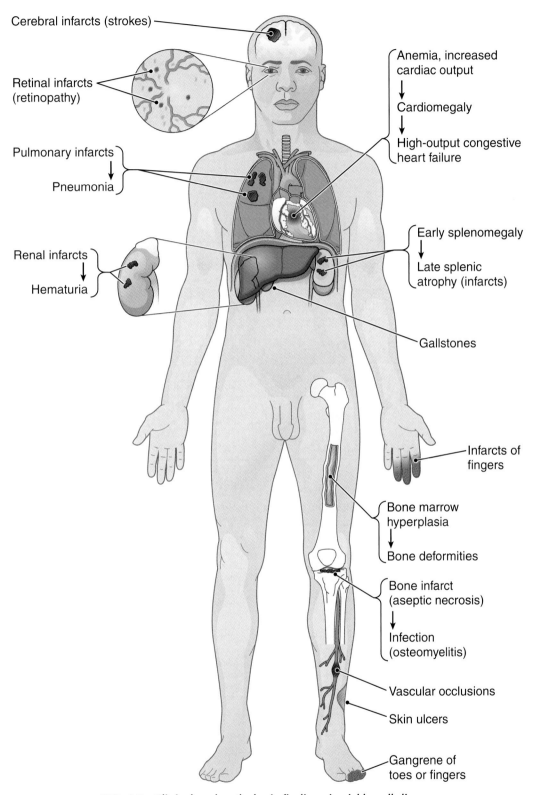

FIG. 4.6. Clinical and pathologic findings in sickle cell disease.

- The athlete should maintain adequate hydration, especially in warm conditions.
- There is also an increased risk of sickling at higher altitudes from lower oxygen concentrations; in these settings oxygen should be administered.

Prognosis/Return to Play

There is no absolute contraindication to athletic involvement in those athletes with a sickle cell trait, but they should be monitored closely in high-risk situations such as heat and altitude.

Complications/Indications for Referral

Dehydration, extreme heat, and altitude are associated risk factors for an adverse event, so the athlete should be closely monitored when competing in these conditions.

KEY POINTS
• EIA generally refers to the chronic asthmatic who has exercise as one of his or her triggers and can be seen in 80% to 90% of asthmatics.
• Diagnosis can be made with exercise and pharmacologic provocative tests. Spirometry and metalcholine challenge being most useful testing methods.
• Treatment consists of avoidance of triggers and pharmacologic therapy. Inhaled corticosteroids and short-acting β-agonists are the mainstay of pharmacologic treatment.
• Athletes with EIB experience their symptoms only with the trigger of exercise and do not have evidence of chronic asthma. Diagnosis is difficult, and treatment consists of modifying activities to avoid the triggers.
• Anemia is often present in young athletes and needs to be considered in part of the workup for shortness of breath or fatigue.
• Anemia can be caused by iron deficiency, dilutional pseudoanemia, and intravascular hemolysis or by genetic causes, that is, sickle cell disease.

REFERENCES

1. O'Byrne P, Bateman ED, Fitzgerald M, et al. Global Initiative for Asthma-Global Strategy for Asthma Management and Prevention 2007 (update). www.ginasthma.org.
2. Storms WW. Asthma associated with exercise. *Immunol Allergy Clin North Am.* 2005;25:31–43.
3. McFadden ER, Gilbert IA. Vascular responses and thermally induced asthma. In: Holgate ST, Austen KF, Lichtenstein AM, et al., eds. *Asthma: Physiology, Immunopharmacology and Treatment.* San Diego: Academic Press; 1993:337–355.
4. Anderson SD, Argyros J, Magnussen H, et al. Provocation by eucapnic voluntary hyperpnoea to identify exercise-induced bronchoconstriction. *Br J Sports Med.* 2001;35:344–347.
5. Johnson MB. A review of overtraining syndrome-recognizing the signs and symptoms. *J Athl Train.* 1992;27:352–354.
6. Kawabori I, Pierson WE, Conquest LL, et al. Incidence of exercise-induced asthma in children. *J Allergy Clin Immunol.* 1976;58:447–455.
7. Sonna LA, Angel KC, Sharp MA, et al. The prevalence of exercise-induced bronchospasm among US Army recruits and its effects on physical performance. *Chest.* 2001;119:1676.
8. Kukafka DS, Lang DM, Porter S, et al. Exercise-induced bronchospasm in high school athletes via a free running test: incidence and epidemiology. *Chest.* 1998;114:1613.
9. Di Santolo M, Stel G, Banfi G, et al. Anemia and iron status in young fertile non-professional female athletes. *Eur J Appl Physiol.* 2008;102(6):703–709.
10. Rundell KW. Exercise and other indirect challenges to demonstrate asthma or exercise-induced bronchoconstriction in athletes. *J Allergy Clin Immunol.* 2008;122:238–246.
11. Hunter CJ, Brightling CE, Woltmann G, et al. A comparison of the validity of different diagnostic tests in adults with asthma. *Chest.* 2002;121(4):1051–1057.
12. Kyle JM, Walker RB, Hanshaw SL, et al. Exercise-induced bronchospasm in the young athlete: guidelines for routine screening and initial management. *Med Sci Sports Exerc.* 1992;24:856–859.
13. Gotshall RW. Exercise Induced Bronchoconstriction. *Drugs.* 2002;62:1725–1739.
14. National Asthma Education and Prevention Program. Expert Panel Report 3 (EPR-3): Guidelines for the Diagnosis and Management of Asthma-Summary Report 2007. *J Allergy Clin Immunol.* 2007;120(5):S94–S138.
15. McKenzie DC, McLuckie SL, Stirling DR. The protective effects of continuous and interval exercise in athletes with exercise-induced asthma. *Med Sci Sports Exerc.* 1994;26:951–956.
16. Mercer KW, Densmore JJ. Hematologic disorders in the athlete. *Clin Sports Med.* 2005;24:599–621.
17. Zlotkin S, Arthur P, Antwi KY, et al. Randomized, controlled trial of single versus 3-times-daily ferrous sulfate drops for treatment of anemia. *Pediatrics.* 2001;108(3):613–616.
18. Adams WB, Birrer RB, O'Connor FG, et al. Hematologic concerns in the athlete. In: *Sports Medicine for the Primary Care Physician.* CRC Press; 2004:761–763.
19. Steinberg MH. Management of sickle cell disease. *N Engl J Med.* 1999;340:1021–1030.
20. Kark JA, Posey DM, Schumacher HR, et al. Sickle-cell trait as a risk factor for sudden death in physical training. *N Engl J Med.* 1987;317:781–787.

Female Athlete

Lee A. Mancini

INTRODUCTION

It has been over 35 years since the passage of Title IX in 1972, which prohibited sex discrimination in sports. There are now almost 2.5 million female athletes competing in high school sports, in addition to nearly 200,000 female athletes at the collegiate level. With increase in number of female athletes, there have also come increased examinations into conditions specific to the female athlete.

The "female athlete triad" is a term used to describe the combination of amenorrhea, disordered eating, and osteoporosis in physically active girls and women. It was first defined at the Triad Consensus Conference in 1992 by the American College of Sports Medicine. More recently, it has been recognized that energy imbalance likely plays the underlying role resulting in the findings of amenorrhea and osteoporosis.[1] This is the approach to the female athlete suspected to having the female athlete triad. Other conditions commonly encountered in female athletes that are addressed in other chapters include patello–femoral syndrome, stress fractures, and anterior cruciate ligament (ACL) tears.

PATHOPHYSIOLOGY

Eating Disorders

Anorexia nervosa is an eating disorder characterized by restrictive eating in which the individuals view themselves as overweight and are afraid of gaining weight even though they are at least 15% below expected weight for age and height. Amenorrhea is a diagnostic criterion for anorexia nervosa.[2] In this instance, amenorrhea is defined as the lack of three consecutive menstrual cycles. Anorexia nervosa can be further divided into restricting or purging subtypes.

Bulimia nervosa is another eating disorder where the affected individuals are usually in the normal weight range. In Bulimia, individuals repeat a cycle of overeating (binge eating) and then purging. The purging may be from induced vomiting, restricted eating, excessive exercise, misuse of laxatives or medications, or other compensatory behaviors. An individual must have at least two episodes per week for 3 months to meet the criteria for bulimia.

The *Diagnostic and Statistical Manual of Mental Diseases*, 4th Edition (DSM-IV), outlines the criteria for anorexia nervosa and bulimia nervosa. Athletes who do not meet all the DSM-IV criteria are given the diagnosis of eating disorder not otherwise specified (EDNOS). Disordered eating includes any abnormal eating pattern and is not limited to anorexia nervosa or bulimia. It can include food restriction, fasting, binging, using laxatives, diuretics, and diet pills, or excessive exercise.

Menstrual Function

Eumenorrhea is defined as a menstrual cycle that lasts 28 days with a standard deviation of 7 days. This is the median interval for young adult women. Oligomenorrhea is defined as having a menstrual cycle occur at intervals longer than 35 days.[3] Amenorrhea can consist of either primary or secondary amenorrhea. Primary amenorrhea is defined as the absence of menarche after the athlete has reached 15. Secondary amenorrhea refers to the absence of menses for 3 consecutive months or longer.

Bone Mineral Density

With respect to the female athlete triad, there is recognition of a spectrum of bone mineral density (BMD) ranging from optimal bone health to osteoporosis.[1] Osteoporosis is defined as a skeletal disorder characterized by compromised bone strength, predisposing a person to an increased risk of fracture. Osteoporosis is not always caused by accelerated bone mineral loss in adulthood. It can also be due to not accumulating optimal BMD during childhood and adolescence. The World Health Organization (WHO) uses T and Z scores for defining osteoporosis and osteopenia. The T score compares an individual's BMD to the average adult peak BMD. In the nonathlete population, osteopenia is defined as a T score between -1 and -2.5. Osteoporosis is defined as a T score less than -2.5. With a reduction of BMD of 1 standard deviation, the fracture rate doubles.[4] The Z score compares an individual's BMD to age and sex-matched controls. The Z score is a more accurate measure of BMD in athletes, because the evidence has shown that weight-bearing sport athletes have a BMD 5% to 15% higher than nonathletes.[5] The American

College of Sports Medicine (ACSM) position statement on female athlete triad defines low BMD as a Z score between −1.0 and −2.0. The term "low BMD" is defined as a history of nutritional deficiencies, hypoestrogenism, stress fractures, and other secondary clinical risk fractures for fractures. With respect to the female athlete triad, osteoporosis is defined as a Z score less than −2.0. Low BMD can result from premature bone resorption, impaired bone formation, or both. Deficiencies in calcium, vitamin D, and caloric intake lead to increased bone resorption.

Low Energy Balance

A low energy balance whether or not the athlete has an eating disorder affects both BMD and menstrual function. Athletes at greatest risk are those who are vegetarians, who limit the variety of foods they eat, and who exercise for prolonged periods of time. Animal models have shown that a 30% reduction in caloric intake causes both infertility and skeletal demineralization.[1] Low energy availability disrupts the gonadotropin-releasing hormone (GnRH) and luteinizing hormone (LH) pulsatility. It also increases the rate of bone resorption and decreases the rate of bone formation.[1]

EPIDEMIOLOGY

Individuals diagnosed with anorexia nervosa have a six times greater mortality rate compared with the general population.[6] One study showed that 5.4% of athletes with eating disorders had attempted suicide.[7] There is an increased risk of female athlete triad, and it is greatest in endurance sports emphasizing leanness such as cross-country, in sports emphasizing body image such as gymnastics or dance, or in sports where weight classes are used such as lightweight crew. Eating disorders are found in 31% of these thin-build sports compared with 5.5% of the general population.[8] Another study showed 25% of these thin-build sports athletes compared with 9% of the general population.[9] Disordered eating occurs in nearly two thirds of all female athletes.[10] The prevalence of primary amenorrhea is less than 1% in the general population, but more than 22% in cheerleading, diving, and gymnastics.[11,12] Secondary amenorrhea has been seen as high as 69% in dancers and 65% in long-distance runners.[2] Overall the female athlete triad is seen in 2.7% of college athletes and 1.2% of high school athletes.[13,14] In both of these studies, the examiners used more narrow guidelines than the accepted ACSM position stand guidelines.

NARROWING THE DIFFERENTIAL DIAGNOSIS

History

The preparticipation physical should be used to screen for the female athlete triad. Female athletes should be asked about caloric intake, dietary habits, weight fluctuations, body image, fear of weight gain, and menstrual dysfunction. Athletes should be asked about a history of stress fractures, family history of osteoporosis or osteopenia, and family or personal history of vitamin D deficiency. Any athlete who is found to have one component of the female athlete triad should be assessed further. Athletes who are discovered to have disordered eating should be referred to a mental health practitioner for further evaluation.[1]

Evidence-based Physical Examination

Physical examination should include height, weight, and vital signs. Orthostatic hypotension is a finding often seen in female athlete triad as is both bradycardia and tachycardia. Physicians should pay attention to cold or discolored hands and feet, hypercarotenemia, lanugo hair, and parotid gland enlargement. Dental examination can evaluate for oral erosions seen with frequent purging.

Diagnostic Testing

Laboratory

Laboratory tests that should be done to work up secondary amenorrhea should include a pregnancy test, follicle-stimulating hormone (FSH) and LH, serum cortisol, estradiol, and a progesterone challenge. The FSH/LH ratio is important for ruling out polycystic ovary syndrome (PCOS). Also free testosterone and dehydroepiandrosterone sulfate (DHEA) levels should be done if the female athlete has any evidence of androgenic examination findings. A prolactin test should be ordered to determine if the athlete has a lactotrophic-secreting tumor. Other necessary lab work should include thyroid function tests, urinalysis, erythrocyte sedimentation rate, calcium, vitamin D, electrolytes, chemistry profile, and complete blood count with differential.[1]

Imaging

If an athlete has had the criteria of the female athlete triad for 6 months or more, then a bone density (dual-energy x-ray absorptiometry [DEXA]) scan should be ordered. A repeat DEXA scan is recommended in 12 months.

Other Testing

An electrocardiogram (ECG) should be ordered to assess for prolonged QT interval or another arrhythmia.

APPROACH TO THE ATHLETE WITH FEMALE ATHLETE TRIAD

HISTORY AND PHYSICAL EXAMINATION

Physicians should ask about frequent fluctuations in weight. Look for both weight gain and weight loss. Does the athlete have a history of stress fractures? Does the athlete have a history of menstrual irregularities? At what age did menarche occur? Has the athlete ever gone more than 3 months without menses? Has the athlete ever menstruated less than six times in a year?

Physicians should monitor vital signs, including orthostatic blood pressure readings. The athlete's height and weight should be documented. The athlete's extremities should be examined to look for circulation issues, including cold or discolored hands and feet. Additional findings may include hypercarotenemia, lanugo hair, and parotid gland enlargement. Dental examination can evaluate for oral erosions seen with frequent purging.

Diagnostic Testing

Laboratory

Lab work should include thyroid function tests, urinalysis, erythrocyte sedimentation rate, calcium, vitamin D, electrolytes, chemistry profile, and complete blood count with differential. To further work up amenorrhea, laboratory tests may include FSH, LH, prolactin test, free testosterone, DHEA, serum cortisol, estradiol, and a progesterone challenge.[1]

Imaging

If an athlete has the criteria of the female athlete triad for 6 months or more, then a bone density (DEXA) scan should be ordered. A repeat DEXA scan is recommended in 12 months.

Other Testing

An ECG should be ordered to assess for prolonged QT interval or another arrhythmia.

TREATMENT

General Measures

- Treatment of female athlete triad should focus on education and prevention
- Treatment should include a physician, a registered dietitian, and a mental health counselor
- Primary goal is to restore normal *energy balance* via an increase in caloric intake and/or to decrease energy expenditure
- Athletes with the female athlete triad must agree with the following:
  - To comply with all treatment strategies
  - To be closely monitored by health care professionals
  - To place precedence on treatment over training and competition

- To modify the type, duration, and intensity of training and competition
- A written contract may be necessary to specify these agreements
  - If the athlete does not accept treatment, breaks contract, eating behavior does not improve, or weight does not improve then the athlete may be removed from practice or game participation
- Athletes with eating disorders should meet minimal established criteria to continue exercising and competing
- Nutritional recommendations include
  - Vitamin D 400 to 800 IU daily (greater if vitamin D deficient)
  - Calcium 1,000 to 1,300 mg daily
  - Protein 1.6 g/kg body weight daily
  - Caloric intake between 30 and 45 kcal/kg daily
  - Optimization of overall nutritional status

Pharmacologic Treatment

- No pharmacologic agent adequately restores bone loss or corrects the hormonal or metabolic deficiencies.
- Bisphosphonates should not be used in young female athletes because they can remain in a woman's bone for many years, causing harm to a developing fetus during pregnancy.
- There is no documented benefit to hormone replacement therapy.
- Athletes should take the recommended nutritional supplements such as vitamin D, calcium, and adequate protein.
- Oral contraceptive pills (OCPs) may be considered in athletes with functional hypothalamic secondary amenorrhea, especially in athletes over the age of 16.
- Antidepressants are often used for bulimia nervosa, anorexia nervosa, EDNOS, depression, and anxiety disorders.

Prognosis/Return to Play

- An athlete can return to sports participation once the following conditions are met:
  - If there is no evidence of end-organ injury from the female athlete triad—for example:
    - Stress fracture
    - Cardiac arrhythmias
    - Orthostatic hypotension
    - Bradycardia or tachycardia at rest
  - Athletes should meet the weight and nutritional guidelines set forth in their contract

Complications/Indications for Referral

In severe cases, athletes may need inpatient treatment. If an ECG shows a cardiac arrhythmia secondary to an eating disorder, then the athlete may need inpatient treatment.

KEY POINTS
• Disordered eating, eating disorders, and amenorrhea occur more frequently in sports that emphasize leanness.
• Menstrual irregularities and low BMD increase the risk of stress fractures.
• Screening for the female athlete triad should occur at the preparticipation physical examination (PPE).
• BMD should be assessed after a stress fracture and after 6 months of amenorrhea, disordered eating, or an eating disorder.

REFERENCES

1. Nattiv A, Loucks AB, Manore MM, et al. American College of Sports Medicine position stand. The female athlete triad. *Med Sci Sports Exerc.* 2007;39(10):1867–1882.
2. American Psychiatric Association Work Group on Eating Disorders. Practice guidelines for the treatment of patients with eating disorders (revision). *Am J Psychiatry.* 2000;157(1):1–39.
3. Marcus R, Cann C, Madvig P, et al. Menstrual function and bone mass in elite women distance runners. Endocrine and metabolic features. *Ann Intern Med.* 1985;102:158–163.
4. Hui SL, Slemenda CW, Johnston CC Jr. Baseline measurement of bone mass predicts fracture in white women. *Ann Intern Med.* 1989;111:355–361.
5. Fehling PC, Alekel L, Clasey J, et al. A comparison of bone mineral densities among female athletes in impact loading and active loading sports. *Bone.* 1995;17:205–210.
6. Neilsen S, Miller-Madsen S, Isager T, et al. Standardized mortality in eating disorders – a quantitative summary of previously published and new evidence. *J Psychosom Res.* 1998;44:413–434.
7. Sundgot-Borgen J. Risk and trigger factors for the development of eating disorders in female elite athletes. *Med Sci Sports Exerc.* 1994;26: 414–419.
8. Byrne S, McLean N. Elite athletes: effects of the pressure to be thin. *J Sci Med Sport.* 2002;5:80–94.
9. Sundgot-Borgen J, Torstveit MK. Prevalence of eating disorders in elite athletes is higher than in general population. *Clin J Sport Med.* 2004;14: 25–32.
10. Lerand SJ, Williams JF. The female athlete triad. *Pediatr Rev.* 2006;27: e12–e13.
11. Beals KA, Manore MM. Disorders of the female athlete triad among collegiate athletes. *Int J Sports Nutr Exerc Metab.* 2002;12:281–293.
12. Chumlea WC, Schubert CM, Roche AF, et al. Age at menarche and racial comparisons in US girls. *Pediatrics.* 2003;111:110–113.
13. Beals KA, Hill AK. The prevalence of disordered eating, menstrual dysfunction, and low bone mineral density among US collegiate athletes. *Int J Sports Nutr Exerc Metab.* 2006;16:1–23.
14. Nichols J, Rauh MJ, Lawson MJ, et al. Prevalence of the female athlete triad syndrome among high school athletes. *Arch Pediatr Adolesc Med.* 2006;160:137–142.

Athlete with Rash

Christopher J. Lutrzykowski

INTRODUCTION

There are a multitude of exanthems that affect the athlete. The number and breadth of rashes mimic the general population, and the primary care provider must have a sound foundation in diagnosing and treating those conditions. There are eruptions, however, that bear specific emphasis for the provider caring for athletes due to their morbidity and communicability. The presence of certain rashes may also exclude the athlete from sports participation unless properly covered and/or treated. This chapter will focus on four types of skin infections commonly found in athletes that can affect their participation: tinea, herpes, cellulitis/furunculosis, and molluscum contagiosum. Special attention will be addressed to community-acquired methicillin-resistant *Staphylococcus aureus* (cMRSA) due to the recent rise in incidence and significant deleterious effects on athletes.

PATHOPHYSIOLOGY

For a variety of reasons, athletes are at risk for particular skin disorders. The athletes' dermis is under constant stress due to their sport exposure as well as microenvironmental conditions (moisture, heat) and unique macroenvironmental conditions (heat, cold, water, sun). Additionally, the dermis can be affected by systemic stress from exercise, including decreased immunity and alterations in blood supply. The normal skin barrier can be easily compromised with close skin contact, abrasions, and cuts. Furthermore, the metabolic stress of exercise may compromise an athlete's short-term immunity and increase their risk of skin infections. Team sports also present a risk for athletes in that they are often sharing space and personal items among themselves.[1-3]

EPIDEMIOLOGY

There are no formal data on the incidence or prevalence of skin disorders or exanthems in athletes as outbreaks can occur sometimes in sporadic fashion. Prevalence can also vary by geography and patient population.

NARROWING THE DIFFERENTIAL DIAGNOSIS

History

It is paramount to obtain an adequate history when an athlete presents with a rash. In addition to location, noting the time of onset and precipitating factors is important in narrowing the differential diagnosis. Pertinent questions include the following: Was there a prodromal symptom complex? Was there fever? Did any other team member present with a rash? Was the rash in a shaved area? Is the rash painful, itchy, and raised? Were any new creams, detergents, or topical ointments used? Is there any comorbid medical illness? A good history will help the clinician to a narrower differential diagnosis and streamlined care.

Evidence-based Physical Examination

With clues taken from a thorough history, the physical examination guides the clinician to an appropriate diagnosis and treatment. The athlete may present with multiple types of rash, and careful skin examination is important. Rashes cannot be adequately diagnosed through clothing; thus, adequate visualization is important. Is the rash macular or papular? Is it red? Where is it located? Are there satellite lesions? Is it vesicular? Is there a scale? Are there lesions in various states of healing? Are there areas of central clearing? Does the rash vary in size and shape? These questions among many also may help the clinician arrive at the correct diagnosis.

Diagnostic Testing

Laboratory

Lab testing may be appropriate for specific diseases, including serologies. While not explicitly listed below, Lyme titers are helpful in the diagnosis of Lyme disease, in particular if IgM levels are elevated.

Imaging

Imaging is rarely useful in the diagnosis of rash. It may prove beneficial in the presence of a cellulitis if osteomyelitis is a considered diagnosis.

Other Testing

Skin scrapings, shavings, and biopsy can prove useful in the diagnosis and treatment of rashes, in particular in recalcitrant cases. Polymerase chain reaction (PCR) (see later in the chapter) may prove a useful adjunct as well. Wound cultures are always recommended when accessible or clinically indicated. This is particularly true with the rise of cMRSA.

APPROACH TO THE ATHLETE WITH TINEA

Tinea refers to dermatophyte infections that predominantly stem from three different genera. Risk factors for tinea include direct contact with soil, infected humans and animals, and fomites.[3] Dermatophytes invade and proliferate in keratinized tissue, including skin, hair, and nails.[3] Tinea clinically are subdivided and named based on location. Several locations have been described and include tinea capitis, tinea corporis, tinea cruris, and tinea pedis. Each will be discussed separately.

APPROACH TO THE ATHLETE WITH TINEA CAPITIS

No incidence data are available for tinea capitis among athletes, but it can occur in epidemic form.[4,5] Athletes may present with alopecia, desiring treatment.

HISTORY AND PHYSICAL EXAMINATION

Multiple clinical presentations exist for tinea infections of the scalp. Black dot type is named after the fractured hair follicles from tinea infection (Fig. 6.1). Gray patch type, which is most common, is noted for circular areas of alopecia (Fig. 6.2). A

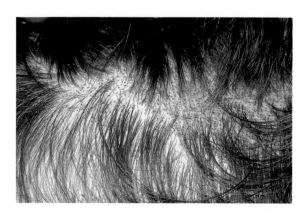

FIG. 6.1. Tinea capitis: black dot type. Reprinted with permission from Goodheart HP. *Goodheart's Photoguide of Common Skin Disorders.* 2nd ed. Philadelphia: Lippincott Williams & Wilkins; 2003.

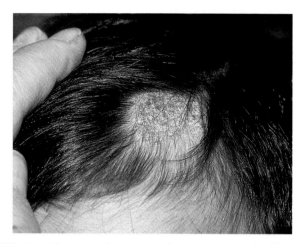

FIG. 6.2. Tinea capitis: gray patch type. Reprinted with permission from Goodheart HP. *Goodheart's Photoguide of Common Skin Disorders.* 2nd ed. Philadelphia: Lippincott Williams & Wilkins; 2003.

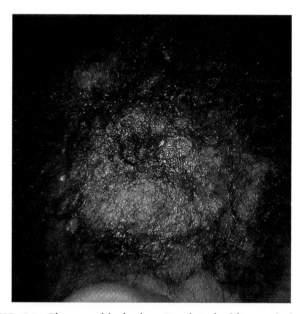

FIG. 6.3. Tinea capitis: kerion. Reprinted with permission from Fleisher GR, Ludwig S, Baskin MN. *Atlas of Pediatric Emergency Medicine.* Philadelphia: Lippincott Williams & Wilkins; 2004.

kerion may be present, which is a slightly erythematous boggy mass with alopecia that may progress to scarring (Fig. 6.3).

DIAGNOSTIC TESTING

Skin scrapings may be isolated on a slide for microscopic examination with 10% potassium hydroxide (KOH). Tinea have characteristic hyphae with septate branching and when present can confirm the diagnosis. Scrapings and hair may also be sent for fungal culture.

TREATMENT

General Measures

- Tinea may be spread by fomites, and cleansing mats, headgear, and clothing may decrease spread among other athletes.
- Showering directly after practice may help limit the spread of the disease.[6–12]

Pharmacologic Treatment

- Topical therapy alone with selenium sulfide and ketoconazole shampoos is often not enough to clear infection but may be used as an adjunct to oral therapy.
- Mainstay of treatment is oral therapy with griseofulvin, itraconazole, or terbinafine.[3]
- Treatment must continue until clinically and microscopically clear.[3]

Prognosis/Return to Play

- Overall prognosis is excellent, but recurrence rates are high in affected individuals. For return-to-play guidelines in athletes with close skin contact, see the "Approach to the Athlete with Tinea Corporis (Gladiatorum)" section.

Complications/Indications for Referral

Scar and alopecia may be permanent. Referral is indicated for recalcitrant cases and treatment failures.

APPROACH TO THE ATHLETE WITH TINEA CORPORIS

Tinea corporis is a common skin dermatophyte seen in all age groups. Tinea corporis, common among wrestlers, is also known as tinea gladiatorum and is discussed in greater detail in the following sections.

HISTORY AND PHYSICAL EXAMINATION

This dermatophyte infection starts clinically as a round, erythematous plaque that expands radially with eventual central clearing (Fig. 6.4). The infection may be an isolated lesion or multiple lesions involving a variety of skin surfaces. Tinea corporis may have an atypical presentation with vesicles, pustules, or crusts.

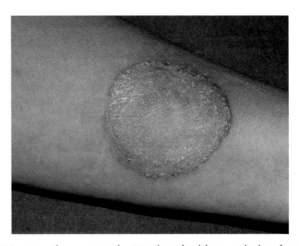

FIG. 6.4. Tinea corporis. Reprinted with permission from Goodheart HP. *Goodheart's Photoguide of Common Skin Disorders.* 2nd ed. Philadelphia: Lippincott Williams & Wilkins; 2003.

DIAGNOSTIC TESTING

Skin scraping, shaving, or biopsy may be necessary to diagnose the rash.

TREATMENT

General Measures

- As listed in the "Approach to the Athlete with Tinea Corporis (Gladiatorum)" section.

Pharmacologic Treatment

- Treatment is topical in isolated cases, but oral therapy is necessary for disseminated cases.[3] See later in the chapter for tinea corporis gladiatorum.

Prognosis/Return to Play

- Overall prognosis is excellent, but recurrence rates are high in affected individuals. For return-to-play guidelines in athletes with close skin contact, see the "Approach to the Athlete with Tinea Corporis (Gladiatorum)" section.

Complications/Indications for Referral

Referral is indicated for recalcitrant cases and treatment failures.

APPROACH TO THE ATHLETE WITH TINEA CRURIS

This is very common among athletes of all sports and ages. Absolute incidence data are lacking.

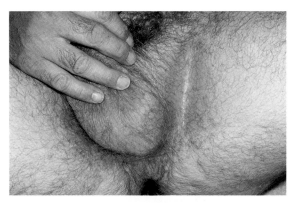

FIG. 6.5. Tinea cruris. Reprinted with permission from Goodheart HP. *Goodheart's Photoguide of Common Skin Disorders.* 2nd ed. Philadelphia: Lippincott Williams & Wilkins; 2003.

HISTORY AND PHYSICAL EXAMINATION

Tinea cruris typically presents as a red, variably pruritic rash with a raised scaly border (Fig. 6.5). It spares the scrotum, which helps distinguish this rash from other entities such as *Candida* sp.[3] and erythrasma. Risk factors for the development of tinea cruris include sweating, warm moist environment, tinea pedis, and toenail onychomycosis.[3]

TREATMENT

General Measures

- Tinea cruris advances in warm moist environments; thus, prevention strategies include drying the groin with a separate towel than used for the feet, putting on socks before undergarments, and treating other areas (tinea pedis) infected with dermatophytes.

Pharmacologic Treatment

- Treatment is usually topical, but oral systemic therapy may be needed for severe or recalcitrant cases.

Prognosis/Return to Play

- Overall prognosis is excellent, but recurrence rates are high in affected individuals. No specific return-to-play guidelines are available, but for athletes with close skin contact, one may want to refer to the guidelines listed under the "Approach to the Athlete with Tinea Corporis (Gladiatorum)" section.

Complications/Indications for Referral

Referral is indicated for recalcitrant cases and treatment failures.

APPROACH TO THE ATHLETE WITH TINEA PEDIS

As with other tinea infections, this common rash presents in all ages and sports.

HISTORY AND PHYSICAL EXAMINATION

Tinea pedis is a dermatophyte infection of the feet that presents in various forms. The most common presentation is in the web spaces between the toes (Fig. 6.6). The skin appears macerated, scaly, and cracked, and the rash tends to be intensely pruritic. Bacterial superinfection causes the classic "athlete's foot."[3] The infection can also present in a "moccasin" distribution as well as a pustular pruritic form.

DIAGNOSTIC TESTING

See the "Approach to the Athlete with Tinea Corporis (Gladiatorum)" section.

TREATMENT

General Measures

- Adjunctive agents to decrease sweating and antifungal powders may be useful.
- Frequent sock changes and a dry environment may also prove useful for clearing the infection.

Pharmacologic Treatment

- Topical agents are effective but may need to be used for up to 4 weeks to achieve eradication.[3]

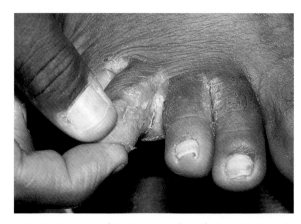

FIG. 6.6. Tinea pedis. Reprinted with permission from Goodheart HP. *Goodheart's Photoguide of Common Skin Disorders.* 2nd ed. Philadelphia: Lippincott Williams & Wilkins; 2003.

Prognosis/Return to Play

Prognosis/Return to Play

- Overall prognosis is excellent, but recurrence rates are high in affected individuals. No specific return-to-play guidelines are available, but for athletes with close skin contact, one may want to refer to the guidelines listed under the "Approach to the Athlete with Tinea Corporis (Gladiatorum)" section.

Complications/Indications for Referral

Referral is indicated for recalcitrant cases and treatment failures.

APPROACH TO THE ATHLETE WITH TINEA VERSICOLOR

Tinea versicolor is caused by organisms different from those that cause other tinea infections. Etiologic species include *Pityrosporum orbiculare* and *Pityrosporum ovale*. The incidence of this rash is unknown among the athletic population.

HISTORY AND PHYSICAL EXAMINATION

The lesions can present as either hyper- or hypopigmented macules on the trunk and upper extremities and may be pruritic (Fig. 6.7). Lesions begin as multiple small, circular macules of white, pink, or brown color that enlarge radially.[13] These may present in various forms and may be nearly indistinguishable in white athletes in the winter. In black athletes the lesions may appear hyperpigmented. The lesions are most common on the upper trunk but may appear on any skin surface.[13]

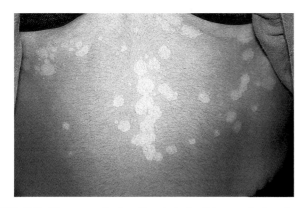

FIG. 6.7. Tinea versicolor. Reprinted with permission from Goodheart HP. *Goodheart's Photoguide of Common Skin Disorders.* 2nd ed. Philadelphia: Lippincott Williams & Wilkins; 2003.

DIAGNOSTIC TESTING

The dermatophyte can be obtained from skin scrapings and identified under microscopy with the characteristic "spaghetti and meatballs" appearance of budding yeast and branched hyphae.[3]

TREATMENT

General Measures

- Once-weekly application of ketoconazole 2% shampoo, applied as a lotion to the neck, trunk, and upper extremities 5 to 10 minutes before showering, may help prevent recurrences.[13]

Pharmacologic Treatment

- Hypopigmentation may remain for months despite adequate treatment.[3]
- Treatment is usually topical with selenium sulfide or ketoconazole shampoo but may occasionally need oral systemic therapy.
- Oral therapy does not include griseofulvin, as it has insufficient activity against tinea versicolor. Recurrence rates are as high as 40% to 60%.[13]

Prognosis/Return to Play

- Overall prognosis is excellent, but recurrence rates are high in affected individuals. No specific return-to-play guidelines are available, but for athletes with close skin contact, one may want to refer to the guidelines listed under the "Approach to the Athlete with Tinea Corporis (Gladiatorum)" section.

Complications/Indications for Referral

Referral is indicated for recalcitrant cases and treatment failures.

APPROACH TO THE ATHLETE WITH DERMATOPHYTE FOLLICULITIS

P. orbiculare yeast folliculitis (yeast form of malassezia) may mimic bacterial folliculitis and acne. It is less common than bacterial infections, although true incidence is unknown. Risk factors include heat, sweating, and poor hygiene.

HISTORY AND PHYSICAL EXAMINATION

P. orbiculare folliculitis will usually spare the face and has a predilection for warm moist areas under friction (upper shoulders under pads in football).[3]

DIAGNOSTIC TESTING

Yeast forms may be seen on microscopy, further distinguishing it from bacterial infections.

TREATMENT

General Measures

- Good hygiene practices and prompt showering may limit spread and recurrence.

Pharmacologic Treatment

- This dermatophyte can be treated with ketoconazole 2% shampoo or selenium sulfide 2.5% shampoo.
- Recalcitrant or severe cases may require oral treatment with antifungal agents.
- There is a high rate of reoccurrence, and suppressive therapy with ketoconazole shampoo weekly may be necessary.[1]

Prognosis/Return to Play

- Overall prognosis is excellent, but recurrence rates are high in affected individuals. No specific return-to-play guidelines are available, but for athletes with close skin contact, one may want to refer to the guidelines listed under the "Approach to the Athlete with Tinea Corporis (Gladiatorum)" section.

Complications/Indications for Referral

Referral is indicated for recalcitrant cases and treatment failures.

APPROACH TO THE ATHLETE WITH TINEA CORPORIS (GLADIATORUM)

Tinea corporis gladiatorum refers to outbreaks among athletes where there is close contact among participants, most notably in wrestling. There are three genera that are responsible for tinea corporis: *Trychophyton tonsurans*, *Trychophyton rubrum*, and *Trychophyton mentagrophytes*. The most common etiologic agent for tinea corporis gladiatorum is *T. tonsurans*, accounting for the vast majority of outbreaks.[14] *T.*

mentagrophytes has been described as a rare source and may come from an animal vector.[15]

Tinea gladiatorum is the second most common skin infection among National Collegiate Athletic Association (NCAA) wrestlers and has prevalence rates among wrestling teams from 20% to 77%.[14,16] Wrestling is the most common sport associated with tinea gladiatorum, but prevalence rates among other combatant sports such as judo are also high.[17] Tinea, unlike other infections, may be isolated from wrestling mats and can be a source for the infection.[14] It can also rapidly spread from team participants to nonathletes via close contact (i.e., sexual partners).[17] Outbreaks of tinea capitus gladiatorum have also been reported, and wrestling boarding schools are particularly at risk with younger-age combatants.[4,5] Risk factors for developing tinea include heat, moisture, friction, and close skin-to-skin contact.

HISTORY AND PHYSICAL EXAMINATION

Diagnosis of tinea gladiatorum is clinical, with the characteristic rash recognizing that the rash presents with the usual appearance described earlier but also as plaques and scaling papules.[16] Usual locations of involvement are upper extremities, shoulders, face, and head and neck reflecting areas of greatest contact among athletes in combat sports.

DIAGNOSTIC TESTING

Skin scraping or hair follicle KOH prep under microscopy usually assists in the diagnosis. PCR for rapid detection has been tested and is highly accurate, but not yet commercially available.[18]

TREATMENT

General Measures

- Prevention includes showering directly after practice, refraining from towel/clothes sharing, and bleaching mats with chlorine.
- Prophylaxis has been studied and is effective, but no definitive recommendations exist to treat unaffected team members due to the cost of the medications, potential side effects of the medications, and the potential development of resistant organisms.[16]

Pharmacologic Treatment

- Treatment for isolated lesions is usually topical with the azole, allylamine, or pyradone class of agents.
- The cream is applied to the entire lesion plus a 2-cm perimeter of normal skin twice weekly for a minimum of 2 weeks.[19]

- Disseminated disease, tinea capitus, inflammatory lesions, or failure of clearance with topical agents necessitate oral systemic therapy.
- Athletes have been reported to be infectious for up to 3 weeks on treatment and may account for epidemic outbreaks of tinea gladiatorum.[4,14,17,20–23]

Prognosis/Return to Play

- Restricting the athlete with active infection is paramount to limit spread, and included are the recommendations for NCAA division I wrestling and for high school wrestling.
- Readers are encouraged to review the specific guidelines published for the sport in question, but when in doubt, use of the following restrictions are reasonable.
- According to the 2006 NCAA division I wrestling handbook and National Federation of State High Schools (NFHS) Sports Medicine Advisory Committee rules, a minimum of 72 hours of topical therapy is required for skin lesions.[24]
- A minimum of 2 weeks of systemic antifungal therapy is required for scalp lesions. The NCAA further stipulates that "the fungicidal topical antifungals terbinafine or naftifine are suggested for treatment.
- Wrestlers with extensive and active lesions will be disqualified. Activity of treated lesions can be judged either by the use of KOH preparation or by a review of therapeutic regimen.
- Wrestlers with solitary, or closely clustered, localized lesions will be disqualified if lesions are in a body location that cannot be "adequately covered."
- Covering routine should include selenium sulfide washing of lesion or ketoconazole shampoo, followed by application of naftifine gel or cream or terbinafine cream, and then gas-permeable dressing such as Op-Site or Bioclusive, followed by ProWrap and stretch tape.
- Dressing changes should be done after each match so that lesions can air dry. The disposition of tinea cases will be decided on an individual basis, as determined by the examining physician or certified athletic trainer."[25]

Complications/Indications for Referral

Referral is indicated for recalcitrant cases and treatment failures.

APPROACH TO THE ATHLETE WITH HERPES GLADIATORUM

Herpes infection is the most common skin infection among combatant sports.[14] Multiple documented outbreaks have been reported in medical literature as well as lay press.[26–29] Herpes gladiatorum is caused by herpes virus and is thought to be transmitted from skin to skin by close contact. No transmission has been reported from towels, mats, or other fomites.[30] Incidence of new cases may be as high as 47%

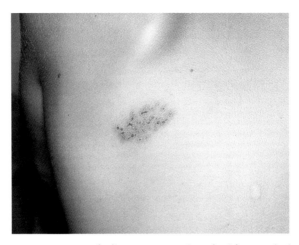

FIG. 6.8. Herpes gladiatorum. Reprinted with permission from Goodheart HP. *Goodheart's Photoguide of Common Skin Disorders.* 2nd ed. Philadelphia: Lippincott Williams & Wilkins; 2003.

among herpes naive wrestlers.[29] The incubation period is problematic in that it ranges from 4 to 10 days, making control of outbreaks challenging.[30] As with any of the infections in the herpes family, herpes gladiatorum may remain latent in the dorsal sensory root ganglia and reactivate during periods of physical or emotional stress.[3]

HISTORY AND PHYSICAL EXAMINATION

The painful rash appears as grouped vesicles on an erythematous base that will eventually rupture to produce the characteristic ulcerated base (Fig. 6.8). The eruption also may present with a straw-colored crust similar to impetigo. Prior to the presence of the lesions, athletes may have a prodromal symptom complex including systemic symptoms of fever and chills with new infections.[3,29,30] Abrasions or open wounds may facilitate transfer of the virus. Diagnosis is both clinical and by culture.

DIAGNOSTIC TESTING

A culture of a vesicle or a wound may aid in diagnosis.[13] A Tzanc smear may also be used to assist in diagnosis, but should not be relied upon, as it is insensitive and nonspecific.[13] PCR for herpes is available in some centers and may prove the most accurate.

TREATMENT

General Measures

- Prophylaxis has been studied and appears effective.
- Valacyclovir and acyclovir have been studied, and in initial studies the former appears to be superior.[29,31]
- This may be used in advance of the season in susceptible individuals.

Pharmacologic Treatment

- Treatment is by antiretrovirals to limit the duration of the disease. Antivirals should be started early in the course of the disease, as effectiveness wanes after 48 hours of lesion presentation.[3]
- Multiple medications now exist for the treatment of herpes outbreaks and include acyclovir, valacyclovir, and famciclovir.
- Famciclovir and valacyclovir regimens for primary herpes infection are of shorter durations than acyclovir, but more expensive. Usual regimens for primary herpes outbreak include acyclovir 200 mg five times a day for 10 days, valacyclovir 1,000 mg twice daily for 7 days, or famciclovir 500 mg three times daily for 7 days.[30]
- Recurrent infections are treated similarly, but with shorter duration: 7 days for acyclovir, 5 days for famciclovir (twice daily), and 7 days for valacyclovir.[30]
- Treatment regimens depend on the most recent outbreak of herpes. If lesions were present less than 2 years prior to the season, 1,000 mg daily of valacyclovir is recommended.
- If more than 2 years has passed since the most recent outbreak, 500 mg appears to be an effective preventative dose.[29,30]

Prognosis/Return to Play

National Federation of State High School Associations (NFHS) Sports Medicine Advisory Committee recommendations for herpes infection are very similar to the NCAA recommendations listed below. Covering an active herpes lesion is inadequate. Skin checks before every match could provide the best prevention, but are unrealistic, particularly at the high school level. Many states now require skin checks before large meets and tournaments.[29]

NCAA herpes simplex infection guidelines are as follows:

- Primary infection:
  - Wrestler must be free of systemic symptoms of viral infection (fever, malaise, etc.).
  - Wrestler must have developed no new blisters for 72 hours before the examination.
  - Wrestler must have no moist lesions; all lesions must be dried and surmounted by a firm adherent crust.
  - Wrestler must have been on appropriate dosage of systemic antiviral therapy for at least 120 hours before and at the time of the meet or tournament.
  - Active herpetic infections shall not be covered to allow participation. See above-mentioned criteria when making decisions for participation status.
- Recurrent infection:
  - Blisters must be completely dry and covered by a firm adherent crust at the time of competition, or wrestler shall not participate.

- Wrestler must have been on appropriate dosage of systemic antiviral therapy for at least 120 hours before and at the time of the meet or tournament.
- Active herpetic infections shall not be covered to allow participation.
- See above-mentioned criteria when making decisions for participation status.[25]

Complications/Indications for Referral

Serious sequela with ocular involvement has been reported and requires prompt attention to avoid corneal injury.[32] Early referral is indicated with ocular involvement.

APPROACH TO THE ATHLETE WITH CELLULITIS/FURUNCULOSIS

Cellulitis is defined as an inflammatory painful erythematous infection of the skin. Furuncles are follicular-based inflammatory nodules that may progress to abscess formation. Carbuncles are a confluence of multiple furuncles that form a deep connecting purulent mass. All of these infections may cause systemic as well as local symptoms. The causative agents are usually streptococci and staphylococci. Traditionally, these infections were well treated by first-generation cephalasporins of semisynthetic penicillins. After 2000 the incidence of cMRSA began to climb.

MRSA had previously only been recognized as a potentially devastating hospital-acquired infection (hMRSA); however, recent estimates of 60% incidence of isolates in metropolitan emergency departments probably undershoot the true incidence of the infection.[33] cMRSA is genetically distinct from hMRSA, but can be just as devastating. Rapid recognition with prompt appropriate treatment is essential in treatment and avoidance of systemic complications.

HISTORY AND PHYSICAL EXAMINATION

Cellulitis and furunculosis are commonly seen in training rooms. Lesions may present as furuncles or carbuncles, may progress rapidly, and rarely can be fatal.[34] Multiple outbreaks have been recorded in the literature.[35] Presumed risk factors include poor hygiene, towel/clothes sharing, open wounds, shaving, and close contact. Contact may not always be obvious, as an outbreak did occur among fencers who were sharing the same sensor.[35]

As noted, due to the rise of cMRSA with outbreaks reported commonly among teams, a high suspicion for cMRSA should exist for all acute skin infections (Fig. 6.9). Any skin abscess should be presumed to be cMRSA till proven otherwise. Prompt recognition and treatment are paramount in preventing further spread from the affected host to other athletes as well as systemic involvement of the athlete.

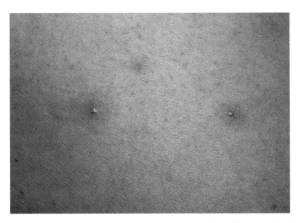

FIG. 6.9. Abscess with cMRSA. Reprinted with permission from Goodheart HP. *Goodheart's Photoguide of Common Skin Disorders.* 2nd ed. Philadelphia: Lippincott Williams & Wilkins; 2003.

DIAGNOSTIC TESTING

Diagnosis is clinical. Prompt incision and drainage with culture should be obtained for all pustular lesions, abscess, or fluctuant lesions due to potential risk of cMRSA.

TREATMENT

General Measures

- Cleaning equipment with antibacterial solutions or bleach is also very effective in limiting outbreaks.
- Carrier status through nares swab cultures and subsequent eradication may be necessary, but as yet are not recommended due to limited effectiveness and high rate of recurrence.[36]

Pharmacologic Treatment

- Treatment for cMRSA at the time of publication includes incision and drainage with culture followed by antibiotics.
- The combination of a cephalosporin with good Gram-positive coverage and trimethoprim/sulfamethoxazole until cultures return is currently recommended.
- cMRSA in most communities is still sensitive to trimethoprim/sulfamethoxazole. If the patient is sulfa allergic, alternatives include doxycycline or clindamycin.
- Questions exist regarding clindamycin due to the cross-resistance with erythromycin (microbiology lab must perform D-diffusion test) and its ability to penetrate deep into an abscess.[36]
- Rifampin may be a helpful adjunct, but is not to be used alone.

As cellulitis and furunculosis can be common among wrestlers, the NCAA and NFHS have guidelines that can be generally followed for other contact sports:

- NCAA division I wrestling and NFHS both require that the wrestler be free of new lesions for 48 hours and all existing lesions are crusted over.
- Wrestler must have completed at least 72 hours of antibiotics prior to an event with no exudative lesions.
- NFHS recommends at least 10 days of treatment and all lesions crusted prior to participation, whichever comes *last.*
- Recurrent cases of cMRSA can occur, and close monitoring of affected athletes after resolution is recommended.

APPROACH TO THE ATHLETE WITH MOLLUSCUM CONTAGIOSUM

Molluscum contagiosum is a viral infection of the skin and mucous membranes (rare) that is caused by a member of the poxvirus family. The incidence in the general population is 1.2/100.[37] It is aptly named as it is very contagious and is spread by skin-to-skin contact. Transmission has also been reported from fomites. Bath sponges, towels, beauty parlors, and swimming pools have all been reported to be sources of infection.[38] The incubation period ranges from 2 to 50 days, rendering outbreaks difficult to control.[37]

HISTORY AND PHYSICAL EXAMINATION

Molluscum usually has a characteristic appearance of flesh-colored papules with central umbilication, but occasionally can mimic other skin lesions such as verrucae and basal cell cancers (Fig. 6.10). The lesions are often in clusters and can

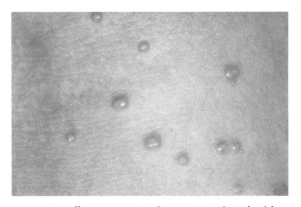

FIG. 6.10. Molluscum contagiosum. Reprinted with permission from Goodheart HP. *Goodheart's Photoguide of Common Skin Disorders.* 2nd ed. Philadelphia: Lippincott Williams & Wilkins; 2003.

range in size from 1 to 6 mm. The infection is usually self-limited but may take up to 18 months to clear.[3]

DIAGNOSTIC TESTING

Diagnosis is usually made clinically, but contents of the lesion can be examined microscopically for evidence of the poxvirus. A recent report for rapid detection uses a technique similar to tinea microscopy. Crushed contents are applied to a KOH-prepped slide and examined microscopically for Henderson–Patterson bodies.[39,40]

TREATMENT

General Measures

- Lesions may spontaneously resolve, but can be treated by curettage, cryotherapy, cantharidin application, or KOH application.[39,40]

Pharmacologic Treatment

- Podophylin and imiquimod cream have been used successfully to eradicate molluscum.[3]

Prognosis/Return to Play

- Restrictions for high school and NCAA division I wrestling are listed and can be applied to other contact sports.
- According to the NCAA division I wrestling handbook, "lesions must be curetted or removed before the meet or tournament.
- Solitary or localized, clustered lesions can be covered with a gas-permeable membrane such as Op-Site or Bioclusive, followed by ProWrap and stretch tape."
- High school participants must have the lesion removed 24 hours prior to participation.[24]

KEY POINTS

- Athletes that participate in a contact sport may not compete until tinea lesions are adequately treated and covered
- Athletes that participate in a contact sport may not compete until herpetic lesions are crusted, no appearance of new lesions for 72 hours, treatment has been initiated for 120 hours, and no systemic symptoms are present
- The etiologic agent for cellulitis/furunculosis must be assumed to be cMRSA and treated as such until culture confirmation

- Cleansing of equipment and wrestling mats may be useful in preventing the spread of tinea and cMRSA
- Prophylaxis appears to be beneficial in preventing the spread of herpes gladiatorum in susceptible athletes
- Valacyclovir may be superior to acyclovir in the treatment of herpes gladiatorum

REFERENCES

1. Freeman A, Barankin B, Elpern DJ. Sports dermatology part 1: common dermatoses. *CMAJ.* 2004;171(8):851–853.
2. Freeman A, Barankin B, Elpern DJ. Sports dermatology part 2: swimming and other aquatic sports. *CMAJ.* 2004;171(11):1339–1341.
3. Cordoro KM, Ganz JE. Training room management of sports conditions: sports dermatology. *Clin Sports Med.* 2005;24:565–598.
4. El Fari M, Gryser Y, Presber W, et al. An epidemic of tinea corporis caused by *Trichophyton tonsurans* among children (wrestlers) in Germany. *Mycoses.* 2000;43:191–196.
5. Ergin S, Ergin C, Erdoğan BS, et al. An experience from an outbreak of tinea capitis gladiatorum due to *Trichophyton tonsurans. Clin Exp Dermatol.* 2006;31:212–214.
6. Mohammad H, et al. A study on tinea gladiatorum in young wrestlers and dermatophyte contamination from wrestling mats from Sari, Iran. *BJSM* 2007;41:331–334.
7. Piqu E, Copado R, Cabrera A, et al. An outbreak of tinea gladiatorum in Lanzarote. *Clin Exp Dermatol* 1999;24:7–9.
8. Beller M, Gessner BD. An outbreak of tinea corporis gladiatorum on a high school wrestling team. *J Am Acad Dermatol* 1994;31(Pt 1):197–201.
9. Adams BB. Tinea corporis gladiatorum: a cross-sectional study. *J Am Acad Dermatol* 2000;43:1039–1041.
10. Stiller MJ, Klein WP, Dorman RI. Tinea corporis gladiatorum: an epidemic of Trichophyton tonsurans in student wrestlers. *J Am Acad Dermatol* 1992;27:632.
11. El Fari M, Gryser Y, Presber W, et al. An epidemic of tinea corporis caused by Trichophyton tonsurans among children (wrestlers) in Germany. *Mycoses* 2000;43:191–196.
12. Poisson DM, Rousseau D, Defo D, et al. Outbreak of tinea corporis gladiatorum, a fungal skin infection due to Trichophyton tonsurans, in a French high level judo team. *Euro Surveill* 2005;10:187–190.
13. Habif TP. *Clinical Dermatology.* 4th ed. Mosby 2004:350–351, 451.
14. Hedeyati MT, Afshar P, Shokohi T, et al. A study on tinea gladiatorum in young wrestlers and dermatophyte contamination from wrestling mats from Sari, Iran. *BJSM.* 2007;41:331–334.
15. Skořepová M, Stork J, Hrabáková J, et al. Case reports. Tinea gladiatorum due to *Trychophyton mentagrophytes. Mycoses.* 2002;45:431–433.
16. Adams B. Tinea corporis gladiatorum. *J Am Acad Dermatol.* 2002;47:286–290.
17. Poisson DM, Rousseau D, Defo D, et al. Outbreak of tinea corporis gladiatorum, a fungal skin infection due to *Trichophyton tonsurans,* in a French high level judo team. *Euro Surveill.* 2005;10:187–190.
18. Yoshida E, Makimura K, Mirhendi H, et al. Rapid identification of *Trichophyton tonsurans* by specific PCR based on DNA sequences of nuclear ribosomal internal transcribed spacer (ITS) 1 region. *J Dermatol Sci.* 2006;42(3):225–230.
19. Drake LA, Dinehart SM, Farmer ER, et al. Guidelines of care for superficial mycotic infections of the skin: tinea corporis, tinea cruris, tinea faciei, tinea manuum, and tinea pedis. Guidelines/Outcomes Committee. American Academy of Dermatology. *J Am Acad Dermatol.* 1996;34:282–286.
20. Piqu E, Copado R, Cabrera A, et al. An outbreak of tinea gladiatorum in Lanzarote. *Clin Exp Dermatol.* 1999;24:7–9.
21. Beller M, Gessner BD. An outbreak of tinea corporis gladiatorum on a high school wrestling team. *J Am Acad Dermatol.* 1994;31(pt 1):197–201.
22. Adams BB. Tinea corporis gladiatorum: a cross-sectional study. *J Am Acad Dermatol.* 2000;43:1039–1041.
23. Stiller MJ, Klein WP, Dorman RI. Tinea corporis gladiatorum: an epidemic of *Trichophyton tonsurans* in student wrestlers. *J Am Acad Dermatol.* 1992;27:632.

24. The National Federation of State High School Associations. Available at: http://www.nfhs.org. Accessed April 2009.

25. *National Collegiate Athletic Association 2006 Division I wrestling Handbook 2005.* 3rd ed. NCAA, Indianapolis Indiana 2006:16–19.

26. Centers for Disease Control. Herpes gladiatorum at a high school wrestling camp—Minnesota. *MMWR Morb Mortal Wkly Rep.* 1990; 39(5):69–71.

27. Belongia EA, Goodman JL, Holland EJ, et al. An outbreak of herpes gladiatorum at a high school wrestling camp. *N Engl J Med.* 1991; 325(13):906–910.

28. Rosenbaum GS, Strampfer MJ, Cunha BA. Herpes gladiatorum in a male wrestler. *Int J Dermatol.* 1990;29(2):141–142.

29. Johnson R. Herpes gladiatorum and other skin diseases. *Clin Sports Med.* 2004;23:473–484.

30. Anderson BJ. The epidemiology and clinical analysis of several outbreaks of herpes gladiatorum. *Med Sci Sports Exerc.* 2003;35(11): 1809–1814.

31. Anderson B. Prophylactic valacyclovir to prevent outbreaks of primary herpes gladiatorum at a 28 day wrestling camp. *Jpn J Infect Dis.* 2006;59: 6–9.

32. Holland EJ, Mahanti RL, Belongia EA, et al. Ocular involvement in an outbreak of herpes gladiatorum. *Am J Ophthalmol.* 1992;114:680–684.

33. Boyce JM, Cookson B, Christiansen K, et al. Methicillin-resistant *Staphylococcus aureus. Lancet Infect Dis.* 2005;5:653–663.

34. Cohen PR, Grossman ME. Management of cutaneous lesions associated with an emerging epidemic: community acquired methicillin-resistant *Staphylococcus aureus* skin infections. *J Am Acad Dermatol.* 2004;51: 132–135.

35. Barrett TJ, Moran GJ. Update on emerging infections: news from the Centers for Disease Control and Prevention. *Ann Emerg Med.* 2004; 43(1):43–47.

36. Gorwitz RJ, Jernigan DB, Powers JH, et al. Strategies for the clinical management of MRSA in the community: summary of an experts meeting convened by the Centers for Disease Control and Prevention. March 2006. Available at: http://www.cdc.gov. Accessed November 2006.

37. Pannell RS, Fleming DM, Cross KW. The incidence of molluscum contagiosum, scabies and lichen planus. *Epidemiol Infect.* 2005;133: 985–991.

38. Dohil MA, Lin P, Lee J, et al. The epidemiology of molluscum contagiosum in children. *J Am Acad Dermatol.* 2006;54(1):47–54.

39. Bauer JH, Miller OF, Peckham SJ, et al. Medical pearl: confirming the diagnosis of molluscum contagiosum using 10% potassium hydroxide. *J Am Acad Dermatol.* 2007;56(5):s104–s105.

40. Short KA, Fuller LC, Higgins EM, et al. Double-blind, randomized, placebo-controlled trial of the use of topical 10% potassium hydroxide solution in the treatment of molluscum contagiosum. *Pediatr Dermatol.* 2006;23(3):279–281.

Febrile/Sick Athlete

Pierre Rouzier

INTRODUCTION

Caring for the sick athlete is both rewarding and challenging. In general your patient is healthier and more motivated to get well. However, because of training and competition needs, athletes or their coach may have an unrealistic expectation of when they can participate in their sport or training routine.

PATHOPHYSIOLOGY

Exercise and the Immune System

Components of the immune system include the innate system and the acquired system. Innate components include the skin, mucous membranes, phagocytes, natural killer (NK) cells, cytokines, and complement factors. The acquired components of the immune system include T and B lymphocytes and plasma-secreted antibodies. Moderate exercise and intense, prolonged exercise can have different effects on the immune system. Persons who engage in regular moderate physical activity have been shown to have fewer respiratory illnesses than those who do not exercise.[1,2] However, athletes with a vigorous training schedule or those who overtrain are at risk for more illness.[3] Changes that occur with bouts of prolonged, intense exercise include a decrease in ciliary action, mucosal IgA levels, NK cell count and activity, T lymphocyte count, and T helper ($CD4^+$) to T suppressor ($CD8^+$) ratio. During this period an athlete may be more susceptible to infection. Endurance athletes may be at an increased risk for upper respiratory infections (URIs) during peak training and during the 2-week period after a marathon.[4]

College athletes in particular can be more susceptible to illness due to several factors, including high-density living (dormitories), exposure to sick teammates and classmates, less sleep than previously experienced, practice and competition in adverse environmental conditions, and possible overtraining.

EPIDEMIOLOGY

A 3-year analysis of college athletes' visits to team physicians showed that athletes are more likely to seek medical care for an illness in comparison to injury.[5] This chapter will look at common illnesses that athletes are likely to get and help give guidelines on return to play.

NARROWING THE DIFFERENTIAL DIAGNOSIS

The history and physical examination will be tailored to the affected systems. Appropriate diagnostic testing may be needed when indicated. Some general factors to consider in treating the sick athlete are as follows.

Should Athletes Train or Compete When They Are Sick?

Athletes should not train when they have a fever greater than 100.5 °F, significant malaise, myalgias, weakness, or shortness of breath or severe cough, or are dehydrated. Fever has been shown to compromise aerobic power, strength, endurance coordination, and concentration.[6] Moderate exercise training during a rhinovirus URI does not appear to affect illness symptom severity or duration.[7]

The "neck check"[8,9] has been a useful guideline in making a determination if athletes can participate. The basic premise is that if symptoms are above the neck (sore throat, nasal congestion, runny nose) and are not associated with symptoms below the neck (severe cough, malaise, gastrointestinal, or fever), then the athlete can have a trial of exercise at half intensity for 10 minutes, and if not worse, can continue as tolerated. When athletes resume training after recovery from an illness, it is important that they start at a moderate pace and gradually increase their intensity to the preillness level over 1 to 2 days of every training day missed.[9,10]

Nonmedical Factors

Unfortunately, there can be nonmedical factors contributing to or interfering with the care of the sick athlete. Elite-level athletes (professional and collegiate) as well as athletes in high school may feel that they must practice or compete despite their illness. They may feel pressure from their coaches or peers. Athletes may even underreport their illnesses to athletic trainers or team physicians because of these factors.

If athletes believe that you as a provider will return them to their sport as soon as is safely possible, they will be more willing to be compliant and honest about their symptoms.

Reducing the Risk of Infection[1]

1. Keep other life stresses to a minimum
2. Eat a well-balanced diet
3. Avoid overtraining and chronic fatigue
4. Obtain adequate sleep
5. Avoid rapid weight loss
6. Avoid putting the hands to the eyes and nose
7. Before major competition avoid sick people and large crowds if possible
8. Get the influenza vaccine

APPROACH TO THE ATHLETE WITH UPPER RESPIRATORY INFECTIONS

Viral URIs are the most common medical ailments facing the athlete. The average adult has one to six episodes of the common cold each year, with 40% caused by rhinoviruses. In the United States, URIs are associated with major socioeconomic expense, with time lost from work and school, medical visits, and cost of medications. Though moderate exercise training may decrease the risk of getting URIs, heavy exercise may increase the risk of getting a URI. Despite this, athletes and exercise enthusiasts remain active during bouts of URI.[11]

HISTORY AND PHYSICAL EXAMINATION

URIs commonly present with complaints such as nasal congestion, runny nose, sore throat, cough, malaise, and fever. Physical examination is usually unremarkable except for potential rhinorrhea, pharyngeal erythema, and coarse upper respiratory breath sounds.

Pharyngitis and tonsillitis can be caused by group A streptococcus and viruses, including mononucleosis. The athlete will present with a sore throat, fever, and cervical lymphadenopathy. Tonsils will be enlarged and erythematous and may have exudate. A full description of mononucleosis and the athlete is reviewed below.

DIAGNOSTIC TESTING

Lab tests are rarely needed for viral URIs unless influenza is suspected. In those situations, a rapid influenza test may be indicated. For suspected strep pharyngitis, a throat culture or rapid strep test should be obtained. Patients with clinical suspicion of mononucleosis should have a monospot or appropriate Epstein–Barr virus (EBV) serology checked, as noted in the section "Approach to the Athlete with Mononucleosis."

TREATMENT

General Measures

- The mainstay of treatment for viral URIs is symptomatic, including fluids, analgesia, decongestants, and cough suppressants, as needed.
- Where relevant, care must be taken to document medical indication for decongestant use by athletes, as several are banned substances by various governing bodies, including pseudoephedrine.

Pharmacologic Treatment

- Positive throat cultures or high clinical suspicion for group A strep pharyngitis should be treated with appropriate antibiotic.
- Current recommendation for treatment of group A strep pharyngitis is penicillin V 500 mg two to three times per day for 10 days.[12]
- For penicillin-allergic patients, treatment options include erythromycin or cephalosporin.

Prognosis/Return to Play

- Current recommendations for uncomplicated viral URI are fever less than 100.5 °F, no significant malaise, myalgias, weakness, shortness of breath or severe cough, or signs of dehydration.
- Affected individuals with streptococcus are usually not infectious after 24 hours of antibiotic treatment and may return to sport as tolerated if afebrile and fluid status normalized.

Complications/Indications for Referral

The most common complication from continued activity during a viral illness is simply feeling and performing poorly while sick. More significant cardiac complications, myocarditis and pericarditis, can occur as an aftermath of viral illnesses. Cardiotropic viruses, in particular Coxsackie B virus, have been implicated as the most common cause of myocarditis in the United States. Myocarditis is an inflammation of the myocardium accompanied by cellular necrosis. Athletes with myocarditis can present with chest pain or shortness of breath on exertion. They may present with congestive heart failure (CHF), syncope, or sudden death. Physical examination can show tachycardia, tachypnea, S4 gallop, edema, or other signs of CHF. An electrocardiogram (ECG) may show ST elevation and atrioventricular (AV) block. An echocardiogram can reveal left ventricular (LV) dysfunction, abnormal septal thickness, or diastolic dimensions.[13]

Athletes with pericarditis will frequently have an antecedent viral illness, pleuritic chest pain, hypotension, and a friction rub on clinical examination. Their ECG can show tachycardia, ST elevation, PR segment depression, and low-voltage QRS complex. An echocardiogram should be performed and can show pericardial fluid in sac, decreased ejection fraction and global hypokinesis, and normal septal size and diastolic dimensions. Treatment can include anti-inflammatory medications, and in some cases, pericardiocentesis may need to be performed.[14,15] Concern for myocarditis and pericarditis warrants a cardiology consultation.

APPROACH TO THE ATHLETE WITH OTITIS MEDIA

Common ear complaints in athletes include otitis media (OM) and otitis externa (OE). OM can be a common complication of a viral URI. Subclassification of OM includes acute OM, recurrent OM, OM with effusion, and chronic OM.

HISTORY AND PHYSICAL EXAMINATION

Symptoms of acute OM include ear pain, muffled hearing, and occasionally drainage. OM can be associated with a URI. Physical findings of OM include an erythematous, bulging tympanic membrane with decreased mobility (Fig. 7.1).

TESTING

Testing is usually not required in acute cases. Cases of chronic serous OM may require audiology evaluation to assess for hearing loss.

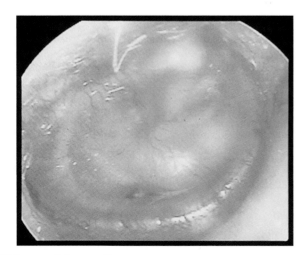

FIG. 7.1. Otits media.

TREATMENT

General Measures

- Over-the-counter (OTC) analgesia and decongestants will typically offer symptomatic improvement, as the majority of cases will resolve on their own.

Pharmacologic Treatment

- Current recommendations for antibiotic treatment are amoxicillin or amoxicillin–clavulonic acid.
- Alternative choices for penicillin-allergic patients include cefdinir, cefpodoxime, cefuroxime, azithromycin, clarithromycin, erythromycin–sulfisoxazole, or trimethoprim–sulfamethoxazole[16].

Prognosis/Return to Play

- The swimmer with OM should remain out of the water until treatment has been initiated and symptoms begin to improve.
- The swimmer with a perforated tympanic membrane who has begun treatment may swim with ear plugs in chlorinated water (not fresh or ocean water) and be cautioned to swim on the surface and not at a depth greater than 3 ft.

Complications/Indications for Referral

Potential complications include perforation and otorrhea. Rare complications include acute mastoiditis, meningitis, and hearing loss.

APPROACH TO THE ATHLETE WITH OTITIS EXTERNA

OE is an infection of the external auditory canal commonly caused by pseudomonas, but may be due to *Staphylococcus aureus* or epidermidis, and rarely fungal or yeast. A variant may be eczematous OE. OE is a common condition found in swimmers and divers as well as athletes participating in wet and humid environments.

HISTORY AND PHYSICAL EXAMINATION

Symptoms of acute OE include ear pain, muffled hearing, and occasionally drainage. Common physical examination findings include pain while moving pinna, swelling, and erythema of canal and possible purulent discharge (Fig. 7.2). OE can sometimes be secondary to OM with perforation.

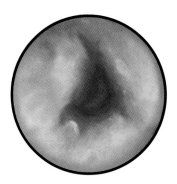

FIG. 7.2. Otitis externa. Reprinted with permission from Bickley LS, Szilagyi P. *Bates' Guide to Physical Examination and History Taking.* 8th ed. Philadelphia: Lippincott Williams & Wilkins; 2003.

DIAGNOSTIC TESTING

Diagnostic tests are usually not required, but cultures can be obtained if pathogen remains unclear.

TREATMENT

General Measures

- The athlete needs to avoid swimming and humid or moist environments.
- The ear canal can be kept dry be using a blow dryer at a low setting held 1 ft from the ear.

Pharmacologic Treatment

- Topical antibiotic drops such as combination neomycin, polymyxin B, and hydrocortisone or topical fluoroquinolones can be used.
- Sometimes a wick needs to be inserted in the ear canal to keep it open and to allow drainage.
- Nonantibiotic drops containing acetic acid and alcohol can also be effective.
- Athletes prone to OE may use several drops of a preparation of 50% rubbing alcohol and 50% vinegar at the earliest onset of symptoms before seeking medical attention.

Prognosis/Return to Play

- The swimmer with OE should remain out of the water until treatment has been initiated and symptoms and physical findings show resolution.

Complications/Indications for Referral

Complications of OE include stenosis of the ear canal, cellulitis, chondritis, and persistent disease.

APPROACH TO THE ATHLETE WITH LOWER RESPIRATORY TRACT INFECTIONS

Lower respiratory tract infections include pneumonia, bronchitis, and influenza. They are common conditions that can result in potential significant morbidity for the athlete.

HISTORY AND PHYSICAL EXAMINATION

The athlete with a lower respiratory tract infection (pneumonia, bronchitis, influenza) will typically present with cough, shortness of breath, fever, fatigue, and malaise. Aerobic capacity and exercise tolerance will be diminished. Physical examination may reveal rhonchi, rales, or wheeze and may have a decrease in oxygen saturation or pulmonary function.

DIAGNOSTIC TESTING

Useful laboratory tests may include a complete blood count (CBC), rapid influenza test, sputum culture, and Gram stain and chest x-ray (Fig. 7.3).

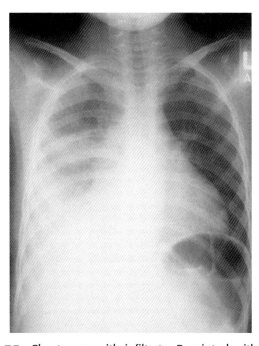

FIG. 7.3. Chest x-ray with infiltrate. Reprinted with permission from Fleisher GR, Ludwig W, Baskin MN. *Atlas of Pediatric Emergency Medicine.* Philadelphia: Lippincott Williams & Wilkins; 2004.

TREATMENT

General Measures

- Athletes with lower respiratory tract infections have usually been ill and attempting to continue their sport for several days prior to their presentation.
- Appropriate rest is imperative in their treatment plan.

Pharmacologic Treatment

- Accurate determination of the pathology is important in deciding if an athlete should be treated with antibiotics.
- It is felt that athletes, especially at the more elite level, may be treated with antibiotics more frequently than is necessary.
- Antitussives and bronchodilators may be helpful.
- Influenza prophylaxis with oseltamivir (Tamiflu) may be considered for teams with members not properly immunized or at high risk for complications of pneumonia. Medication must be started within 48 hours of exposure and given for minimum of 10 days.

Prognosis/Return to Play

- Athletes with lower respiratory infections may need a prolonged recovery time for return to play.
- Their symptoms and clinical examination must return to normal before resuming training, which may take several weeks.

Complications/Indications for Referral

Complications from pneumonia can include sepsis and acute respiratory failure.

APPROACH TO THE ATHLETE WITH MONONUCLEOSIS

Infectious mononucleosis (IM) is a common illness among athletes and young adults. Mononucleosis is caused by the EBV (Fig. 7.4). The peak incidence in the United States is between 15 and 24 years of age. Approximately 1% to 3% of college students become infected each year. Many people have had subclinical infections to IM at an early age and have developed protective antibodies.

HISTORY AND PHYSICAL EXAMINATION

The incubation period for IM is 30 to 50 days. The source of contact is rarely known. Neither roommates nor boyfriends/girlfriends are commonly the source of infection.[17,18] The presentation of IM can be variable, and there may be times when very few of the classic findings are present.

Prodromal nonspecific symptoms, such as headache, malaise, and loss of appetite, usually last 3 to 5 days. Typical presenting complaints are fever, pharyngitis, lymphadenopathy, and fatigue. Physical examination usually shows erythematous enlarged tonsils (sometimes exudative) and cervical lymphadenopathy (posterior cervical chain can be indicative of IM). Splenomegaly may be present (Table 7.1).

DIAGNOSTIC TESTING

A CBC can show an increase in white blood cells (WBCs) and a rise in lymphocytes with 10% to 20% atypical lymphocytes. A mild rise in transaminases commonly occurs. The heterophile antibody test ("monospot") will be positive after 5 to 7 days of symptoms. In 10% to 15% of cases, the monospot remains negative and Epstein–Barr serology can be useful. An EBV panel includes viral capsid antigen (VCA),

TABLE 7.1 Symptoms and Findings in Adolescents and Young Adults with Infectious Mononucleosis

Common	Less Common
Lymphadenopathy (cervical or generalized) 94%	Myalgia 20%
Pharyngitis 84%	Hepatomegaly 12%
Malaise 82%	Rash 10%
Fever 76%	Jaundice 9%
Splenomegaly 52%	Arthralgia 2%
Atypical lymphocytosis (>10%) 90%	Heterophile negative 10–15%
Mild elevation in transaminases (2–3 times normal) 90%	
Heterophile antibody positive 85–90%	
Lymphocytosis 70%	

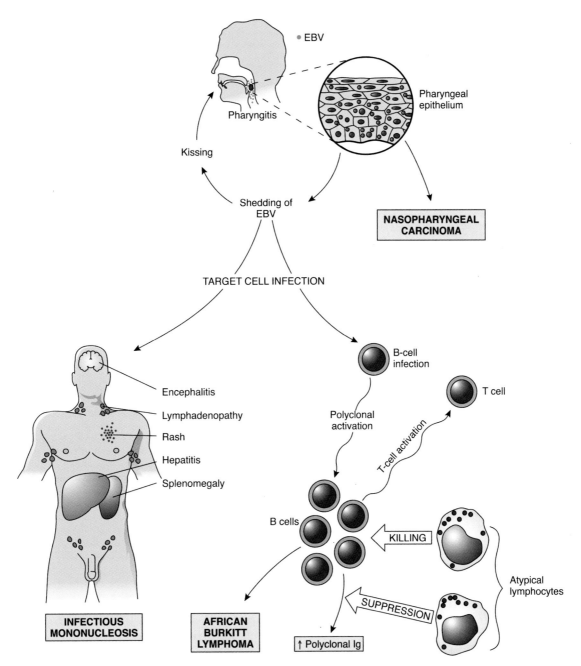

FIG. 7.4. Epstein–Barr virus pathway and manifestations. Reprinted with permission from Rubin E, Farber JL. *Pathology.* 3rd ed. Philadelphia: Lippincott Williams & Wilkins; 1999.

IgM and IgG antibodies, and EBV nuclear antigen (EBNA) antibodies. IgM antibodies are present in the acute phase of illness and remain positive for 1 to 2 months; IgG antibodies then form and remain positive for life; EBNA appear 6 to 12 weeks after onset of symptoms. The profile of IM within the first 4 weeks of symptoms should be VCA IgM positive, VCA IgG positive, and EBNA negative.[19]

Group A beta strep can be positive in 7% to 30% of patients diagnosed with mononucleosis and needs to be appropriately treated.[20] Treatment of streptococcus with amoxicillin can result in a rash.

TREATMENT

General Measures

- Mononucleosis is a self-limited illness, with full recovery expected within several weeks. The mainstays of treatment are rest, hydration, and pain control.
- Pain control can usually be obtained with acetaminophen or nonsteroidal anti-inflammatory medication, though sometimes narcotic medication is needed.

- The dehydrated patient may need intravenous fluids.
- Concomitant illnesses such as beta strep need to be treated.

Pharmacologic Treatment

- Acetaminophen or nonsteroidal anti-inflammatory medication may be used for pain control.
- Narcotic medication may be needed for more severe pain.
- Corticosteroids may be indicated for more advanced tonsillar enlargement as noted below.

Prognosis/Return to Play

- Athlete must be asymptomatic and have no evidence of splenomegaly to prevent the uncommon complication of spleen rupture.
- Athletes who return to activity too soon often will experience a relapse with prolonged fatigue and poor performance.
- Most spleens in IM are enlarged, but many are not palpable, and many studies have documented that the clinical examination of the spleen is highly variable.[21]
- Many clinicians advocate imaging the spleen before return to contact sports.
- The most commonly used imaging study is ultrasound.
- The upper limit of normal spleen length is 12 cm, but spleen size increases with height and body surface area.
- Eichner has summarized four guidelines:
  - A 3-week rest after diagnosis, then if no splenomegaly, a 4-week graded return to full activity.[22]
  - If spleen size is normal, return 3 to 5 weeks after onset of symptoms, beginning with 1 week of graded exercise.[23]
  - If spleen size is normal, return 4 weeks after onset of illness.[19]
  - If spleen size is normal, noncontact 3 weeks after illness, full play after 1 month.[24]

Complications/Indications for Referral

The most serious complication in mononucleosis is splenic rupture. Nearly all cases of splenic rupture occur during the first 21 days of illness; very few have been reported beyond 4 to 5 weeks.[8] Lymphocytic infiltration of the spleen distorts its normal tissue anatomy and support structures, increasing its fragility. Splenic ruptures occur in 0.1% to 0.5% of cases[21]; 80% of ruptures are under the age of 25. Most splenic ruptures are spontaneous and *not* the result of contact.

Airway obstruction can occur due to significant tonsillar enlargement and edema. This can be treated with systemic corticosteroids. Patients warrant hospitalization and may require emergency tracheostomy.

Neurologic complications, such as encephalitis and meningitis, can occur but are not common.

APPROACH TO THE ATHLETE WITH GASTROENTERITIS

Gastroenteritis (GE) is most commonly caused by viruses (norwalk, rotavirus, enterovirus) and sometimes by bacteria (*Salmonella, Shigella, Campylobacter, Escherichia coli*). If the athlete has had recent travel to endemic areas, appropriate etiologies should be considered. This is of particular relevance to athletes involved in international competitions. The Centers for Disease Control and Prevention (CDC) has the most up-to-date reference for foreign travel.

HISTORY AND PHYSICAL EXAMINATION

Athletes with GE will present with abdominal pain, diarrhea, nausea, and vomiting. They may be febrile and be dehydrated. Physical examination may reveal abdominal tenderness and increased bowel sounds. Abdominal guarding or high fevers should warrant consideration of alternative etiology.

DIAGNOSTIC TESTING

Usually diagnostic tests are not needed. If there is travel to endemic areas, if stools are purulent or bloody, or if diarrhea remains persistent, stool tests for WBCs, culture, and ova and parasites may be warranted.

TREATMENT

General Measures

- Viral GE can be treated with fluid and electrolyte replacement.
- If the athlete exhibits signs of dehydration and is unable to tolerate oral fluids, intravenous rehydration may be necessary.
- It is important that good hand washing techniques be used along with avoidance of shared water bottles and minimal contact with other athletes to avoid spread of illness.

Pharmacologic Treatment

- Antidiarrheals such as immodium and bisthmuth subsalycylate may provide benefit for the athlete.
- Antibiotic treatment is reserved for cases of traveler's diarrhea and bacteria-induced diarrhea.
- The vomiting athlete may be treated in an office setting with parenteral medications such as promethazine, prochlorperazine, and others.

Prognosis/Return to Play

- For athletes to return to play, they should be afebrile, without signs of dehydration, and have resolution of symptoms.

Complications/Indications for Referral

Severe symptoms, prolonged symptoms, moderate to severe dehydration may require more intensive therapy. Bloody stools and/or significant weight loss may require more in-depth evaluation.

KEY POINTS
• Athletes with a vigorous training schedule or those who overtrain are at risk for more illness[1]
• Persons who engage in regular moderate physical activity have been shown to have fewer respiratory illnesses than those who do not exercise[1,2]
• Moderate exercise training during a rhinovirus URI does not appear to affect illness symptom severity or duration[7]
• Febrile athlete may be at increased risk of dehydration and heat illness
• Rare but serious complications from viral illnesses include myocarditis and pericarditis
• Return to play 4 to 6 weeks after onset of mononucleosis symptoms with normal spleen

REFERENCES

1. Nieman DC. Is infection risk linked to exercise workload? *Med Sci Sports Exerc.* 2000;32(7):S406–S411.
2. Matthews CE, Ockene IS, Freedson PS, et al. Moderate to vigorous physical activity and risk of upper-respiratory tract infection. *Med Sci Sports Exerc.* 2002;34(8):1242–1248.
3. Nieman DC. Current perspective on exercise immunology. *Curr Sports Med Rep.* 2003;2:239–242.
4. Nieman DC. Upper respiratory tract infections and exercise. *Thorax.* 1995;50(12):1229–1231.
5. Rouzier P. Healthcare of College Athletes. *Am J Sports Med.* Publication pending.
6. Mellion MB, Walsh WM, Madden C, et al. *Team Physician's Handbook.* 3rd ed. Philadelphia: Hanley & Belfus; 2002:225–243.
7. Weidner TG, Cranston T, Schurr T, et al. The effect of exercise training on the severity and duration of a viral upper respiratory illness. *Med Sci Sports Exerc.* 1998;30(11):1578–1583.
8. Eichner ER. Infection, immunity, and exercise: what to tell your patients. *Phys Sportsmed.* 1993;21:125.
9. Primos WA. Sports and exercise during acute illness. Recommending the right course for patients. *Phys Sportsmed.* 1996;24:44–53.
10. Metz JP. Upper respiratory tract infections: who plays, who sits? *Curr Sports Med Rep.* 2003;2:84–90.
11. Weidner TG, Anderson BN, Kaminsky LA, et al. Effect of a rhinovirus-caused upper respiratory illness on pulmonary function test and exercise responses. *Med Sci Sports Exerc.* 1997;29(5):604–609.
12. Hayes CS, Williamson H. Management of group A beta-hemolytic streptococcal pharyngitis. *Am Fam Physician.* 2001;63(8):1557–1564.
13. Brennan FH, Stenzler B, Oriscello R. Diagnosis and management of myocarditis in athletes. *Curr Sports Med Rep.* 2003;2:65–71.
14. Goyle KK, Walling AD. Diagnosing pericarditis. *Am Fam Physician.* 2002;66(9):1695–1702.
15. Seidenberg PH, Haynes J. Pericarditis: diagnosis, management, and return to play. *Curr Sports Med Rep.* 2006;5:74–79.
16. American Academy of Pediatrics, American Academy of Family Physicians. Diagnosis and management of acute otitis media. Clinical practice guidelines: 1–36.
17. Sawyer RN, Evans AS, Neiderman JC, et al. Prospective studies of a group of Yale University freshman. I. Occurrence of infectious mononucleosis. *J Infect Dis.* 1971;123:263–270.
18. Halle TJ, Evans AS, Neiderman JC, et al. Infectious mononucleosis at the United sates Military Academy: a prospective study of a single class over 4 years. *Yale J Biol Med.* 1974;3:183–195.
19. Auwaerter PG. Infectious mononucleosis: return to play. *Clin Sports Med.* 2004;23:485–497.
20. Rush MC, Simon MW. Occurrence of Epstein–Barr virus illness in children diagnosed with group A streptococcal pharyngitis. *Clin Pediatr (Phila).* 2003;42(5):417–420.
21. Farley DR, Zietlow SP, Bannon MP, et al. Spontaneous rupture of the spleen due to infectious mononucleosis. *Mayo Clin Proc.* 1992;67(9) 846–853.
22. MacKnight JM. Infectious mononucleosis: ensuring a safe return to sport. *Phys Sportsmed.* 2002;30:27–32.
23. Kinderknecht JJ. Infectious mononucleosis and the spleen. *Curr Sports Med Rep.* 2002;1:116–120.
24. Waninger KN, Harcke HT. Determination of safe return to play for athletes recovering from infectious mononucleosis. *Clin J Sport Med.* 2005;25(6):410–416.

Athlete with Diabetes

Gregory Czarnecki and Jake D. Veigel

INTRODUCTION

For patients with both type 1 and type 2 diabetes mellitus, exercise has been and continues to be an integral component of disease management. While exercise has shown improvements in comorbidities often associated with diabetes, including improved cholesterol profile, reduced blood pressure, and weight control or reduction, knowledge of the effects of exercise on glucose regulation is imperative for both the physician and the athlete. In high-risk subjects, lifestyle modifications have been shown to prevent type 2 diabetes.[1] Exercise improves insulin sensitivity and thus may be of great benefit in most diabetics; however, this increased sensitivity may also put a diabetic athlete at increased risk of a hypoglycemic event. While tight glycemic control is paramount in preventing long-term complications of diabetes, caution must be taken during exercise.

PATHOPHYSIOLOGY

Type 1 diabetes is characterized by insulin deficiency from destruction of the pancreatic β cells, most commonly from an autoimmune process. Typical presentation and diagnosis is before age 30, but this is not absolute. Progression to requirement of exogenous insulin is the natural course of type 1 diabetes. Because of the ultimate reliance on exogenous insulin, hypoglycemic events are common, and despite aggressive management, such events may place the athlete at significant risk. While exercise may be of limited benefit in reducing hemoglobin A1c values, in part due to risk of hypoglycemia, in the type 1 diabetic it may provide significant benefits, including improved cardiovascular fitness, reduced resting systolic and diastolic blood pressures, and improved lipid profile.[2,3]

Type 2 diabetes is characterized by insulin resistance, impaired insulin secretion, and increased glucose production. A period of impaired glucose tolerance may be present for months to years preceding type 2 diabetes. Progression to requirement of exogenous insulin is not always the case in type 2 diabetes. Exercise has been shown in part to prevent or delay progression from insulin resistance to overt type 2 diabetes.[4,5] A recent Cochrane review on exercise in type 2 diabetics showed significant improvements in glycemic control as well as reductions in plasma triglycerides and visceral fat with exercise programs irrespective of weight loss.[6]

Serum blood glucose levels in an otherwise healthy individual remain tightly controlled through the actions of both insulin and its counterregulatory hormones including glucagon, adrenaline, cortisol, and growth hormone. Fatty acids give greatest fuel contribution to skeletal muscle at rest. Initial fuel source during exercise begins with glycogen stores in skeletal muscle, followed by blood glucose and increasing fatty acid utilization. As serum blood glucose levels fall in response to tissue uptake, insulin secretion decreases. As this happens, there is an increase in the counterregulatory hormones, most notably glucagon and epinephrine. Through liver gluconeogenesis and glycogenolysis, there is increased glucose production to maintain serum levels as skeletal muscle continues its glucose uptake. Fatty acid mobilization is also increased through actions of the counterregulatory response, increasing through hepatic production.[7]

Two concerns that arise in diabetic athletes, type 1 or those with type 2 on insulin or secretagogue therapy, are of exercise-induced hypoglycemia and late-onset hypoglycemia. The first effect may occur as early as 30 minutes with exercise or for several hours following exercise. This occurs in part due to the inability to suppress insulin that has already been administered and alteration of the counterregulatory response as described in the following paragraphs. The second effect may continue to be realized up to 24 hours following the exercise activity and is due to enhanced insulin sensitivity.

GLUT4, a transport protein in skeletal muscle, is upregulated with both exercise and insulin and is responsible for increased uptake of blood glucose, thus improving sensitivity. Following exercise, glycogen stores need replenishment in both the liver and skeletal muscle. In this state, there is a period of hyperglycemia and hyperinsulinemia. GLUT4 contributes to the increased insulin sensitivity. It is important to avoid aggressive correction of blood glucose during this time due to the enhanced action of insulin. Following prolonged exercise, complete replacement of muscle glycogen may take up to 24 hours.[8] Exogenous glucose is often necessary during prolonged or moderate–high-intensity exercise and in the recovery period.

Failure of the regulatory system in maintaining euglycemia and preventing hypoglycemia is a common concern and reality in the diabetic athlete. In type 1 diabetics and type 2 patients on insulin therapy, there is an inability to suppress exogenous insulin levels once administered. With an insulin excess, the body's initial response of lowering serum insulin in the setting of falling blood glucose levels during exercise is lost. On the other hand, insulin deficiency during exercise may lead to further augmentation of the counterregulatory response with resultant hyperglycemia. This, in turn, may lead to precipitating diabetic ketoacidosis or a hyperosmolar nonketotic state.

Type 1 diabetics have been shown to lose the counterregulatory glucagon response to hypoglycemia early in the course of the disease. However, this glucagon response in type 1 diabetics is preserved with exercise, but this may also be lost with recent hypoglycemia prior to exercise.[9] With the loss of the glucagon response to hypoglycemia, an increase in serum epinephrine becomes the next defense in the setting of decreasing serum glucose levels. This response may additionally become blunted in the setting of recent hypoglycemia. As noted earlier, through exercise with upregulation of GLUT4, insulin's action is enhanced, and this effect may last hours after exercise. Two concepts that have been introduced to explain failed counterregulatory mechanisms in those with diabetes include hypoglycemia-associated and exercise-associated autonomic failures.

Hypoglycemia-associated autonomic failure occurs in response to recent hypoglycemia and puts the athlete at significant risk of precipitating further hypoglycemia, especially with repeated exercise. This failure has been shown in clinical studies in both nondiabetics and type 1 diabetics. The first failure as noted earlier is the loss of glucagon response to hypoglycemia. This may be followed by diminished epinephrine response to repeated hypoglycemia. With this blunted response, there is a decreased manifestation of autonomic symptoms that may present, and with this an unawareness by the patient of their hypoglycemia. With repeated exposures to hypoglycemia, this hypoglycemia unawareness edges to a lower and lower threshold. This counterregulatory failure has also been shown in moderate-intensity exercise following a period of hypoglycemia the previous day.[9] Exercise-associated autonomic failure has been demonstrated with impaired counterregulatory response following prolonged exercise and next-day hypoglycemia, with the recent bout of exercise leading to impaired response to exposure of hypoglycemia.[10] Counterregulatory failure may occur as early as 30 minutes into exercise with recent experience of hypoglycemia.[9,10]

EPIDEMIOLOGY

The prevalence of diabetes is estimated at 20.8 million in the United States, with 6.2 million of these being yet undiagnosed. Even more staggering is the 54 million estimated to have prediabetes, or insulin resistance. One in six overweight adolescents aged 12 to 19 are prediabetic, while 1 in 400 to 600 children and adolescents have type 1 diabetes. For those aged 60 years and older, roughly one in five have diabetes.[11] Athletes with diabetes have successfully competed and succeeded at the highest levels in their sports. Successes include Olympic gold medals in swimming, grand slam titles in tennis, heavyweight boxing championships, and competitions in the Major League Baseball (MLB), the National Hockey League (NHL), and the National Football League (NFL) to name a few sports.[12]

NARROWING THE DIFFERENTIAL DIAGNOSIS
History

History in the diabetic patient should focus not only on duration of disease, current level of glycemic control, and medications but also on potential complications of diabetes. Neuropathy, retinopathy, and microvascular disease are well-known complications of diabetes. Duration of disease is helpful in the screening of such conditions as is long-term and current level of glycemic control. Questioning should include a thorough history of hypoglycemic events including frequency, setting/timing, associated symptoms, severity, and level of treatment required, that is, self-administered or reliance on another individual. Patients on insulin or insulin secretagogues are at the greatest risk for hypoglycemic events with or without exercise. A history of diabetic ketoacidosis or hyperglycemic nonketotic coma is equally important. Is the athlete up to date on routine screenings such as ophthalmologic examinations and urine microalbumin? Symptoms associated with hypoglycemia may vary from patient to patient and include palpitations, anxiety, tremor, sweating, hunger, and possibly paresthesias. Fatigue, behavioral change, seizure, and loss of consciousness may occur. Additional symptoms that may be suggestive of hypoglycemia include decreased self-confidence, vivid dreams/nightmares, and disturbed sleep.[7,10] These latter symptoms are especially important in obtaining history for nocturnal hypoglycemic events of which the athlete may be unaware. Has the athlete noted a change in or lack of symptoms of hypoglycemia?

When managing a diabetic athlete, an important start is determining the athlete's current level of self-monitoring of blood glucose, exercise, and dietary regimens. Does the athlete have a sugar source readily available when exercising? Do they keep their glucometer nearby? What other medications is the athlete taking, including supplements? Medications such as β-blockers may blunt the adrenergic symptoms associated with hypoglycemia. What does the athlete know about foot care? Does the athlete routinely inspect their feet, preferably daily and before and after exercise? The physician should inquire about history of callus, ulcerations, blisters, or fissures. Symptoms of nausea and vomiting or early satiety may indicate underlying gastroparesis.

Is there a known history of diabetic retinopathy or nephropathy? Are there symptoms of peripheral or autonomic neuropathy? A well-known complication of microvascular disease is erectile dysfunction, which may give clues to the presence of other neuropathic diseases. Additionally, comorbidities, especially hypertension and hyperlipidemia, and smoking and family histories should be ascertained.

Evidence-based Physical Examination

Inspection should include assessment of skin integrity, especially at injection sites and the feet. Pay particular attention to identifying callus, ulcerations, blisters, or fissures. Acanthosis nigricans (Fig. 8.1) is associated with insulin resistance.

Perform a fundoscopic examination looking for microaneurysms, deep hemorrhages, or hard exudates that may be found with nonproliferative stage of retinopathy (Fig. 8.2).

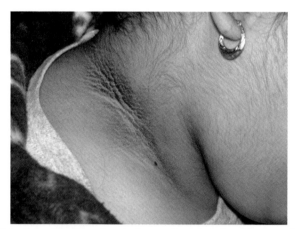

FIG. 8.1. Acanthosis nigricans. Reprinted with permission from Goodheart HP. *Goodheart's Photoguide of Common Skin Disorders.* 2nd ed. Philadelphia: Lippincott Williams & Wilkins; 2003.

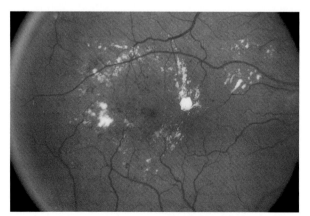

FIG. 8.2. Nonproliferative retinopathy. Reprinted with permission from Gold DH, Weingeist TA. *Color Atlas of the Eye in Systemic Disease.* Baltimore: Lippincott Williams & Wilkins; 2001.

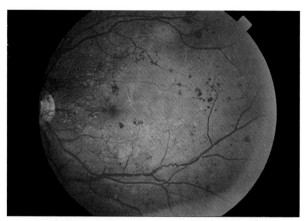

FIG. 8.3. Proliferative retinopathy with neovascularization. Reprinted with permission from Tasman W, Jaeger E. *The Wills Eye Hospital Atlas of Clinical Ophthalmology.* 2nd ed. Philadelphia: Lippincott Williams & Wilkins; 2001.

In the proliferative stage, findings may include neovascularization, vitreous hemorrhage, and proliferating fibrous tissue[13] (Fig. 8.3).

Thyroid palpation should also be routine. A thorough cardiac examination should be done, including blood pressure and, when indicated, orthostatic testing. Assess neurovascular status, noting strength of peripheral pulses and presence or absence of sensation via light touch, vibratory testing, or 10-g monofilament. Proprioception sense and reflexes should also be noted.[14]

Diagnostic Testing

Laboratory

Laboratory tests include measurement of serum creatinine, glucose, hemoglobin A1c, urinalysis, urine microalbumin, fasting lipid profile, liver function, and thryroid-stimulating hormone.[14] Blood glucose monitoring for those athletes on insulin therapy is recommended before and after exercise in addition to premeal (includes morning fasting) and prior to bedtime. With prolonged moderate or vigorous exercise, testing may need to be done during the activity. An example is in marathon training. Ultimately, an athlete needs to understand his/her glycemic response to varying activities and the accompanying duration and intensity. Unplanned activities may require closer monitoring as suggested by the counterregulatory failure described earlier. In addition, more frequent monitoring is recommended when altering training regimen in both new activities and/or increasing intensity of exercise training.

Imaging

Imaging studies are usually unnecessary unless complications from diabetes arise.

Other Testing

Consider resting electrocardiogram (ECG) as indicated by history and physical and underlying comorbidities. Preparticipation screening ECGs remain controversial in athletes due to the high rate of false positives and associated costs of additional testing to explore such findings. Currently, "there are no evidence-based guidelines for screening the diabetic patient for coronary artery disease."[14] Exercise tolerance/cardiac stress testing should be considered for sedentary individuals older than 35 years who are planning a vigorous exercise program and those with type 2 diabetes of more than 10 years or type 1 diabetes of more than 15 years. Additional consideration is recommended with the presence of peripheral vascular disease, autonomic neuropathy, microvascular disease, or additional coronary artery disease risk factors.[15]

The American College of Sports Medicine (ACSM) recommends exercise testing for moderate-risk patients planning vigorous-intensity exercise ($\geq$60% VO_{2max}) and for high-risk patients planning moderate- or high-intensity programs. Impaired fasting glucose, hypertension, dyslipidemia, obesity, and sedentary lifestyle are all considered coronary artery disease risk factors, with two or more factors putting the patient in the moderate-risk category. Men older than 45 and women older than 55 are considered moderate risk with recommendations for testing.[15]

APPROACH TO THE DIABETIC ATHLETE

HISTORY AND PHYSICAL EXAMINATION

Please refer to the "History" and "Evidence-based Physical Examination" sections earlier in text for a thorough approach to the evaluation of the diabetic athlete.

DIAGNOSTIC TESTING

Please refer to the "Diagnostic Testing" section earlier in text for a thorough approach to the evaluation of the diabetic athlete.

TREATMENT

General Measures

- During exercise an athlete should have a simple-sugar source and glucometer available and ensure adequate hydration.
- A medical ID bracelet should be worn.

- Those on insulin therapy are advised to exercise at the same time of day, preferably in the morning, for added predictability of glycemic response and monitoring for postexercise and delayed-onset hypoglycemia.
- Evening exercise is discouraged in type 1 diabetics. Injection site for insulin should also be considered.
- The general recommendation is to inject away from major exercising muscle groups due to increased absorption at these sites.
- Monitor blood glucose before and after exercise.[7]
- If blood sugar is greater than 250 mg/dL with ketones or greater than 300 mg/dL, then avoid exercise and use appropriate pharmocology.[7]
- Adjust for heat, cold, winds, intense game, weight loss, or activity.
- If blood sugar is less than 100 mg/dL, then ingest extra carbohydrate and avoid prolonged exercise unless there is an established protocol. Provide readily available absorbable glucose.[7]
- Allow for delayed gastric emptying for glucose absorption and discomfort.[7]

Pharmacologic Treatment

- For moderate- or high-intensity exercise for type 1 diabetics or type 2 diabetics on insulin therapy, either insulin reduction or glucose supplementation is necessary to prevent exercise-induced hypoglycemia.
- There are guidelines for such adjustments, but therapy must be individualized and will change with duration and intensity of exercise.
- Recommended modifications for planned exercise for those on insulin therapy include reducing long-acting insulin by 20% to 50% for most athletes and up to 70% for elite athletes.[7]
- Reduce insulin by 50% for moderate-intensity workouts and 70% to 90% for high-intensity or prolonged exercise.[7]
- Premeal insulin also should be reduced or even eliminated prior to planned moderate- or greater-intensity exercise.
- Carbohydrate source should be available during and after exercise.
- Carbohydrate is recommended prior to exercise if blood glucose is less than 100 mg/dL. If preexercise glucose is greater than 250 mg/dL with ketosis or greater than 300 mg/dL, exercise should be avoided.[15]
- For unplanned exercise with insulin already administered, exogenous glucose supplementation is often needed to prevent hypoglycemia.
- Recommended supplementation for moderate-intensity exercise is 20 to 30 g carbohydrate prior to exercise and every 30 minutes of continued exercise.
- A recent study suggests that 40 g carbohydrate 15 minutes prior to a 60-minute bout of moderate-intensity exercise can be effective without alteration in insulin regimen.[16]

- Ultimately, the glucose supplementation will need to be individualized and based on known responses to varying activities and duration of exercise.
- Hyperglycemia may be present following exercise due to counterregulatory response, but because of the increased insulin sensitivity and depleted glycogen stores, insulin dosing for meals following exercise also needs caution, with likely reduction in short-acting insulin, as mentioned earlier (20% to 50%).
- Further caution is given for nocturnal hypoglycemia, and an evening snack (complex carbohydrate) may be necessary.

Prognosis/Return to Play

- Prognosis can be quite favorable for those athletes with frequent blood glucose monitoring and learning to adjust insulin dosing and glucose supplementation to varying training schedules.
- There are diabetic athletes competing in a wide range of professional sports throughout the world.
- Caution is advised for participation in setting of recent hypoglycemia, as counterregulatory response may be impaired.
- If hypoglycemia unawareness is present, it may take up to 2 weeks of hypoglycemia-free period for recovery to baseline. In this setting, tolerance of mild hyperglycemia is suggested.

Complications/Indications for Referral

A multidisciplinary approach is recommended, with patient involvement and education at the forefront. Medical nutritional therapy is an integral component of this care. Specific complications are addressed in the following sections.

APPROACH TO THE DIABETIC ATHLETE WITH AUTONOMIC NEUROPATHY

HISTORY AND PHYSICAL EXAMINATION

History may vary from asymptomatic to heat intolerance, symptoms of orthostatic hypotension, gastroparesis, recurrent dehydration, diarrhea, constipation, or bladder or erectile dysfunction. Erratic glucose control can be seen with gastroparesis due to impaired carbohydrate absorption. Physical examination findings may include resting tachycardia, decreased heart rate variability, and eventual orthostatic hypotension. During exercise, there may be an exaggerated blood pressure response and/or decreased maximum heart rate.[14] Autonomic

neuropathy may also be associated with a prolonged QT interval.[8] Impaired thermoregulation is possible and places the individual at greater risk for heat illness and hypothermia and may have an impaired response to dehydration.[15]

DIAGNOSTIC TESTING

Exercise tolerance test is recommended for those with autonomic neuropathy.[14] EPS/tilt-table testing is rarely needed unless there is an atypical presentation.[14] A gastric-emptying study may be useful to confirm gastroparesis, and an EGD may be indicated to exclude other pathology. Colonoscopy may be warranted when further bowel involvement is present, that is, persistent or recurrent diarrhea or constipation. Urologic studies may also be indicated.

TREATMENT

General Measures

- Avoiding exercise in extremes of temperatures.
- Ensuring proper clothing and maintaining adequate hydration.
- Maintaining tight glycemic control, which is the mainstay of therapy to prevent or slow progression of disease.[14]

Pharmacologic Treatment

- Pharmacologic treatment targets the underlying symptoms, but does not alter the course of disease.
- Maintaining tight glycemic control is imperative to prevent or slow progression of disease.

Prognosis/Return to Play

- If long QT syndrome is present, return to exercise should be restricted and the guidance of an experienced cardiologist may be warranted.
- For other conditions listed earlier, safety of the patient should be of utmost importance, and the risk of athletic participation must be minimal to allow participation.

Complications/Indication for Referral

Complications may ensue as outlined earlier in the "History and Physical Examination" section. Indications for referral will be based on presenting symptoms and need for diagnostic testing as outlined earlier. Often, such patients will require multidisciplinary care.

APPROACH TO THE ATHLETE WITH PERIPHERAL NEUROPATHY

Diabetic athletes are in general at greater risk of developing foot complications as a result of peripheral vascular disease and associated peripheral neuropathy. Both small and large nerve fibers may be affected. Loss of small fibers leads to decreased pain and temperature sensation, while large fiber loss may alter light-touch sensation and proprioception, putting the athlete at increased risk of further injury. It is interesting to note that up to 50% of patients with diabetic peripheral neuropathy may be asymptomatic.[14] With microvascular disease, healing is impaired or delayed. When autonomic neuropathy is present, the skin loses elasticity with decreased sweating, and the skin of the foot is prone to fissures. If a simple blister, callus, or fissure goes undetected, secondary infection may ensue or progressive damage may occur.

HISTORY AND PHYSICAL EXAMINATION

Symptoms of peripheral neuropathy can vary greatly from relatively asymptomatic to extremely painful. Loss of or reduction in sensation is an early indicator of disease. Is the patient aware of sensory loss? Important to the history is any prior or current callus, fissures, or blisters. Physical examination should search for the same. Testing should also include 10-g monofilament for sensation, as well as vibratory and position sense, and deep tendon reflexes. Skin findings may include hair loss due to microvascular disease. Peripheral pulses may also be diminished in macrovascular disease, and symptoms of claudication may be present.

DIAGNOSTIC TESTING

Electromyogram/nerve conduction study may be useful in confirming neuropathy or ruling out separate conditions.

TREATMENT

General Measures

- Education for the patient includes daily and pre- and postexercise inspection of the feet.
- Dry feet should be moisturized with exception of between the toes (risk of fungal infection).
- Nails should be trimmed and edges smoothed.
- Pumice stone or file for callus should be used.
- Proper footwear is important in maintaining support, without constricting blood flow or causing abrasive lesions due to improper fit.

- Caution is advised for those with peripheral neuropathy for weight-bearing activities.[17]
- Endurance or high-impact events receive greatest caution with suggestion of alternate forms of physical activity in advanced disease.
- Optimizing glycemic control is imperative in slowing or preventing progression of disease.

Pharmacologic Treatment

For symptomatic diabetic peripheral neuropathy, medications include:
- Tricyclic drugs such as amitriptyline, nortriptyline, and imipramine
- Anticonvulsants including gabapentin, carbamazepine, and pregabalin duloxitine, a 5-hydroxytryptamine norepinephrine uptake inhibitor
- Substance P inhibitor, namely, capsaicin[14]

Prognosis/Return to Play

- If sensation deficits limit awareness of foot propioception or other altered sensations, then activity modifications should be made.
- Activities such as running, racquet sports, and hiking may need to be replaced with stationary bicycle, swimming, and golf.

Complications/Indications for Referral

Recurrent ulcers or nonhealing wounds should be comanaged with a foot care specialist. Red flags include any signs or symptoms of infection.

APPROACH TO THE ATHLETE WITH DIABETIC RETINOPATHY

Diabetic retinopathy is the leading cause of blindness in adults aged 20 to 74 years. There is strong evidence (level A) that tight glycemic control and optimal blood pressure control can reduce risk and progression of diabetic retinopathy.[14,18] It is generally recommended for any patient with proliferative diabetic retinopathy to avoid strenuous activities, especially those that involve Valsalva, such as heavy weight lifting, because of potential risk of vitreous hemorrhage or retinal detachment.[18] Epidemiologic studies of physical activity in those with insulin-dependent diabetes have not demonstrated an association of increased or decreased risk of developing or progressing proliferative retinopathy.[19,20] The balance appears to lie between the benefits of chronic exercise and physiologic risks of acute exercise, namely, elevated blood pressure.

HISTORY AND PHYSICAL EXAMINATION

Diabetic retinopathy is relatively asymptomatic prior to the onset of vision loss. Screening and monitoring through ophthalmologic examinations remain the mainstay of surveillance. On dilated eye examination, findings may include neovascularization, macular edema, and retinal thickening or distortion[18] (see Fig. 8.3).

DIAGNOSTIC TESTING

Standard of care is dilated funduscopic examination annually, preferably by an ophthalmologist.

TREATMENT

General Measures

- Ensure proper breathing techniques with weight lifting, that is, no breath holding.
- Physicians should stress the importance of maintaining optimal glycemic and blood pressure control as well as yearly ophthalmologic examinations.

Pharmacologic Treatment

Proper glycemic control with medications as discussed earlier.

Prognosis/Return to Play

For those with proliferative diabetic retinopathy, strenuous/vigorous activity should be avoided.

Complications/Indications for Referral

Refer any patient with macular edema, severe nonproliferative diabetic retinopathy, or any proliferative diabetic retinopathy.

APPROACH TO THE ATHLETE WITH DIABETIC NEPHROPATHY

Diabetic nephropathy is the leading cause of end-stage renal disease; 20% to 40% of those with diabetes will develop nephropathy.[14] There are limited prospective data on exercise in the setting of diabetic nephropathy. From available literature, there is no evidence that exercise induces or leads to progression of nephropathy. While physical activity may help control other factors associated with nephropathy such as blood pressure and glycemic control, high-intensity exercises are generally discouraged[21] (level C). There is no consensus for specific limitations. Screening recommendations include obtaining annual urine microalbumin in type 1 diabetics starting 5 years after diagnosis and annually in all patients with type 2 diabetes (level C). Annual serum creatinine/calculated glomerular filtration rate (GFR) (level C).

TREATMENT

General Measures

- Exercise within 24 hours of testing may elevate urinary albumin excretion, and retesting after 24-hour relative rest may yield more accurate assessment of proteinuria.
- Treatment is mainly directed at optimizing blood glucose and blood pressure control[14] (level A).
- Though some studies have shown that protein restriction helps slow progression of proteinuria and eventual ESRD, this has not been studied in athletes with diabetic nephropathy.

Pharmacologic Treatment

- Angiotensin-coverting enzyme (ACE) inhibitor or Angiotensin Receptor Blocker (ARB) is recommended to slow progression in both micro- and macroalbuminuria[14] (level A).
- For those athletes on ACE/ARB, ensure adequate hydration, especially with concomitant nonsteroidal anti-inflammatory drugs (NSAID) use, to avoid precipitating acute renal failure.

Prognosis/Return to Play

- The ACSM position stand on exercise and type 2 diabetes recommends for those with nephropathy to avoid activities that cause the systolic blood pressure to rise to 180 to 200 mm Hg, and exercise testing is recommended to measure such limits in those with advanced disease (level C).

Complications/Indications for Referral

Nephrology consultation is warranted if GFR is less than 30 mL/min.

<table>
<tr><td>

KEY POINTS

- Duration and intensity of exercise as well as preexercise blood glucose levels and insulin supply are contributing factors to exercise's effect on serum blood glucose concentration, both during and after exercise

- Individualized therapy and patient education are crucial

- Frequent blood glucose (BG) monitoring (ideally before, during, and after exercise). An athlete must learn to adapt insulin-dosing or carbohydrate supplementation according to varying training schedules and intensities

- For those on insulin therapy, avoid aggressive correction of blood glucose in period following exercise due to increased insulin sensitivity

- Appropriate screening prior to initiating exercise program

- Consider exercise testing for those with advanced nephropathy for exercise limits to maintain systolic blood pressure under 180 to 200 mm Hg

</td></tr>
</table>

REFERENCES

1. Tuomilehto J, Lindstrom J, Eriksson JG, et al.; for the Finnish Diabetes Prevention Study Group. Prevention of type 2 diabetes mellitus by changes in lifestyle among subjects with impaired glucose tolerance. *N Engl J Med.* 2001;344:1343–1350.
2. American College of Sports Medicine. *ACSM's Guidelines for Exercise Testing and Prescription.* 7th ed. Philadelphia: Lippincott Williams & Wilkins; 2006.
3. Laaksonen DE, Atalay M, Niskanen LK, et al. Aerobic exercise and the lipid profile in type 1 diabetic men: a randomized controlled trial. *Med Sci Sports Exerc.* 2000;32(9):1541–1548.
4. Pan X, Li G, Hu Y, et al. Effects of diet and exercise in preventing NIDDM in people with impaired glucose tolerance: the DaQing IGT and diabetes study. *Diabetes Care.* 1997;20:537–544.
5. Diabetes Prevention Program Research Group. Reduction in the incidence of type 2 diabetes with lifestyle intervention or metformin. *N Engl J Med.* 2002;346:393–403.
6. Thomas DE, Elliott EJ, Naughton GA. Exercise for type 2 diabetes mellitus (Review), The Cochrane Collaboration, Hoboken: NJ; Wiley & Sons, Ltd. Issue 3, 2007.
7. NS Pierce. Diabetes and exercise. *Br J Sports Med.* 1999;33:161–172.
8. Chipkin SR, Klugh SA, Chasan-Taber L. Exercise in secondary prevention and cardiac rehabilitation. *Cardiol Clin.* 2001;19(3):489–505.
9. Galassetti P, Tate D, Neill RA, et al. Effect of antecedent hypoglycemia on counterregulatory responses to subsequent euglycemic exercise in type 1 diabetes. *Diabetes.* 2003;52:1761–1769.
10. Cryer PE, Davis SN, Shamoon H. Hypoglycemia in diabetes. *Diabetes Care.* 2003;26(6):1902–1912.
11. American Diabetes Association. Total prevalence of diabetes and pre-diabetes. Available at: http://www.diabetes.org.
12. Inspiration and expert advice: famous people. Available at: http://www.dlife.com/dLife/do/ShowContent/inspiration_expert_advice/famous_people/sports.html.
13. Bates B. *A Guide to Physical Examination and History Taking.* 6th ed. Philadelphia: J.B. Lippincott Company; 1995.
14. ADA Position Statement. Standards of medical care in diabetes—2007. *Diabetes Care.* 2007;30:S4–S41.
15. Diabetes Mellitus and Exercise. ADA/ACSM diabetes mellitus and exercise joint position paper. *Med Sci Sports Exerc.* 1997;29(12):1–6.
16. Dube MC, Weisnagel SJ, Prud'homme D, et al. Exercise and newer insulins: how much glucose supplementation to avoid hypoglycemia? *Med Sci Sports Exerc.* 2005;37(8):1276–1282.
17. Lemaster JW, Reiber GE, Smith DG, et al. Daily weight-bearing activity does not increase the risk of diabetic foot ulcers. *Med Sci Sports Exerc.* 2003;35(7):1093–1099.
18. ADA Position Statement. Retinopathy in diabetes. *Diabetes Care.* 2004; 27(Suppl 1):S84–S87.
19. Cruickshanks KJ, Moss SE, Klein R, et al. Physical activity and proliferative retinopathy in people diagnosed with diabetes before age 30 yr. *Diabetes Care.* 1992;15(10):1267–1272.
20. Cruickshanks KJ, Moss SE, Klein R, et al. Physical activity and the risk of progression of retinopathy or the development of proliferative retinopathy. *Opthalmology.* 1995;102(8):1177–1182.
21. Albright A, Franz M, Hornsby G, et al. American College of Sports Medicine position stand. Exercise and type 2 diabetes. *Med Sci Sports Exerc.* 2000;32(7):1345–1360.

CHAPTER

9

Athlete with Neck Pain

Vasilios Chrisostomidis and Jake D. Veigel

INTRODUCTION

Acute and overuse neck injuries are common conditions encountered among athletes. Approximately 8.7% of all new cases of spinal cord injuries in the United States result from sports.[1] It is important for medical providers who care for an athletic population to be familiar with the various causes of neck pain, which may range from mild cervical strains to catastrophic spinal cord injuries. This is accomplished by an understanding of the anatomy of neck, a working knowledge of the common causes of neck pain, and an understanding of the signs and symptoms of a serious cervical injury.

When dealing with a possible cervical emergency during an athletic event, basic cardiopulmonary resuscitation and trauma management guidelines should be followed. It is important to keep the injured athlete immobilized until cervical spine injury is ruled out. Unconscious athletes should always be assumed to have a cervical spine injury until proven otherwise. Shoulder pads and helmets should always be left on in evaluation of football and hockey athletes. The facemask may be cut away if needed for airway management, and jaw thrust maneuver applied if necessary. The helmet should only be removed if the airway cannot be maintained or if the helmet prevents cervical immobilization. Patient should be log rolled on a backboard and transported to the nearest hospital. If one functions as a team physician, it may be prudent to practice this type of drill with your athletic training staff so that everyone is aware of his or her role.

FUNCTIONAL ANATOMY

The function of the vertebral column is to protect the spinal cord. The vertebrae of the cervical spine are smaller and more delicate than those of the thoracic and lumbar spine. Despite this, they are often required to dissipate a significant amount of force, especially in collision sports.

The atlas and axis (C1 and C2) work together as a unit to permit 50% of cervical spine motion. The atlanto-occipital joint permits flexion and extension, while the atlantoaxial joint permits the majority of rotation.[2] Varying amounts of flexion, extension, lateral bending, and rotation occur from C3 to C7.

The vertebral bodies form the anterior aspect of the spinal column. A bony lip on the lower surface of the vertebral body forms the uncovertebral joint with the adjacent vertebrae. There are intervertebral discs below C2 to provide shock absorption and cushioning for the vertebral column.

The anterior and posterior longitudinal ligaments provide stabilization for the vertebral bodies. The posterior column is made up of the pedicles, laminae, facets, and spinous processes. The facet joints are the posterior articulations of the vertebrae. The posterior column is stabilized by the nuchal ligament complex, which is made up of the supraspinous, interspinous, and infraspinous ligaments, in addition to the ligamentum flavum and capsular ligaments. Damage to these may result in cervical spine instability.

The spinal cord originates from the medulla oblongata and travels caudally through the vertebral foramina until it terminates in the lumbar region. The spinal cord is composed of three tracts, whose function and location may help to determine the site of an injury. The posterior columns carry fine touch, vibration sense, proprioception, and pressure from the ipsilateral side. The corticospinal tract is located in the posterolateral spinal cord and carries motor fibers to the ipsilateral side. The spinothalamic tract is located in the anterolateral spinal cord and carries pain and temperature fibers from the contralateral side.

Paired spinal nerve roots containing motor and sensory neurons exit from the spinal cord at each vertebral level via the intervertebral foramina. There are eight pairs of cervical spinal nerves named for the vertebral body above which they exit. Spinal nerves are subject to pressure phenomena from disc herniation or foraminal narrowing. The sensory cervical dermatomes are listed (Fig. 9.1).

The biceps and brachioradialis reflexes are mediated by the C5-6 roots and the triceps reflexes are mediated by the C6-7 nerves roots (Table 9.1).

The muscles of the neck may be subdivided into anterior and posterior divisions. The anterior aspect includes the platysma, sternocleidomastoid, anterior vertebral muscles

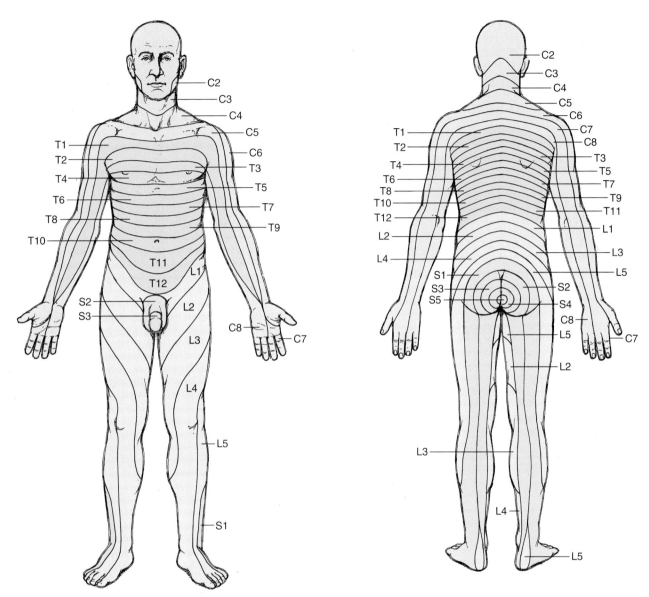

FIG. 9.1. Distribution of dermatomes on the skin. Reprinted with permission from *Stedman's Medical Dictionary.* 27th ed. Baltimore: Lippincott Williams & Wilkins; 2000.

TABLE 9.1   **Peripheral Motor Nerve Innervation**

Nerve Root(s)	Innervation
C3-5	Diaphragm
C5	Deltoid/biceps
C6	Wrist extensors, abductor/extensors of thumb
C7	Triceps/wrist flexors/finger extensors
C8	Finger flexors
T1	Intrinsic hand muscles

(longus colli, longus capitis, rectus capitis anterior, and rectus capitis lateralis), and the lateral vertebral muscles (scalene muscles).

The sternocleidomastoid muscle allows for flexion, lateral bending, and neck rotation. The anterior vertebral muscles assist in neck flexion, rotation, and lateral bending.

The posterior division includes the trapezius, splenius capitis, semispinalis capitis, and levator scapulae. The posterior group is stronger than the anterior group and is important in maintaining posture as well as providing neck stabilization.

The important vessels in the neck include the common carotid arteries, vertebral arteries, jugular veins, and vertebral veins. The common carotid further separates into the external and internal carotids. The vertebral arteries join together to form the basilar artery of the brain. Damage to the vertebral arteries associated with cervical spine or neck trauma can result in death.[3]

EPIDEMIOLOGY

It is estimated that 10% to 15% of football players experience an injury to the cervical spine; fortunately, a majority of these are self-limited stingers/burners. The overall incidence of spinal cord injury in the high school and college population is around 1 in 100,000.[4] Most are incomplete with preservation of varying degrees of neurologic function. In an analysis of football players from 1977 to 1989, catastrophic spinal cord injuries were secondary to fracture/dislocations or burst fractures in 33% and 22% of the cases, respectively.[2] Cervical spine injuries are also seen in ice hockey, rugby, wrestling, gymnastics, and water sports (e.g., diving).[5]

The prevalence of degenerative disc disease is about 10% in the second decade of life and progresses linearly to 95% to 100% by age 70 years.[6]

NARROWING THE DIFFERENTIAL DIAGNOSES

History

This should include the full characterization of the neck pain as well as its duration and distribution. Any significant past medical history should be reviewed, especially any previous neck pain or neck surgery. Important questions include the following factors:

- Location of pain
- Onset/duration of pain
- Radiation of pain
- Numbness/tingling in extremities
- Decreased motor strength
- Exacerbating/alleviating factors
- Previous examination/treatment/diagnostic tests
- Mechanism of injury
  - Flexion injuries (including spearing) compress the anterior elements and disrupt the posterior elements, causing vertebral body fractures, dislocations, and rupture of the posterior ligaments or posterior discs.
  - Extension injuries compress the posterior elements and disrupt the anterior elements, causing damage to the spinous process, facets, and anterior ligaments or discs.
  - Cervical spine in neutral results in dissipation of energy into the cervical muscles—if the force is great enough, compression fractures may result.

Evidence-based Physical Examination

The physical examination plays a crucial role in narrowing your differential diagnosis by assessing for structural as well as neurologic deficits. A thorough and organized examination as outlined in the following sections is very important and will help in consistency.

Inspection

Perform from anterior, posterior, and lateral views. Note posture as well as muscle atrophy or deformity. Check for normal cervical lordosis—its absence may be consistent with cervical spasm. Inspection may reveal ecchymosis or swelling at the level of injury.

Palpation

One should evaluate for point tenderness over the spinous processes and lateral processes. Note any hypertonicity of the musculature on examination consistent with muscle spasm. Note for any step off if there was a history of trauma.

Range of Motion

- Perform active range of motion (ROM) prior to passive ROM.
- Evaluate flexion and extension by asking the patient to touch his or her chin to the chest and then look up at the ceiling.
- Evaluate lateral bending of the neck, with normal being 45 degrees.
- Evaluate lateral rotation, with normal being from 60 to 80 degrees.

Strength Testing

Strength should be tested in all planes (flexion, extension, lateral bending, and rotation).

Special Tests

Spurling Maneuver

Patient's neck is extended and rotated toward the involved side as axial compression is applied. If there is pathology at the root or foramen, symptoms are recreated because this position narrows the intervertebral foramen on the affected side. Early studies have shown the sensitivity to be 40% to 60% with a specificity of 92% to 100%.[7] More recent studies have shown Spurling test to have a sensitivity of 92% and specificity of 95% with positive predictive value of 96.4% and negative predictive value of 90.9%.[8]

Distraction Test

Manual vertical cervical traction is applied to confirm the diagnosis of radiculopathy. This maneuver temporarily relieves pressure at the level of the disc and facet joints, which may in turn temporarily relieve the patient's symptoms. This test is reported to have a sensitivity of 40% to 43% and sensitivity of 100%.[7]

Neurologic

Neurologic symptoms may suggest a central lesion, radiculopathy, or peripheral nerve entrapment. A detailed neurologic examination includes upper extremity strength testing, deep tendon reflexes at the triceps, brachialis and brachioradialis, sensation testing, and cranial nerve evaluation. Sensation should be evaluated and any deficits correlated with appropriate peripheral nerve distribution or dermatome.

Diagnostic Testing

Laboratory

Routine laboratory studies are generally not required with acute or overuse neck pain or injuries. If suspected autoimmune etiology for overuse neck pain exists, sedimentation rate along with rheumatoid factor, antinuclear antibody test, and human leukocyte antigen B27 may be considered based on pretest probability and clinical scenario.

Imaging

Athletes with suspected cervical spine injury often require radiologic evaluation. Three views, including anteroposterior (AP), open-mouth odontoid, and cross-table lateral, are usually recommended. In addition, one may consider flexion and extension radiographs of the spine if instability is suspected and acute fracture excluded. Oblique views may be included to assess for facet degenerative joint disease in the appropriate setting/age of athlete.

Computed tomography (CT) may be indicated when suspicion of cervical fracture exits despite negative radiographs. It may also play a role when area of the cervical and upper thoracic spine may not be visualized with plain radiographs.

Magnetic resonance imaging (MRI) may be helpful in evaluation for nerve or disc injury and should be considered in any athlete that has spinal cord symptoms (transient quadriplegia, burning hands syndrome, or other bilateral sensory or motor deficits).

Other Testing

Electrodiagnostic testing may be indicated for evaluation of peripheral nerve injury. Complete details are outlined in Chapter 23, "Athlete with Peripheral Nerve Injuries."

APPROACH TO THE ATHLETE WITH CERVICAL STRAIN

Cervical strains are the most common type of cervical injury in athletes and may occur from both acute and overuse mechanisms. Common mechanisms in athletics include whiplash force secondary to a fall or being tackled. Cervical strains can also occur from weight lifting or repetitive strain to the cervical and trapezius muscle groups. Primary goal is differentiating simple cervical strain from more serious etiologies including cervical disc or cord conditions as well as occult fractures.

HISTORY AND PHYSICAL EXAMINATON

Pain is usually localized with some stiffness and decreased ROM. There are no radicular symptoms and no neurologic deficits by history or physical examination.

DIAGNOSTIC TESTING

Radiologic studies are usually not indicated in the acute management unless pain is secondary to trauma. They may play a role ruling out underlying degenerative changes as well as occult fractures or instability in the appropriate clinical setting. MRI or electrodiagnostic studies are rarely needed unless radicular symptoms are present or symptoms persist despite conservative management.

TREATMENT

Nonoperative

- Management is usually conservative and includes ice, heat, nonsteroidal anti-inflammatory drugs (NSAIDs), and relative rest.
- Manual manipulation and physical therapy are helpful in resolving symptoms.

Operative

- Operative intervention plays no role for cervical strains.

Prognosis/Return to Play

- Prognosis is generally excellent. The athlete may return to play when examination reveals painless full ROM and full strength.

Complications/Indications for Referral

If symptoms persist, consider further evaluation with radiographs, MRI, and specialist referral.

APPROACH TO THE ATHLETE WITH CERVICAL DISC DISEASE

Cervical disc disease is a common source of neck pain that can occur from degeneration of the cervical discs (degenerative disc disease), acute disc herniation, or a combination of both. The incidence of cervical disease increases with age and is seen commonly in sports such as football, wrestling, and rugby. These sports may actually increase the incidence of cervical disc problems over the lifetime of the athlete.[9] Disc herniation is more common in the younger athlete. The prevalence of degenerative disc disease is about 10% in the second decade of life and progresses linearly to 95% to 100% by age 70 years.[6] The challenge for the clinician is in differentiating acute discherniation from degenerative disc disease.

HISTORY AND PHYSICAL EXAMINATION

Acute disc protrusion or herniation will most often result in sudden onset of pain with radicular symptoms that radiate down the arm. There is often numbness, tingling, and/or loss of strength in that extremity. These symptoms may or may not be preceded by symptoms of degenerative disc disease with diffuse, dull neck pain, generally without radiculopathy. There often is no history of trauma with acute disc herniation, but an inciting event may be noted.

Physical examination reveals decreased ROM, spasm, and tenderness of the neck. Neurologic examination may reveal sensory or motor deficits. The Spurling maneuver may be positive.

DIAGNOSTIC TESTING

Radiologic examination usually includes radiographs to evaluate for bony injury and degenerative changes. MRI is the test of choice to evaluate for cervical disc disease that can run the spectrum of pathology from disc bulge to protrusion to herniation.

TREATMENT

Nonoperative

- Treatment is usually conservative and involves management of pain with NSAIDs, ice/heat, massage, manual manipulation, and physical therapy.
- A soft cervical collar may help with symptoms.
- Epidural injections may be of benefit if radicular symptoms are present and lack of response to first-line conservative measures.

Operative

- Indications for surgical intervention include severe neurologic symptoms, failure to improve with conservative treatment, or worsening of symptoms.
- Surgical options include a discectomy/fusion as indicated. In nonathletes, surgery resulted in better outcomes when

compared with medical management,[10] although randomized studies have yet to be performed.

Prognosis/Return to Play

- Return to play is dictated by the absence of symptoms and presence of full strength.
- Most return when they have painless full ROM and full strength.
- Contact sports: criteria and guidelines are as follows.
- Athletes who require cervical one-level fusion are permitted to return to activity gradually, with a progression of walking to floor exercises in the first month.
- Postoperative weight training and swimming can begin in the second month. In the third month, treadmill workouts can be allowed, with progression to aerobic exercises in the fourth month.
- Athletes in collision and contact sports should not participate until the next season after a cervical fusion or laminectomy and in consultation with the orthopaedic surgeon or neurosurgeon.[11]
- Athletes with stable two- or three-level fusions are rarely permitted to return to contact sports. Return to play with these athletes should be determined in consultation with an orthopaedic spine or neurosurgery specialist.[12]

Spinal injuries in sports: criteria and guidelines for return/nonreturn to play in contact and other high-risk sports and recreational activities are as follows.[11]

Allow return to play under following conditions:

- Neurologic injuries with no persistent neurologic symptoms or deficits, which recover to normal, persist related to root injury only, or single transient spinal cord injury or spinal cord concussion
- Spinal column injuries that are stable, stability restored by conservative or operative treatment, minor fracture, or no instability in flexion and extension radiographs
- Congenital lesions with minor spinal stenosis or congenital or operative fusion of one motion segment
- Acquired lesions with mild cervical spondylosis or other arthropathy
- MRI findings show normal cord signal

Disallow return to play under following conditions:

- Neurologic injuries with residual neurologic deficits, repeated transient cord injury, or chronic myelopathy
- Spinal column injuries with unstable spinal column, major fractures, or instability present in flexion and extension radiographs
- Congenital lesions with major spinal stenosis, atlantoaxial dislocation, fusion (congenital or operative) of two or more motion segments
- Acquired lesions with severe cervical spondylosis
- MRI findings with T2 signal changes in cord or syrinx

Complications can include progression to disc herniation with nerve root compression with neurologic deficits.

Worsening of pain and neurologic symptoms, severe neurologic symptoms, and failure of conservative management are indications for referral.

APPROACH TO THE ATHLETE WITH CERVICAL FRACTURE

Fractures of the cervical spine include but are not limited to atlas (C1)—Jefferson fractures, axis (C2)—odontoid or Hangman's fracture, cervical compression fractures (types I to IV), and cervical spinous process fractures.

HISTORY AND PHYSICAL EXAMINATION

The most common finding on history and physical examination is pain and tenderness with loss of ROM.

DIAGNOSTIC TESTING

Radiographs should be performed on any athlete in whom there may be a fracture. CT scan is often utilized to assess for suspected occult fracture that may not be seen on plain films.

FUNCTIONAL TREATMENT

Nonoperative

- Nonoperative management is usually a halo brace or semirigid cervical collar.
- Cervical fractures treated nonoperatively include
  - Majority of altas fractures
  - Stable and healed odontoid fractures
  - Hangman's fractures
  - Types I and II compression fractures
- Clay shoveler's fractures usually heal well spontaneously

Operative

- Fractures usually requiring surgery include
  - Unstable and nonhealed odontoid fractures
  - Hangman's fractures with nonunion of the C2-3 disc
  - Types III and IV compression fractures

Prognosis/Return to Play

Return to play depends on the type of fracture (Table 9.2) and whether there is any inherent instability. This should be determined in conjunction with a spine specialist. Players may be permitted to return in the following situations:[12]

- Fracture is fully healed with normal alignment
- Single-level fusion has been performed below the level of C2

TABLE 9.2 **Spinal Injuries in Sports: Criteria and Guidelines for Return/Nonreturn to Play in Contact and other High-Risk Sports and Recreational Activities**

	Allow return to play	Advise never to return to play
Neurologic injury	• No persisting neurologic symptoms or deficit attributable to cord injury • Neurologic deficit that recovers to normal • Persisting neurologic deficit related to root injury only • Single transient SCI or spinal cord concussion	• Residual neurologic deficit related to SCI • Repeated transient cord injury or spinal cord concussion • Chronic myelopathy
Spinal column injury	• Stable spinal column • Spinal column stability restored by conservative or operative treatment • Minor fracture (e.g., spinous process, single body compression fracture) • No instability in flexion-extension radiographs	• Unstable spinal column • Major fracture (e.g., burst fracture with canal compromise) • Instability present in flexion-extension radiographs
Congenital lesions	• Minor spinal stenosis • Congenital or operative fusion of one motion segment	• Major spinal stenosis • Atlantoaxial dislocation • Congenital or operative fusion of two or more motion segments
Acquired lesions	• Mild cervical spondylosis or other arthropathy	• Severe cervical spondylosis or other arthropathy
MRI findings	• Normal cord signal	• T2 signal changes in cord • Syrinx

From Tator CH, Recognition and management of spinal cord injuries in sports and recreation. Neurol Clin. 2008; 26(1):79–88.

- There is no residual canal compromise, pain, or neural deficit
- There is no instability on dynamic radiographs

Complications/Indications for Referral

Specialist consultation should be made in any cervical spine fracture as death, permanent disability, or extreme morbidity could result. In any athlete who loses consciousness, an unstable cervical fracture or dislocation of the spine should be assumed.

APPROACH TO THE ATHLETE WITH LIGAMENTOUS INSTABILITY

Cervical vertebral subluxation may occur when there is axial compression combined with cervical flexion, which is seen when a tackler leads with his helmet. This may result in anterior translation of the vertebral body.

HISTORY AND PHYSICAL EXAMINATION

Patient will usually complain of neck pain and stiffness without neurologic deficits. ROM may or may not be limited.

DIAGNOSTIC TESTING

After cervical fracture has been ruled out, dynamic radiographs should be performed with the athlete in active flexion and extension in addition to the standard cervical radiographs. The patient should be alert and cooperative and actively flex and extend only to the point of pain. Motion of the vertebral body relative to the plain views, displacement of the vertebral body, or angulation of the vertebral body should prompt urgent MRI and neurosurgical consultation.

FUNCTIONAL TREATMENT

Nonoperative

- If ligamentous instability exists, there is little role for nonoperative management, except the proper stabilization in the acute setting, as with all suspected cervical injuries.

Operative

- The treatment is usually aggressive in the form of cervical fusion to avoid chronic instability and future risk of injury.

Prognosis/Return to Play

- Return to play is decided on the nature of the injury and the nature of the activity, though serious consideration should be given to avoid all contact/collision sports with a history of this type of injury.

Complications/Indications for Referral

Athlete should avoid all contact/collision sports with this type of injury. Urgent neurosurgical referral is indicated.

APPROACH TO THE ATHLETE WITH SPEAR TACKLER'S SPINE

This was originally described in 1993 in football players that recurrently tackled using the top of the head as an initial point of contact. The main result is loss of normal cervical lordosis as a result of axial loading and microtrauma to the spinal structures. This may or may not be reversible. Prevention involves teaching appropriate tackling technique. When the straightened cervical spine is subjected to an axial loading force, it behaves like a segmented column. This axial force compresses the intervertebral discs, and the spine flexes with maximum compressive force and then buckles, resulting in fracture, subluxation, or dislocation. The combination of headfirst tackling with spear tackler's spine is extremely dangerous.

HISTORY AND PHYSICAL EXAMINATION

Symptoms usually include pain and stiffness with the absence of neurologic signs.

DIAGNOSTIC TESTING

Radiographs reveal developmental narrowing of the cervical spinal canal, posttraumatic changes, and loss of the normal cervical lordotic curve. MRI is often ordered to further evaluate the cervical spinal canal and the amount of functional reserve space (i.e., amount of surrounding spinal fluid in relation to cord diameter).

FUNCTIONAL TREATMENT

Nonoperative

- The athlete is excluded from all contact sports unless the condition is reversed (i.e., return of normal cervical lordosis).
- Physical therapy program involves relative rest, neck and shoulder ROM stretches, heat and massage, and a progressive neck-strengthening program.

Operative

- Surgical methods of correcting abnormal cervical lordosis of spear tackler's spine are currently unavailable.

Prognosis/Return to Play

- Return to play is possible if the condition is reversed with the use of physical therapy and change in tackling technique.
- If the condition is not reversible, then the athlete is excluded from all contact and collision sports due to the risk of catastrophic neurologic damage.

Complications/Indications for Referral

The combination of spear tackler's spine and headfirst tackling is extremely dangerous as fracture, dislocation, or subluxation may result. Should complications arise, then cervical stabilization with transport to hospital and urgent surgical consultation is indicated.

APPROACH TO THE ATHLETE WITH CERVICAL CORD NEURAPRAXIA

Cervical cord neurapraxia is a transient neurologic event that may cause neurologic symptoms in bilateral arms, legs, all extremities, or the ipsilateral arm and leg from site of injury. The key feature that differentiates cervical cord neurapraxia from a cervical burner/stinger is the bilateral involvement or the involvement of both upper and lower extremity symptoms.

HISTORY AND PHYSICAL EXAMINATION

Symptoms may be both motor and sensory in nature. An athlete may describe "burning of the hands," numbness, or tingling. Motor weakness may be mild or may include transient quadriparesis. The usual mechanism of injury is the axial loading of the spine when flexed or extended. This is believed to cause transient narrowing of the cervical canal, which in turn may cause a transient injury to the spinal cord. By definition, this is transient and symptoms resolved within 48 hours, though often in 10 to 15 minutes.

DIAGNOSTIC TESTING

Radiographs and MRI should be urgently obtained along with appropriate specialist consultation. MRI may be normal or show reversible spinal cord signal abnormalities.

FUNCTIONAL TREATMENT

Nonoperative

- Nonoperative treatment largely involves stabilization in the setting of an acute injury per cervical spine injury protocol.

Operative

- By definition, cervical cord neuropraxia is transient and treated nonsurgically. Should MRI show an entity with potential for permanent symptoms, then urgent surgical consultation is indicated, including but not limited to spinal instability, spinal stenosis, significant disc disease, spinal cord lesion, or cervical fracture.

Prognosis/Return to Play

- Return to play is determined on a case-by-case basis in conjunction with the neurosurgeon or spine specialist and is controversial.
- Any athlete who has had this should be treated as one with a serious spinal injury with immobilization and transport to a local hospital.
- Restriction from contact sports is recommended in athletes who have a documented episode of[13]
  - Cervical cord neuropraxia associated with ligamentous instability
  - Intervertebral disc disease with cord compression
  - Significant degenerative changes
  - MRI evidence of cord defect or swelling
  - Symptoms of positive neurologic findings lasting more than 36 hours
  - More than one recurrence

Complications/Indications for Referral

Because of the symptoms, urgent neurosurgical consultation is warranted.

APPROACH TO THE ATHLETE WITH SPINAL STENOSIS

Spinal stenosis or narrowing of the cervical spinal canal may be congenital or acquired. The stenosis may be caused by cervical disc protrusion, spondylolisthesis, osteophytic narrowing, or even ligamentous calcification. A correlation between spinal stenosis and cervical cord neuropraxia has been found.[14] However, the question of spinal stenosis predisposing an athlete to increased risk for permanent neurologic injury or even transient quadriparesis is unknown.

HISTORY AND PHYSICAL EXAMINATION

Symptoms and physical examination are variable, but athletes may feel pain, weakness, or numbness on the shoulders, arms, and legs. Hand clumsiness or gait disturbance may occur. Physical examination reveals decreased ROM, spasm, and tenderness of the neck. Neurologic examination may reveal sensory or motor deficits. The Spurling maneuver may be positive.

DIAGNOSTIC TESTING

Evaluation includes radiographs and MRI of the cervical spine. Special attention is paid to the sagittal canal diameter in the lateral view of the radiograph.

FUNCTIONAL TREATMENT

Nonoperative

- Nonoperative therapies include the following:
  - Nonsteroidal anti-inflammatories or epidural steroid injection may be used to treat to reduce pain and swelling
  - Activity modification at times of acute pain
  - Physical therapy to increase strength and flexibility

Operative

- Operative care is usually determined on an individual basis, persistent symptoms after conservative therapy
- Surgery options include anterior cervical discectomy and fusion, cervical corpectomy, and laminoplasty

Prognosis/Return to Play

- Return to play is determined on a case-by-case basis.
- The Torg ratio is controversial but calculated as follows:
  - This is a ratio comparing the sagittal diameter to the midbody diameter of the vertebral body at the same level.[15]
  - This ratio is commonly referred to as the Torg ratio, and a value of less than 0.8 has been found to be predictive of spinal stenosis.[16]
  - Although this ratio is considered sensitive by some, it has some utility when counseling patients who have had an episode of cervical cord neuropraxia.
  - A Torg ratio of less than 0.5 correlates with an estimated risk of 75% of recurrence of cervical cord neuropraxia.
- The term "functional stenosis" has arisen, which denotes the loss of cerebrospinal fluid (CSF) surrounding the spinal cord on midsagittal MRI and has been used as a contraindication to play.[17]
- Return to play after surgical treatment is discussed in the section "Approach to Patient with Cervical Disc Disease."

Complications/Indications for Referral

Team physicians should be aware of functional cervical spinal stenosis, especially in the setting of normal Torg ratios in the athlete. Return to play in the setting of severe stenosis, functional or otherwise, could result in quadriplegia.

APPROACH TO THE ATHLETE WITH BURNERS/STINGERS (TRANSIENT BRACHIAL PLEXOPATHY)

This injury is named after the symptoms the athlete experiences upon injury and is one of the most common cervical injuries sustained in American football. It usually occurs after the athlete strikes his or her head against another athlete, a wall, or a mat, resulting in a transient brachial plexopathy or cervical root compression. This most commonly occurs at the C5 and C6 levels. Acute brachial plexopathies in the younger athlete are usually a result of lateral neck deviation away from the sight of injury, thus causing traction neurapraxias. Recurrent or chronic brachial plexopathies, typically in the older player, result from compression of the nerve root, causing symptoms on the contralateral side of the impact.

HISTORY AND PHYSICAL EXAMINATION

The diagnosis is usually made by history and physical examination. Mechanism of injury reveals trauma to the neck or shoulder with resultant pain that radiates down the upper extremity in addition to numbness, paresthesias, or weakness. These symptoms do not follow a dermatomal pattern. It is seen most often in football. Symptoms are usually transient and related to a brachial plexopathy or cervical root compression. The true incidence in sports is unknown, probably in part to underreporting.[18] Physical examination will often show weakness of shoulder abductors and external rotators as well as biceps, while athlete is symptomatic. Larger/stronger athletes may require the examiner to fatigue the affected muscle groups to detect weakness on examination. This can be performed by repeating manual resistance testing several times.

DIAGNOSTIC TESTING

Diagnostic testing is not usually indicated. In select cases, electrodiagnostic studies may confirm the diagnosis and x-ray may be indicated to rule out any bony injury. Note that electrodiagnostic studies may demonstrate no abnormalities for 4 to 6 weeks post-injury (refer to Chapter 23 "Athlete with Peripheral Nerve Injuries" for a complete review). MRI may be indicated with prolonged symptoms or recurrent symptoms to rule out more central etiology, including nerve root, spinal canal, or cervical disc injury.

FUNCTIONAL TREATMENT

Nonoperative

- The management is conservative and involves addressing predisposing factors, correcting strength deficits, and enhancing protective equipment.[12]
- Improving flexibility and strength are important to decrease stiffness and weakness, which may predispose to injury.[12]
- Technique in playing style should be evaluated and corrected if it is putting the athlete at risk for repeat injury.
- Protective equipment such as cowboy collars, neck rolls, or custom orthoses may limit excess cervical motion and prevent recurrence.[15]

Operative

- In the absence of underlying cervical spine instability or cervical disc disease, there is generally no indication for surgical intervention.

Prognosis/Return to Play

- Athletes may return to play when their symptoms have completely resolved and they have full strength.
- Abnormalities may persist long term on electromyography (EMG), so it is not a useful tool in determining clearance to return to play.
- Burners have a high rate of recurrence, and the risk of permanent nerve injury has not been elucidated.[16]

Complications/Indications for Referral

Referral to a neurologist may be considered if the athlete's symptoms do not resolve with rest or if the symptoms continue to be recurrent despite the treatment measures listed earlier. Although rare, symptoms may last up to months, with muscle weakness supported by EMG.[19] Athletes with chronic burner syndrome should alert the clinician to further imaging, as there is a high incidence of cervical disc disease in these athletes.[20]

KEY POINTS
• Cervical injuries occur most commonly in collision/contact sports
• Unconscious athletes should be suspected to have a cervical spine injury until proven otherwise
• Helmets and shoulder pads should be left on for spine boarding transport with a suspected cervical spine–injured athlete as long as the patient is stable

• Evaluate in emergency department (ED) with radiographs and potential CT if there is any uncertainty regarding severity of acute cervical injury
• Cervical burners (transient brachial plexopathy) typically resolve within seconds to minutes. Chronic or recurrent burners warrant further workup
• Cervical disc disease and other causes of spinal stenosis are contraindications to play. Be wary of functional cervical spinal stenosis
• The combination of spear tackler's spine and contact sport is an absolute contraindication to contact/collision sports

REFERENCES

1. Boden BP, Jarvis CG. Spinal injuries in sports. *Neurol Clin.* 2008; 26(1):63–78.
2. Cantu RC, Mueller FO. Catastrophic spine injuries in football (1977–1989). *J Spinal Disord.* 1990;3:227–231.
3. Wu WQ, Lewis RC. Injuries of the cervical spine in high school wrestling. *Surg Neurol.* 1985;23:143–147.
4. Torg JS, Vesgo JJ, O'Neill MJ, et al. The epidemiologic, pathologic, biomechanical, and cinematographic analysis of football induced cervical spine trauma. *Am J Sports Med.* 1990;18:50–57.
5. Kiwerski J. Cervical spine injuries caused by diving into water. *Paraplegia.* 1980;18:101–106.
6. Maroon JC. "Burning hands" in football spinal cord injuries. *JAMA.* 1977;238:2049–2051.
7. Viikari-Juntura E, Porras M, Laasonen EM. Validity of clinical tests in the diagnosis of root compression in cervical disease. *Spine.* 1989;14: 253–257.
8. Shah KC, Rajshekhar V. Reliability of diagnosis of soft cervical disc prolapse using Spurling's test. *Br J Neurosurg.* 2004;18(5):480–483.
9. Torg JS, Sennett B, Pavlov H. Spear tackler's spine: an entity precluding participation in tackle football and collision activities that expose the cervical spine to axial energy inputs. *Am J Sports Med.* 1993;21: 640–649.
10. Sampath P, Bendebba M, Davis JD, et al. Outcome of patients treated for cervical myelopathy: a prospective, multicenter study with independent clinical review. *Spine.* 2000;6:670–676.
11. Tator CH. Recognition and management of spinal cord injuries in sports and recreation. *Neurol Clin.* 2008;26(1):79–88.
12. Torg JS, Ramsay-Emrhein JA. Cervical spine and brachial plexus injuries: return-to-play recommendations. *Phys Sportsmed.* 1997;25: 61–88.
13. Torg JS, Pavlov H, Genuario SE, et al. Neuropraxia of the cervical spinal cord with transient quadriplegia. *J Bone Joint Surg Am.* 1986;68: 1354–1370.
14. Torg JS. Cervical spinal stenosis with cord neuropraxia and transient quadriplegia. *Sports Med.* 1995;20:429–434.
15. Meyer SA, Schulte KR, Callaghan JJ, et al. Cervical spinal stenosis and stingers in collegiate football players. *Am J Sports Med.* 1994;22: 158–166.
16. Thomas BE, McCullen GM, Yuan HA. Cervical spine injuries in football players. *J Am Acad Orthop Surg.* 1999;7:338–347.
17. Cantu RC. Functional cervical spinal stenosis: a contraindication to participation in contact sports. *Med Sci Sports Exerc.* 1993;25(3): 316–317.
18. Haight RR, Shiple BJ. Sideline evaluation of neck pain: when is it time for transport? *Phys Sportsmed.* 2001;29:8–15.
19. Toth C. Peripheral nerve injuries attributable to sport and recreation. *Neurol Clin.* 2008;26:89–113.
20. Levitz CL, Reilly PJ, Torg JS. The pathomechanics of chronic, recurrent cervical nerve root neurapraxia, the chronic burner syndrome. *Am J Sports Med.* 1997;25:73–76.

Athlete with Shoulder Dislocation and Instability

Amy Abbot

INTRODUCTION

The shoulder is the least constrained joint in the body, which affords it an incredible range of motion but also leaves it vulnerable to instability. Shoulder stability is dependent both on static stabilizers, including the glenohumeral articulation, the glenoid labrum, the capsule, and its associated glenohumeral ligaments, and on dynamic stabilizers consisting of the rotator cuff and the periscapular musculature. Instability itself should be thought of as a continuum of abnormal motion ranging from joint laxity to subluxation to frank dislocation. It is important to remember that just because a shoulder demonstrates excess motion does not mean that this motion is pathologic; on the contrary, it may be requisite for performance in certain sports.

Clinical presentation can be highly variable from complaints of vague shoulder pain to acute dislocation, and it is imperative to perform an in-depth history and physical examination to rule out other sources of shoulder pain. If instability is present, these will also be essential in guiding the choice of treatment options.

FUNCTIONAL ANATOMY

Static stabilizers in the shoulder consist of bony articulations, labrum, and capsuloligamentous structures (Fig. 10.1). The bony conformity of the glenohumeral joint alone generally does not play a large role in gross shoulder stability but rather works in concert with other static and dynamic stabilizers to keep the humeral head centered and compressed into the glenoid (adhesion–cohesion, concavity–compression, finite joint volume). The exception to this is when bone deficiency (either traumatic or dysplastic) of the glenoid or humeral head exceeds 20%, which can result in decreased force required for dislocation and lead to primary and recurrent subluxation and dislocation[1–4] (Fig. 10.2).

The importance of soft-tissue restraints for recurrent shoulder instability was first described in the early 1900s, with Bankart describing detachment of the anteroinferior labrum as the "essential lesion."[5–7] More recently, in-depth biomechanical studies have further elucidated the synergistic roles of the labrum, capsule, and the associated glenohumeral ligaments in maintaining shoulder stability.

The labrum is a fibrocartilaginous ring that is attached to the glenoid rim and to which the glenohumeral ligaments insert. The labrum assists in stability by adding up to 50% to the glenoid depth and to the conformity of the glenohumeral articulation. This allows the labrum to act as a bumper to glenohumeral translation, resisting translational forces by as much as 60%.[3] It is important to remember that there is considerable natural variability to the labral attachment, particularly superior where it is attached much more loosely versus inferiorly where it is nearly confluent with the glenoid cartilage surface. Inability to recognize normal variants such as a sublabral foramen or Buford complex can result in inappropriate treatment. Labral lesions in isolation, though, have not been demonstrated to be sufficient to cause dislocation without a concomitant injury to the shoulder capsule and/or glenohumeral ligaments.[1,8,9]

The stabilizing action of the capsule and the associated glenohumeral ligaments is dependent on the position of the humerus in space and the force going through the glenohumeral joint. The superior glenohumeral ligament in concert with the coracohumeral ligament and rotator interval is the primary restraint to inferior translation when the arm is adducted and externally rotated. The middle glenohumeral ligament becomes the major anterior stabilizer as the arm is moved into increasing abduction and elevated to 45 degrees. The inferior glenohumeral ligament serves a wide variety of functions as a stabilizer since it spans like a hammock from the anteroinferior glenoid through the axillary pouch to the posteroinferior glenoid. As the humerus is abducted to 90 degrees, the inferior glenohumeral ligament becomes the major restraint to inferior translation. The anterior band tightens as the arm is placed in abduction and external rotation, resisting anterior translation, while the posterior band tightens with abduction and internal rotation, providing posterior instability.[1,9]

Dynamic stability is primarily provided by the rotator cuff, which compresses the humeral head into the glenoid and through coordinated contraction assists in keeping the humeral head well located on the glenoid face.[8] The biceps also contribute to shoulder stability by resisting excessive rotatory forces, tending to stabilize anteriorly with the arm in external rotation and posteriorly in internal rotation.[8,10,11] The other periscapular muscles that cross the glenohumeral

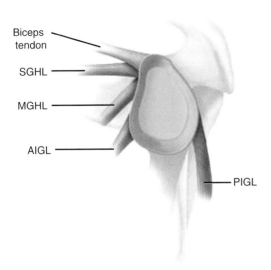

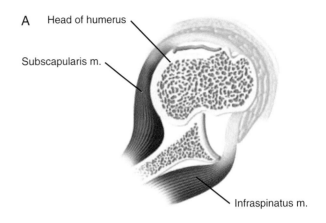

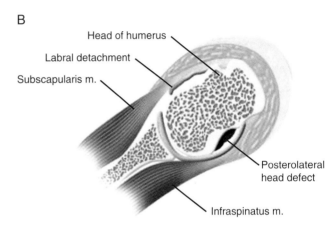

FIG. 10.1. The labrum serves as an attachment for the biceps tendon and also as the attachment point of various stabilizing ligaments, including the superior glenoid humeral ligament (SGHL), the middle glenohumeral ligament (MGHL), the inferior glenohumeral ligament (IGHL) and its bands, the anterior band of the inferior glenohumeral ligament (AIGHL), and the posterior band of the inferior glenohumeral ligament (PIGHL). Reprinted with permission from Burkhart SS, Lo IKY, Brady PC. *Burkhart's View of the Shoulder: A Cowboy's Guide to Advanced Shoulder Arthroscopy.* Philadelphia: Lippincott Williams & Wilkins; 2006.

FIG. 10.2. Typical pathology of traumatic anterior glenohumeral instability. **A:** A traumatic dislocation. **B:** Anatomic defects persisting after reduction.

joint may also play a significant role in the maintenance of stability, but this has yet to be demonstrated scientifically. What has been demonstrated is that shoulder laxity and instability are associated with rotator cuff weakness and fatigue, and this may put the capsulolabral complex at risk.[8,12]

When the circumferential capsulolabral complex is disrupted and the delicate balance between static and dynamic restraints is altered, instability can result. The classic Bankart lesion is an anteroinferior capsulolabral injury, while a reverse Bankart is similarly located in the posteroinferior glenoid. If there is capsulolabral detachment without rupture of the periosteum of the glenoid, the complex can displace medially and scar down, resulting in an ALPSA (anterior labral periosteal sleeve avulsion) lesion.[8,13] More recently, injuries superiorly on the glenoid known as SLAP (superior labral anterior to posterior) lesions have been implicated in shoulder instability, but before considering such lesions as pathologic, it is important to remember that there is significant natural variability of the labral anatomy in this area.[8,14] Recent biomechanical studies have demonstrated that lesions in the 1 to 3 o'clock region typically showed no increase in instability, but when the lesion extended across the entire superior rim (10 to 3 o'clock), there was significant translation.[8,14] Even without actual labral detachment,

the capsule and ligaments can become elongated and attenuated and result in functional instability. Finally, the function of the capsuloligamentous complex can be compromised in a much less common avulsion of the ligaments from the humeral attachment site known as a HAGL (humeral avulsion of glenoid labrum) lesion.

EPIDEMIOLOGY

The vast majority (96%) of shoulder dislocations are the result of acute traumatic events such as a fall on an outstretched hand/arm (FOOSH), a forceful wrenching of the arm, or a direct collision. Only 4% are atraumatic in origin, typically secondary to genetically increased capsular laxity or to recurrent traumatic dislocation.[9,15] Patients with capsular laxity secondary to genetic factors are much more likely to have multidirectional instability (MDI) and may experience more microinstability or subluxation versus frank dislocation. This distinction can be very useful in deciding on a treatment plan and determining the likelihood of recurrence. In fact, this has led to the TUBS (traumatic unidirectional Bankart surgery) versus AMBRI (atraumatic multidirectional bilateral rehabilitation inferior capsular shift) classification, which combines diagnosis and treatment.

Age is also a critical factor in both the type of injury sustained during primary dislocation and the development of recurrent dislocation with nonsurgical management. A study by Rowe demonstrated that shoulder dislocations occur with a bimodal distribution with peaks in the 20s and 60s.[15] In patients under age 40 years with primary dislocation, the most common injury is to the capsulolabral attachments (intracapsular), while in those above 40 years the most common injury is a tear of the rotator cuff (extracapsular).[9,15] The development of recurrent dislocation has been widely demonstrated to be highly age dependent. In patients 20 years or younger with primary dislocation, the recurrence rate approaches 90%; in those between 20 and 40 years, this drops to around 60%; and in those over 40 years, this drops even further to 10% to 16%. This is a very important factor when deciding on options for management.[9,15,16]

NARROWING THE DIFFERENTIAL DIAGNOSIS

The differential diagnosis of an athlete presenting with shoulder instability may include traumatic dislocation, voluntary dislocation, glenohumeral subluxation, MDI, glenoid or humeral bone loss, HAGL lesion, and ALPSA lesion.

History

A thorough history is crucial to defining the etiology of instability and planning treatment. The history can often be directed by using a simple classification that divides instability into four major categories: (1) *degree of instability*—microinstability, subluxation, or dislocation; (2) *frequency of instability*—primary versus chronic; (3) *etiology*—traumatic, atraumatic, or acquired; and (4) *direction of instability*—unidirectional, bidirectional, or multidirectional.[17]

It is important to assess whether there is a history of a specific traumatic event or is the description more consistent with generalized laxity and repetitive microtrauma resulting in instability. The patient may complain of a "dead-arm syndrome," the sensation that the arm went "dead" during an episode of contact, abduction, and external rotation or during throwing secondary to stretch of the brachial plexus as the humeral head subluxes. Determining the position of the extremity during instability events and location of pain about the shoulder can also provide important information about the direction of instability and the probability of associated pathology.

Important questions include the following: (1) What was the magnitude of trauma? (2) Was a reduction required? (3) How long was the disability after the event? (4) What activity or arm positions does the patient avoid? (5) How many episodes has the patient had? These questions will assist the surgeon in determining the direction of instability, whether the patient had a true traumatic episode with capsulolabral disruption, whether bone deficiency is likely, or whether the patient has generalized laxity as the primary etiology for the instability.[18]

The patient's age, activity level, and arm dominance as well as direction and frequency of dislocation should be assessed. Younger age (<25 years) has consistently been demonstrated to be a risk factor for developing recurrent dislocation with conservative management alone. High rates of recurrence have been observed in collision and contact sports, but the exact correlation has not been defined. It is also important to ascertain whether the patient has previously tried a rehabilitation protocol and how successful this conservative management was in controlling instability events.[19,20]

Evidence-based Physical Examination

As with all shoulder complaints, physical examination should begin with a complete general shoulder examination, including assessment of the cervical spine, inspection of the shoulder to identify altered contour or muscular atrophy, location of tenderness (e.g., glenohumeral joint, acromioclavicular joint), neurologic evaluation, and assessment of shoulder motion (passive and active) and strength compared to the opposite shoulder. In acute dislocation, the normal shoulder contour can be lost. Anterior dislocations tend to exhibit a hollow in the deltoid, with the humeral head medially and inferiorly displaced. The arm is held in an abducted and externally rotated position. Posterior dislocations can be more difficult but may show posterior prominence with the humerus held in adduction and internal rotation. After reduction, neurologic deficit may be present, particularly of the axillary nerve. This can manifest acutely as weakness and decreased sensation in the axillary distribution and chronically with muscular wasting and weakness. Weakness, loss of motion, or dyskinesis can also indicate disruption of the rotator cuff.

There is also a group of specific tests to evaluate laxity and instability in the shoulder. These include the sulcus sign, anterior/posterior load shift, apprehension, and relocation (Jobe) tests. It is also important to examine other joints to assess for generalized ligamentous laxity; for example, thumb to forearm flexion, elbow recurvatum, and knee hyperextension.

Diagnostic Testing

Sulcus Sign

This test was first described by Neer and Foster as an assessment of inferior instability and can be performed with the patient seated, standing, or supine (most commonly seated) by applying inferior traction to the humerus.[21] The test is considered positive if a dimple appears between the lateral acromion and the humeral head. Grading has been described by several authors as follows: grade I < 1 cm, grade II = 1 to 2 cm, and grade III > 2 cm.[1,22,23] A sulcus sign of 2 cm or more has been shown to have a high likelihood of instability (likelihood ratio 6:1).[9,24]

Anterior/Posterior Load and Shift

Descriptions as to how to perform this test vary – for example, seated versus supine, varying degrees of abduction, flexion, and rotation from 0 to 90 degrees – but the general principles are the same.[1,24–28] The examiner grasps the patient's arm and humerus and applies a force into the glenoid to center the humeral head. The examiner then applies an anterior and posterior force in an attempt to shift the humeral head on the glenoid surface. Grading for this test has also undergone evolution with time, but is generally described as follows: grade 0 = humeral head does not move to glenoid rim; grade 1 = humeral head moves to glenoid rim but not over it; grade 2 = humeral head goes over glenoid rim, but spontaneously reduces; and grade 3 = humeral head goes over glenoid rim, but does not spontaneously reduce.[27,29] This test has been shown to have a high specificity (98% to 100%) but low sensitivity (41% for unidirectional instability and 26% for multidirectional). This may be due to the high level of intra- and interobserver variability observed. Levy et al. demonstrated that this variability is improved when grades 0 and 1 are combined (agreement of 74% to 78%), and this is further improved if the examination is performed under anesthesia.[30,31]

A variation of this test can be performed with one hand stabilizing the scapula while the other grasps the humeral head and attempts to shift it anteriorly or posteriorly over the glenoid. A similar grading system is applied.

Apprehension and Relocation (Jobe)

This test can be performed with the patient either standing or supine. The patient's shoulder is then passively brought into maximal external rotation with the arm abducted, traditionally to 90 degrees. An anterior force is then applied to the humerus. A positive test elicits sudden apprehension with or without pain in the patient's shoulder.[32,33] In a modification of this test proposed by Jobe and Kvitne, after eliciting apprehension a posterior force is applied to the humeral head, "relocating" it into the glenoid and relieving the patient's apprehension and pain.[34] With this modification and use of apprehension as the diagnostic criterion rather than pain, sensitivity was found to be 68%, specificity 100%, and a positive predictive value of 100%.[32,35]

Another version of this test is known as the anterior release. In this test, the humeral head is stabilized with a posterior force as the shoulder is brought into abduction and maximal external rotation. The pressure on the humeral head is then released, and the test is positive if the patient experiences pain and apprehension. In a series of 82 patients, the sensitivity of this test was 92%, specificity was 89%, and positive predictive value was 87%.[23,32,36] Apprehension is the key criterion for instability, and this may or may not be accompanied by pain. Pain alone is more indicative of rotator cuff pathology.[32,36]

SLAP Tests

Clinical evaluation of SLAP lesions is controversial at this time. At least eight tests have been described for the diagnosis of SLAP lesions (e.g., active compression, biceps load, Kim and Crank tests), but no test or combination of tests have been shown to be consistently reliable. Although the primary authors have reported high sensitivity and specificity, their results have not been reproducible by other clinicians, and no anatomic studies have been performed to assess their ability to test the biceps/labral complex.[32]

Imaging

Radiographic examination should include the standard shoulder trauma series with a true anteroposterior (AP) view of the shoulder (beam aimed 30 degrees from the sagittal plane), scapular Y, and axillary lateral. The axillary lateral is useful in assessing head location on the glenoid surface (concentric vs. eccentric) and any bony glenoid deficiency.[37] Other specific views that may prove useful include the apical oblique view, the West Point view, and the Stryker Notch view. The apical oblique view is a true AP view with the beam tilted 45 degrees caudally. The West Point view is taken with the patient prone, arm 90 degrees abducted, and the beam aimed from inferior, 25 degrees from medial, and 25 degrees from the horizontal. This view is useful for visualizing bony Bankart lesions. The Stryker Notch view is taken supine with the arm 90 degrees forward elevated (hand on head), with the beam directed 10 degrees cephalad and centered over the coracoid. This view provides good visualization of Hill–Sachs lesions on the humerus.

Magnetic resonance imaging (MRI) with or without arthrography can be useful to further define soft-tissue pathology, including labral injury, rotator cuff tears, and HAGL lesions. Noncontrast MRI is most useful in evaluating rotator cuff lesions and bony abnormalities (e.g., Hill–Sachs lesions), but **MRI arthrography** has been shown to have increased sensitivity (88% to 90%) in identifying labral lesions and increased joint volume associated with capsular attenuation. This is improved even further with positioning the upper extremity in abduction and external rotation during the scan.[38] Computed tomography (CT) scanning, particularly with three-dimensional reconstruction, can also be useful in further defining bony deformities, especially the extent and location of glenoid deficiency and/or Hill–Sachs lesions.

The question arises when the adjunctive imaging modalities are required in evaluating symptomatic patients. Multiple instability events and those that occur with lower degrees of abduction and external rotation may indicate significant bone loss. Instability during sleep, history of seizure disorder, and failed previous stabilization procedures are also useful indications that a bone defect is present. During the physical examination, marked apprehension in less abduction and external rotation typically indicates bone loss. These imaging studies can be very important for preoperative planning and proper selection of procedure including potential bone grafting or transfers.

APPROACH TO THE ATHLETE WITH INSTABILITY (DISLOCATION, SUBLUXATION, MULTIDIRECTIONAL INSTABILITY)

HISTORY AND PHYSICAL EXAMINATION

It is important to take a comprehensive approach for the athlete with instability. Major areas to be addressed when taking the history are as follows: (1) *degree of instability*—microinstability, subluxation, or dislocation; (2) *frequency of instability*—primary versus chronic; (3) *etiology*—traumatic, atraumatic, or acquired; and (4) *direction of instability*—unidirectional, bidirectional, or multidirectional.[17] Demographics such as age, hand dominance, level of athletic participation, timing in the season, presence of any neurologic symptoms (e.g., axillary nerve deficits), demands of the work environment, and perhaps most importantly, patient demands and expectations all affect the treatment protocol.

Craig et al. suggested a series of useful questions to be addressed when considering shoulder instability in the athlete.[39] First, it is important to determine whether the affected shoulder is truly unstable. Patients' descriptions of instability can often describe other shoulder disorders, so particular attention must be paid to the history and whether pain or apprehension is the predominant symptom. Also, laxity is not necessarily pathologic and in fact is often requisite for sports performance. Objective laxity may be observed in both shoulders while only one may be symptomatic. It is important to assess whether this is generalized or traumatic laxity and what level of energy is required to produce instability (e.g., was there a single forceful collision vs. repetitive microtrauma). It is also important to recognize whether the laxity is unidirectional, bidirectional, or multidirectional, and from there what is the source of instability (e.g., trauma, ligamentous laxity, glenoid dysplasia).

Lastly, it is important to consider who the patient is. As has been discussed, patients under the age of 20 have a near 100% probability of having a repeat dislocation, so treatment of traumatic instability in young, active individuals is frequently recommended, whereas conservative treatment can frequently be successful in patients over the age of 40. Level of activity is also an important consideration. Participation in high-level and in a particular action or contact sport increases the risk of recurrence. At the

same time an athlete in midseason may be a candidate for a trial of conservative management and bracing prior to proceeding to surgical management. It is important to thoroughly discuss with the athlete the risks and benefits of nonoperative and operative management, including all the available options.

The patient's history will help direct a focused physical examination and development of a differential diagnosis. A witnessed primary and/or recurrent dislocation will have a strong influence on clinical evaluation and in the acute setting may significantly limit the ability to assess the shoulder. In these cases, it is frequently necessary to allow the shoulder to "cool down" with short-term sling immobilization and gentle range-of-motion exercises until pain and range of motion are improved. Once the shoulder is ready to be assessed, the **anterior and posterior load and shift** tests can be useful to determine the direction and extent of instability. This is frequently important in cases of recurrent instability where labral damage and possible bone loss (bony Bankart) can be progressive. **Jobe apprehension and relocation** tests can also be useful in this situation of acute and/or recurrent dislocations. Frequently, in this acute situation, it is difficult or impossible to perform the apprehension test directly, because the patient will not allow the shoulder to be brought into a position of instability. In these cases the **anterior release** is very useful, since the humeral head is stabilized with a posteriorly directed force while the shoulder is brought into a position of abduction and external rotation. As the stabilizing force is released, the patient experiences apprehension with or without pain.

Complaints by patients that are more consistent with subluxation can be of either traumatic instability or MDI. Athletes with MDI will often present with chronic recurrent mild subluxation or gradual-onset diffuse shoulder pain. MDI largely affects the young and adolescent overhead (baseball, softball, tennis, swimming) or tumbling athlete (gymnastics, cheering) under the age of 25. Pain is described as diffuse in the deltoid region and exacerbated primarily with overhead sporting activities (throwing, tennis serve, gymnastics, tumbling). Athletes with MDI will often demonstrate signs of generalized joint laxity on examination, including **elbow or knee recurvatum** as well as **thumb-to-forearm sign.** The differentiation of MDI from acute traumatic instability is important because the surgical treatment of instability in these individuals is much less successful. The **anterior and posterior load and shift tests** and **the sulcus sign** can be useful in determining the direction and extent of subluxation, or in some cases dislocation. Any neurologic deficit should also be noted since not only injuries to the brachial plexus and in particular the axillary nerve can occur with shoulder dislocation but also disorders of the cervical spine can affect the shoulder and upper extremity and confound assessment of shoulder disorders.

DIAGNOSTIC TESTING

Imaging

- Radiographic evaluation: A true AP, scapular lateral (Y view), and axillary view are essential
  - Can provide the direction of dislocation and can frequently demonstrate bony injuries to the glenoid and humeral head
  - Can demonstrate the size of any bony Bankart or Hill–Sachs lesion
  - Can evaluate glenoid dysplasia
  - West Point—visualizes bony Bankart lesions
  - Stryker Notch—better elucidates Hill–Sachs lesions
- MRI
  - Valuable for identifying type, location, and extent of capsuloligamentous injuries
  - MRI arthrography generally provides the clearest visualization of these capsulolabral lesions
- CT scanning
  - Useful when bony injury to the glenoid rim and/or humeral head is present
  - Better for surgical planning, and must weigh risks versus benefits, given the relatively large radiation exposure

TREATMENT

Nonoperative

- Acute dislocations require
  - Expeditious reduction
  - Gentle maneuvers to avoid further damage
    - Traction is applied inferiorly to the humerus, with the arm in slight abduction
    - Countertraction is applied by a sheet around the body
  - Performing open reduction if closed reduction fails
  - Immobilization ranging from 3 to 6 weeks[40]
  - Immobilization in external rotation, which may decrease the risk for recurrent anterior dislocation[37,41,42]
  - Passive range of motion and pendulum, after the initial period of immobilization
  - A following rehabilitation program focusing on dynamic rotator cuff and periscapular strengthening
    - Limiting external rotation beyond neutral for 6 weeks
    - Limiting abduction to beyond 90 degrees for 6 weeks after an anterior dislocation
  - Rotator cuff strength and endurance, which are essential for maintaining dynamic stabilization of the shoulder
  - Advancing the strength gradually with the goal to attain full range of motion by week 10[20,43]
- MDI
  - Nonoperative management is mainstay of treatment
  - Focus of treatment involves strengthening the rotator cuff and supporting periscapula muscle groups
  - Progression to upper-extremity propioception (balance/stability) as well as plyometric (explosive change of direction) exercises recommended for the athlete involved in overhead (throwing sports, tennis) or upper-extremity weight-bearing sports (gymnastics, wrestling)

Operative

- Indication for operative management is irreducible or fixed acute shoulder dislocation
  - Timing and procedure are less clear
- Risk of recurrent dislocation is inversely related to age[9,15,16]
- Active patients in their early 20s or younger have a very high risk of redislocation, with a low probability to be able to return to the same level of activity, and they generally have poor outcome[44]
- Primary early repair in young, active patients is done with clinical and MRI evidence for a Bankart lesion[19,20]
  - Better functional outcome than rehabilitation
- Surgical management is suggested for middle-aged patients
  - Failed rehabilitation
  - Recurrent dislocation
- Patients over the age of 40 are less likely to develop recurrent instability
  - Injury is more often to the rotator cuff
  - Patients do much better with rehabilitation alone or with primary treatment of their rotator cuff pathology
- Goal of surgery
  - Repair the labral lesion and restore the bumper effect
  - Address stretching of the capsulolabral complex
  - Perform capsular shift with imbrication with or without rotator interval closure, which has proved to be successful for MDI[45]
- Examination under anesthesia
  - Range of motion, sulcus sign, and anterior/posterior load and shift should be tested
  - Increases the sensitivity and specificity of these tests, and it is a useful adjunct for surgical planning[46]
- Diagnostic arthroscopy can also be useful
- Most instability repairs can be done either arthroscopically or open
  - Outcomes for arthroscopic and open repairs have become comparable[40]
  - Arthroscopic repair has the advantage of not necessitating taking down the subscapularis

Prognosis/Return to Play

- A recent study suggests that many athletes with acute shoulder dislocation/subluxation may be able to return and finish the season following a dislocation.[47]

- After a very brief period of immobilization, early range of motion, and cuff strengthening, most athletes returned to play in an average of less than 2 weeks.
- Use of a brace or harness to limit external rotation is recommended when the player returns.
- More than half underwent operative stabilization at the end of the season.
- Athletes with chronic subluxation or MDI who have failed conservative management may often defer surgical treatment till the end of their competitive season based on symptoms and function.

Complications/Indications for Referral

The most common complication associated with unstable shoulders is continued episodes of subluxation and dislocation, leading to further damage to the structures within the shoulder joint. Axial nerve and brachial plexus injuries should also be considered in the setting of shoulder dislocations. Postsurgical degenerative joint disease secondary to overconstraint of the glenohumeral joint has been reported with open procedures.

KEY POINTS
• Surgical repair recommended for shoulder dislocations in patients under the age of 25 to prevent further episodes of anterior dislocation and arthritic changes
• If there is a Hill–Sachs defect, then surgical treatment is recommended
• MRI arthrography is the most appropriate study to visualize the soft-tissue damage associated with acute and recurrent shoulder instability
• Arthroscopic Bankart repair may have higher redislocation rates when compared with open procedures (7% to 17% versus 5%)
• Midseason athletes may return to sport after a brief period of immobilization with the use of a brace or harness for acute subluxation or dislocation
• Physical therapy focused on strengthening exercises is mainstay of treatment for athletes with shoulder MDI

REFERENCES

1. Bahk M, Keyurapan E, Tasaki A, et al. Laxity testing of the shoulder: a review. *Am J Sports Med.* 2007;5(1):131–144.
2. Lippitt S, Matsen F. Mechanisms of glenohumeral joint stability. *Clin Orthop Relat Res.* 1993;291:20–28.
3. Lippitt SB, Vanderhooft JE, Harris SL, et al. Glenohumeral stability from concavity-compression: a quantitative analysis. *J Shoulder Elbow Surg.* 1993;2:27–35.
4. Itoi E, Lee SB, Berglund LJ, et al. The effect of a glenoid defect on anterior-inferior stability of the shoulder after Bankart repair: a cadaveric study. *J Bone Joint Surg Am.* 2000;82:35–46.
5. Bankart ASB. The pathology and treatment of recurrent dislocation of the shoulder joint. *Br J Surg.* 1938;26:23–29.
6. Perthes G. Uber operationen bei habitueller schulterluxation. *Deutsch Zischr Chir.* 1906;85:199–227.
7. Thomas TT. The reduction of old unreduced dislocations of the shoulders. *Ann Surg.* 1913;57:217–243.
8. Levine WN, Flatow EL. The pathophysiology of shoulder instability. *Am J Sports Med.* 2000;28(6):910–917.
9. Walton J, Paxionos A, Tzannes A, et al. The unstable shoulder in the adolescent athlete. *Am J Sports Med.* 2002;30(5):758–767.
10. Pagnani MJ, Deng XH, Warren RF, et al. Role of the long head of the biceps brachii in glenohumeral stability: a biomechanical study in cadavera. *J Shoulder Elbow Surg.* 1996;5:255–262.
11. Rodosky MW, Harner CD, Fu FH. The role of the long head of the biceps muscle and superior glenoid labrum in anterior stability of the shoulder. *Am J Sports Med.* 1994;22:121–130.
12. Warner JJ, Micheli LJ, Arslanian LE, et al. Patterns of flexibility, laxity and strength in normal shoulders and shoulders with instability and impingement. *Am J Sports Med.* 1990;18(4):366–375.
13. Neviaser TJ. The anterior labroligamentous periosteal sleeve avulsion lesion: a cause of anterior instability of the shoulder. *Arthroscopy.* 1993;9:17–21.
14. Warner JJP, Kann S, Marks P. Arthroscopic repair of combined Bankart and superior labral detachment anterior and posterior lesions: technique and preliminary results. *Arthroscopy.* 1994;10:383–391.
15. Rowe CR. Prognosis in dislocations of the shoulder. *J Bone Joint Surg Am.* 1956;38:957–977.
16. McLaughlin HL, Cavallaro WU. Primary anterior dislocation of the shoulder. *Am J Surg.* 1950;80:615–621.
17. Backer M, Warren RF. Glenohumeral instabilities. In: *The Shoulder.* 3rd ed. Philadelphia, PA: WB Saunders; 2004:1020–1033.
18. DeAngelis NA, Busconi BD, Mazzocca AD, et al. Recurrent anterior shoulder instability. In: *Orthopaedic Knowledge Update: Shoulder and Elbow.* 3rd ed. Rosemont, IL: American Academy of Orthopaedic Surgeons; 2008.
19. Kirkley A, Werstine R, Ratjek A, et al. Prospective randomized clinical trial comparing the effectiveness of immediate arthroscopic stabilization versus immobilization and rehabilitation in first traumatic anterior dislocations of the shoulder: long-term evaluation. *Arthroscopy.* 2005;21(1):55–63.
20. Kirkley A, Griffin S, Richards C. Prospective randomized clinical trial comparing the effectiveness of immediate arthroscopic stabilization versus immobilization and rehabilitation in first traumatic anterior dislocations of the shoulder. *Arthroscopy.* 1999;15:507–514.
21. Neer CS II, Foster CR. Inferior capsular shift for involuntary inferior and multidirectional instability of the shoulder: a preliminary report. *J Bone Joint Surg Am.* 1980;62:897–908.
22. Hawkins RJ, Schutte JP, Janda DH, et al. Translation of the glenohumeral joint with the patient under anesthesia. *J Shoulder Elbow Surg.* 1996;5:286–292.
23. Silliman JF, Hawkins RJ. Classification and physical diagnosis of instability of the shoulder. *Clin Orthop Relat Res.* 1993;291:7–19.
24. Tzannes A, Murrell GAC. Clinical examination of the unstable shoulder. *Sports Med.* 2002;32:447–457.
25. Gerber C, Ganz R. Clinical assessment of instability of the shoulder: with special reference to anterior and posterior drawer tests. *J Bone Joint Surg Br.* 1984;66:551–556.
26. Matsen FA III, Thomas SC, Rockwood CA Jr, et al. Glenohumeral instability. In: Rockwood CA Jr, Matsen FA III, eds. *The Shoulder.* 2nd ed. Philadelphia, PA: WB Saunders; 1998:611–754.
27. McFarland EG, Torpey BM, Curl LA. Evaluation of shoulder laxity. *Sports Med.* 1996;22:264–272.
28. Tzannes A, Paxinos A, Callanan M, et al. An assessment of the interexaminer reliability of tests for shoulder instability. *J Shoulder Elbow Surg.* 2004;13:18–23.
29. McFarland EG. Instability and laxity. In: *Examination of the Shoulder. The Complete Guide.* New York: Theime; 2006:161–212.
30. Levy AS, Lintner S, Kenter K, et al. Intra- and interobserver reproducibility of the shoulder laxity examination. *Am J Sports Med.* 1999;27:460–463.

31. Lerat JL, Chotel F, Besse JL, et al. Dynamic anterior jerk of the shoulder. A new clinical test for shoulder instability [in French]. *Rev Chir Orthop Reparatrice Appar Mot.* 1994;80:461–467.

32. Tennent TD, Beach WR, Meyers JF. A review of the special tests associated with shoulder examination: Part II: laxity, instability, and superior labral anterior and posterior (SLAP) lesions. *Am J Sports Med.* 2003; 31:301–307.

33. Rowe CR, Zarins B. Recurrent transient subluxation of the shoulder. *J Bone Joint Surg Am.* 1981;63:863–872.

34. Jobe FW, Kvitne RS. Shoulder pain in the overhand or throwing athlete. The relationship of anterior instability and rotator cuff impingement. *Orthop Rev.* 1989;18:963–975.

35. Speer KP, Hannafin JA, Altchek DW, et al. An evaluation of the shoulder relocation test. *Am J Sports Med.* 1994;22:177–183.

36. Gross ML, Distefano MC. Anterior release test. A new test for occult shoulder instability. *Clin Orthop.* 1997;339:105–108.

37. Itoi E, Lee SB, Amrami KK, et al. Quantitative assessment of classic anteroinferior bony Bankart lesions by radiography and computed tomography. *Am J Sports Med.* 2003;31(1):112–118.

38. Jensen KL, Rockwood CA Jr. Glenohumeral instability: classification, clinical assessment, and imaging. In: Norris TR, ed. *Orthopaedic Knowledge Update: Shoulder and Elbow.* 2nd ed. Rosemont, IL: AAOS; 2002:69.

39. Craig EV, Warren RF, Ragsdale EK. Decision making in recurrent shoulder instability. In: Warren RF, Craig EV, Altchek DW, eds. *The Unstable Shoulder.* Philadelphia, PA: Lippincott Williams & Wilkins; 1999:189–204.

40. Bottoni CR, Wilckens JH, DeBerardino TM, et al. A prospective randomized evaluation of arthroscopic stabilization versus nonoperative treatment in patients with acute, traumatic, first-time shoulder dislocations. *Am J Sports Med.* 2002;30(4):576–580.

41. Itoi E, Hatakeyama Y, Urayama M. Position of immobilization after dislocation of the shoulder: a cadaveric study. *J Bone Joint Surg Am.* 1999;81(3):385–390.

42. Itoi E, Sashi R, Minagawa H, et al. Position of immobilization after dislocation of the gleno-humeral joint: a study with the use of MRI. *J Bone Joint Surg Am.* 2001;83(5):661–667.

43. Backer M, Warren RF. Glenohumeral instabilities in adults. In: DeLee JC, Drez D Jr, Miller MD, eds. *Orthopaedic Sports Medicine: Principles and Practice.* Philadelphia, PA: WB Saunders; 2003:1020–1034.

44. Burkhead WZ, Rockwood CA Jr. Treatment of instability of the shoulder with an exercise program. *J Bone Joint Surg Am.* 1992;74:890–896.

45. Caprise PA Jr, Sekiya JK. Open and arthroscopic treatment of multidirectional instability of the shoulder. *Arthroscopy.* 2006;22:1126–1131.

46. Oliashirazi A, Manasat P, Cofield RH, et al. Examination under anesthesia for evaluation of anterior shoulder instability. *Am J Sports Med.* 1999;27:464–468.

47. Buss DD, Lynch GP, Meyer CP, et al. Non-operative management of in-season athletes with anterior shoulder instability. *Am J Sport Med.* 2004;32(6):1430–1433.

Athlete with Shoulder Pain during Throwing/Overhead Motion

Lee A. Mancini

INTRODUCTION

Shoulder pain is a common complaint found in the athlete involved in throwing/overhead motions. The throwing motion seen in baseball, softball, and football is an unusual action that places tremendous stress on the shoulder joint complex. This overhead motion is also seen in swimmers, volleyball players, javelin throwers, and tennis players and in a repetitive nature can result in overuse shoulder pain and injury. The spectrum of pathology may range from shoulder multidirectional instability (MDI) with secondary impingement to rotator cuff and/or labral tears. While acute shoulder dislocations, subluxations, and labral tears can occur in the throwing/overhead athlete, the approach is reviewed in Chapter 10 Athlete with Shoulder Dislocation and Instability. The approach to overuse shoulder pain in the general or older athlete is reviewed in Chapter 12 Athlete with Overuse Shoulder Pain. The focus of this chapter is on the evaluation and management of shoulder pain in the throwing or overhead athlete, with center of attention being chronic shoulder instability and superior labral (SLAP) tears.

FUNCTIONAL ANATOMY

The shoulder joint is actually a complex of four articulations: the sternoclavicular joint, the acromioclavicular joint, the glenohumeral (GH) joint, and the scapulothoracic joint (Figs 11.1 and 11.2).

The GH joint has the widest range of motion of any joint in the body. It is a product of the incongruous nature of the GH joint and surrounding soft tissue envelope. This provides dynamic stability as well as varying degrees of passive stability with minimal restriction of motion (Fig. 11.3).

The static constraints of the GH joint include the labrum, the shoulder capsule, the coracohumeral ligament (CHL), the superior glenohumeral ligament (SGHL), the middle glenohumeral ligament (MGHL), and the inferior glenohumeral ligament (IGHL). The shoulder capsule has twice the surface area as the humeral head. All sides of the capsule, except the inferior portion, are reinforced by the rotator cuff.[1] The CHL is a thin capsular fold that stretches from the base of the coracoid process to the transverse humeral ligament. It works together with the SGHL. The SGHL extends from the supraglenoid tubercle to the lesser tuberosity of the humerus. It works with the CHL to prevent inferior instability of the shoulder when the arm is adducted. A secondary role is to assist the shoulder capsule in resisting posterior instability when the shoulder is in the flexed, adducted, and internally rotated position. The MGHL goes from the mid anterior labrum to the lesser tuberosity. It functions as a secondary restraint to anterior translation of the humeral head. The IGHL is the major stabilizer of the GH joint. It is composed of anterior and posterior bands with an interposed axillary pouch. When the shoulder is abducted and externally rotated, the anterior band of the IGHL prevents anterior translation. When the shoulder is internally rotated, the posterior band prevents posterior translation. Which static constraint serves to prevent anterior dislocation depends on the degree of abduction in the shoulder. At 90° abduction it is the IGHL, at 45° it is primarily the MGHL with assistance from the subscapularis and the IGHL, and at 0° it is the subscapularis. The IGHL is the primary anterior stabilizer in throwing athletes.

In the GH joint, the humeral head has a surface area two to four times greater than that of the glenoid and a diameter two times greater than that of the glenoid. The glenoid labrum is a cartilage ring that appears triangular when seen in cross-sectional area. The labrum doubles the anterior–posterior (AP) depth of the glenoid from 2.5 to 5 mm^2 and deepens the concavity of the glenoid. This increase in depth enhances the stability of the GH joint by increasing the contact surface area for the humeral head. A torn labrum results in a 20% loss in resistance to translation from a compressive load. The inferior labrum is a rounded fibrous structure which is firmly attached to the glenoid and is also continuous with the articular cartilage.[2] The superior labrum can have a meniscal appearance and is attached loosely and is mobile. It is also the attachment site of the MGHL and SGHL. The long head of the biceps tendon originates from

Left Shoulder
(Anterior)

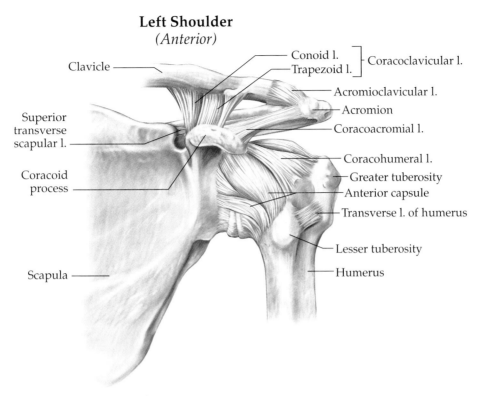

FIG. 11.1. Shoulder anatomy, anterior view. Asset provided by Anatomical Chart Co.

Left Shoulder
(Posterior)

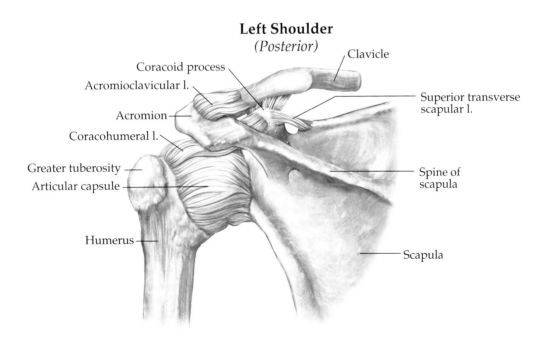

FIG. 11.2. Shoulder anatomy, posterior view. Asset provided by Anatomical Chart Co.

the superior labrum and the supraglenoid tubercle. The Bufford complex, first described by Williams and Snyder in 1994, is a rare anatomic finding where a cord-like MGHL originates directly from the superior labrum at the base of the biceps tendon. The vascular supply of the labrum is bet-

ter peripherally than centrally. The anterior, anterosuperior, and superior portion of the labrum have a decreased blood supply relative to other parts of the labrum.[3]

Detachment of the superior labrum (superior labrum anterior to posterior) SLAP lesion rarely causes frank instability.

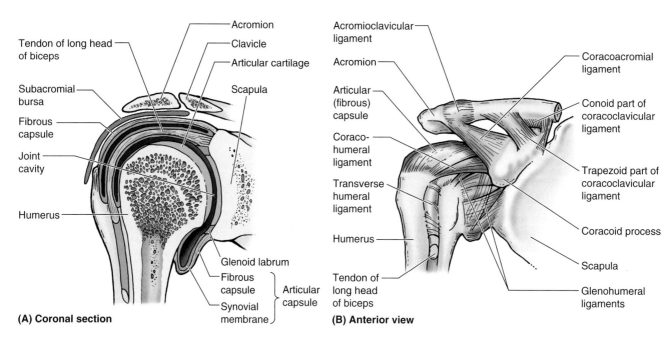

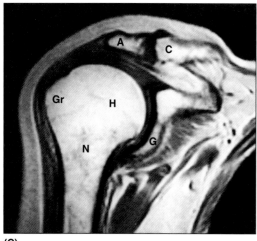

(C)

FIG. 11.3 A, Coronal section of the shoulder region illustrating the articulating bones, the articular capsule and cartilage, and the subacromial bursa. B, Drawing of an anterior view of a dissection of the acromioclavicular (AC), coracohumeral, and glenohumeral ligaments. The glenohumeral ligaments strengthen the anterior aspect of the capsule of the glenohumeral joint, and the coracohumeral ligament strengthens the capsule superiorly. C, Coronal MRI of the right glenohumeral and AC joints. *A,* acromion; *C,* clavicle; *Gr,* greater tubercle of the humerus; *H,* head of humerus; *G,* glenoid cavity; *N,* surgical neck of humerus. (From Moore KL, Dalley AF II. *Clinically Oriented Anatomy.* 4th ed. Philadelphia: Lippincott Williams & Wilkins; 1999.)

SLAP lesions often occur in association with an anterior labral lesion known as a Bankart lesion. SLAP lesions are classified as type I, II, III, and IV primarily.[4] This classification system is based on Snyder's classification system described in 1990 (Table 11.1). A type I SLAP lesion has fraying of the edge of the superior labrum. Type II is the most common type of SLAP lesion. In a type II lesion, there is fraying of the edge of the superior labrum as well as a detached biceps tendon anchor from the superior glenoid tubercle. Type III lesions consist of a bucket-handle tear of a meniscoid superior labrum with an otherwise normal biceps tendon attachment.

Type IV lesions also contain the bucket-handle tear as well as an extension of this tear into the biceps tendon. Combined lesions have also been described usually as type II and III or type II and IV. These are cases where there is a significantly detached biceps tendon anchor, a type II lesion, in addition to either a type III or a type IV lesion[3] (Fig. 11.4).

The dynamic constraints of the shoulder include the rotator cuff, the long head of the biceps tendon, and the scapular rotators. The rotator cuff and long head of the biceps are the most important stabilizers of the GH joint. The GH ligaments serve as passive stabilizers at extremes of motion.

TABLE 11.1	Types of SLAP Tears: Snyder's SLAP Lesion Classification System		
Type I	Type II	Type III	Type IV
Fraying of the edge of the superior labrum	Fraying of the edge of the superior labrum Detached biceps tendon anchor from the superior glenoid tubercle	Bucket-handle tear of a meniscoid superior labrum Normal biceps tendon attachment	Bucket-handle tear of a meniscoid superior labrum Tear extends into biceps tendon

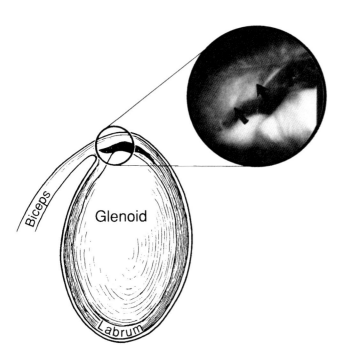

FIG. 11.4. Labral tear, SLAP lesion picture. Reprinted with permission from Bucholz RW, Heckman JD. *Rockwood & Green's Fractures in Adults.* 5th ed. Philadelphia: Lippincott Williams & Wilkins; 2001.

The rotator cuff consists of four muscles: the subscapularis, the supraspinatus, the infraspinatus, and the teres minor. The subscapularis arises from the anterior aspect of the scapula and attaches over the lesser tuberosity. It is innervated by the upper and lower subscapular nerves (C5, C6). Its function is internal rotation. The supraspinatus arises from the supraspinatus fossa of the posterior scapula, under the acromion, and attaches to the superior aspect of the greater tuberosity. It is innervated by the suprascapular nerve (C5, C6). The function of the supraspinatus is humeral head depression. The infraspinatus originates from the infraspinatus fossa of the posterior scapula and inserts on the posterior lateral aspect of the greater tuberosity. It is innervated by the suprascapular nerve (C5, C6). The function of the infraspinatus is external rotation. The teres minor arises from the lower aspect of the scapula and attaches to the lower aspect of the greater tuberosity. It is innervated by the axillary nerve (C5, C6) and its function is external rotation. Six different arteries supply the rotator cuff: the

posterior humeral circumflex, the suprascapular, the anterior humeral circumflex, the acromial branch of the thoracoacromial, the subscapular branch of the axillary artery, and the suprahumeral branch of the axillary artery (Fig. 11.5).

The long head of the biceps tendon adds to the anterior stability of the shoulder by resisting excessive external rotation forces when the shoulder is abducted and externally rotated. The long head of the biceps tendon helps to decrease the stress on the IGHL. The scapula rotators are a collection of muscles that serve to manipulate the scapula in different directions. The middle division of the trapezius and the rhomboids major and minor promote scapular retraction. The trapezius and the serratus anterior create upward rotation of the scapula. Protraction of the scapula is caused by the serratus anterior. Depression of the scapula is caused by the lower division of the trapezius and the inferior serratus anterior. The levator scapulae and the upper division of the trapezius provide postural support.

Scapulohumeral rhythm is the 2:1 ratio between GH and scapulothoracic motion at the shoulder joint. For every two degrees of motion at the GH joint, there is one degree of motion at the scapulothoracic joint. In the pitching motion, the angular velocity of the shoulder reaches 6,100 degrees/sec. Internal rotation torque is 14,000 inch-pounds prior to the release of the baseball. The kinetic energy generated is 27,000 inch-pounds. The pitching motion is divided into six phases: wind-up, early cocking, late cocking, acceleration, deceleration, and follow through. The first three phases make up 80% of the pitching motion and in these phases the ball does not move forward. In the early cocking phase, the shoulder is flexed and abducted. In the late cocking phase, the shoulder is abducted 90°, extended 30°, and externally rotated 90° up to even 160°. In the acceleration phase, there is derotation of the shoulder (Fig. 11.6).

EPIDEMIOLOGY

Problems with the shoulder joint, specifically impingement and tearing of the rotator cuff tendon, tend to increase with patient age. A study done in 1995 found that only 4% of asymptomatic patients between the ages of 19 and 39 had a partial-thickness tear of the rotator cuff and there were no full-thickness tears. This is in comparison to 28% incidence of full-thickness tears and 26% incidence of partial-thickness tears in asymptomatic patients over the age of 60.[5]

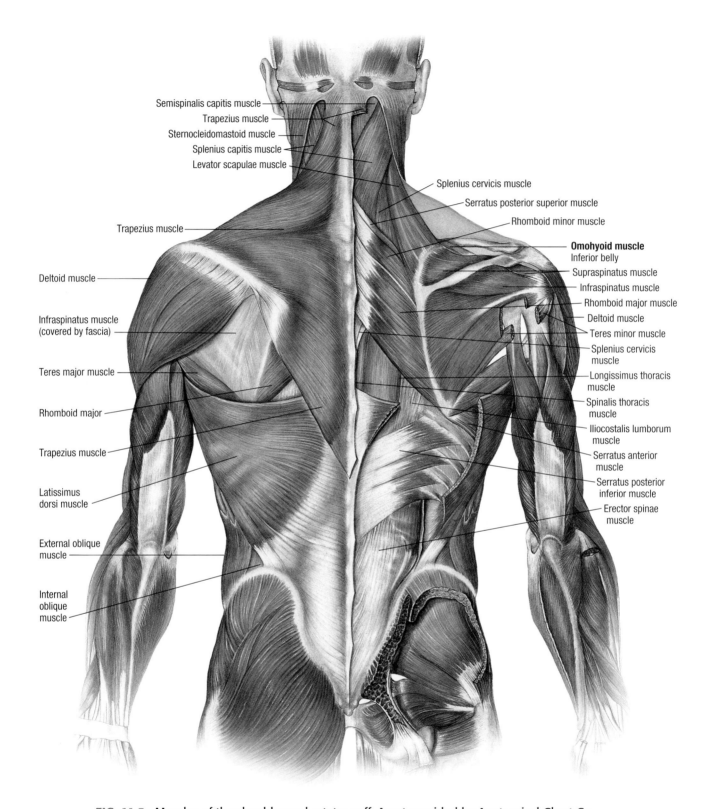

FIG. 11.5. Muscles of the shoulder and rotator cuff. Asset provided by Anatomical Chart Co.

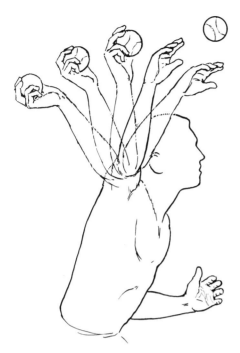

FIG. 11.6. Side view of throwing motion. MediClip image copyright © 2003 Lippincott Williams & Wilkins. All rights reserved.

Any sport that involves overhead activity, including tennis, volleyball, baseball, golf, football (quarterbacks), and swimming, is at increased risk of tendinopathy or rotator cuff tear. Over 50% of elite tennis players have had shoulder pain from rotator cuff or biceps tendon injuries. Nearly 80% of swimmers have reported shoulder pain. Fifty-seven percent of pitchers suffer some form of shoulder injury during a season.[6]

NARROWING THE DIFFERENTIAL DIAGNOSIS

The challenge in evaluating the throwing or overhead athlete with shoulder pain is differentiating pain coming from functional weakness and chronic instability seen in MDI from structural injury including SLAP tears or rotator cuff tears (generally undersurface tears). Primary external impingement causing rotator cuff tendinosis (RCT) and tears are more frequent in older athletes. Secondary external impingement is the most frequent cause of pain in overhead athletes. Microinstability is the term used when overhead athletes have no perceptible instability of the GH joint. In athletes with microinstability, it is an overuse injury caused by weakness in rotator cuff and periscapular musculature. Microinstability can lead to injuries of the anterosuperior labrum.

History

Shoulder pain is a common complaint in the throwing athlete. Often the athlete will have minimal to no pain when not involved in his or her sport. The patient may complain of vague shoulder pain made worse by the overhead or throwing motion. Pain is typically distributed in the deltoid region but may also involve the anterior or posterior aspects of the shoulder joint.

In overhead throwing athletes, the throwing motion can be divided into several stages: wind-up, cocking, acceleration, deceleration, and follow through. Sometimes the cocking phase may be divided into early and late phases. The wind-up is the first part of the pitching motion; it has the most variability from pitcher to pitcher and the there is minimal stress on the shoulder. The early cocking phase starts when the pitcher's hands break and the arm is abducted. The late cocking phase starts when the pitcher's stride leg is planted on the ground and the arm is maximally abducted and externally rotated. In the late cocking phase, there is increased stress on the supraspinatus, infraspinatus, and teres minor. In the acceleration phase, the arm rotates at speeds greater than 7,000 degrees/sec in an explosive action. The late cocking and acceleration phases are the parts of the pitching motion where athletes tend to complain of pain the most. The deceleration phase begins when the ball is released and is the most violent phase of the throwing cycle, with maximal forces on the shoulder joint. The final phase is the follow through where the body moves forward until the arm motion stops.[6] GH joint microinstability causing secondary external impingement occurs during the late cocking and early acceleration phases.

Important Questions

What sport of sports does the athlete play? Participating in any overhead sport such as volleyball, tennis, swimming, javelin, baseball, or softball increases the risk of shoulder pain and rotator cuff pathology. Overhead athletes are more prone to repetitive overuse injuries such as MDI, impingement syndromes, and subluxations. Is your dominant or nondominant shoulder affected? If the athlete is a baseball player, which position does he play? Pitchers are at greater risk than other players, with catchers and shortstops the next most likely positions to develop pain. For pitchers, their age, pitch selection, and arm angle are important. Skeletally immature pitchers throwing breaking pitches such as curveballs and sliders are at increased risk of injury. Pitchers throwing with a three-quarter arm angle instead of straight over the top have an increased risk for shoulder injuries. Previous treatments such as physical therapy, corticosteroid injections, and operative treatments will dictate how best to proceed in this situation.

Evidence-based Physical Examination

The challenge for most providers in evaluation of the shoulder is the large number of examination maneuvers available. Additionally, the overall sensitivity and specificity of each maneuver is generally low. Most maneuvers are better at ruling out a specific condition than ruling it in. Of note, most tests gain greater significance when several tests point toward a specific condition rather than a single isolated test.

The shoulder examination should progress in an organized and coordinated fashion as detailed below to minimize the above issues and arrive at an accurate diagnosis. A thorough neck and neurologic examination should be performed to rule out any potential referred or neurologic source of pain.

Inspection

The first part of the shoulder examination should be inspection of the injured athlete. This should take place with the male athlete's shirt removed or the female athlete in a tank top or sports bra. Inspect the deltoid for lateral flattening which is a sign of atrophy. Inspect the athlete from behind to look for atrophy of the rotator cuff muscles and atrophy of the periscapular muscles. Also look for asymmetry of scapular alignment.

Palpation

Palpate the acromioclavicular joint, subacromial space, biceps tendon, and the shoulder joint capsule for any tenderness.

Range of Motion (ROM)

Normal ROM of forward flexion of the shoulder is from 0° to 170–180°. Normal ROM for shoulder abduction is from 0° to 170–180°. External and internal rotation is evaluated in neutral position. From the posterior view of the patient, observe scapulohumeral rhythm and symmetry of scapular movement (Fig. 11.7).

Strength Testing

The empty can test is a test for supraspinatus weakness. The athlete forward flexes his or her shoulder to 90°, then abducts 30° to the plane of the scaula, and finally internally rotates until his or her thumbs are pointing at the ground. Weakness in the infraspinatus and teres minor is tested in external rotation in neutral against resistance. Internal rotation in neutral against resistance tests for weakness in the

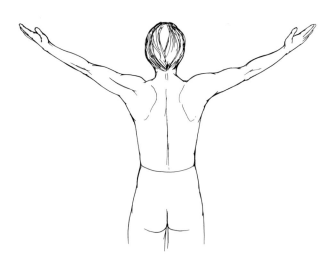

FIG. 11.7. Abduction of the shoulder from posterior view.

subscapularis. Other tests for subscapularis injury/pathology include the lift-off or belly-press tests.

Laxity Tests

Load and Shift Test

The load and shift test is used to confirm anterior and posterior shoulder laxity as well as the amount of translation of the humeral head on the glenoid. This test can be performed with the athletes in the seated or supine position. In the seated position, the athlete places his or her arm on the examiner's hip. The examiner places one hand on the posterior shoulder GH joint and provides an AP force on the humeral head. The examiner's other hand is placed on the athlete's axilla. In the supine position, the patient is placed on the examining table with his or her scapula on the edge of the bed. The humeral head is off the bed to facilitate GH rather than scapulothoracic translation. In either position, the examiner grabs the athlete's arm with both hands—one near the humeral head and one on the forearm near the elbow. The distal hand loads the humeral head. The proximal hand applies an AP force to shift the humeral head. Athletes are given a grade based on the amount of humeral head movement. The modified Hawkins grading is the most common grading method.[7] Grade 0 means there is little or no humeral head movement. Grade 1 is when the humeral head rides up onto the glenoid rim. Grade 2 is when the humeral head can be dislocated but spontaneously relocates. Grade 3 is when the humeral head does not relocate when pressure is removed. It is rare for athletes with stable shoulders to have a positive result of Grade 2 or higher. It is the only test that has been validated to assess anterior and posterior laxity.[7] The load and shift test has a specificity of 100% and a sensitivity of 8% to 50%.[7] It has poor sensitivity in clinical setting, only 41% with unidirectional instability and 26% with bilateral multidirectional instability.[8]

Sulcus Sign

The sulcus test was initially described by Neer and Foster.[7] This test is an indicator of shoulder capsule laxity and laxity of the SGHL. The athlete is in seated position with his or her arm relaxed down the side. The examiner grabs the athlete's elbow and pulls it inferiorly. In a positive test, a dimple appears beneath the acromion as the humeral head moves inferiorly. If the sulcus size is greater than 2 cm, it means the athlete is highly likely to have MDI of shoulder. If the sulcus sign is greater than 1 cm, this test has a sensitivity of 72% and a specificity of 85%. If the sulcus sign is greater than 2 cm, it has a sensitivity of 82% and a specificity of 97%.[7] The likelihood ratio of shoulder instability is 6:1.[8]

Impingement Tests

Neer Impingement Test

The Neer impingement test is a test for impingement of the rotator cuff. The athlete is in seated position and the athlete's arm starts in full internal rotation and in 0° of forward

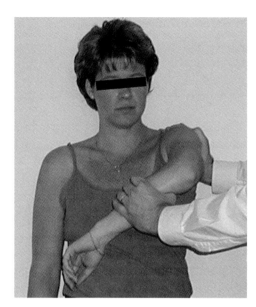

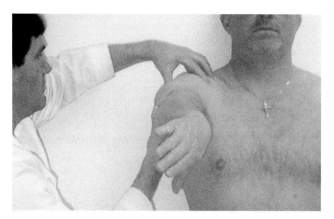

FIG. 11.9. Hawkins impingement test. Reprinted with permission from Berg D, Worzala K. *Atlas of Adult Physical Diagnosis.* Philadelphia: Lippincott Williams & Wilkins; 2006.

FIG. 11.8. Neer impingement test. From Koval KJ, Zuckerman, JD. *Atlas of Orthopaedic Surgery: A Multimedia Reference.* Philadelphia: Lippincott Williams & Wilkins; 2004.

flexion. The examiner passively forward flexes the athlete's arm while in full internal rotation. A positive test produces pain with this motion. A positive test can indicate impingent. It has a low specificity, however, as it can also be positive with tears of the rotator cuff, other rotator cuff pathology, as well as a SLAP lesion (Fig. 11.8).

Hawkins Test

The Hawkins test is primarily a test for impingement of the rotator cuff. The athlete is in seated position with his or her arm forward flexed to 90° and elbow flexed to 90°. The examiner passively internally and externally rotates the athlete's arm while in this position. A positive test produces pain with internal rotation. A positive test indicates impingement of the rotator cuff, other rotator cuff pathology, or a SLAP lesion (Fig. 11.9).

Instability Tests

Apprehension Test

The apprehension test is also known as crank test, fulcrum test, and Feagin maneuver. It was originally described by Rowe and Zarins in 1981.[7] It is used to confirm anterior shoulder instability. The athlete can be sitting or supine. In the starting position, the athlete's shoulder is in 90° of shoulder abduction with elbow bent in 90° of flexion. The examiner places stress on the GH joint by applying an anterior force or an externally rotary force. The examiner progressively externally rotates the shoulder. A positive test is one where the athlete feels the shoulder coming out of the

joint. A positive test is also if the athlete feels pain with this maneuver, which is also a sign of anterior instability.[9] This is a better test for anterior instability when examiner uses apprehension than pain.[10] The sensitivity of this test is 53%. The specificity is 99%. The positive predictive value (PPV) is 98% and the negative predictive value (NPV) is 73%.[9] If the apprehension test is positive for pain, it has 50% sensitivity, 56% specificity, 14% PPV, and 88% NPV.[11] However, if the apprehension test is positive for apprehension, it has 72% sensitivity, 96% specificity, a PPV of 75%, and an NPV of 96%.[10]

Relocation Test

The relocation test is used to differentiate pain secondary to instability and pain for other reasons. It is used to test for anterior shoulder stability. The relocation test was originally described by Jobe in 1989. The athlete can be either seated or supine. It is the second of three instability tests performed after the apprehension test and before the surprise test. The examiner keeps the shoulder in the abducted and maximally externally rotated position. A posteriorly directed force is then applied to the proximal humerus. A negative test is one where the athlete has no difference in symptoms with or without posteriorly directed force. A positive test causes the athlete to have pain prior to application of force and a decrease in the pain or apprehension and tolerance to increased external rotation after application of force.[9] The relocation test fails to differentiate between anterior instability and RCT. The relocation test has a higher specificity or high PPV if the athlete has a positive apprehension test.[10]

The relocation test is a better test for anterior instability when examiner uses relief of apprehension than relief of pain.[10] If the relocation test is positive for relief of pain, it has 49% sensitivity, 90% specificity, a PPV of 19%, and an

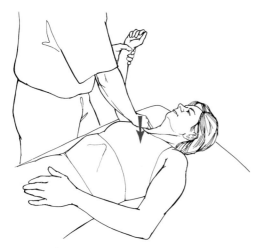

FIG. 11.10. Relocation test.

NPV of 94%. If the relocation test (Fig. 11.10) is positive for relief of apprehension, it has 85% sensitivity, 96% specificity, a PPV of 53%, and an NPV of 98%.[8]

Surprise Test

The surprise test is also known as release test and is the third part of the apprehension/relocation/surprise test series. It was originally described by Silliman and Hawkins in 1993. This test is used to test for anterior shoulder instability. The athlete starts in the same position as that during the end of the relocation test. The examiner quickly removes the posteriorly directed force from the relocation test. It is considered a positive test if the athlete reports pain or apprehension after sudden removal of posteriorly directed force. It is considered to be the most accurate individual examination maneuver.[9] It has 64% sensitivity, 99% specificity, 98% PPV, and 78% NPV. When all three instability tests, apprehension, relocation, and surprise tests, are positive this is highly specific for anterior GH instability.

Shoulder Anterior Drawer Test

The anterior drawer test of the shoulder tests for shoulder laxity. It can be used as a provocative maneuver for anterior shoulder instability. The athlete starts in supine position with the examined shoulder being placed over the edge of the table. The examiner places one hand on athlete's wrist and the other hand on the athlete's proximal humerus. The athlete's shoulder is abducted to 80° and 0° of rotation. An axial load is applied to the arm and the humeral head is translated anteriorly over the glenoid rim. Amount of translation of the humeral head over the glenoid rim is then measured. Translation of the humerus to the glenoid rim but not over it is classified as Grade I. Grade II is translation of the humerus over the glenoid rim that spontaneously reduces. Translation of the humerus over the glenoid rim and the humeral head remaining dislocated when the hand on the humerus is removed is Grade III. A positive test is a Grade II or III translation with reproduction of symptoms of instability.[8] If the test is positive for pain only, it is 28% sensitive, 71% specific, and has a 13% PPV and an 86% NPV for shoulder instability. If the test is positive for Grade II or III laxity, then it is 60% sensitive, 74% specific, and has a 26% PPV and a 92% NPV for anterior shoulder instability.[8]

Shoulder Posterior Drawer Test

The posterior drawer test of the shoulder tests for shoulder laxity (Table 11.2). It is used as a maneuver for posterior shoulder instability. The athlete starts in supine position and the examiner grabs the athlete's forearm with one hand. The athlete's arm is abducted 80° to 120° and the elbow is flexed to 120°. The examiner's other hand is placed on the athlete's scapula. The athlete's arm is flexed to 60° to 80° while the examiner tries to sublux the humeral head posteriorly. Amount of translation of the humeral head over the glenoid rim is then measured. Translation of the humerus to the glenoid rim but not over it is classified as Grade I. Grade II is

TABLE 11.2 **Accuracy of Shoulder Tests for Instability**

Test Name	Sensitivity (%)	Specificity (%)	PPV (%)	NPV (%)
Load and shift test	8–50	100		
Sulcus sign test − >1 cm	72	85		
Sulcus sign test − >2 cm	82	97		
Apprehension test	53	99	98	73
Apprehension test – positive for apprehension	72	96	75	96
Apprehension test – positive for pain	50	56	14	88
Relocation test – relief of pain	49	90	19	94
Relocation test – relief of apprehension	85	96	53	98
Surprise test	64	99	98	78
Anterior drawer test – positive for pain only	28	71	13	86
Anterior drawer test – Grade II or III laxity	60	74	26	92

PPV, positive predictive value; NPV, negative predictive value.

translation of the humerus over the glenoid rim that spontaneously reduces. Translation of the humerus over the glenoid rim and the humeral head remaining dislocated when the hand on the humerus is removed is Grade III. A positive test is a Grade II or III translation with reproduction of symptoms of instability.[8]

SLAP Tear Tests

Active Compression/O'Brien's Test

While there are numerous tests in the literature, the O'Brien's test is one of the most technically easier tests for labral pathology. The athlete starts in seated position and the athlete's arm is positioned in 90° of forward flexion, 10–20° of adduction, and the thumb pointed down in internal rotation. The examiner applies downward pressure on athlete's arm testing for pain in this position. The athlete's arm is then externally rotated until his or her palm is facing upwards. Again the examiner applies downward pressure testing for pain in this position. A positive test produces pain in initial internally rotated position and reduction or elimination of pain in externally rotated palm-up position.[7] Initially, the test was believed to be very accurate for labral pathology and the sensitivity was 100% and specificity was 98%.[7] However, more recent studies have shown that the O'Brien's or active compression test (Fig. 11.11) is only about 40% to 60% sensitive and 50% to 60% specific.[11] This has a better correlation with type II SLAP lesions than with other types of SLAP lesions.[3]

Biceps Tendon Tests

Speed's Test

The Speed's test (Fig. 11.12) is a test for biceps tendon pathology as well as a SLAP lesion. The athlete starts in seated or standing position with his or her arm forward

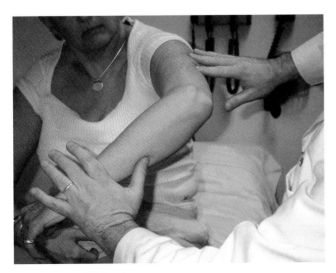

FIG. 11.11. O'Brien's test.

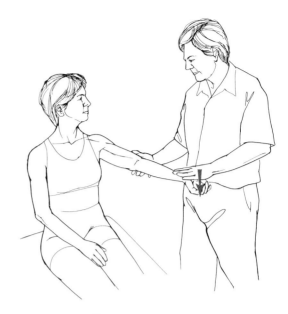

FIG. 11.12. Speed's test.

flexed to 90° with the elbow fully extended and forearm supinated. The examiner provides downward pressure on the arm. A positive test produces pain at the proximal shoulder where the biceps tendon attaches to the superior labrum. A positive test is more suggestive of biceps tendon inflammation or damage; it also can show that there has been damage at the anchor site on the superior labrum.[3]

Putting the tests together, one can start to see patterns consistent with specific conditions found in the overhead or throwing athlete:

SLAP Tears

A positive O'Brien's test indicates a high likelihood of SLAP lesion. A positive Speed's test indicates the possibility of SLAP lesion and biceps tendon damage.

Anterior Instability

The examination indicates anterior instability if there is a positive load and shift test, a positive apprehension test, a positive relocation test, a positive anterior drawer test, and if in the acute presentation the athlete has the arm in abduction and external rotation. With anterior instability also look for axillary nerve injuries.

Posterior Instability

The examination indicates posterior instability if in the acute presentation, the athlete has his or her arm in external rotation, there is posterior joint line tenderness on palpation, there is posterior rotator cuff weakness, there is positive posterior drawer test, there is positive load and shift test for posterior popping and displacement, and there are negative apprehension and relocation tests.

Multidirectional Instability

The examination indicates MDI if there is evidence of generalized ligamentous laxity, there is rotator cuff weakness, there is posterior rotator cuff weakness, there is a positive sulcus test, there are positive anterior and posterior drawer tests with displacement in both directions, and there are positive load and shift tests in both directions.

Diagnostic Testing

Laboratory

Laboratory tests are not indicated in the routine evaluation of shoulder pain in the throwing athlete unless systemic or infectious etiology is suspected.

Imaging

Standard plain radiograph views of the shoulder include a true AP film, an axillary film, and a supraspinatus outlet view or scapular Y view (Fig. 11.13). In the absence of trauma, most radiographs will be normal.

Magnetic resonance imaging (MRI) is indicated when alternative diagnosis is not evident and plain films are negative. A plain MRI will often miss labral injuries or partial rotator cuff tears that can occur in throwing/overhead athletes. A plain MRI has been shown to have a sensitivity between 30% and 50% and a specificity of around 70% to 80% for labral pathology.[12] Therefore, an MRI arthrogram (MRA) is the imaging test of choice in the throwing or overhead athlete with shoulder pain. An MRA involves the injection of contrast agent intra-articularly to better visualize labral pathology. An MRA is 89% sensitive and 91% specific for detecting labral pathology. It also has a 90% PPV for detecting labral pathology.[3]

Other Testing

Examination of shoulder under anesthesia is the ultimate "gold standard" for assessing shoulder laxity. Under anesthesia, the passive stabilizers of the shoulder are tested in isolation. Arthroscopy is the gold standard for assessing labral pathology. Electrodiagnostic testing may be indicated in suspected cases of peripheral nerve injuries about the shoulder as detailed in Chapter 23 Athlete with Peripheral Nerve Injuries.

APPROACH TO THE THROWING OR OVERHEAD ATHLETE WITH A ROTATOR CUFF TEAR

Rotator cuff tears in the throwing/overhead athlete are most commonly seen in older athletes over the age of 40 or athletes participating in collegiate/professional sports. These can be a diagnostic challenge as most are partial or undersurface rotator cuff tears. A high degree of clinical suspicion is necessary in the appropriate population as they may be missed even on MRA. The evaluation and treatment of rotator cuff tears in the athlete is detailed in Chapter 12 Athlete with Overuse Shoulder Pain.

APPROACH TO THE ATHLETE WITH THROWING OR OVERHEAD INTERNAL IMPINGEMENT

Internal impingement is an overuse injury seen almost exclusively in the throwing or overhead athlete. It results from the compression of the articular side of the rotator cuff tendon between the greater tuberosity and the posterosuperior edge of the glenoid. This typically takes place when the shoulder is abducted and is in maximally externally rotated position as seen in the late cocking and early acceleration phase of the throwing cycle. The result of repetitive internal impingement can be undersurface tears of the rotator cuff as well as posterior SLAP fraying and tears. Internal impingement is more closely related to other injuries associated with overhead athletes, such as SLAP lesions (SLAP tears) and anterior laxity/instability, than to subacromial impingement or acromial-sided cuff tears as seen in older patients with overuse syndromes. The evaluation and treatment of internal impingement is reviewed in Chapter 12 Athlete with Overuse Shoulder Pain.

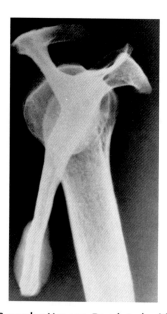

FIG. 11.13. Scapular Y x-ray. Reprinted with permission from Bucholz RW, Heckman JD. *Rockwood & Green's Fractures in Adults.* 5th ed. Philadelphia: Lippincott Williams & Wilkins; 2001.

APPROACH TO THE THROWING OR OVERHEAD ATHLETE WITH CHRONIC INSTABILITY

HISTORY AND PHYSICAL EXAMINATION

If the overhead or throwing athlete complains of chronic instability, it should be asked if there was a history of traumatic dislocation or subluxation in the past. The athlete should report insidious onset of shoulder pain. The direction of instability can be unidirectional, bidirectional, or multidirectional. Often the athlete does not need to stop participating in his or her sport because the pain is not significant enough. Laxity is not necessarily pathologic and in fact is often requisite for sports performance. Objective laxity may be observed in both shoulders while only one may be symptomatic. It is important to assess whether this is generalized or traumatic laxity and what level of energy is required to produce instability. The patient's history will help direct a focused physical examination and development of a differential diagnosis.

Athletes with microinstability often have a normal physical examination. These athletes only have GH translation during high-velocity overhead or throwing motions. If there is some secondary impingement of the rotator cuff, the athlete may have a positive Neer or Hawkins impingement test. One should also perform the laxity tests: sulcus test, load and shift tests, and apprehension, relocation, and surprise tests.

Athletes with MDI will often present with chronic recurrent mild subluxation or gradual onset diffuse shoulder pain. MDI largely affects the young and adolescent overhead (baseball, softball, tennis, swimming) or tumbling athlete (gymnastics, cheering) under the age of 25 years. Pain is described as diffuse in the deltoid region and exacerbated primarily with overhead sporting activities (throwing, tennis serve, gymnastic tumbling). Athletes with MDI will often demonstrate signs of generalized joint laxity on examination including elbow or knee recurvatum as well as thumb to forearm sign. The anterior and posterior load and shift and sulcus tests are used to determine the direction and extent of instability. Apprehension, relocation, and surprise tests are also important for determining the degree of MDI. Neer and Hawkins impingement tests should be performed to see if there is any secondary impingement of the rotator cuff.

DIAGNOSTIC TESTING

Imaging

- Radiographic evaluation
  - A true AP, scapular lateral (Y view), and axillary view are essential

- MRI – not usually necessary for microinstability and MDI
  - Valuable for identifying type, location, and extent of capsuloligamentous injuries
  - Helpful in determining rotator cuff impingement
  - MRI arthrography generally provides the clearest visualization of these capsulolabral lesions

TREATMENT

Nonoperative

- Athletes do not need to be placed in a sling for treatment of shoulder MDI or microinstability
- MDI and microinstability have better success with shoulder-strengthening protocols for nonoperative treatment
- Focus on progressive strength and flexibility reconditioning

Rehabilitation Plan

- Four phases
  - Phase I
    - Rest
    - Nonsteroidal anti-inflammatory drugs (NSAIDs)
    - Ice
  - Phase II
    - Isometric strengthening
    - Isotonic strengthening
    - Begin exercises with shoulder in adduction and forward flexion and progress
  - Phase III
    - Muscular endurance building along with strengthening exercises
    - Goal to progress shoulder strength to 90% of uninjured shoulder
  - Phase IV
    - Increase activity to sport-specific activities
- Strengthen dynamic stabilizers in the shoulder
- In the transverse plane, strengthen
  - Subscapularis
  - Infraspinatus
  - Teres minor
- In the coronal plane, strengthen
  - Anterior head of the deltoid
  - Rotator cuff
- Theraband exercises have been shown to strengthen the rotator cuff
- Improve reactive neuromuscular control
  - Exercise shoulder in positions that maximally challenge the dynamic stabilizers
  - Shoulder in 90° abduction and 90° external rotation

- This position allows for enhanced recruitment of the infraspinatus and teres minor
- Plyometric exercises are one method of achieving this
- Strengthen the periscapular stabilizers such as the trapezius and serratus anterior
  - Four key exercises in scapular strengthening
    - Rowing exercises
    - Scapular plane elevation exercises
    - Press-up with accentuated scapular protraction
    - Push-up with accentuated scapular protraction
- Many overhead athletes also have tight posterior shoulder capsule so rehab should also focus on restoring capsule length by increasing posterior capsule ROM
- For throwing athletes, see Appendix C Interval Throwing Program

Operative

Multidirectional Instability

- Anterior capsular shift – most commonly performed and most successfully reported surgical procedure for MDI
  - Open procedure that involves imbricating the capsular interval between the subscapularis and supraspinatus tendons
  - Has been reported to be successful in small series of patients with subluxation[8]
- Capsular shrinkage
  - Thermal denaturation of collagen
  - Mixed results
- Studies have shown 15% to 40% reduction in length of collagenous tissue when subjected to heat in 65 to 72°C range
- Studies have also shown a loss in load-to-failure strength in thermally denatured collagen fibers
  - Complications
- Transient axillary nerve palsies
- Capsular disruption
  - Long-term evaluation necessary to evaluate this technique[8]
- Most instability repairs can be done either arthroscopically or open
  - Outcomes for arthroscopic and open repair have become comparable
  - Arthroscopic repair has the advantage of not necessitating taking down the subscapularis.
- Examination under anesthesia

Prognosis/Return to Play

- Good prognosis with compliance to physical therapy and home exercise program
- Athletes with MDI who have failed conservative management may often defer surgical treatment till the end

of their competitive season based on symptoms and function
- When athlete has pain-free full ROM
- When athlete has strength at least 90% of uninjured shoulder if unilateral symptoms

Complications/Indications for Referral

The most common complication associated with unstable shoulders is continued episodes of subluxation and dislocation, leading to further damage to the structures within the shoulder joint. Chronic MDI can lead to labral pathology.

APPROACH TO THE THROWING OR OVERHEAD ATHLETE WITH SLAP TEARS

HISTORY AND PHYSICAL EXAMINATION

The throwing athlete with a SLAP tear complains of pain during the acceleration phase of the throwing motion. The pain may have flared up from one specific pitch or may have been more gradual in onset. Athletes with SLAP tears do not complain of pain at rest or at night. The athlete complains of pain moving the arm through the entire ROM.

On examination the athlete tends to have a positive O'Brien's test or active compression test which increases the likelihood of SLAP lesion. The examiner should also perform the tests for laxity and impingement.

DIAGNOSTIC TESTING

Imaging

Plain radiographs are the initial radiograph of choice and should include the AP views with the shoulder in internal and external rotation. The modified axillary view is important in ruling out posterior dislocation. It is also known as the "West Point" view. It has a better visualization of glenoid rim. A fracture of anterior glenoid is bony Bankart lesion. The Stryker notch view is good at showing the presence of a Hill–Sachs defect.

An MRI is indicated when alternative diagnosis is not evident and plain films are negative. A plain MRI will often miss labral injuries or partial rotator cuff tears that can occur in throwing/overhead athletes. A plain MRI has been shown to have a sensitivity between 30% and 50% and a specificity of around 70% to 80% for labral pathology.[12] Therefore, an MRA is the imaging test of choice in the throwing or overhead athlete with shoulder pain. An MRA involves the injection of contrast agent intra-articularly to better visualize labral pathology. An MRA is 89% sensitive and 91% specific for detecting labral pathology. It also has a 90% PPV for detecting labral pathology.[3]

FUNCTIONAL TREATMENT

Nonoperative

For athletes with a documented SLAP tear

- Focus on progressive strength and flexibility reconditioning
- Avoidance of aggravating factors

Rehabilitation Plan

- Four phases
  - Phase I
    - Rest
    - NSAIDs
    - Ice
  - Phase II
    - Isometric strengthening
    - Isotonic strengthening
    - Begin exercises with shoulder in adduction and forward flexion and progress
  - Phase III
    - Muscular endurance building along with strengthening exercises
    - Goal to progress shoulder strength to 90% of uninjured shoulder
  - Phase IV
    - Increase activity to sport-specific activities
- Strengthen dynamic stabilizers in the shoulder
- In the transverse plane, strengthen
  - Subscapularis
  - Infraspinatus
  - Teres minor
- In the coronal plane, strengthen
  - Anterior head of the deltoid
  - Rotator cuff
- Theraband exercises have been shown to strengthen the rotator cuff
- Improve reactive neuromuscular control
  - Exercise shoulder in positions that maximally challenge the dynamic stabilizers
  - Shoulder in 90° abduction and 90° external rotation
  - This position allows for enhanced recruitment of the infraspinatus and teres minor
  - Plyometric exercises are one method of achieving this

- Strengthen the periscapular stabilizers such as the trapezius and serratus anterior
  - Four key exercises in scapular strengthening
    - Rowing exercises
    - Scapular plane elevation exercises
    - Press-up with accentuated scapular protraction
    - Push-up with accentuated scapular protraction
- Many overhead athletes also have tight posterior shoulder capsule so rehab should also focus on restoring capsule length by increasing posterior capsule ROM
- For throwing athletes, see Appendix C Interval Throwing Program

Operative

Labral Pathology/Tears

- Type I SLAP lesions – conservative debridement of frayed labrum
- Type II SLAP lesions – single-anchor, double-suture technique
- Type III SLAP lesions – initial resection of unstable bucket-handle labral fragment and insertion of biceps anchor attachment for stability
- Type IV SLAP lesions– initial resection of unstable bucket-handle labral fragment and insertion of biceps anchor attachment for stability
  - If biceps tendon slip is severe, more than 30% of tendon included with displaced labral tear
  - May need to consider either
    - Repairing the tendon
    - Releasing the tendon and repairing the labral
    - Performing a biceps tenodesis
  - Decision depends on the age and activity of the patient[3]

Prognosis/Return to Play

- Prognosis – fair with nonoperative treatment
- Prognosis – good with surgical intervention
- When athlete has pain-free full ROM
- When athlete has strength at least 90% of uninjured shoulder if unilateral symptoms
- When postsurgical patient has progressed through rehabilitation protocol

Complications/Indications for Referral

Complications are rare but may include numbness and tingling with weakness of deltoid—make sure to evaluate for axillary nerve injury.

KEY POINTS
• Apprehension and relocation tests are more accurate when the definition of a positive test result is apprehension and not pain
• Positive sulcus test is indicative of MDI
• Physical therapy focused on strengthening exercises is mainstay of treatment for athletes with shoulder MDI
• MRA has better sensitivity and specificity than plain MRI for assessing SLAP tears

REFERENCES

1. Burkart AC, Debski RE. Anatomy and function of the glenohumeral ligaments in anterior shoulder instability. *Clin Orthop Relat Res.* 2002;400: 32–39.
2. Luime JJ, Verhagen AP, Miedema HS, et al. Does this patient have an instability of the shoulder or a labrum lesion? *JAMA.* 2004;292(16): 1989–1999.
3. Nam EK, Snyder SJ. Clinical sports medicine update. The diagnosis and treatment of superior labrum, anterior and posterior (SLAP) lesions. *Am J Sports Med.* 2003;31(5):798–810.
4. Maurer SG, Rosen JE, Bosco JA III. SLAP lesions of the shoulder. *Bull Hosp Joint Dis.* 2003–2004;61(3–4):186–192.
5. Sher JS, Uribe JW, Posada A, et al. Abnormal findings on magnetic resonance images of asymptomatic shoulders. *J Bone Joint Surg Am.* 1995;77:10–15.
6. Ouellette H, Labis J, Bredella M, et al. Spectrum of shoulder injuries in the baseball pitcher. *Skeletal Radiol.* 2008;37:491–498.
7. Tzannes A, Murrell GAC. Clinical examination of the unstable shoulder. *Sports Med.* 2002;32(7):447–457.
8. Walton J, Paxinos A, Tzannes A, et al. The unstable shoulder in the adolescent athlete. *Am J Sports Med.* 2002;30:758–767.
9. Lo IKY, Nonweiler B, Woolfrey M, et al. An evaluation of the apprehension, relocation, and surprise tests for anterior shoulder instability. *Am J Sports Med.* 2004;32:301–307.
10. Hegedus E, Goode A, Campell S, et al. Physical examination tests of the shoulder: a systematic review with meta-analysis of individual tests. *Br J Sports Med.* 2008;42:80–92.
11. Dessaur W, Magarey M. Diagnostic accuracy of clinical tests for superior labral anterior posterior lesions: a systematic review. *J Orthop Sports Phys Ther.* 2008;38(6):341–352.
12. Jbara M, Chen Q, Marten P, et al. Shoulder MR arthrography: how, why, when. *Radiol Clin North Am.* 2005;43(4):683–692.

12 Athlete with Overuse Shoulder Pain

Michael Brown

INTRODUCTION

Shoulder pain is one of the most common complaints encountered in a sports medicine clinic. Subacromial or internal impingement and tears of the rotator cuff are the most common causes for shoulder pain. Isolated acromioclavicular (AC) joint degeneration may also cause shoulder pain similar to that of impingement syndrome or rotator cuff tendonopathy. There are many factors that may be related to the development of shoulder pain in the athlete, including anatomy, repetitive motion, fatigue, or altered mechanics of the shoulder.

FUNCTIONAL ANATOMY

At the most basic level, the shoulder is composed of the humerus, the clavicle, and the scapula, which is further divided into the acromion, the coracoid, and the glenoid. The shoulder consists of four different articulations: the sternoclavicular (SC), the AC, the glenohumeral, and the scapulothoracic. The combination of motion at these articulations allows for the greatest range of motion of any joint in the body, with the majority of the stability of the joints coming from the surrounding soft-tissue elements.

The clavicle serves to connect the upper extremity with the axial skeleton. The SC joint is the only true synovial joint in the shoulder complex and lacks bony stability. The AC joint also has a combination of capsular and ligamentous stabilizers, consisting of the joint capsule to prevent anterior/posterior translation, with the named AC ligaments being thickenings of this capsule. The trapezoid coracoclavicular ligament prevents posterior translation and contributes to superior stability with the conoid coracoclavicular ligament.[1]

The scapula has many muscular attachments that secure its position on the thorax and is otherwise only held in position by the AC and coracoclavicular ligaments. The muscles involved include the trapezius, levator scapulae, serratus anterior, pectoralis minor, and the rhomboids. The motion achieved by these muscles allows the scapula to be positioned for maximal stability of the glenohumeral joint during upper extremity motion, namely maintaining the glenoid under the humeral head. The scapulothoracic rhythm is defined as the relative motion between the scapulothoracic articulation and the glenohumeral joint during abduction of the arm. Over the entire arc of abduction, the glenohumeral joint moves more, but the difference is far greater at the beginning of abduction than at the end.[2]

The glenohumeral joint is surrounded by the rotator cuff muscles, which are the primary dynamic stabilizers of this joint (Fig. 12.1). The supraspinatus originates in the posterior–superior scapula, just superior to the scapular spine, and runs under the acromion to insert onto the greater tuberosity of the humerus.

It is active throughout scapular-plane abduction of the arm, and loss of innervation by the suprascapular nerve will lead to a 50% loss in abduction torque.[3] The infraspinatus and teres minor run together from their origination on the posterior scapula, just inferior to the scapular spine, to their insertion on the posterior aspect of the greater tuberosity. They work together during external rotation and extension of the humerus. The infraspinatus is primarily involved when the arm is at the side, and the teres minor is the major muscle for external rotation when the shoulder is elevated 90 degrees.[4] The tendinous insertions of these three muscles, the supraspinatus, infraspinatus, and teres minor, are not separate at the level of the greater tuberosity. The subscapularis is the fourth rotator cuff muscle. It originates on the anterior surface of the scapula and inserts on the lesser tuberosity of the humerus. Contraction leads to internal rotation and flexion of the humerus.

The deltoid is the largest of the glenohumeral muscles. It has a tripennate origin from the clavicle, acromion, and scapular spine and inserts midway down the lateral humerus on the deltoid tubercle. The anterior portion of the deltoid performs forward flexion and contributes to abduction. The posterior portion extends and adducts the humerus, while the middle portion abducts the arm. It is possible for the deltoid to fully abduct the arm without supraspinatus involvement. Loss of the deltoid through paralysis of the axillary nerve results in a 50% loss of abduction torque.[3]

The biceps brachii originate from the scapula, with the long head originating from the superior articular margin of the glenoid, where it joins with the labrum within the

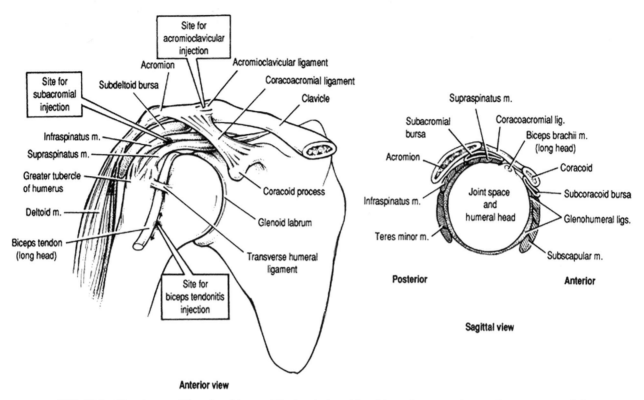

FIG. 12.1. Structures of the shoulder and their relationships. Note the acromion and coracoacromial ligaments, which may impinge on the supraspinatus tendon on abduction of the arm. Note the location for subacromial injection into the bursa and about the rotator cuff tendons. Adapted from Pansky B. *Review of Gross Anatomy.* New York: Macmillan; 1979.

synovial sheath; the short head originates from the coracoid, where it joins with the tendon of the coracobrachialis to form the conjoined tendon. Because the muscle extends from the scapula to the elbow, it traverses both the shoulder and the elbow and can therefore have effects at both joints. At the elbow, the biceps are the primary supinators and have a large role in flexion as well. The long head of the biceps serves as an active stabilizer of the glenohumeral joint as it passes along the bicipital groove on the humeral head and onto the glenoid.[5] This position allows it to act as a restraint to superior migration of the humeral head as well as anterior migration of the head.[6] This action becomes extremely important in the presence of a massive rotator cuff tear.

The bony anatomy of the glenohumeral joint itself is what allows for such a large range of motion, but it provides only minimal stability. The humeral head is slightly elliptical and is larger in the vertical dimension. The articular surface typically forms a 150- to 160-degree arc; it is 45 degrees from the shaft and is retroverted 30 degrees relative to the transcondylar axis of the distal humerus.[7–9] The glenoid is also larger in the vertical dimension and is angled slightly superiorly and posteriorly to the plane of the scapula.

The glenohumeral capsular and ligamentous structures provide the majority of the static stability for the glenohumeral joint. The joint capsule has nearly twice the surface area of the humeral head, which allows for a large range of motion.[10] Depending on the position of the arm, selective portions of the capsule become taut to provide support for

the humeral head; when the arm is by the side, the superior capsule is tight and the inferior capsule is loose. There are three anterior glenohumeral ligaments (GHLs), which provide reinforcement for the anterior capsule; they are named for their humeral insertions: superior, middle, and inferior. The superior GHL prevents inferior subluxation when the arm is at the side.[11] The middle GHL resists anterior translation with the arm in 45 degrees of abduction and external rotation.[12] The inferior GHL acts as a sling for the humeral head; with the arm abducted and externally rotated, the anterior band limits anterior translation as well as inferior subluxation; the posterior band becomes helpful in limiting inferior subluxation when the arm is abducted more than 45 degrees.[11,13]

The labrum is the final soft-tissue structure important for glenohumeral joint stability through its wide range of motion. It is positioned on the periphery of the glenoid and is the insertion point for the capsuloligamentous structures discussed earlier.[14] Through its position, it increases the surface area of the glenoid and deepens the socket by 50%.[15]

EPIDEMIOLOGY

Problems with the shoulder joint, specifically impingement and tearing of the rotator cuff tendon, tend to increase with patient age. A study done in 1995 found that only 4% of asymptomatic patients between the age of 19 and 39 had a partial-thickness tear of the rotator cuff and there were no full-thickness tears. This is in comparison to 28% incidence of full-thickness tears and 26% incidence of partial-thickness tears in asymptomatic patients over the age of 60.[16]

Patients at increased risk of developing impingement syndrome and rotator cuff tendonopathy include both athletes and laborers. Any sport that involves overhead activity will place a player at risk; these include tennis, volleyball, baseball, golf, football (quarterbacks), and swimming. Laborers, such as carpenters, mechanics, or painters, who perform the majority of their work overhead are also at increased risk.

NARROWING THE DIFFERENTIAL DIAGNOSIS

The differential diagnosis of shoulder pain includes rotator cuff disorders (tendonopathy, partial-thickness or full-thickness tears), glenohumeral instability (more common in younger overhead athletes), cervical radiculopathies, calcific tendonitis, adhesive capsulitis, degenerative joint disease of the glenohumeral or AC joints, and peripheral nerve compression.[17]

History

Common complaints related to the shoulder will include feelings of stiffness, weakness, pain (typically anterolateral or posterolateral), or sleep disturbance. Pain is typically exacerbated by any sort of overhead activity, such as putting things away in overhead cabinets/shelves. Decreased endurance, accuracy, or speed is a common complaint among overhead athletes. Many women will report difficulty styling their hair. Any or all of these symptoms may be found in patients with AC joint arthritis, subacromial impingement, internal impingement, or tears of the rotator cuff tendon.

Patients with isolated AC joint arthritis present with symptoms that are consistent with all of the most common shoulder pathologies: dull ache over the deltoid area and pain with motion of the shoulder. Reaching for something in front of the opposite shoulder (cross-body adduction) is the most irritating to patients with as yet isolated AC joint arthritis.

In subacromial impingement, patients typically complain of pain, generally in the anterior/superior aspect of the shoulder. Depending on the time course, they may also report weakness and/or stiffness of the affected shoulder. Subacromial impingement is typically insidious in onset. However, some patients may report an acute event that led to traumatic bursitis that eventually develops into a chronic impingement syndrome. A complete history will be helpful in the diagnosis: location of pain, timing of pain (day or night), activities that exacerbate/alleviate pain, treatment modes already attempted (therapy, medications, injections, activity modifications, operations). Remember, true subacromial impingement is typical in patients over the age of 40. In younger patients, other diagnoses, such as glenohumeral instability, labral pathology, or internal impingement, should be considered.

Internal impingement is a source of posterior shoulder pain and can mimic both subacromial impingement as well as rotator cuff tears. However, internal impingement most frequently occurs in overhead athletes younger than 40 years of age. Symptoms of internal impingement are similar to those of subacromial impingement, with a slow, insidious onset of shoulder pain eventually leading to subjective weakness and stiffness of the affected shoulder. The major difference, however, is the location of the pain. Internal impingement typically presents with posterior shoulder pain, as opposed to anterior pain associated with subacromial impingement. Pain is usually associated only with the specific activity that brings the shoulder into the offending position of external rotation, abduction, and extension. Pitchers may specifically report an increase in the time required for warm-up or decreased endurance.[18]

Tears of the rotator cuff may be partial- or full-thickness. Interestingly, a recent study found that 73% of patients with partial-thickness tears reported significant and severe pain at night, as compared to only 50% of patients with full-thickness tears. Comparing preoperative patients' complaints with intraoperative findings, this same study also found that bursal-sided tears tended to cause more pain than intratendinous or articular-sided tears.[19] Patients over the age of 40 who suffer a traumatic dislocation are at high risk for having an acute rupture of the rotator cuff. Typically, however, rotator cuff tears are more indolent and chronic in nature, with a progression from subacromial or internal impingement to partial tears to full-thickness tears. Patients may have waxing and waning symptoms depending on their activity levels, and many patients will have made lifestyle adaptations to avoid the pain associated with the pathology.

Evidence-based Physical Examination

Examination of the shoulder should always include examination of both shoulders and begins with simple inspection. The shoulders should be exposed as much as possible while maintaining patient modesty. Standing behind the patient, inspect the scapula and periscapular muscles. Look for any evidence of scapular winging or muscle atrophy in the supraspinatus or infraspinatus fossa. Obvious muscle atrophy in the rotator cuff muscles can be helpful in the diagnosis of a full-thickness tear of the tendon but may also be linked to peripheral nerve compression syndromes, such as the infraspinatus wasting seen in patients with glenoid notch cysts. In a study of 400 patients, it was found that patients who had supraspinatus weakness, weakness in external rotation, and a positive impingement sign had a 98% probability of having a rotator cuff tear.[20]

Ask the patient to raise his or her arms over the head and observe the motion of the scapulae in relation to each other as well as in relation to the glenohumeral joint—is it a smooth motion or does the patient have to manipulate his or her shoulder to be able to achieve maximal elevation? Notice if any local muscles, such as the trapezius, have been recruited to help with shoulder motion. During this time you should also examine the skin for any overlying lesions or changes or any obvious masses. In AC joint arthritis, a painful arc will be noted in a range that is higher in elevation (120 to 180 degrees) compared to the painful arc noted with cuff impingement (60 to 120 degrees).[21]

Next, palpate potential areas of pain and inflammation to see if this will recreate or elicit the patient's pain. These areas include the long head of the biceps as it passes along the anterior humeral head in the bicipital groove, the tendinous insertion of the rotator cuff muscles on the greater tuberosity, the AC joint, and the posterior shoulder. Leaving a hand over the shoulder while passively or actively moving the shoulder will allow the examiner to assess for crepitus related to degenerative joint disease, which will often accompany shoulder impingement to some degree. This is again an important time to rule out any underlying masses or abnormalities that would need to be investigated further.

There are multiple tests described to attempt to diagnose shoulder impingement or to highlight weakness in the various rotator cuff muscles. However, they are not all equal in terms of their sensitivity and specificity and, therefore, their clinical usefulness. In 2005, Park et al.[22] tested eight different common examination techniques in patients with varying degrees of rotator cuff pathology: bursitis without a tear,

partial-thickness cuff tear, and full-thickness cuff tear. There have been a few studies to compare the accuracy of these tests in patients with simple bursitis versus any degree of cuff tear, but Park's study is the only one that divided the cuff tear group into partial or complete tears based on intraoperative findings. The tests, described in subsequent paragraphs, include the Neer impingement sign, Hawkins impingement sign, painful arc sign, supraspinatus muscle strength test, Speed test, cross-body adduction test, drop-arm sign, and infraspinatus muscle strength test (Fig. 12.2).

The Neer impingement sign (Fig. 12.2A) is defined as pain with passive forward flexion of the arm until either full elevation is reached or the patient expresses pain in the anterior/lateral shoulder. It is considered a positive test if the pain arises during forward flexion of 90 to 140 degrees.[23]

The Hawkins–Kennedy impingement sign (Fig. 12.2B) starts with the arm at 90 degrees of forward flexion and the elbow bent. The arm is then brought into internal rotation until either the patient describes pain or rotation of the scapula is observed. This test is considered positive when the patient expresses pain during the maneuver.

The painful arc sign asks the patient to actively elevate the arm in the scapular plane until full elevation is achieved and

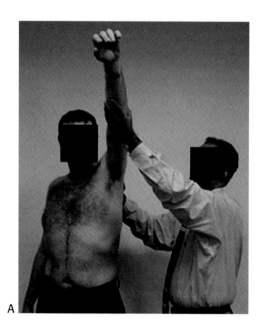

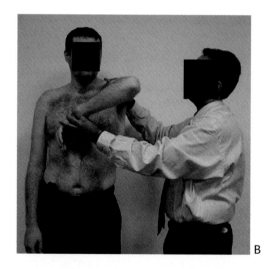

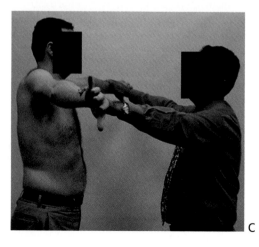

FIG. 12.2. Provocative maneuvers for rotator cuff pathology. **A.** Neer impingement test performed by forward flexing the arm, with the scapula stabilized, until pain is experienced or full flexion is achieved. **B.** Hawkins–Kennedy sign performed with the arm flexed to 90 degrees and then being forcibly internally rotated. **C.** Supraspinatus strength testing performed with the arm elevated to 90 degrees within the scapular plane and being in internal rotation or neutral. Forced abduction is resisted by the physician.

then lower the arm in the same plane. It is considered positive if the patient notices pain or catching between 60 and 120 degrees of elevation.

Next, the supraspinatus muscle test (Fig. 12.2C) attempts to isolate this muscle from the other cuff muscles. The patient is asked to elevate his or her arm to 90 degrees and either maintain neutral or slight internal rotation. The examiner then attempts to resist the patient's active abduction of the arm. This test is positive if the patient is unable to sustain the contraction due to pain/weakness.

The Speed test starts with the patient fully extending his or her elbow and then elevating the arm to 90 degrees of forward flexion. The forearm is maintained in full supination while the examiner applies a downward force. Again, pain, or inability to resist the downward force, is considered positive.

The cross-body adduction test brings the arm to 90 degrees of forward flexion and then adducts the arm across the body. A positive test is defined by pain during this maneuver.

The drop-arm sign begins with the patient elevating the arm to full forward flexion and then slowly reversing the same arc against gravity. If the arm drops abruptly or, again, the patient expresses pain during this maneuver, the test is positive.

The infraspinatus muscle strength test tries to isolate out a specific cuff muscle. The arms are left down by the side and the elbows are flexed to 90 degrees. The patient is asked to externally rotate his or her forearms against the examiner's resistance, while keeping the elbows locked at his or her side. Again, weakness against resistance or pain during the maneuver defines a positive test. Alternatively, the patient may be asked to keep his or her elbows bent at the side as described and then to maximally externally rotate the forearms and hold this position. It is also a positive test if the patient is unable to hold this position.

The results of Park's study show that for patients with tendonitis or bursitis, but no cuff tear, the Neer impingement sign was most sensitive (85.7%); it also had the highest positive predictive value at 20.9% and the highest negative predictive value at 95.7%. The cross-body adduction test had the best overall accuracy, 73.1%, and the highest specificity, 79.7%.

In patients with a partial-thickness rotator cuff tear, the Neer and the Hawkins–Kennedy signs had the best sensitivity at 75.4%, but poor overall specificity at 48% and 44%, respectively. The Neer sign also had the highest positive predictive value (18.1%) and the highest negative predictive value (92.6%). Again, however, the cross-body adduction test had the highest specificity (78.5%) and the best overall accuracy at 70.8%. All of the positive predictive values were below 20%, but the negative predictive values were all above 86%.

Finally, in the patients found to have full-thickness rotator cuff tears at the time of surgery, the drop-arm sign was the most specific test, with a specificity of 87.5%. The painful arc sign remains very helpful, with a sensitivity of 75.8% and a high negative predictive value of 76.4%. The specific tests for the supraspinatus and the infraspinatus had the highest positive predictive values, 68.0% and 69.1%,

respectively, as well as the best overall accuracy in this group, both around 70%.

Regression analysis helped the authors to determine that if a patient has a positive Hawkins–Kennedy impingement sign, a painful arc sign, and a positive infraspinatus muscle test, the posttest probability of the patient having any degree of impingement syndrome was 0.95. If these tests are all negative, the likelihood of that patient having any degree of impingement syndrome is less than 24%. If a patient has a positive painful arc sign, drop-arm sign, and infraspinatus muscle test, the likelihood of the patient having a full-thickness rotator cuff tear was greater than 91%. If these three tests are negative, then the likelihood of the presence of a full-thickness tear is less than 9%.

Diagnostic Testing

Imaging

There are multiple studies available to aid in determining the etiology of shoulder pain. Evidence of fracture or dislocation can be seen on plain radiographs, and these are critical diagnoses to rule out before proceeding with the development of treatment plans. Plain radiographs are also helpful to determine the type of acromion present or to diagnose an os acromiale, which may predispose patients to subacromial impingement. A diagnosis of calcific tendonitis can also be made on plain x-ray.

Magnetic resonance imaging (MRI) is a common imaging modality currently used for evaluation of shoulder pain (Fig. 12.3). A recent meta-analysis looked at 29 different

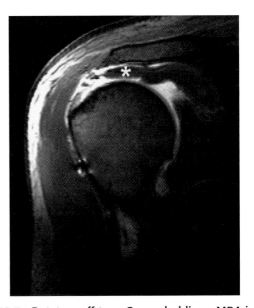

FIG. 12.3. Rotator cuff tear. Coronal oblique MRA image demonstrating shredding and atrophy of the supraspinatus tendon (*) with extravasation of contrast into the subdeltoid bursa. Reprinted with permission from Daffner RH. *Clinical Radiology: The Essentials.* 3rd ed. Philadelphia: Lippincott Williams & Wilkins; 2007.

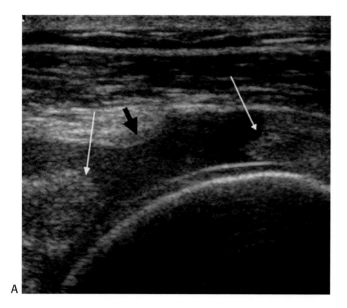

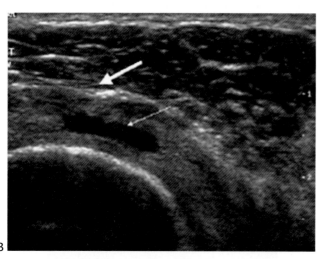

FIG. 12.4. Ultrasound of the rotator cuff. **A.** Transverse scan of full-thickness supraspinatus tear. Tear margins (*white arrows*) are irregular but well defined. The edge of the articular cartilage (*thin curved white line*) deep to the defect. **B.** Partial-substance tear (*thin arrow*) of supraspinatus.

cohort studies and found that for a full-thickness rotator cuff tear, MRI had a sensitivity of 0.89 and a specificity of 0.93. For partial-thickness tears, however, the sensitivity dropped to 0.44, and specificity remained high at 0.90.[24] However, the use of MR arthrography (MRA) increased the sensitivity to 0.84 and the specificity to 0.96 in another study on partial-thickness tears.[25] MRI, including arthrogram, should be used when a tear of the rotator cuff tendon is suspected or when there is concern of additional pathologies, such as superior labral (SLAP) tears or Bankart lesions, based on history and physical examination. However, MRI are not necessary in the setting of isolated degenerative disease or impingement syndrome.

Ultrasound has also been described in the diagnosis of partial-thickness and full-thickness rotator cuff tears (Fig. 12.4). It can offer an inexpensive alternative but does not provide the same amount of information regarding possible concomitant pathologies of the shoulder. Results using ultrasound have also been found to be extremely dependent on the skills of the operator.[26] A 2005 study found that the preoperative accuracy of ultrasound was similar to that of MRI, with 70% and 73% accuracy, respectively.[27] Ultrasound does offer the unique ability to perform functional imaging of the rotator cuff to assess for impingement.

APPROACH TO THE ATHLETE WITH ARTHRITIS OF THE ACROMIOCLAVICULAR JOINT

HISTORY AND PHYSICAL EXAMINATION

The AC joint is a diarthrodial joint, with the concave articular surface of the acromion articulating with the convex distal clavicle. There is an intra-articular disc, but this is frequently incomplete or absent.[28] Degeneration of this joint is a natural consequence of aging and has been found to begin as early as in the second decade.[29] Also, the inferior surface of the joint directly contacts the subacromial bursa and rotator cuff and can therefore play a role in the development of subacromial impingement.[21] Biomechanical studies have demonstrated that at 60 degrees of shoulder abduction, the rotator cuff begins to contact the undersurface of the AC joint, and by 70 degrees, it is directly underneath the joint.[30] It is easy to understand, then, why inferior osteophytes resulting from degeneration of the AC joint will cause pain when elevating the arm and irritation and tearing to the supraspinatus tendon.

DIAGNOSTIC TESTING

- Radiographic evaluation
  - Subchondral cysts, sclerosis, osteophyte formation, and joint-space narrowing consistent with degeneration of the joint
  - Findings may also be present in asymptomatic patients
  - Weighted stress views for acute injury are helpful to diagnose and classify an injury to the AC ligaments and resulting joint instability
- MRI
  - AC joint arthritis presents as capsular hypertrophy, effusions, and subchondral edema on an MRI
- Interventional testing
  - Injection of local anesthetic can be used as a diagnostic aid. If AC joint arthritis is the source of the pain, the patient's symptoms are completely alleviated within minutes of the injection

• It is most important to remember that the patient needs to be symptomatic at the time of the injection for it to be useful

TREATMENT

Nonoperative

• Anti-inflammatory medication
  • Activity modification
  • Physical therapy—strengthen surrounding musculature
  • Correct joint mechanics
• Corticosteroid injections—indicated if relief provided by local anesthetic injection
  • Evidence suggests bridging solution[31]
  • 93% initial relief
  • 67% ultimately required surgical intervention

Operative

• Both open and arthroscopic distal clavicle excision have proven successful at relieving AC joint arthrosis

Prognosis/Return to Play

• Pain is the only impediment to return to activity

Complications/Indications for Referral

Alterations in joint mechanics related to pain may lead to increased risk for other injuries.

APPROACH TO THE ATHLETE WITH SUBACROMIAL IMPINGEMENT SYNDROME

HISTORY AND PHYSICAL EXAMINATION

Subacromial impingement is understood to be the pathologic or painful contact between the rotator cuff, the subacromial bursa, and the undersurface of the anterior acromion. It is typically a combination of overuse and early degenerative changes and therefore is typically a disease of patients over the age of 40. It is one of the most common causes of shoulder pain and is one of the most frequent reasons patients seek medical attention.

Subacromial impingement syndrome is thought to be the beginning of a continuum of disease states that ultimately ends with a complete tear of the rotator cuff tendon. Neer described three different stages of impingement: (i) edema and hemorrhage of bursa and tendon found in younger patients; (ii) irreversible changes of fibrosis and tendonitis found in patients 25 to 40 years of age; and (iii) partial or complete tears of the rotator cuff tendon, typically in patients greater than 40 years of age.[32] Neer felt that 90% to 95% of rotator cuff tears resulted from a narrowing of the supraspinatus outlet due to a hooked acromion or spur formation at the acromion or AC joint that forced this pathologic contact between bone and tendon. Bigliani described three different types of acromion based on lateral radiographs and direct observation of cadaveric dissections. A type I acromion (17%) is flat, type II (43%) is curved, and type III (40%) is hooked. His group found a substantially higher number of full-thickness rotator cuff tears in the shoulders with a type III acromion.[33]

It has also been proposed, however, that in the setting of a repetitive motion/activity, subacromial impingement has a multifactorial etiology, including patient age, work conditions, and shoulder mechanics, in addition to patient anatomy as described by Neer. Work-related factors are always important to consider when entertaining a diagnosis of subacromial impingement syndrome. Things to investigate are the arm position during work, the amount of weight lifted on a regular basis, and the number of daily repetitions.[34]

Biomechanical studies have demonstrated that in a shoulder with impingement syndrome, active elevation of the arm causes greater superior migration of the humeral head, which contributes to the propagation of the disease. Between 60 and 90 degrees of elevation, the humeral head is most likely to migrate superiorly due to contraction of the deltoid. This is the range, therefore, where the rotator cuff muscles/tendons must work the hardest to prevent superior migration and are therefore at greatest risk for injury.[35] Repetitive overhead activities require a significant amount of endurance from the scapular rotators/stabilizers to maintain efficient glenohumeral mechanics. Fatigue of these muscles may cause increased force transmission to the rotator cuff muscles and therefore contribute to the development of tendonitis/bursitis and resultant subacromial impingement syndrome. Dysrhythmic scapulothoracic motion also compounds the issue by failure of the acromion to rotate with the humerus, which causes further diminution of space available in the subacromial area.[36] Repetitive overhead activities, either work- or sport-related, will likely produce soft-tissue inflammation, particularly in the setting of poor mechanics or inappropriate conditioning. This decreases the amount of space available for the cuff tendon and contributes to friction and increasing wear and microtrauma to the tendon; this is the most likely etiology of impingement syndrome in a younger patient/athlete.[33]

A complete examination of the affected and unaffected shoulder should be performed as described previously in this chapter. As mentioned, there are multiple tests to help differentiate the diagnosis from the spectrum of impingement through rotator cuff tears, but none are especially sensitive or specific. The result of each test, considered in concert, helps to formulate the diagnosis. A specific examination of the neck and associated nerve roots should be carried out to rule out a cervical etiology for shoulder pain or a concomitant problem. The Neer impingement sign and cross-body adduction maneuver have the best statistical results for diagnosing bursitis/tendonitis and the absence of a cuff tear. The pain associated with impingement syndrome can sometimes cloud the picture and mimic the weakness typically found in rotator cuff tears. In addition, patients typically avoid activities that cause pain, and this can lead to stiffness and loss of range of motion in the affected shoulder.

DIAGNOSTIC TESTING

- Radiographic evaluation
  - Complete plain radiographs of the shoulder should be performed and the type of acromion identified on the lateral projection
  - An axillary view may demonstrate an unfused acromial epiphysis, or os acromiale, which can be a cause of impingement syndrome
- MRI
  - An MRI will be useful to ensure that a rotator cuff tear is not missed
- Interventional testing
  - An injection of local anesthetic can be helpful in the diagnosis of subacromial impingement
  - Alleviation of the patient's pain and, possibly, improvement in his or her strength after injection of lidocaine into the subacromial space can be diagnostic
- Alternative imaging
  - Ultrasound and CT arthrography can be used as alternative imaging studies if MRI is not tolerated or is contraindicated

TREATMENT

Nonoperative

- Initial treatment
  - Activity modification
  - Anti-inflammatory medication
  - Physical therapy
  - Scapular stabilization
  - Rotator cuff strengthening
- Corticosteroid injection
  - 6 to 7 months relief[37]
  - Pain control
  - Improved range of motion

Operative

- Surgical consultation recommended if nonoperative measures fail at 6 months

- Subacromial decompression
- Removal/flattening of the anterior acromion
- Excision of subacromial bursa
- Creation of more space for the rotator cuff tendon
- Predictable return to activities[38]

Prognosis/Return to Play

- Pain-free full range of motion
- Full strength

Complications/Indications for Referral

Untreated or undertreated impingement syndrome can potentially lead to shoulder stiffness, recurrence or chronic pain, and ultimately progression to a full rotator cuff tear.

APPROACH TO THE ATHLETE WITH INTERNAL IMPINGEMENT

HISTORY AND PHYSICAL EXAMINATION

Internal impingement occurs when the articular side of the rotator cuff tendon is compressed between the greater tuberosity and the posterosuperior edge of the glenoid. This typically takes place when the shoulder is abducted 60 to 90 degrees and in maximal external rotation and horizontal extension, as in the cocking/acceleration phase of the pitching cycle.[39] With improper conditioning of the antagonizing subscapularis and laxity of the anterior stabilizers, namely the inferior GHL and anterior capsule, or with simple overuse and fatigue, this contact between the glenoid and the articular surface of the rotator cuff becomes pathologic.[40] Because of this, internal impingement is more closely related to other injuries associated with overhead athletes, such as SLAP lesions (SLAP tears) and anterior laxity/instability, than with subacromial impingement or acromial-sided cuff tears as seen in older patients with overuse syndromes. It has also been suggested that subtle instability is actually a major contributing factor to the development of internal impingement and articular-sided rotator cuff lesions.[41]

Physical examination and radiographic studies are carried out as usual for shoulder pain. However, the most specific sign of internal impingement is eliciting the same pain experienced by the patient by bringing the arm into the position of injury. By observing scaption, the abduction of the arms in the scapular plane, the examiner may notice significant alteration in the motion of the affected shoulder. The patient with more advanced internal impingement will compensate for pain/weakness of the rotator cuff muscles by "hiking" the shoulder and using more scapular motion than normal to elevate the arm. The Jobe relocation test may also be positive, suggesting that anterior laxity and instability are leading contributors to the pathogenesis of internal impingement.[40] The history and symptoms described by the patient are very useful in diagnosing internal impingement.

DIAGNOSTIC TESTING

- See section "Approach to the Athlete with Subacromial Impingement Syndrome"

TREATMENT

Nonoperative

- Initial treatment
  - Activity modification
  - Anti-inflammatory medication
  - Intra-articular glenohumeral cortisone injection
    - Useful in initial management in inflammation reduction[42]
- Physical therapy
  - Initiated once pain and inflammation under control
  - Restoration of normal shoulder mechanics
  - Synchronization of scapulothoracic and glenohumeral motion
  - Rotator cuff strengthening—subscapularis and periscapular muscles
  - Posterior capsule stretching of critical importance[40]

Operative

- Reserved for patients who have failed rigorous nonoperative management
- Examination under anesthesia[40]
  - Diagnose instability as underlying cause for internal impingent
  - Guide postoperative rehabilitation
- Arthroscopic evaluation and possible debridement of pathologic structures

Prognosis/Return to Play

- Completion of the rehabilitation program
- Full range of motion and strength

Complications/Indications for Referral

Similar to external impingement, untreated internal impingement can lead to stiffness, pain, and full-thickness rotator cuff tears.

APPROACH TO THE ATHLETE WITH TEARS OF THE ROTATOR CUFF TENDON

HISTORY AND PHYSICAL EXAMINATION

Next, in this spectrum of disease states that affect the shoulder of an athlete is a rotator cuff tear, either partial or complete. Ellman developed a classification and grading system for partial-thickness tears based on findings at the time of arthroscopy. He classified partial tears as bursal, articular, or interstitial depending on their location and assigned a grade based on the depth of the tear. A grade I tear is less than 3 mm deep, a grade II tear is 3 to 6 mm deep, and a grade III tear is greater than 6 mm deep.[43]

At this time, it is typically accepted that there are intrinsic and extrinsic factors that lead to partial rotator cuff tears. The first is the extrinsic etiology as described by Neer, where patients with subacromial narrowing and impingement eventually develop tearing in the supraspinatus tendon.[32] Recently, the increased understanding of internal impingement has led many to believe that there are specific intrinsic factors that lead to the articular-sided tears. In older patients, this would be related to osteophyte formation and degenerative changes of the glenohumeral joint; and in younger patients, this is related to the pathologic association between the tendon and the superoposterior glenoid associated with excessive external rotation, extension, and abduction.[26]

The current understanding of partial rotator cuff tears is that they typically do not heal and will likely progress over time. A study evaluating articular-sided partial tears with arthrography found that 53% of the tears grew bigger, while 28% became complete full-thickness tears. Surprisingly, 10% of patients had a decrease in the size of the tear, and an additional 10% had their tear "disappear."[44]

Physical examination of a patient with a rotator cuff tear will reveal weakness in the rotator cuff muscles, specifically the supraspinatus, with associated weakness of external rotation. Patients also typically have positive impingement signs. It is often difficult to distinguish between a partial-thickness and full-thickness tear. Atrophy of the rotator cuff muscles is one sure sign of disuse of these muscles related to a chronic full-thickness tear of the tendon. Frank inability to actively raise the arm above the level of the shoulder is also indicative of a full-thickness tear in the setting of normal passive motion.

DIAGNOSTIC TESTING

Radiographic Imaging

- Anteroposterior (AP), lateral, axillary, and supraspinatus outlet views are recommended

- MRI should be obtained in all patients suspected of having a rotator cuff tear (Fig. 12.3)
  - Provides the most information about the shoulder joint
- Ultrasound can be helpful if MRI is not possible due to implantable devices in diagnosing rotator cuff pathology (Fig. 12.4)
- CT arthrogram is an alternative if MRI and ultrasound are unavailable

TREATMENT

Nonoperative

- Initial treatment
  - Activity modification
  - Anti-inflammatory medication
  - Physical therapy
    - Scapular stabilization
    - Rotator cuff strengthening
    - Regain/retain full range of motion
  - Partial-thickness tears may require 12 to 18 months of therapy for a completely successful outcome[26]
  - Nonoperative modalities yield unpredictable results for full-thickness tear
    - Should be considered for initial management in all patients
    - Less likely to succeed in long-standing disease[45]
- Corticosteroid injection
  - No evidence-based indication for management in rotator cuff disease[46]

Operative

- Surgical consultation recommended if nonoperative measures fail or pain worsens
- Surgery should be considered in the face of objective weakness and substantial functional limitations
- Arthroscopic evaluation
- Debridement of tear
  - Repair if tear is complete or felt to be nearly complete
- Subacromial decompression with acromioplasty
  - If external impingement thought to be a factor

Prognosis/Return to Play

- Postoperative rehabilitation will depend largely on the findings at surgery
  - 6 weeks to 6 months
- Phase I (0 to 6 weeks)
  - Protecting the repair
  - Gradually increasing passive range of motion
  - Pendulum exercises
- Phase II (week 6 to week 12)
  - Progress to active range of motion
  - Avoid strengthening exercises

- Phase III (week 12 to week 16)
  - Strengthening exercises can begin
  - Weights less than 5 lb
  - Scapulothoracic motion and shoulder stability are emphasized
  - Return to functional activities is encouraged
- Phase IV
  - Sport-specific exercises
  - Improve strength and endurance
  - Return to full activity assuming successful pain-free completion of each phase[47]

Complications/Indications for Referral

Prognosis for patients whose symptoms have been present for greater than 1 year, who have large full-thickness tears, and who present with functional weakness or significant disability in the affected shoulder will be poor. Therefore, in the setting of objective weakness and substantial functional limitations, surgical repair is indicated sooner rather than later regardless of the duration of symptoms to achieve the best possible outcome. Unlike the results for surgical intervention in subacromial impingement, workman's compensation status appeared to have a negative impact on the results of surgical repair of rotator cuff tears.

KEY POINTS
• Internal impingement occurs in overhead athletes younger than 40 years of age due to pathologic contact between the articular surface of the rotator cuff tendon and the posterosuperior glenoid (intrinsic)
• Subacromial impingement is an overuse injury associated with overhead activity in patients older than 40 years of age that causes a narrowing of the subacromial space related to chronic bursitis and inflammation as well as acromion morphology (extrinsic)
• Management should begin with conservative measures: rest, activity modification, physical therapy, and anti-inflammatory medications, with or without corticosteroid injection
• Presentation with objective weakness, significant disability, and symptom duration of greater than 1 year predicts poor prognosis in the repair of rotator cuff tears
• Restoration/maintenance of full range of motion and normal joint kinematics are the mainstays of treatment for shoulder pain
• Results and recovery from rotator cuff repair involve intensive physical therapy and effort on the part of the patient, and it can often take up to a year before return to full activity

REFERENCES

1. Lee KW, Debski RE, Chen CH, et al. Functional evaluation of the ligaments at the acromioclavicular joint during anteroposterior and superoinferior translation. *Am J Sports Med.* 1997;25:858–862.
2. Poppen NK, Walker PS. Normal and abnormal motion of the shoulder. *J Bone Joint Surg Am.* 1976;58:195–201.
3. Colachis SC, Strohm BR. Effect of suprascapular and axillary nerve blocks on muscle force in upper extremity. *Arch Phys Med Rehabil.* 1971;52:22–29.
4. McMahon PJ, Tibone JE. Functional anatomy and biomechanics of the shoulder. In: *DeLee and Drez's Orthopaedic Sports Medicine: Principles and Practice.* 2nd ed. Philadelphia: Saunders; 2003.
5. Andrews JR, Carson WG Jr, McLeod WD. Glenoid labrum tears related to the long head of the biceps. *Am J Sports Med.* 1985;13:337–341.
6. Rodosky MW, Rudert MJ, Harner CH, et al. Significance of a superior labral lesion of the shoulder: a biomechanical study. *Trans Orthop Res Soc.* 1990;15:276.
7. Jobe CM, Iannotti JP. Limits imposed on glenohumeral motion by joint geometry. *J Shoulder Elbow Surg.* 1995;4:281–285.
8. Iannotti JP, Gabriel JP, Schneck SL, et al. The normal glenohumeral relationships. An anatomical study of one hundred and forty shoulders. *J Bone Joint Surg Am.* 1992;74:491–500.
9. Inman V, Saunders M, Abbott L. Observations on the function of the shoulder joint. *J Bone Joint Surg Am.* 1944;27:1–30.
10. DePalma A. *Surgery of the Shoulder.* Philadelphia: JB Lippincott; 1983.
11. Warner JJP, Deng XH, Warren RF, et al. Static capsuloligamentous anatomy of the glenohumeral joint. *J Shoulder Elbow Surg.* 1993;2:115–133.
12. Turkel SJ, Panio MW, Marshall JL, et al. Stabilizing mechanisms preventing anterior dislocation of the glenohumeral joint. *J Bone Joint Surg Am.* 1981;63:1208–1217.
13. Warner JJP, Deng XH, Warren RF, et al. Superior–inferior translation in the intact and vented glenohumeral joint. *J Shoulder Elbow Surg.* 1993;2:99–105.
14. Moseley HF, Overgaard B. The anterior capsular mechanism in recurrent anterior dislocation of the shoulder: morphological and clinical studies with special reference to the glenoid labrum and glenohumeral ligaments. *J Bone Joint Surg Br.* 1962;44:913–927.
15. Howell SM, Galinat BJ. The glenoid-labral socket. A constrained articular surface. *Clin Orthop Relat Res.* 1989;243:122–125.
16. Sher JS, Uribe JW, Posada A, et al. Abnormal findings on magnetic resonance images of asymptomatic shoulders. *J Bone Joint Surg Am.* 1995;77:10–15.
17. Bigliani LU, Levine WN. Current concepts review: subacromial impingement syndrome. *J Bone Joint Surg Am.* 1997;79:1854–1868.
18. Jobe CM. Superior glenoid impingement. Current concepts. *Clin Orthop Relat Res.* 1996;330:98–107.
19. Fukuda H. Partial-thickness rotator cuff tears: a modern view on Codman's classic. *J Shoulder Elbow Surg.* 2000;9:163–168.
20. Murrell GA, Walton JR. Diagnosis of rotator cuff tears. *Lancet.* 2001;357:769–770.
21. Chen AL, Rokito AS, Zuckerman JD. The role of the acromioclavicular joint in impingement syndrome. *Clin Sports Med.* 2003;22:343–357.
22. Park HB, Yokota A, Gill HS, et al. Diagnostic accuracy of clinical tests for the different degrees of subacromial impingement syndrome. *J Bone Joint Surg Am.* 2005;87:1446–1455.
23. Neer CS II. Anterior acromioplasty for the chronic impingement syndrome in the shoulder: a preliminary report. *J Bone Joint Surg Am.* 1972;54:41–50.
24. Dinnes J, Loveman E, McIntyre L, et al. The effectiveness of diagnostic tests for the assessment of shoulder pain due to soft tissue disorders: a systematic review. *Health Technol Assess.* 2003;7:1–166.
25. Meister K, Thesing J, Montgomery WJ, et al. MR arthrography of partial thickness tears of the undersurface of the rotator cuff: an arthroscopic correlation. *Skeletal Radiol.* 2004;33:136–141.
26. Wolff AB, Sethi P, Sutton KM, et al. Partial-thickness rotator cuff tears. *J Am Acad Orthop Surg.* 2006;14:715–725.
27. Iannotti JP, Ciccone J, Buss DD, et al. Accuracy of office-based ultrasonography of the shoulder for the diagnosis of rotator cuff tears. *J Bone Joint Surg Am.* 2005;87:1305–1311.
28. Buttaci CJ, Stitik TP, Yonclas PP, et al. Osteoarthritis of the acromioclavicular joint: a review of anatomy, biomechanics, diagnosis, and treatment. *Am J Phys Med Rehabil.* 2004;83:791–797.
29. DePalma AF. The role of the disks of the sternoclavicular and acromioclavicular joints. *Clin Orthop Relat Res.* 1959;13:222–233.
30. Cuomo F, Kummer FJ, Zuckerman JD, et al. The influence of acromioclavicular joint morphology on rotator cuff tears. *J Shoulder Elbow Surg.* 1998;7:555–559.
31. Jacob AK, Sallay PI. Therapeutic efficacy of corticosteroid injections in the acromioclavicular joint. *Biomed Sci Instrum.* 1997;34:380–385.
32. Neer CS II: Impingement lesions. *Clin Orthop Relat Res.* 1983;173:70–77.
33. Bigliani LU, Morrison DS, April EW. The morphology of the acromion and its relationship to rotator cuff tears. *Orthop Trans.* 1986;10:228.
34. Cohen RB, Williams GR Jr. Impingement syndrome and rotator cuff disease as repetitive motion disorders. *Clin Orthop Relat Res.* 1998;351:95–101.
35. Deutsch A, Altchek DW, Schwartz E, et al. Radiologic measurement of superior displacement of the humeral head in the impingement syndrome. *J Shoulder Elbow Surg.* 1996;5:186–193.
36. Warner JJ, Micheli LJ, Arslanian LE, et al. Scapulothoracic motion in normal shoulders and shoulders with glenohumeral instability and impingement syndrome. *Clin Orthop Relat Res.* 1992;285:191–199.
37. Blair B, Rokito AS, Cuomo F, et al. Efficacy of injections of corticosteroids for subacromial impingement syndrome. *J Bone Joint Surg Am.* 1996;78:1685–1689.
38. Nicholson GP. Arthroscopic acromioplasty: a comparison between workers' compensation and non-workers' compensation populations. *J Bone Joint Surg Am.* 2003;85:682–689.
39. Walch G, Liotard JP, Boileau P, et al. Postero-superior glenoid impingement. Another impingement of the shoulder. *J Radiol.* 1993;74:47–50.
40. Jobe CM. Posterior superior glenoid impingement: expanded spectrum. *Arthroscopy.* 1995;11:530–536.
41. Davidson PA, Elattrache NS, Jobe CM, et al. Rotator cuff and posterior–superior glenoid labrum injury associated with increased glenohumeral motion: a new site of impingement. *J Shoulder Elbow Surg.* 1995;4:384–390.
42. Krishnan SG, Hawkins RJ. Rotator cuff and impingement lesions in adult and adolescent athletes. In: *DeLee and Drez's Orthopaedic Sports Medicine: Principles and Practice.* 2nd ed. Philadelphia: Saunders; 2003.
43. Ellman H. Diagnosis and treatment of incomplete rotator cuff tears. *Clin Orthop Relat Res.* 1990;254:64–74.
44. Yamanaka K, Matsumoto T. The joint side tear of the rotator cuff. A follow up study by arthrography. *Clin Orthop Relat Res.* 1994;304:68–73.
45. Oh LS, Wolf BR, Hall MP, et al. Indications for rotator cuff repair. *Clin Orthop Relat Res.* 2007;455:52–63.
46. Koester MC, Dunn WR, Kuhn JE, et al. The efficacy of subacromial corticosteroid injection in the treatment of rotator cuff disease: a systematic review. *J Am Acad Orthop Surg.* 2007;15:3–11.
47. Millett PJ, Wilcox RB III, O'Holleran JD, et al. Rehabilitation of the rotator cuff: an evaluation-based approach. *J Am Acad Orthop Surg.* 2006:14:599–609.

Athlete with Elbow Pain

Michelle Mariani and Ethan Healy

INTRODUCTION

Elbow pain is a common complaint among athletes that can result from acute or chronic conditions. From a diagnostic standpoint, the majority of elbow injuries in athletes occur from chronic processes with an insidious onset; however, some may be acutely exacerbated by a distinct insult. Building a differential diagnosis will depend on the site of the elbow pain and what activities the patient is involved in. A significant proportion of throwing athletes may experience elbow pain, which must be taken seriously and expands the differential significantly. Athletes involved in racquet or stick-based sports are also prone to overuse injuries, while contact and collision sports see the majority of acute elbow injuries.

FUNCTIONAL ANATOMY

Osteology of the Elbow

The elbow joint is a hinge (ginglymus) joint formed by the articulation of the distal humerus and the two bones of the forearm, the radius, and the ulna. The trochlea of the humerus, medially, forms an intrinsically stable hinge joint with the trochlear notch of the proximal ulna. The olecranon process proximally and the coronoid process distally form the trochlear notch. Laterally, the radioulnar joint is made up of the articulation of the capitellum of the humerus and the radial head. This joint is important for supination and pronation of the forearm. The elbow has a slight valgus configuration (5 to 7 degrees), referred to as the "carrying angle."

Ligaments of the Elbow

Although the bony structures of the elbow confer an inherently stable joint, the collateral ligaments account for roughly half of the elbow's varus–valgus stability. The medial (or ulnar) collateral ligament (MCL or UCL) contains a strong anterior bundle and is important in resisting valgus deformation at the elbow (Fig. 13.1). The lateral (or radial) collateral ligament (LCL or RCL) stabilizes against varus force at the elbow and contains the lateral UCL, important for rotational stability of the elbow (Fig. 13.2).

Muscles at the Elbow

The muscles responsible for flexion of the elbow are anterior and include the brachialis, biceps brachii, and brachioradialis. Elbow extension is controlled by the triceps and anconeus, posteriorly. Supination of the forearm is accomplished by the extensor–supinator complex, arising from the lateral epicondyle of the humerus. This muscle group includes the extensor digitorum, extensor digiti minimi, extensor carpi ulnaris, and the "mobile wad of three" (extensor carpi radialis longus [ECRL], extensor carpi radialis brevis [ECRB], and brachioradialis). The flexor–pronator mass arising from the medial epicondyle includes the flexor carpi radialis, flexor carpi ulnaris, flexor digitorum superficialis, and pronator teres and is important in pronation of the forearm.

Vasculature at the Elbow

The arterial supply to the hand and forearm passes anterior to the elbow. The brachial artery travels anterior to the brachialis muscle and branches into the ulnar and radial arteries in the cubital fossa. The ulnar artery enters the forearm deep to the pronator teres, while the radial artery follows underneath the medial border of the brachioradialis.

Nerves at the Elbow

The radial nerve lies between the brachialis and the brachioradialis along the anterolateral aspect of the elbow. It divides into the posterior interosseous nerve (PIN) and the superficial radial nerve as it crosses the elbow. The PIN dives between the two heads of the supinator, or arcade of Frohse, and the superficial radial branch follows the undersurface of the brachioradialis distally. The median nerve lies anterior to the elbow joint and enters the forearm by diving between the two heads of the pronator teres. The ulnar nerve lies posterior to the elbow joint, along the medial aspect of the humerus, in the cubital tunnel. It enters the anterior compartment of the forearm by passing posterior to the medial epicondyle and through the two heads of the flexor carpi ulnaris.

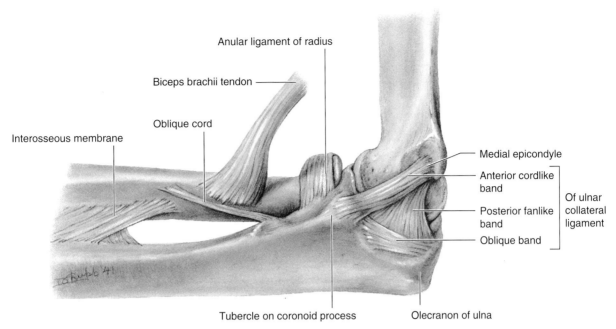

Medial view

FIG. 13.1. Ulnar (medial) collateral ligament. Reprinted with permission from Moore KL, Dalley AF II. *Clinical Oriented Anatomy.* 4th ed. Baltimore: Lippincott Williams & Wilkins; 1999.

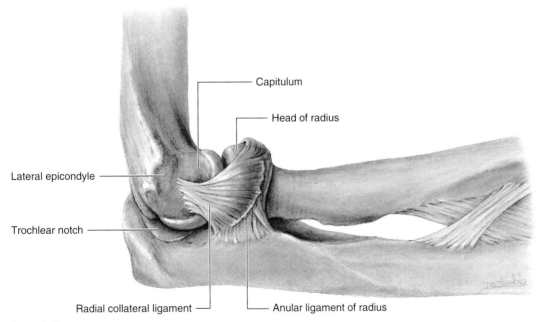

Lateral view

FIG. 13.2. Radial (lateral) collateral ligament. Reprinted with permission from Moore KL, Dalley AF II. *Clinical Oriented Anatomy.* 4th ed. Baltimore: Lippincott Williams & Wilkins; 1999.

EPIDEMIOLOGY

Elbow injuries are becoming more common as more people participate in throwing and racquet sports. The type of injury that is encountered depends, to some extent, on the type of athletic pursuit. The injuries can be roughly grouped into the enthesopathies/tendinopathies (lateral and medial epicondylitis and other rarer similar conditions), valgus stress injuries from repetitive throwing, and peripheral nerve injuries (from repetitive compression or tension). The epidemiology and incidence of specific conditions are detailed under the particular diagnosis in the second half of the chapter.

NARROWING THE DIFFERENTIAL DIAGNOSIS

History

The hallmark of an athletic elbow injury is pain at the elbow. The pain frequently radiates distally and is accentuated by palpation over the area of maximal tenderness. Those affected typically may complain of a "cramping" pain in the dorsal forearm over the flexor or extensor muscles. In addition, neurologic symptoms may be present. Weakness may be present in the muscles innervated by the posterior interosseous, including the digital, thumb, and wrist extensors. A throwing athlete with UCL instability will present with a history of medial-sided pain often associated with the late-cocking and acceleration phase of throwing. Pitchers may report a loss of "pop" on the ball. A history of grinding, catching, or locking may indicate the presence of loose bodies, posterolateral impingement, or chondromalacia. Ulnar nerve symptoms have been associated with chronic medial instability.

Evidence-based Physical Examination

Inspection

The elbow should first be inspected for any gross abnormalities or deformities. The entire upper extremity should be exposed to search for any signs of previous trauma, deformity, muscular tone, and skin changes. The carrying angle is the angle made by the upper arm and forearm when the patient stands with palms facing forward. This should be a valgus angle of roughly 11 degrees in men and 13 degrees in women. Overhand pitchers may have a significant increase in this angle as compared to the nondominant arm.[1] A decrease in this angle is referred to as cubitus varus or a "gunstock" deformity, while an increase in the angle is called cubitus valgus.

Palpation

The four major bony landmarks should be palpated to look for tenderness, swelling, and crepitus. The medial epicondyle is found along the medial aspect of the distal humerus and is the insertion of the flexor–pronator mass as well as the UCL. The olecranon is a subcutaneous bony process at the posterior aspect of the ulna. Check this structure for any overlying swelling or bogginess that would suggest an inflammation in the overlying bursa. Posterior to the medial epicondyle and lateral to the olecranon, the ulnar nerve can be palpated in its groove known as the cubital tunnel. In addition, palpate the olecranon fossa just proximal to the olecranon as well as the proximal border of the olecranon for osseous irregularities. Along the lateral border of the distal humerus, the lateral epicondyle can be palpated. This is the site of insertion of the extensor–supinators including the "mobile wad of three." Two to three centimeters distal to the lateral epicondyle, the radial head can be palpated. The examiner can ask the patient to pronate and supinate the forearm to palpate most of its surface.

Range of Motion

The normal range of motion of the elbow is as follows: flexion of 135 degrees or above, extension to at least 0 degree, supination to 90 degrees, and supination to 90 degrees.[2] Strength testing should be employed in all planes of motion at the elbow, in addition to at the wrist, hand, and digits to examine for the presence of neurologic deficits or muscular weakness.[3]

Special Tests

There are several examination maneuvers that are important in diagnosing specific injuries to the elbow joint. These will be explained in order to construct a more thorough examination.

Tinel Test

The ulnar nerve can be assessed at the cubital tunnel. Tapping over the nerve along the groove of the cubital tunnel resulting in distal conduction of pain, paresthesias, or numbness is considered a positive test. A positive test suggests nerve irritation and/or inflammation from compression at the elbow.[4]

Valgus Stress Test

The valgus stress test is important in assessing the competency of the UCL of the elbow. The elbow must be placed at 15 to 25 degrees of flexion in order to unlock the olecranon from the olecranon fossa. The test is performed by cupping the patient's elbow with one hand, while holding the distal forearm/wrist with the other hand and applying a valgus-producing force across the elbow. A positive test is confirmed when gapping is detected along the medial aspect of the elbow, as compared to the unaffected side. Medial-sided pain without excessive gapping may be elicited when a UCL sprain is present.[2,5]

Test for Tennis Elbow

The test for the presence of lateral epicondylitis involves attempting to reproduce the discomfort of this elbow injury. Stabilize the patient's elbow and proximal forearm while palpating the lateral epicondyle with one hand. With the other hand, resist wrist extension. The test is considered positive when pain is reproduced at the lateral epicondyle approximately 0.5 cm distal, medial, and anterior to the midpoint of the condyle.[6,7] Medial epicondylitis can be tested for in a similar way, by palpating the medial epicondyle while resisting wrist flexion/pronation.

Valgus Extension Overload Test

The valgus extension overload test is employed to determine the presence of an olecranon osteophyte impinging on the olecranon fossa. With the elbow in full extension, a valgus-directed force is imparted across the elbow. Posteromedial pain signifies a positive test. In addition, tenderness or crepitus along the posteromedial olecranon suggests the presence of osteophytes or loose bodies in this area.[6]

Diagnostic Testing

Laboratory

Routine serology is not required unless an autoimmune etiology is suspected. Lyme titers should be considered for an atraumatic effusion in endemic areas. Fluid analysis including cell count and cultures is often indicated in the setting of a suspected intra-articular infection. Fluid analysis for crystals should be obtained if clinical presentation is suspicious for gout.

Imaging

Plain radiographs are the initial imaging test, particularly in the setting of potential acute fracture and dislocation. X-ray may also show evidence of bony ligament avulsion on the anterior, medial, or lateral sides. The lateral radiograph lends information about the congruency of the joint. Radiographs may show osteophytes or calcific bodies.

Computerized topography (CT) is also very useful in the evaluation of the acute elbow injury. It gives very fine definition of the bony structures of the elbow and can confirm evidence of an effusion. It is also helpful for the evaluation of an occult fracture.

Magnetic resonance imaging (MRI) has shown to be useful in many acute elbow injuries. MRI gives outstanding detail and the precise location of ligament and chondral injuries. It is useful in delineating the presence of a discrete macroscopic tear versus the presence of microscopic damage and inflammation, as evidenced by high signal intensity on T2 images. MRI study can be helpful in preoperative planning. MRI examination can be helpful in identifying a space-occupying lesion, can show mass effect on the nerve atrophy and diffuse hyperintensity of the muscles affected on T2 imaging.

MRI arthrography is the test of choice in evaluating for potential UCL injury, articular cartilage injury, or presence of a loose body.

Musculoskeletal ultrasound is growing in popularity due to its high resolution of tendon and ligament structures about the elbow. It can be used in a dynamic fashion to assess for UCL injury. Its high resolution of superficial structures allows for superior imaging of the tendons about the elbow, including the diagnosis of tendinosis and partial tendon tears. Its use is limited by access to trained physicians and sonographers.

Other Testing

Electromyography (EMG) studies may confirm the diagnosis of a peripheral nerve injury about the elbow, although neurodiagnostics early in the course of the disorder are frequently normal.

APPROACH TO THE ATHLETE WITH MEDIAL EPICONDYLITIS (GOLFER'S ELBOW)

Medial epicondylitis, or "golfer's elbow," is a tendinosis of the origin of the flexor–pronator mass at the medial epicondyle of the distal humerus. It is the most common cause of medial elbow pain, with an annual incidence of four to seven cases per 1,000 patients.[8,9] It is twice as common in men as women, has a typical age range of 35 to 54 years, and has a propensity to occur in throwers, racquet sport athletes, golfers, swimmers, and bowlers.[5]

HISTORY AND PHYSICAL EXAMINATION

Athletes will typically complain of pain over the proximal, medial forearm, centered at the medial epicondyle. Grip strength may be reduced. Onset is usually insidious. Palpation just distal and anterior to the medial epicondyle will elicit pain. In addition, resisted wrist flexion and pronation will reproduce the patient's symptoms.

DIAGNOSTIC TESTING

Diagnostic imaging is typically unnecessary. Plane radiographs are usually normal, although traction spurs at the medial epicondyle can be seen on rare occasions. MRI findings include thickening and increased signal intensity of the common flexor tendon and soft tissue edema around the common flexor tendon.[10] Musculoskeletal ultrasound is excellent at demonstrating tendon thickening and hypoechoic areas consistent with tendinosis as well as tendon partial tears.

TREATMENT

Nonoperative

- Conservative measures are commonly reported to be successful in 85% to 90% of cases
- Splinting
- Activity modification
- Nonsteroidal anti-inflammatory drugs (NSAIDs)
- Counterforce bracing
- Physical therapy
- Corticosteroid injections (care must be taken to avoid the ulnar nerve)[11]
- Ultrasound (not shown to be effective)[12]

- Shock-wave therapy (not shown to be effective)[12]
- Laser therapy (early results are promising)[13]

Operative

- Surgical referral should be considered if conservative management is unsuccessful after 6 months.
- Surgical treatment involves removing the diseased portion of tendon, repairing the defect, and securing the tendon to its insertion at the medial epicondyle.

Prognosis/Return to Play

- Most athletes with medial epicondylitis will recover with nonoperative methods of treatment.
- If surgical treatment is needed, most patients can expect a full recovery and a return to sport. Most authors report successful surgical results in over 85% of cases.[14,15]

Complications/Indications for Referral

It is important not to miss a more serious derangement of the elbow such as an UCL injury or an ulnar nerve entrapment at the elbow. Ulnar nerve pathology at the elbow can be concomitant with medial epicondylitis.

APPROACH TO THE ATHLETE WITH LATERAL EPICONDYLITIS (TENNIS ELBOW)

Lateral epicondylitis, commonly known as "tennis elbow," is a tendinosis at or near the origin of the extensor–supinator muscles at the lateral epicondyle. Tennis elbow is the most common cause of lateral elbow pain and typically has an incidence reported to be one to three per 100. The ECRB insertion is usually cited as the culprit and may be damaged by abrasion against the lateral capitellum.[16] This damage in the form of microscopic tears to the ECRB results in fibroblastic and vascular proliferation and disordered repair of the tendon.[17] Lateral epicondylitis has a high incidence in racquet athletes (up to 50%), equal frequency among men and women, and a typical age range of 35 to 55 years.

HISTORY AND PHYSICAL EXAMINATION

The hallmark of lateral epicondylitis is pain at the lateral elbow, usually 5 mm distal and anterior to the lateral epicondyle. The pain frequently radiates distally and is accentuated by palpation over the area of maximal tenderness.

Extending the elbow and resisting the wrist extension and/or supination reproduces the discomfort.

DIAGNOSTIC TESTING

Radiographs are typically normal, but may show osteophytes or calcification at the lateral epicondyle in one fifth of patients.[5] MRI is useful in delineating the presence of a discrete macroscopic tear in the common extensor insertion versus the presence of microscopic damage and inflammation at the origin, as evidenced by high signal intensity on T2 images. MRI study can be helpful in preoperative planning and can identify the presence of a tear in the extensor origin, although the significance of this finding has not been established in the literature. Musculoskeletal ultrasound is excellent at demonstrating tendon thickening and hypoechoic areas consistent with tendinosis as well as tendon partial tears.

TREATMENT

Nonoperative

- Conservative measures are successful in approximately 90% of cases
- Rest
- Ice
- Activity modification
- NSAIDs[18]
- Counterforce bracing[19]
- Physical therapy[20]
- Acupuncture (short-term benefit in pain improvement)[21]
- Shock-wave therapy[22]
- Autologous blood injection or platelet rich plasma injection

Operative

- If nonoperative treatments fail after 6 months, surgical referral should be considered.
- Operative management typically involves excision of the diseased area of tendon, with or without a limited lateral epicondylectomy (Fig. 13.3).
- Rehabilitation should include an active physical therapy regimen, similar in nature to the nonoperative protocol. Results from case series show success in roughly 80% of cases, although there are currently no controlled trials comparing surgical intervention to another treatment available in the literature.[23]

Prognosis/Return to Play

- Return to sport is determined on a case-by-case basis.
- Athletes may return to their respective sports when they can actively grip a racquet or similar object.

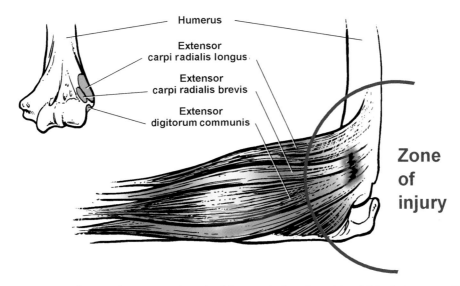

FIG. 13.3. Tennis elbow release. Reprinted with permission from Koval KJ, Zuckerman JD. *Atlas of Orthopaedic Surgery: A Multimedial Reference.* Philadelphia: Lippincott Williams & Wilkins; 2004.

- The vast majority of athletes are able to return to their sports after completing a conservative course of treatment.
- Most authors suggest a gradual return to sport after an initial 12-week postoperative recovery phase is complete.

Complications/Indications for Referral

It is important to recognize a more serious problem concomitant with tennis elbow. PIN entrapment syndrome may mimic or occur simultaneously with lateral epicondylitis. In addition, radiocapitellar pathology can account for symptoms similar to tennis elbow.

APPROACH TO THE ATHLETE WITH POSTERIOR INTEROSSEOUS NERVE ENTRAPMENT SYNDROME

PIN syndrome is caused by compression of the PIN as it passes the proximal edge of the supinator muscle, at the arcade of Frohse (Fig. 13.4). This peripheral nerve entrapment is uncommon and can be found to occur in athletes who perform repetitive supination and pronation cycles of the forearm, such as racquet athletes, discus throwers, and rowers.[24]

HISTORY AND PHYSICAL EXAMINATION

PIN entrapment can often be confused with lateral epicondylitis. To further cloud the picture, the two disorders can occur concomitantly in up to 5% of patients. Those affected typically complain of a "cramping" pain in the dorsal forearm, over the extensor muscles. The pain is usually significantly *distal* to the lateral epicondyle and lacks the classical maximally tender pressure point seen in tennis elbow. In addition, neurologic symptoms may be present. Weakness may be present in the muscles innervated by the posterior interosseous, including the digital, thumb, and wrist extensors. The ECRL is always spared, while the extensor carpi ulnaris is always affected.[25]

DIAGNOSTIC TESTING

Plain radiographs are generally normal. MRI examination can be helpful in identifying a space-occupying lesion that could account for a PIN entrapment, but usually shows mass effect on the nerve atrophy and diffuse hyperintensity of the muscles affected on T2 imaging. EMG is of limited utility due to the deep location of the PIN.[25]

TREATMENT

Nonoperative

- Rest
- NSAIDs
- Activity modification
- Physical therapy

Operative

- If symptoms persist without improvement for 3 months or if motor symptoms worsen, referral should be made to an upper extremity surgeon.

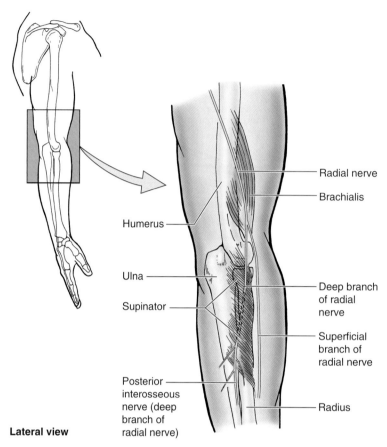

Lateral view

FIG. 13.4. Posterior interosseous nerve. Reprinted with permission from Moore KL, Dalley AF II. *Clinical Oriented Anatomy.* 4th ed. Baltimore: Lippincott Williams & Wilkins; 1999.

- A recent surgical release of the radial nerve/PIN at the elbow resulted in excellent outcomes in 77% of patients, while recovery was considered good in 20%.[26]

Prognosis/Return to Play

- Duration of symptoms, and therefore avoidance of sports, can be somewhat unpredictable in nonoperative patients.
- It is common to allow a graduated resumption of activities after symptoms have ceased.
- A return to sport after surgical release is typically acceptable after the affected extremity regains 80% strength as compared to the unaffected side.
- Eight to twelve weeks is a reasonable time period to expect this return of strength and should include a brief period of immobilization, restoration of range of motion, followed by strengthening.

Complications/Indications for Referral

A patient with motor weakness of the wrist and digital dorsiflexors should be taken seriously, and close clinic follow-up is important. Progression of motor symptoms and/or the presence of a PIN palsy are indications for surgical referral.

APPROACH TO THE ATHLETE WITH CUBITAL TUNNEL SYNDROME

Ulnar nerve entrapment at the elbow, commonly referred to as cubital tunnel syndrome, occurs from pressure placed on the ulnar nerve as it crosses the medial side of the elbow. The ulnar nerve becomes compressed at the cubital tunnel, which is located between the medial epicondyle and the olecranon. The arcuate ligament, or Osborne's ligament, forms the roof of the tunnel. Flexion at the elbow narrows the cubital tunnel by 55% and subsequently increases intraneural pressure.[27] Cubitus valgus increases the risk of cubital tunnel syndrome because the extra length the nerve must travel places increased stretch on the ulnar nerve. This disorder is associated with overhead throwing and is produced by traction injury to the nerve during valgus deformation of the elbow during the late-cocking and early acceleration phases. Cubital tunnel syndrome is the second most common nerve compression syndrome of the upper extremity, behind carpal tunnel syndrome. Men are more likely to be affected. Throwers with UCL injury/insufficiency will often present with symptoms of cubital tunnel syndrome. It is essential, therefore, in throwing athletes with cubital tunnel syndrome to rule out coexisting UCL injury.

HISTORY AND PHYSICAL EXAMINATION

Patients with cubital tunnel syndrome will typically complain of numbness and/or paresthesias in the ulnar-most digits (small and ring fingers) and medial elbow pain. On examination, sensory changes in the ring and small digits and weakness of the intrinsic muscles may be detected, especially with finger abduction.[4] Tinel test at the cubital tunnel is frequently positive. It is also important to palpate for subluxation of the ulnar nerve at the elbow during flexion–extension cycles. Careful ligamentous examination is also important to rule out any valgus laxity, which increases the incidence of ulnar neuropathy at the elbow.

DIAGNOSTIC TESTING

Plane radiographs are helpful in identifying any structural abnormalities or osteophytes at the cubital tunnel. EMG studies may confirm the diagnosis, although neurodiagnos-

tics early in the course of the disorder are frequently normal.

TREATMENT

Nonoperative

- Rest.
- Activity modification.
- Avoidance of inciting events (prolonged periods of elbow flexion, throwing) is important in conservative management. Overhead athletes such as baseball pitchers, racquet athletes, and volleyball players must avoid these activities temporarily.
- NSAIDs.
- Splinting (especially at night) in near extension.
- Physical therapy.

Operative

- Surgical release of the cubital tunnel is indicated.
- Open or endoscopic decompression in situ.
- Subcutaneous transposition of the ulnar nerve, intramuscular or submuscular transposition, and submuscular transposition with medial epicondylectomy (Fig. 13.5).
- In situ decompression has a higher incidence of recurrence, while transpositions are associated with a greater chance of secondary instability.[27]

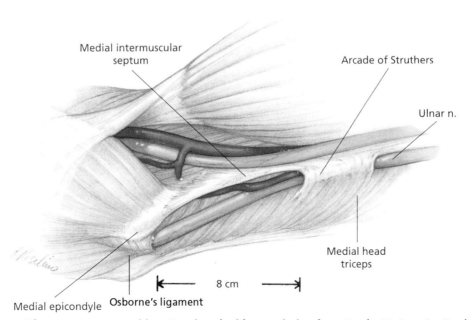

FIG. 13.5. Ulnar nerve transposition. Reprinted with permission from Doyle JR. Arm. In: Doyle JR, Botte MJ, eds. *Surgical Anatomy of the Hand and Upper Extremity.* Philadelphia: Lippincott Williams & Wilkins; 2003:389.

- Duration of symptoms is somewhat unpredictable in non-operative management protocols, but generally results in a return to the patient's sport of choice.
- In patients managed surgically, good to excellent results are typical, with a return to activity following a brief period of immobilization and physical therapy regimen.
- Usual return to sports is 8 to 12 weeks. Patient satisfaction rates after surgery, regardless of technique, are commonly reported to be greater than 80%.

Complications/Indications for Referral

A patient with a physical examination consistent with cubital tunnel syndrome in addition to valgus laxity or frank instability should be referred to an appropriate surgeon, as conservative management is unlikely to allow return to previous activities, especially baseball pitching. In addition, the physical examination findings of constant paresthesias, intrinsic weakness, and muscle atrophy suggest a severe and/or long-standing nerve compression and may be best managed by surgical decompression. Coexisting UCL injury must be ruled out in the overhead or throwing athlete.

APPROACH TO THE ATHLETE WITH DISTAL BICEPS TENDON RUPTURE

Rupture of the distal biceps was once thought to be an uncommon injury but is being seen with increasing frequency. However, a distal biceps rupture is still significantly less common than proximal biceps ruptures and makes up only 3% of all biceps tendon ruptures. This injury is most likely to occur in the dominant arm of middle-aged men during heavy work or lifting.

Avulsion typically occurs during a heavy lift with the elbow flexed approximately 90 degrees and is the result of a sudden or prolonged contracture of the biceps against high load resistance.[28] In most instances, a single traumatic event is recalled by the patient.[28] Prodromal or prerupture symptoms are uncommon.[29] The tear usually occurs at the tendoosseous insertion and notably leaves no distal tendon at the tuberosity.[28] The lacertus fibrosus attachment is damaged to a varying degree but is usually left intact. In fact, the distal biceps tendon may rupture in stages, first with avulsion of the distal biceps tendon proper from the radial tuberosity and then by a second tearing from the lacertus fibrosus.

Pre-existing degenerative changes within the distal tendon at the radial tuberosity are thought to predispose the tendon to rupture. It is unusual to see radiographic changes in the radial tuberosity before tendon avulsion, but Davis and Yassine[30] did identify degenerative changes at the volar aspect of the radial tuberosity. They postulated that these hypertrophic changes could cause tears in the tendon during pronation and supination of the forearm.

HISTORY AND PHYSICAL EXAMINATION

A distal biceps rupture occurs when an unexpected force is applied to the flexed elbow. A patient usually reports a history of lifting or catching a heavy object with a flexed elbow. They may have an audible pop or tearing sensation in the elbow and develop swelling and ecchymosis in the antecubital fossa. Further physical examination will demonstrate tenderness over the antecubital fossa and pain with resisted flexion and supination. Palpation of the distal biceps may be difficult, but the hook test has been described by O'Driscoll as a reliable way to detect a complete distal biceps rupture.[31] The hook test is performed by asking the patient to actively supinate with the elbow flexed 90 degrees while the examiner attempts to hook his or her index finger under the intact biceps tendon from the lateral side. The inability to hook your finger around the cord-like structure indicates distal biceps avulsion.[31]

DIAGNOSTIC TESTING

A good history and physical examination are all that is usually needed to diagnose a distal biceps tendon rupture. Plain radiographs of the elbow may be beneficial in showing hypertrophic bone formation at the radial tuberosity. An MRI is usually ordered to further delineate between partial and complete tears. The MRI will also allow for operative planning if there is significant retraction. Musculoskeletal ultrasound may also be utilized to rule out a distal biceps tendon tear.

TREATMENT

Nonoperative

- There are reports of satisfactory results with nonoperative treatments.[32]
- Partial tendon ruptures are more amenable to conservative management, but most would agree that complete tendon ruptures should have a surgical repair of the distal biceps to the radial tuberosity.
- This will allow the patient to regain the strength and endurance in supination and flexion of the elbow.
- Nonoperative intervention should be reserved for elderly, sedentary patients, and patients who are too ill to undergo surgery.
- Patients who do not wish to have surgical intervention should be informed that they will lose some strength in supination and flexion.
- These patients may also have activity-related forearm pain.

Operative

- Surgical fixation is the recommended treatment for complete biceps tendon ruptures and yields superior results to conservative treatment.
- This should be done within 2 weeks of the injury. Earlier intervention will allow for an easier repair.
- There are many techniques described to repair a distal biceps tendon rupture.
- A single- or two-incision technique may be used, and the tendon may be repaired using bone tunnels, anchors, buttons, or screws.
- All of these techniques have the same objective of returning flexion and supination strength.

Prognosis/Return to Play

- Distal biceps ruptures diagnosed early are easily treated surgically with predictably good results.
- Rehabilitation will vary depending on technique and surgeon preference. Most rehab protocols begin with a short 7 to 10 days of immobilization after surgery followed by gradual increase in range of motion.
- Gentle strengthening is usually begun at 8 weeks with return to unrestricted activities at 3 to 5 months after surgery.

Complications/Indications for Referral

Complications of surgical repair of the distal biceps tendon include nerve and vessel injury, heterotopic bone formation, and elbow stiffness. Nerve injuries usually involve the radial nerve or lateral antebrachial cutaneous nerve. Fortunately, most nerve injuries are the result of traction injury and usually resolve completely. Synostosis of the radius and ulna is less common but more debilitating as it usually prevents rotation of the forearm. All suspected distal biceps ruptures should be referred to a specialist for surgical intervention.

APPROACH TO THE ATHLETE WITH VALGUS EXTENSION OVERLOAD INJURIES (UCL AND ASSOCIATED INJURIES)

Valgus extension injuries of the elbow are common in throwing athletes and can range from inflammatory changes to incompetence of the UCL. The medial structures of the elbow are subjected to significant valgus stresses during overhead throwing activities, which result in a specific pattern of injuries. The repetitive valgus forces during throwing can exceed the tensile strength of the UCL and allow subluxation of the elbow and subsequent posteromedial impingement and bony changes. Throwers may also have a more acute injury to the UCL.

HISTORY AND PHYSICAL EXAMINATION

A throwing athlete with UCL instability will present with a history of medial-sided pain often associated with the late-cocking and acceleration phase of throwing. Pitchers may report a loss of "pop" on the ball as well as a loss of control. A history of grinding, catching, or locking may indicate the presence of loose bodies, posterolateral impingement, or chondromalacia. Ulnar nerve symptoms have been associated with chronic medial instability.

In addition to a routine elbow examination, the physical examination of valgus extension injuries should include valgus stress testing of the elbow as well as evaluating the shoulder range of motion. Often overhead throwers will have shoulder tightness that can lead to increased stresses across the medial side of the elbow. Identifying this shoulder tightness is important as this should be addressed in the treatment. Valgus instability can be assessed by a number of described examinations. With the patient's elbow flexed to about 30 degrees to unlock the olecranon from the fossa, a valgus stress can be applied to the elbow by bracing the patient's forearm between the examiner's forearm and torso. Increased joint space opening and loss of a firm end point when compared to the contralateral side is consistent with UCL incompetence.

More subtle findings of instability may be picked up by the "milking test" or moving valgus test. During the milking test, the patient externally rotates and flexes the affected arm and using the contralateral arm supports the humerus while using the contralateral hand to pull on the affected thumb and recreate a valgus stress. O'Driscoll described the moving valgus stress test, which replicates the dynamic valgus torque that the UCL must resist during throwing. The patient's shoulder is abducted to 90 degrees with the elbow hyperflexed and then the examiner applies a valgus stress to the elbow while extending the arm. Reproducible medial elbow pain in the range of 120 to 70 degrees of flexion is considered a positive test.[33] Lastly, any loss of motion, catching, or crepitation may indicate chondromalacia, arthritis, or loose bodies.

The valgus extension overload test can help determine the presence of an olecranon osteophyte impinging on the olecranon fossa. With the elbow in full extension, a valgus-directed force is imparted across the elbow. Posteromedial pain signifies a positive test. In addition, tenderness or crepitus along the posteromedial olecranon suggests the presence of osteophytes or loose bodies in this area.[6] The test will often recreate medial elbow pain similar to the milking test suggestive of a UCL injury or chronic insufficiency.

DIAGNOSTIC TESTING

Plain radiographs will offer some clues to the stresses the elbow has seen in a throwing athlete. Traction spurs on the medial side of the elbow and calcification within the UCL, as well as radiocapitellar joint space narrowing and osteophyte formation may be seen on an anteroposterior radiograph. Osteophytes may also be seen on the posteromedial olecranon as part of the valgus extension overload syndrome and are best visualized on the hyperflexion lateral and oblique radiographs.[34] Stress anteroposterior radiographs of the elbow may demonstrate gapping along the medial ulnohumeral joint line. A gap of greater than 0.5 mm may indicate complete UCL tear,[35] but stress radiographs have a reported sensitivity of only 46%.[36] MR arthrography is much more sensitive at detecting UCL injuries, with a reported 95% and 86% sensitivity for complete and partial tears, respectively.[37] MR arthrogram will also identify any chondral injury or loose bodies that may be present. Musculoskeletal ultrasound adds the benefit of directly visualizing the UCL while placing a dynamic valgus stress as well as the ability to measure joint space narrowing.

TREATMENT

Nonoperative

- The goal of conservative treatment is to relieve pain and inflammation and to increase the functional strength of the elbow.
- The throwing athlete needs specific attention to strengthening the flexor–pronator muscles in the forearm, as well as capsular stretching and scapular stabilizer strengthening in the shoulder.
- Pitchers need to limit the number of pitches or even rest from pitching for up to 6 weeks.
- NSAIDs.
- Interval Throwing Program (see Appendix B).[38]
- Proper throwing mechanics are imperative to rehabilitation and prevention of future injury.

Operative

- Arthroscopy can be useful in patients that have chondromalacia with loose bodies or for debridement of posteromedial osteophyte formation of the olecranon.
- UCL incompetence in high-level throwing athletes can be reconstructed using palmaris longus autograft or allograft tendon.

Prognosis/Return to Play

- There is a wide spectrum of valgus extension injuries, and prognosis depends on the specific injury and severity.
- Overuse inflammatory conditions and partial UCL tears may improve quickly with conservative measures with return to throwing by 6 weeks.
- Patients usually have excellent results following arthroscopic removal of loose bodies and debridement and can usually return to play by 3 months.

- Elbow pain is usually relieved by removal of posteromedial osteophytes.
- UCL reconstruction has good results, but rehabilitation and return to play may take up to 1 year.
- Prior to beginning any sport-specific training or throwing program, the patient should have a pain-free joint with functional range of motion and strength of the shoulder and elbow.

Complications/Indications for Referral

Complications of valgus extension injuries are usually related to the surgical intervention. Ulnar nerve paresthesias can occur after UCL reconstruction. Elbow arthroscopy carries a risk of neurovascular injury, and debridement of osteophytes and adhesions should be done with caution to avoid destabilizing the elbow. Patients who fail conservative measures should be evaluated by a surgeon.

KEY POINTS
• Medial epicondylitis is the most common cause of medial elbow pain, with an annual incidence of four to seven cases per 1,000 patients[8,9]
• Tennis elbow is the most common cause of lateral elbow pain and typically has an incidence reported to be 1 to 3 per 100
• In posterior interosseous nerve (PIN) syndrome, the extensor carpi radialis longus (ECRL) is always spared while the extensor carpi ulnaris is always affected[25]
• In cubital tunnel syndrome, sensory changes in the ring and small digits and weakness of the intrinsic muscles may be detected, especially with finger abduction[4]
• Palpation of the distal biceps may be difficult, but the hook test has been described by O'Driscoll as a reliable way to detect a complete distal biceps rupture[31]
• The repetitive valgus forces during throwing can exceed the tensile strength of the UCL and allow subluxation of the elbow and subsequent posteromedial impingement and bony changes

REFERENCES

1. King JW, Brelsford HJ, Tullos HS. Analysis of the pitching arm of the professional baseball pitcher. *Clin Orthop Relat Res.* 1969;67:116.
2. Hoppenfeld S. *Physical Examination of the Spine and Extremities.* Norwalk, CT: Apple-Century-Crofts; 1976:35–58.
3. Askew LJ, An KN, Morrey BF, et al. Functional evaluation of the elbow. Normal motion requirements and strength determinations. *Orthop Trans.* 1981;5:304.
4. Lorei MP, Hershman EB. Peripheral nerve injuries in athletes. Treatment and prevention. *Sports Med.* 1993;16(2):130–147.

5. Kandemir U, Fu FH, McMahon PJ. Elbow injuries. *Curr Opin Rheumatol.* 2002;14:160–167.
6. Andrews JR, Wilk KE, Satterwhite YE, et al. Physical examination of the thrower's elbow. *JOSPT.* 1993;17(6):296–304.
7. Sellards R, Kuebrich C. The elbow: diagnosis and treatment of common injuries. *Prim Care.* 2005;32(1):1–16.
8. Plancher KD, Halbrecht J, Lourie GM. Medial and lateral epicondylitis in the athlete. *Clin Sports Med.* 1996;15(2):283–305.
9. Smidt N, van der Windt DA. Tennis elbow in primary care. *BMJ.* 2006;333(7575):927–928.
10. Kijowski R, De Smet AA. Magnetic resonance imaging findings in patients with medial epicondylitis. *Skeletal Radiol.* 2005;34(4):196–202.
11. Stahl S, Kaufman T. The efficacy of an injection of steroids for medial epicondylitis. A prospective study of sixty elbows. *J Bone Joint Surg Am.* 1997;79(11):1648–1652.
12. Krischek O, Hopf C, Nafe B, et al. Shock-wave therapy for tennis and golfer's elbow–1 year follow-up. *Arch Orthop Trauma Surg.* 1999;119(1–2): 62–66.
13. Simunovic Z, Trobonjaca T, Trobonjaca Z. Treatment of medial and lateral epicondylitis–tennis and golfer's elbow–with low level laser therapy: a multicenter double blind, placebo-controlled clinical study on 324 patients. *J Clin Laser Med Surg.* 1998;16(3):145–151.
14. Gabel GT, Morrey BT. Operative treatment of medial epicondylitis: the influence of concomitant ulnar neuropathy at the elbow. *J Bone Joint Surg Am.* 1995;77:1065.
15. Vangsness CT, Jobe FW. Surgical treatment of medial epicondylitis: results in 35 elbows. *J Bone Joint Surg Br.* 1991;73:409.
16. Bunata RE, Brown DS, Capelo R. Anatomic factors related to the cause of tennis elbow. *J Bone Joint Surg Am.* 2007;89:1955–1963.
17. Nirschl RP. Elbow tendinosis/tennis elbow. *Clin Sports Med.* 1992;11: 851–870.
18. Green S, Buchbinder R, Barnsley L, et al. Non-steroidal anti-inflammatory drugs (NSAIDs) for treating lateral elbow pain in adults. *Cochrane Database Syst Rev.* 2002, Issue 2. Art No.: CD003686. DOI: 10.1002/14651858.CD003686.
19. Struijs PAA, Smidt N, Arola H, et al. Orthotic devices for the treatment of tennis elbow. *Cochrane Database Syst Rev.* 2001, Issue 4. Art. No.: CD001821. DOI: 10.1002/14651858.CD001821.
20. Trudel D, Duley J, Zastrow I, et al. Rehabilitation for patients with lateral epicondylitis: a systematic review. *J Hand Ther.* 2004;17:243–266.
21. Green S, Buchbinder R, Barnsley L, et al. Acupuncture for lateral elbow pain. *Cochrane Database Syst Rev.* 2001, Issue 1. Art No.: CD003527. DOI: 10.1002/14651858.CD003527.
22. Buchbinder R, Green S, Youd JM, et al. Shock wave therapy for lateral elbow pain. *Cochrane Database Syst Rev.* 2005, Issue 3. Art. No.: CD003524. DOI: 10.1002/14651858.CD003524.pub2
23. Buchbinder R, Green S, Bell S, et al. Surgery for lateral elbow pain. *Cochrane Database Syst Rev.* 2008, Issue 1. Art. No.: CD003525. DOI: 10.1002/14651858.CD003525
24. Werner CO. Lateral elbow pain and posterior interosseous nerve entrapment. *Acta Orthop Scand Suppl.* 1979;174:1–62.
25. Bencardino JT, Rosenberg ZS. Entrapment neuropathies of the shoulder and elbow in the athlete. *Clin Sports Med.* 2006;25:465–487.
26. Rinker B, Effron CR, Beasley RW. Proximal radial nerve compression. *Ann Plast Surg.* 2004;52:174–180.
27. Cutts S. Cubital tunnel syndrome. *Postgrad Med J.* 2007;83:28–31.
28. Morrey BF, Askew LJ, An KN, et al. Rupture of the distal tendon of the biceps brachii: a biomechanical study. *J Bone Joint Surg Am.* 1985;67: 418–421.
29. Louis DS, Hankin FM, Eckenrode JF, et al. Distal biceps brachii tendon avulsion: a simplified method of operative repair. *Am J Sports Med.* 1986;14:234–236.
30. Davis WM, Yassine Z. An etiological factor in tear of the distal tendon of the biceps brachii: report of two cases. *J Bone Joint Surg Am.* 1956;38:1365–1368.
31. O'Driscoll SW, Goncalves LB, Dietz P. The hook test for distal biceps tendon avulsion. *Am J Sports Med.* 2007;35(11):1865–1869.
32. Carroll RE, Hamilton LR. Rupture of biceps brachii: a conservative method of treatment. *J Bone Joint Surg Am.* 1967;49:1016.
33. O'Driscoll SW, Lawton RL, Smith MA. The "moving valgus stress test" for medial collateral ligament tears of the elbow. *Am J Sports Med.* 2005;33:231–239.
34. Hyman J, Breazeale NM, Altchek DW. Valgus instability of the elbow in athletes. *Clin Sports Med.* 2001;20:25–45,viii.
35. Rijke AM, Goitz HT, McCue FC, et al. Stress radiography of the medial elbow ligaments. *Radiology.* 1994;191:213–216.
36. Azar FM, Andrews JR, Wilk KE, et al. Operative treatment of ulnar collateral ligament injuries of the elbow in athletes. *Am J Sports Med.* 2000;28:16–23.
37. Schwartz ML, al-Zahrani S, Morwessel RM, et al. Ulnar collateral ligament injury in the throwing athlete: evaluation with saline-enhanced MR arthrography. *Radiology.* 1995;197:297–299.
38. Wilk KE, Arrigo C, Andrews JR. Rehabilitation of the elbow in the throwing athlete. *J Orthop Sports Phys Ther.* 1993;17:305–317.

Athlete with Overuse Wrist and Hand Injuries

Patrick Guerrero and Xinning Li

INTRODUCTION

Chronic overuse injuries in the upper extremity are commonly seen in competitive or recreational athletes. It has been reported that 25% to 50% of all sports-related injuries can be attributed to overuse.[1] Overuse is defined as repetitive microtrauma damage to the tissue that exceeds its ability to adapt. The term has been used in a broad spectrum of diagnosis that includes occupational, recreational, activity, or sports-related injuries. Handball, rowing, gymnastics, racquet sports, and volleyball are common sport activities involved in this injury pattern.[2]

FUNCTIONAL ANATOMY

Extensor Tendons

There are six dorsal compartments at the wrist level where extensor tendons gain entrance to the hand and are surrounded by a retinaculum (Fig. 14.1):

First compartment: Abductor pollicis longus (APL) and extensor pollicis brevis (EPB)
Second compartment: Extensor carpi radialis longus (ECRL) and extensor carpi radialis brevis (ECRB) wrist extensors
Third compartment: Extensor pollicis longus (EPL)
Fourth compartment: Extensor digitorium communis (EDC) and extensor indicis propius (EIP) lying ulnar to the EDC
Fifth compartment: Extensor digiti minimi (EDM)
Sixth compartment: Extensor carpi ulnaris (ECU)

Another important structure is the juncturae tendinae (JT), which are interconnections between the EDC tendons that will allow finger extension in the event of extensor tendon laceration proximal to its insertion. Although there are several variations in the pattern of JT origin and insertion, the most common is from the extensor tendon of the ring finger proximal to the metacarpophlangeal (MCP) joint and inserts onto the middle and little finger extensor tendons.

Also, at this level, extensor tendons are covered by synovium. From the metacarpal heads lies the extensor hood, which blends with the common tendon and lateral bands (medial and lateral) to form the central tendons that insert into the base of the middle phalanx; this in turn affects proximal interphalangeal (PIP) joint extension. The lateral bands join together distally with fibers from the common extensor to form a triangular aponeurosis and attach to the base of the distal phalanx as the terminal tendon.

Flexor Tendons

The carpal tunnel at the level of the wrist comprises nine tendons and the median nerve: four tendons from the flexor digitorum profundus (FDP), four from the flexor digitorum superficialis (FDS), and the flexor pollicis longus (FPL), which is the most radial structure (Fig. 14.2).

The brachialradialis (BR) originates on the lateral supracondylar ridge of the humerus and attaches to the distal radial styloid. The flexor carpi radialis (FCR) and flexor carpi ulnaris (FCU) are both wrist flexors and important during procedures involving tendon transfers or basal joint arthroplasty.

A series of annular (A1–A5) and cruciform (C1–C3) pullies envelop the tendons beginning slightly proximal to the metacarpal heads to maximize lever arm and minimize bowstringing. The odd-numbered pullies arise from the joint, while the even-numbered pullies are associated with the shaft. Preservation of the A2 and A4 pullies during surgery is essential in preventing bowstring of the flexor tendon. A synovial sheath envelops the FDS and FDP tendons to allow easy gliding as well as provide a source of nutrition. The FDS and FDP insert at the volar base of the middle and distal phalanx, respectively. The lumbricals are derived from the tendons of the FDP in the palm and insert on the radial lateral band of each finger. They are prime flexors of MCP joint and principal extensors of the interphalangeal joints. Laceration of the FDP tendon distal to the lumbrical insertion will result in paradoxical extension termed the "lumbrical plus" finger.

Bony and Ligamentous Anatomy

The radius articulates with the ulna via the sigmoid notch (distal radioulnar joint) at the wrist joint with a normal arc of motion ranging between 150 and 180 degrees of supination/

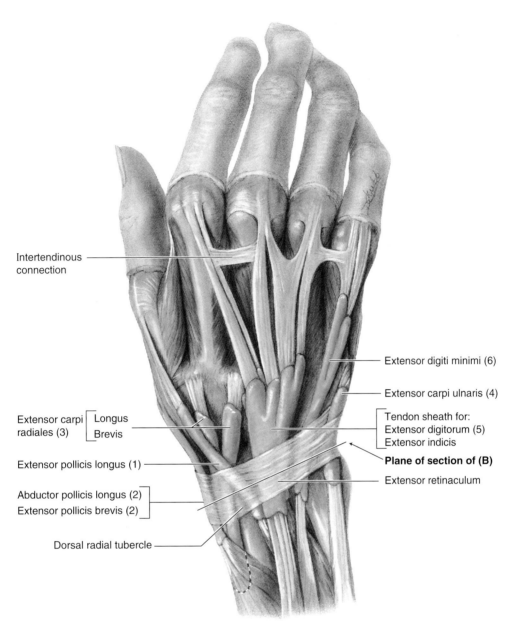

Intertendinous connection

Extensor digiti minimi (6)

Extensor carpi ulnaris (4)

Tendon sheath for:
Extensor digitorum (5)
Extensor indicis

Plane of section of (B)

Extensor retinaculum

Extensor carpi radiales (3) — Longus / Brevis

Extensor pollicis longus (1)

Abductor pollicis longus (2)
Extensor pollicis brevis (2)

Dorsal radial tubercle

FIG. 14.1. Transverse section dorsal compartments. From Moore KL, Dalley AF II. *Clinical Oriented Anatomy.* 4th ed. Baltimore: Lippincott Williams & Wilkins; 1999.

pronation. The normal arc of wrist flexion is 79 degrees, with wrist extension of 59 degrees, radial deviation of 21 degrees, and ulnar deviation of 38 degrees. The triangular fibrocartilage complex (TFCC) is the primary stabilizer of the distal radioulnar joint (DRUJ). The dorsal (Fig. 14.3) and volar (Fig. 14.4) radiocarpal and ulnocarpal (extrinsic) ligaments stabilize the wrist. In addition, multiple intercarpal and interosseous ligaments provide further stability to the wrist and aid in intercarpal motion. The MCP joints as well as the PIP and distal interphalangeal (DIP) joints are CAM shaped with varying degrees of collateral ligament tightness correlating flexion from 0 to 90 degrees

(under maximum stretch with full flexion). A palm/volar plate as well as radial and ulnar collateral ligaments provide ligamentous stability during dorsal/volar and varus/valgus stresses, respectively.

Triangular Fibrocartilage Complex

The TFCC stabilizes the distal radial ulna joint and provides stability at the ulnotriquetral joint. It can be prone to injury with repetitive weight-bearing activities involving ulnar deviation. The TFCC consists of a triangular cartilage disc known as the meniscus homolog as well as the dorsal and

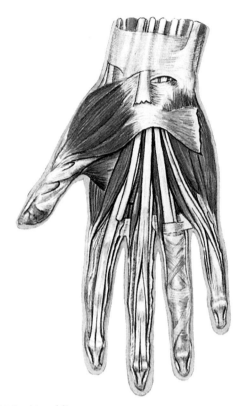

FIG. 14.2. Hand ligaments.

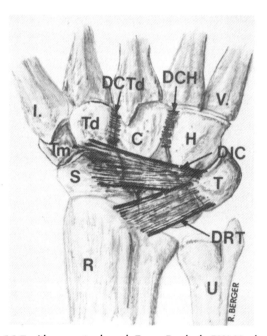

FIG. 14.3. Ligaments dorsal. From Bucholz RW, Heckman JD. *Rockwood & Green's Fractures in Adults.* 5th ed. Philadelphia: Lippincott Williams & Wilkins; 2001.

volar ulnoradial ligaments, the ulnotriquetral and ulnolunate ligaments, and the tendon sheath of the ECU. The vascularity of the meniscus homolog is limited to the peripheral 15% to 20% and therefore prone to chronic tears.

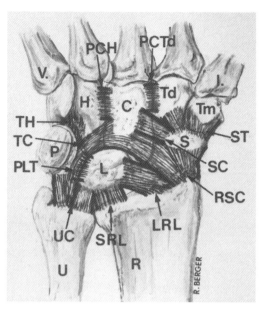

FIG. 14.4. Ligaments volar. From Bucholz RW, Heckman JD. *Rockwood & Green's Fractures in Adults.* 5th ed. Philadelphia: Lippincott Williams & Wilkins; 2001.

Neurovascular Supply

The median nerve runs inside the carpal tunnel superficial and radial to the FDS for the ring and middle fingers and provides motor innervation to the thumb via the recurrent motor branch of median nerve and sensation to the radial three and one half digits. The ulnar nerve traverses the Guyon canal and supplies motor fibers to the hand intrinsics as well as sensation to the ulnar one and a half digits. It also gives a dorsal sensory branch to the dorsum of the hand. The superficial sensory branch of the radial nerve innervates the thumb, index, and occasionally middle fingers, dorsally. Blood supply is via the ulnar and radial arteries.

EPIDEMIOLOGY

Overuse hand and wrist injuries are common injuries sustained in athletes. The repetitive nature of many sports as well as the high degree of force transmitted through the hand and wrist make it particularly vulnerable. Common overuse injuries include de Quervain disease, intersection syndrome, TFCC tears, ECU tendonitis or subluxation, carpal tunnel syndrome, scaphoid fractures that may lead to nonunion, hook of hamate or pisifom fractures, and carpal instability. In the adolescent, overuse injuries may present as apophyseal inflammation. Sports associated with overuse to the hand and wrist include golf, racquet sports, gymnastics, rowing, and activities that require repetitive hand and wrist contact with a ball such as handball or volleyball.[2] It has been estimated that 50% of all athletes will sustain an injury, with 25% to 50% secondary to overuse.[1]

Furthermore, a total of 703 golfers were retrospectively reviewed; 83% of them reported injuries involving overuse and 54% reported injuries involving the upper extremity.[3] Over 85% of 518 recreational cyclists reported injury associated with overuse and 31% reported injury that involved the hand and wrist region.[4] There is also a significant increase in the incidence of overuse injuries in the elite male volleyball players from 16% to 47% over a 10-year period.[5] A recent epidemiology study of injury patterns in recreational rock climbers showed that 33% of 201 active climbers had suffered chronic overuse injuries.[6]

NARROWING THE DIFFERENTIAL DIAGNOSIS

History

A thorough but focused history plays a crucial role in the diagnosis of overuse hand and wrist injuries. Key components include the age of the athlete, mechanism of injury, exacerbating and alleviating factors, as well as any associated symptoms. The age of the athlete is important, as more number of younger patients present with symptoms related to overuse. Also knowledge of the age of growth plate closure is important, as adolescent athlete may present with apophyseal injury. The mechanism and the acuity of onset of symptoms can also help in differentiating between overuse versus acute injuries. Asking about exacerbating and alleviating factors is essential in making the diagnosis, as pain tends to improve with rest in injuries related to overuse. The location of the presenting symptoms along with any neurologic compromise can also help in making the diagnosis. Moreover, acute pain related to a particular event/injury may be able to rule out overuse as a mechanism of injury.

Another important part of the history is asking about the level and practice time the patient spends each week on his/her respective sport. Also knowledge of factors during his/her sports activity that exacerbate his/her symptoms and which factors relieve them will be essential in making the diagnosis and direct treatment. Overuse injuries of the hand and wrist are also associated with more elite-level sports participation and prolonged training time.

Evidence-based Physical Examination

The physical examination plays a key role in the diagnosis of overuse hand and wrist injuries. The progression of one's examination should include the following components as well as special tests:

Inspection

Inspection of the wrist and hand should first focus on visual examination. Particular attention should be paid to the area of the pain and inspection of the skin for lacerations/abrasions, chronic changes/swelling, or any deformities that will help in making the diagnosis. Furthermore, muscle atrophy in a particular region of the hand (thenar or hypothenar) may indicate chronic nerve impingement. A mass seen on the dorsal or volar surface may represent a ganglion cyst, which can indicate an underlying overuse injury to the tendon. It is also important to rule out infection with signs of erythema or warmth over the skin or joint.

Palpation

Palpation of the hand and wrist for overuse injuries involves assessing for deformities, point tenderness, swelling, and crepitus. Attention should be paid to the location of the pain, as ulnar- versus radial- or dorsal- versus volar-sided pain can help narrow the differential diagnosis. Point tenderness directly over a tendon or palpable crepitus can indicate chronic inflammation due to overuse. Tenderness over the hamate or the scaphoid may indicate an acute or stress fracture. Subluxation of the tendon with direct palpation may indicate chronic instability or overuse.

Range of Motion

Normal range of motion at the wrist is 79 degrees of flexion, 59 degrees of extension, 38 degrees of ulnar deviation, 21 degrees of radial deviation, and 80 degrees of forearm supination/pronation. A loss in the range of motion can indicate chronic inflammation of the tendon, restricting its ability to glide smoothly. Arthritis of the wrist or carpal bones due to scaphoid nonunion or lunate advance collapse may also restrict range of motion of the wrist secondary to pain.

Strength Tests

Strength testing should be performed as part of the evaluation with weakness possibility associated with muscle atrophy secondary to chronic nerve entrapment.

Special Tests

Numerous special tests exist in the evaluation of overuse hand and wrist injuries:

- The *Finkelstein test* is a test for de Quervain tenosynovitis and involves adduction of thumb with maximal ulnar deviation of wrist which reproduces symptoms. It has 61% sensitivity and 83% specificity.[7]
- The *piano key sign* involves the examiner performing a dorsal/volar motion of the distal radius and ulna with the wrist in neutral and compares for instability and pain with the contralateral side. This test is mainly for complete tears of the TFCC. It has a sensitivity of 59% and specificity of 96%.[8]
- *Ulna grind test* involves passive ulnar deviation with axial loading by the examiner while the wrist is in neutral position. Pain +/− click may indicate a TFCC tear (chronic or acute).

- The *TFCC shear test* or *ulnomeniscotriquetral dorsal glide test* involves the examiner to stabilize the patient's radius with one hand and glide the pisotriquetral complex dorsally and the ulna volarly. A positive test is when this maneuver reproduces the patient's symptoms and indicates a TFCC tear or lesion. This test has a sensitivity of 66%, specificity of 66%, positive predicative value of 58%, and negative predictive value of 69%.[9]
- The *Watson shift test* for scapholunate dissociation (SLD) involves putting pressure over the scaphoid tubercle while the wrist is brought from ulnar to radial deviation. A painful clunk is felt suggesting a tear of the scapholunate ligament. This test has a sensitivity of 69%, specificity of 66%, positive predictive value of 48%, and negative predictive value of 78%.[9]

Diagnostic Testing

Laboratory

The majority of overuse hand and wrist injuries in athletes do not require laboratory analysis. If an autoimmune etiology is in the differential diagnosis, then sedimentation rate, C-reactive protein (CRP), antinuclear antibody (ANA), and rheumatoid factor may be considered.

Imaging

The majority of overuse hand and wrist injuries can be diagnosed by a thorough history and physical examination. When the diagnosis remains unclear, an understanding of appropriate diagnostic imaging studies is crucial.

Plain radiographs will often be the first imaging modality utilized in the setting of overuse hand and wrist injuries. Plain radiographs play a crucial role by demonstrating any degenerative changes, occult fractures, or bony abnormalities. Ulnar variance is important to assess in the presence of lateral wrist pain and can be associated with ulnar impaction syndrome as well as TFCC injuries. It is a measurement of the relative length of the ulna with respect to the radius. Neutral variance indicates equal length, with negative ulnar variance indicating shorter ulna and positive variance occurring when the ulna is longer than the radius. The mean ulnar variance is 0.9 mm, measured in posteroanterior (PA) radiograph, with the wrist in neutral supination/pronation. A 2.5-mm increase in positive ulnar variance will increase the load bearing of the ulnocarpal joint from 18% to 42%.

Computed tomography (CT) is generally reserved for evaluation of complex fractures or bone pathology (cysts, tumors, etc.) and rarely required in the setting of overuse wrist and hand pathology.

Magnetic resonance imaging (MRI) is often the test of choice with soft-tissue injuries or when the diagnosis remains unclear. Common indications include fullness in the wrist or palm with a history of slowly progressing neurologic deficit without intermittent fluctuations, point bony tenderness without evidence of fracture on plain radiographs to rule out occult or stress fractures, and ligamentous injuries or chronic

wrist pain without specific diagnosis. Occult ganglions, soft-tissue tumors, tendonitis, joint effusions, as well as vascularity of the carpal bones can be accurately visualized with MRI.

Musculoskeletal ultrasound is an excellent modality for many overuse hand and wrist injuries due to the high resolution it provides of superficial soft-tissue structures as well as the dynamic/real-time imaging. Tendonosis, tenosynovitis, tendon nodules (trigger finger), and joint synovitis are common indications that are visualized to a greater degree with ultrasound than on MRI. Musculoskeletal ultrasound's lack of ionizing radiation and relatively quick scanning time make it a good option for pediatric patients. While used extensively worldwide, musculoskeletal ultrasound's utilization is currently limited in the United States by the availability of trained operators.

Other Testing

Electromyogram (EMG) studies may be considered in the setting of suspected peripheral nerve injury or cervical spine radiculopathy.

APPROACH TO THE PATIENT WITH DE QUERVAIN DISEASE

de Quervain disease is a tenosynovitis with inflammation in the first dorsal compartment of the wrist involving the APL and EPB, most often at the radial styloid. It is common in sports with repetitive wrist movements (weight lifters, racquet sports, handball). de Quervain disease tends to correlate with other disorders such carpal tunnel syndrome, trigger digits, epicondylitis, and subacromial bursitis, implicating a more systemic and undefined rheumatic process or predisposition. de Quervain has its highest prevalence among women in the fifth and sixth decades of life.[10]

HISTORY AND PHYSICAL EXAMINATION

There is gradual onset of radial-sided wrist pain exacerbated by ulnar deviation. Patients may complain of associated crepitice. Physical examination is notable for localized tenderness and swelling over the radial styloid as well as pain elicited by stretching of the first dorsal compartment (Fig. 14.5). Finkelstein test with adduction of thumb with maximal ulnar deviation of wrist will often reproduce symptoms and has 61% sensitivity and 83% specificity.[7]

DIAGNOSTIC TESTING

Mainly a clinical diagnosis, but may differentiate between arthritis at the carpometacarpal and scaphotrapezial–trapezoid joints by plain radiographs. Also bone scanning may show increased uptake deep to the first dorsal compartment. MRI and ultrasound may show fluid around the tendons (APL and EPB), and MRI can detect tears on the tendon itself as well as tendinosis.

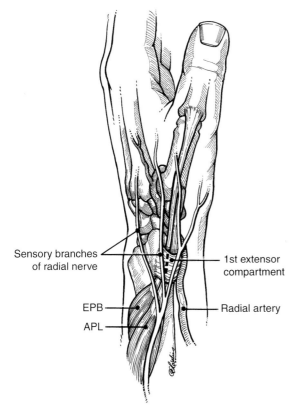

FIG. 14.5. Relevant anatomy for de Quervain's tenosynovitis. The APL and EPB ordinarily share a common fibroosseous canal, but in 33% of cases a separate canal may be present that contains the EPB. Failure to recognize and release this second compartment will result in an incomplete release. Note the relationship of the radial artery and radial nerve to the first extensor compartment. Reprinted with permission from Doyle JR, Tornetta P, Einhorn TA. *Hand and Wrist.* Philadelphia: Lippincott Williams & Wilkins; 2005.

TREATMENT

Nonoperative

- Rest, ice, activity modification, and/or improvement in technique (different bar width, oar size, etc.). Cock-up wrist splint with abducted thumb and nonsteroidal anti-inflammatory drugs (NSAIDs) may also be beneficial.
- For recalcitrant cases, steroid injection may be considered (50% to 60% success between one to two injections).[10]

Operative

- Release of the first dorsal compartment. Of note, the APL has occasionally multiple slips, and the EPB may travel in a separate septa that must be released.[11] The overall success rate has been uniformly excellent, approaching 91%.[7,12]

Prognosis/Return to Play

- Overall prognosis is good, with majority of cases responding to nonoperative treatments.
- Return to activity once symptoms have resolved or significantly improved.
- Splint alone may not be very helpful, and symptoms may return after inciting activity is resumed.
- Proper technique and appropriate gripping should be reviewed with the athlete.

Complications/Indications for Referral

Continued pain despite steroid injections. Steroid induced fat atrophy and skin discoloration following injections (may be seen in 5% to 10% of cases). Radial artery and the superficial branch of the radial nerve can be injured. Tendon subluxation as well as thumb triggering can also occur.[13]

APPROACH TO THE PATIENT WITH INTERSECTION SYNDROME

Intersection syndrome is swelling and entrapment of the second dorsal compartment (ECRL and ECRB). This occurs at about 4 cm proximal to the wrist joint, dorsally characterized by swelling, pain, and crepitice with wrist flexion and extension (Fig. 14.6). This more commonly

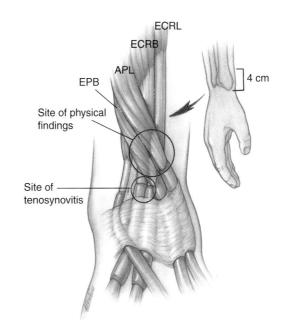

FIG. 14.6. Intersection syndrome. Although the symptoms of swelling and tenderness present in the crossover area 4 cm proximal to the radial styloid, the true pathology is distal in the second extensor compartment. Reprinted with permission from Doyle JR, Tornetta P, Einhorn TA. *Hand and Wrist.* Philadelphia: Lippincott Williams & Wilkins; 2005.

occurs in athletes who perform repetitive wrist motion such as weight lifters and rowers.[14,15] Other conditions to consider with dorsal wrist pain are de Quervain tenosinovitis and neuroma of the superficial branch of the radial nerve.

HISTORY AND PHYSICAL EXAMINATION

This may present with redness, swelling, crepitus, and pain proximal to the wrist. Pain is more proximal (4 cm) than with de Quervain (over the radial styloid). On examination, palpable crepitance may be present as well as pain with resisted extension of the wrist. It is usually brought up by repetitive wrist flexion and extension seen in racquet players.

DIAGNOSTIC TESTING

Diagnosis is usually based on physical examination. Anteroposterior (AP) and lateral radiographs of the wrist including the forearm are indicated, but additional testing including MRI or ultrasound is rarely required.

TREATMENT

Nonoperative

- Majority of intersection syndrome can be treated conservatively. Rest, anti-inflammatory medications, splinting, and occasionally steroid injection may alleviate symptoms.
- A supervised program of physical or occupational therapy can aid in tendon stretching as well as modality implementation.
- Once symptoms are controlled, proper technique especially during "sweep rowing" (excessive and repetitive radial to ulnar deviation as well as wrist extension on the outside hand) and progressive increment in volume (sessions) or amount of weight may aid in prevention of injury.
- Sixty percent to 75% of the patients respond to nonoperative therapy.[16]

Operative

- Release of the second dorsal compartment from the wrist to the level of swelling without repairing the retinaculum.[16]

Prognosis/Return To Play

- Many remain asymptomatic with nonoperative measures.
- The remaining population not responding to conservative measures do improve with surgery.[16]

Complications/Indications for Referral

Complications are rare. Referral for recalcitrant cases unresponsive to nonsurgical management should be considered. If nerve entrapment is believed to be the cause of pain, then EMG studies followed by referral to a specialist is appropriate.

APPROACH TO THE PATIENT WITH TRIANGULAR FIBROCARTILAGE COMPLEX TEARS

TFCC tears are a relatively common source of lateral wrist pain found in athletes with repetitive axial loading or repetitive ulnar deviation at the wrist. These injuries are most commonly found in gymnastics and racquet-based sports. TFCC tears can be acute or chronic and can be associated with ulnar impaction syndrome particularly if there is a history of prior wrist fracture or trauma.

HISTORY AND PHYSICAL EXAMINATION

Athletes with TFCC tears will generally report a history of lateral wrist pain exacerbated by ulnar deviation. There may be a history of an acute event, but more often there may be no history of any specific trauma. Joint swelling, numbness, tingling, or weakness is generally not found with TFCC overuse injuries. History of clicking may point toward carpal instability; a painful click from ulnar to radial deviation may point toward SLD.

On examination, tenderness can often be elicited about the dorsal depression distal to ulnar head and at level of ulnar styloid. Pain is caused by passive motion of the wrist toward ulnar deviation. Also discomfort or pain is noted with resisted radial deviation as well as pain with repeated pronation and supination and strong gripping. A positive piano key sign may indicate a complete tear of the TFCC.

DIAGNOSTIC TESTING

Plain radiographs of the wrist should be obtained. This can provide evidence of positive ulnar variance as well as ulnar styloid fracture or nonuion. A widening of the interval greater than 3 mm between the scaphoid and lunate may point toward SLD. MRI can help determine tears at this location. Arthrography may miss peripheral tears but can also be used (Fig. 14.7). Most physicians use MRI due to the high resolution and anatomic soft-tissue detail that can be visualized.

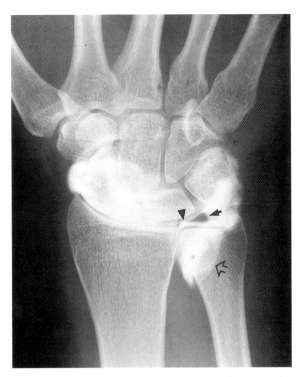

FIG. 14.7. Triangular fibrocartilage complex. Reprinted with permission from Daffner RH. *Clinical Radiology: The Essentials.* 3rd ed. Philadelphia: Lippincott Williams & Wilkins; 2007.

TREATMENT

Nonoperative

- NSAIDs
- Immobilization in slight flexion and ulnar deviation for 4 to 6 weeks
- Long arm cast is advocated by some
- Physical therapy can aid with FCU excursion and inflammation as well as range of motion strength and use of modalities

Operative

- Failure of nonoperative measures warrants surgical evaluation. Techniques vary from percutaneous k-wire fixation to open repair as well as arthroscopic debridement and repair. Ulnar-shortening osteotomy is reserved for cases with continued pain and positive ulnar variance. Careful evaluation should be paid to the DRUJ for signs of instability.

Prognosis/Return to Play

- With positive ulnar variance and traumatic TFCC tears, two thirds (66%) worsen over time symptomatically and

radiologically. It appears that neutral variance reduces the severity of deterioration.
- For chronic problems, modification of activity focusing on avoiding repetitive wrist pronation/supination may help. Splinting also may force the athlete to rest and allow healing to take place.
- A great deal of pain relief may be obtained with a steroid injection.
- Pain-free range of motion with full strength is a good indication to return to play.
- Surgical outcome depends on the type and location of the tear, with traumatic tears having better outcomes than chronic tears.[17]

Complications/Indications for Referral

Failure to diagnose or unrecognized instability of the DRUJ can lead to arthritis, decreased strength, and persistent pain especially with pronation and supination. Surgical complications include infection, nonunion, nerve damage, and hardware failure.

APPROACH TO THE PATIENT WITH EXTENSOR CARPI ULNARIS TENDONITIS/SUBLUXATION

ECU tendonitis is second most common sports-related closed tendon injury at the wrist. It is seen most commonly in racquet sports, basketball, baseball, and rowing. The ECU lies in the six dorsal compartments of the wrist, and at this level it contains a synovial sheath. Inflammation can cause a tenosynovitis. Tear of the ECU sling from repetitive wrist rotation can result in subluxation of the ECU tendon.

HISTORY AND PHYSICAL EXAMINATION

Athletes with ECU tendonitis will complain of dorsal/lateral wrist pain, exacerbated by wrist extension or ulnar deviation. They may also note associated crepitus. Athletes with ECU recurrent subluxation will note a painful pop with forearm rotation.

On examination, tenderness to palpation is noted over the ECU, pain elicited with passive wrist flexion and radial deviation or resisted ulnar deviation and wrist extension. Bony tenderness could indicate traquetrium–pisiform bone or tendon injury; also, one must check for possible ulnar collateral ligament injury as well as potential tear of the TFCC.

DIAGNOSTIC TESTING

X-ray is invaluable to detect a possible fracture, degenerative changes, or possible anatomic congenital anomaly. Ultrasound or MRI can detect tears in the tendon as well as potential tears of the ECU sling that leads to subluxation of the ECU tendon.

FUNCTIONAL TREATMENT

Nonoperative

- In acute setting, rest, ice, splinting, and modification of activity may be sufficient.
- NSAIDs may help diminish swelling and inflammation especially if combined with physical therapy modalities.

Operative

- For chronic conditions that have failed nonoperative treatment, surgical decompression may be an option
- Release of the sixth dorsal compartment
- After surgery, a period of immobilization followed by range of motion and progressive return to play by 6 to 12 weeks

Prognosis/Return To Play

- In acute cases where nonoperative intervention allowed the tendon to heal, 6 to 8 weeks may be all that is needed.
- Near-full strength and range of motion are required for return to play.
- If subluxation is noted, it may require surgical reconstruction of the sling to prevent recurrence of inflammation and pain.

Complications/Indications for Referral

Tendon subluxations as well as tendon rupture are potential complications, particularly with chronic cases.

APPROACH TO THE PATIENT WITH NONUNION SCAPHOID FRACTURES

Nonunion of a scaphoid fracture generally occurs due to a fall on an outstretched hand (FOOSH) with subsequent fracture of the scaphoid that failed to heal or was unrecognized. The blood supply to the scaphoid is mainly retrograde, and fractures often render the waist to proximal pole susceptible to developing a nonunion or avascular necrosis (AVN).

HISTORY AND PHYSICAL EXAMINATION

History of a previous wrist injury with continued pain localized to the snuffbox. Pain often exacerbated with wrist motion and stiffness and tenderness to palpation over the snuffbox (100% sensitivity) may be noted. Reputations and a sense of instability may be noted.[18]

DIAGNOSTIC TESTING

X-rays may demonstrate an area of sclerosis and/or AVN of the proximal pole of the scaphoid (Fig. 14.8). Depending on the stage, radial styloid arthrosis may also be present. In later stages, scaphocapitate arthrosis may be seen along with the radiolunate joint scaphoid arthrosis.

A bone scan may also detect an area of increased uptake; CT may delineate the fracture area if unable to see on plain radiographs. MRI will show bone edema in acute injuries and may show the area of AVN in chronic cases.[19] It is the consensus that continued pain despite a course of

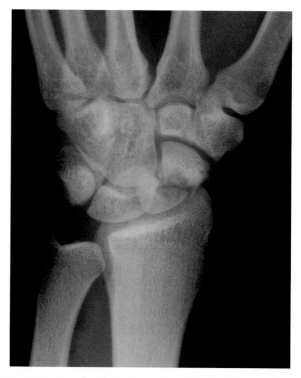

FIG. 14.8. Scaphoid facture. Reprinted with permission from Bucholz RW, Heckman JD. *Rockwood & Green's Fractures in Adults.* 5th ed. Philadelphia: Lippincott Williams & Wilkins; 2001.

nonoperative treatment should alert the provider to the potential of AVN and/or scaphoid nonunion. An MRI is indicated at this point.

TREATMENT

Nonoperative

- Prolonged immobilization – 8 to 10 weeks initially, followed by gentle range of motion. Radiographs should be taken with cast removed. No fracture line should be seen on x-rays.
- No contact sports for 12 weeks.
- In cases of nonunions, a bone stimulator utilizing ultrasound or electrical stimulation may be beneficial.[20]
- Once clinically healed, a course of physical therapy may be indicated to restore strength and range of motion.

Operative

- The approach to the athlete with scaphoid nonunion for the most part is prolonged immobilization, and surgery remains the mainstay treatment after all conservative methods have been exhausted. The gold standard surgical procedure is percutaneous screw fixation with a vascularized pedicle bone graft.

Prognosis/Return to Play

- Prognosis is guarded with majority of nonunion scaphoid fractures requiring surgery.
- Ninety-five percent will heal with vascularized surgery. A repeat procedure may produce only 75% healing.

Complications/Indications for Referral

Pain after closed treatment of a scaphoid fracture even if nondisplaced should be referred to a specialist. During operative intervention, potential complications include failed revision of nonunion, AVN, pain, neurovascular damage, stiffness, infection, and continued nonunion.

APPROACH TO PATIENT WITH NONUNION FRACTURE OF THE HOOK OF THE HAMATE

Hook of the hamate fractures can be a common source of chronic volar/lateral wrist pain, as they can commonly be missed in the acute setting. This type of injury is seen in sports like baseball, golf, tennis, and squash that involve swinging of a club/bat/racquet that abuts the hook of the hamate.[21] If left untreated, some of these fractures progress into nonunion.

HISTORY AND PHYSICAL EXAMINATION

There is generally a previous injury from batting or missing a swing with a golf club hitting the grass. Pain may recur with swinging of a club as well as flexion and ulnar deviation of the wrist. Pain and tenderness occur at the hypothenar eminents 1 cm radial and distal to the pisiform. This pain is also aggravated by grasp. Anatomic location will point toward a hook of the hamate fracture.

DIAGNOSTIC TESTING

Carpal tunnel view x-rays as well as multiple oblique views until a complete profile of the hamulus is obtained are 72% sensitive and 88% specific. A CT scan has 100% sensitivity and 94% specificity.[22]

TREATMENT

Nonoperative

- Ultrasound may alleviate symptoms, initial immobilization, and electrical stimulation. Unfortunately, it is rare for these fractures to heal with conservative management.

Operative

- Excision is usually reserved when continued pain is present despite nonoperative measures. Open reduction and internal fixation offer little advantage over excision.

Prognosis/Return to Play

- Most individuals return to preinjury level with surgical excision.
- Some athletes are able to complete their season with pain control measures and opt for surgery in the off-season.

Complications/Indications for Referral

Continued pain on the hook of hamate and persistent weakness should prompt referral for surgery. Injury to the deep branch of the ulnar nerve can be a complication of surgical excision.

APPROACH TO PATIENT WITH CARPAL INSTABILITY

Unrecognized or undiagnosed injuries to the carpel ligaments can be a cause of a chronic wrist pain in the athlete. The primary mechanism is a FOOSH as well as fall from repetitive weight bearing across the wrist in sports like gymnastics. There are two rows: the proximal row involving the triquetrium, lunate, and pisiform and the distal row involving the trapezium, trapezoid, capitate, and hamate. Bridging the two rows is the scaphoid. These carpal bones are interconnected to each other by a series of ligaments that allow motion to take place. A disruption of these ligaments may produce abnormal kinematics, instability, and pain. The most common interosseous carpel ligament injured is the scapholunate ligament.

HISTORY AND PHYSICAL EXAMINATION

Common complaints in athletes with carpel instability include wrist pain, clicking, or crepitice. Weight bearing or stress to the wrist will often aggravate symptoms. Acute cases will often present with swelling over the dorsum of the wrist. Chronic cases will often result in stiffness and loss or range of motion.

Tenderness with wrist motion, translation, and crepitus may be indicative of ligamentous injury. The Watson shift test for SLD involves putting pressure over the scaphoid tubercle while the wrist is brought from ulnar to radial deviation. A painful clunk is felt, suggesting a tear of the scapholunate ligament. Examination should focus on location of pain and recognize that there are eight carpal bones with multiple interconnecting ligaments.

DIAGNOSTIC TESTING

Radiographs should include PA, lateral, ulnar deviation, and PA clenched-fist views. Additional views may include radial deviation and carpal tunnel views. The clenched-fist view may show widening of the scapholunate joint space (Terry–Thomas sign is >3 mm of widening), while lateral view may show an increased scapholunate angle with tears of the scapholunate ligament.

CT arthrogram may detect ligamentous tears if there is a contraindication to MRI. MRI arthrogram has surpassed CT arthrogram in not only detecting tears but also delineating the extent of these tears.

TREATMENT

Nonoperative

- Splinting may be of moderate benefit, as only 40% of patients remained satisfied with nonoperative treatment.[23] NSAIDs may provide symptomatic relief.

Operative

- Depending on which carpal bones are affected as well as the chronicity, operative intervention may range from pin fixation and immobilization to fusion, carpectomy, and radial or ulnar-shortening osteotomy.

Prognosis/Return to Play

- With closed treatment only 40% of patients remained satisfied.[23] Depending on what procedure was performed, the athlete may return to sports as early as 8 to 12 weeks versus 6 to 9 months for fusions.

Complications/Red Flags/Indications for Referral

Beware of unrecognized perilunate dislocations. Unimproved wrist pain should be referred to a hand specialist or orthopaedic surgeon.

APPROACH TO EPIPHYSEAL INJURIES IN THE WRIST (GYMNAST WRIST)

Chronic injuries to the distal radius epiphysis (gymnast wrist) can commonly occur in skeletally immature gymnasts with repeated axial loading at the wrist. This condition can lead to premature closure of the distal radius epiphysis and subsequent ulna impaction syndrome from resultant positive ulnar variance.[24] Prevalence of positive ulnar variance has been found in 46% to 79% of gymnasts, with 45% of gymnasts having chronic wrist pain for more than 6 months. Anatomically, the radius bears 80% of the load, while the ulna the remaining 20%. Changes in ulnar variance can significantly alter the normal weight-bearing loads across the wrist joint. A positive ulnar variance of 2 mm, for example, will increase the load on the ulna from 20% to 40%. Older gymnasts with dorsal wrist pain may suffer from a distal radius stress fracture or "wrist capsulitis," commonly found in gymnasts.

HISTORY AND PHYSICAL EXAMINATION

The young athlete with chronic epiphyseal injury will complain of dorsal wrist pain exacerbated with weight-bearing activities. Age, activity-related pain (weight bearing vs. torsional), and location are critical questions to narrow the diagnosis. Intersection syndrome, de Quervain tenosynovitis, ulnar impaction syndrome, wrist capsulitis, and wrist stress fracture need to be considered in the differential. Type of activities as well as amount of repetitions and symptoms produced are keys to the diagnosis. The types of mats being used may play a role; if they are too soft, they can cause excessive wrist hyperextension. Examination will reveal tenderness at the distal radius at the level of the physis with dorsal palpation.

DIAGNOSTIC TESTING

X-rays may show widening of the distal radius physis as well as cystic changes of the metaphysic. In chronic cases, radiographs may show premature closure of the distal radius physis with positive ulnar variance and possible ulna impaction syndrome. CT, bone scan, and more importantly MRI may be utilized to detect subtle metaphyseal fractures.[25]

TREATMENT

Nonoperative

- Rest from wrist weight-bearing and aggravating activities
- Splint or short-term casting for symptoms not alleviated with relative rest

Operative

- If ulnar abutement or impaction syndrome is developed, ulnar-shortening osteotomy may be needed.

Prognosis/Return to Play

- Overall prognosis is good if caught early and before physeal changes occur.
- Gradual return to activity once pain free. Typically patient can initiate bar exercises prior to full weight-bearing wrist activity (floor, vault, balance beam).
- Mild cases may return to sport in 3 to 6 weeks.
- Advanced cases may require up to 6 months.

Complications/Indications for Referral

Physeal arrest, continued pain, and decreased range of motion should be indications for referral.

APPROACH TO MALLET FINGER

HISTORY AND PHYSICAL EXAMINATION

Mallet finger is also known as "drop finger" or "baseball finger" and is commonly seen in softball, baseball, basketball, and football receivers.[26] The termination of the extensor tendon attaches to the base of the distal phalanx on the dorsal side. At this point, the tendon narrows and it may be susceptible to ruptures or avulsions. There is weakness or incomplete active extension of the DIP joint.

Axial load on the finger or forced flexion on an extended finger is caused by the ball or collision against another player. It is localized to DIP joint. Weakness in extension is caused by an axial load with forced flexion at the DIP.

DIAGNOSTIC TESTING

If the patient has already had x-rays and this is a chronic case, no need for repeat x-rays.

FUNCTIONAL TREATMENT

Nonoperative

- For the most part nonoperative, as long as no subluxation is present. Extension splint with reported success up to 3 months from the day of injury.[27]

Operative

- If unstable and subluxates, fusion may be the best alternative. Repair may offer return of motion, but may be limited.

Prognosis/Return To Play

- Most return to play without difficulties even with neglect.

Complications/Indications for Referral

Intra-articular fragment and instability should be indications for referral.

APPROACH TO BOUTONNIERE INJURIES

HISTORY AND PHYSICAL EXAMINATION

Chronic untreated disruption of the central tendon more commonly occurs as a consequence of a volar dislocation. The central extensor tendon attaches to the dorsal base of the middle phalanx and provides extension to the PIP. With the wrist and MCP joints flexed, at least to 20 degrees, active extension of the PIP is attempted. Even in acute injuries, extension loss may not be fully appreciated. There is history of previous trauma/dislocation to the digit with loss of extension and weakness at the PIP joint (Fig. 14.9). Progressive decreased range of motion may be a presenting problem. Weakness is seen with PIP joint extension and flexion contracture. Differentiate between a joint contracture from Dupuytren's.

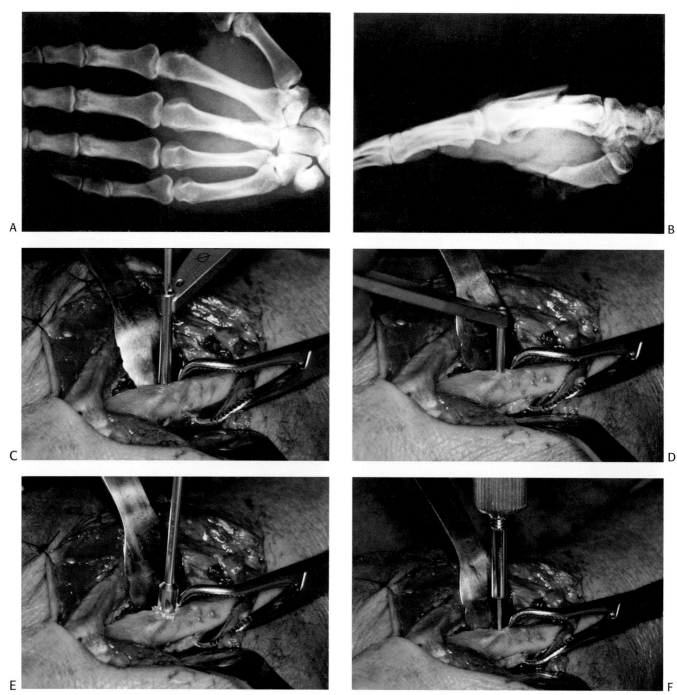

FIG. 14.9. Boutonniere. Reprinted with permission from Strickland JW, Graham TJ. *Master Techniques in Orthopaedic Surgery: The Hand.* 2nd ed. Philadelphia: Lippincott Williams & Wilkins; 2005.

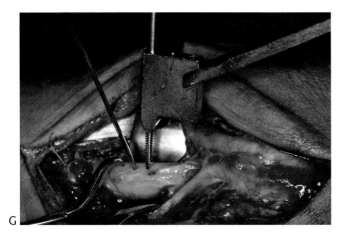

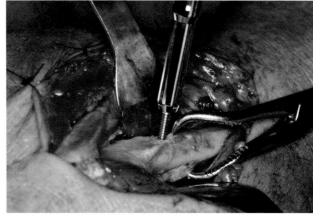

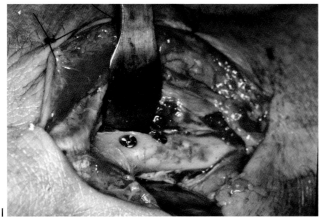

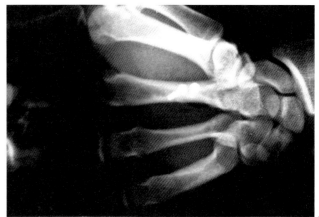

FIG. 14.9. (*Continued*).

Haines–Zancolli test: Positive if unable to passively flex the DIP with an extended PIP.

DIAGNOSTIC TESTING

X-rays and CT may be utilized if considering possible fracture.

FUNCTIONAL TREATMENT

Nonoperative

- Depends on the functional impairment.
- Splinting usually is sufficient. Splint in extension for 6 to 8 weeks.
- In chronic contractures, serial casting may be necessary and for the most time sufficient.
- If nonoperative treatment is followed, then the athlete may return to play as long as the splint is worn at all times.[28]

Operative

- Two-stage procedure, one for a release and the second for repair or reconstruction.
- Haines–Zancolli test can aid in deciding to operate.

Prognosis/Return To Play

- After 6 weeks of treatment, most recover without significant sequelae and can function without impediment.
- Continued incomplete extension may require extension splinting for another 6 weeks versus operative intervention.

Complications/Indications for Referral

Recurrent extension loss or incomplete extension gain, rerupture, and joint instability should be indications for referral.

KEY POINTS
• de Quervain tenosinovitis generally responds well to nonoperative measures
• Have a high suspicion for missed scaphoid fracture with snuffbox tenderness and a history of a FOOSH injury
• Hook of the hamate fractures can be common source of volar wrist pain in sports utilizing a bat or raquet
• Scapholunate ligament tears may be seen with misdiagnosed "wrist sprains". If unrecognized and treated acutely, these ligamenteous injuries can lead to scapholunate instability that may result in persistent pain and disability.
• Distal dorsal radial pain in skeletally immature gymnasts should be suspected for physeal injury
• Mallet finger can be successfully treated with extension splint of the DIP joint. If there is presence of instability/subluxation, then fusion of the DIP joint may be an alternative treatment option

REFERENCES

1. Patel MR, Lipson LB, Desai SS. Conservative treatment of mallet thumb. *J Hand Surg.* 1986;11A:45–47.
2. Fulcher SM, Kiefhaber TR, Stern PJ. Upper extremity tendonitis and overuse syndromes in the athlete. *Clin Sports Med.* 1998;17(3):611–621.
3. Gosheger G, Liem D, Ludwig K, et al. Injuries and overuse syndromes in golf. *Am J Sports Med.* 2003;31(3):438–443.
4. Wilber CA, Holland GJ, Madison RE, et al. An epidemiological analysis of overuse injuries among recreational cyclists. *Int J Sports Med.* 1995;16(3):201–206.
5. Aagaard H, Jorgenson U. Injuries in elite volleyball. *Scand J Med Sci Sports.* 1996;6(4):228–232.
6. Jones G, Asghar A, Llewellyn DJ. The epidemiology of rock-climbing injuries. *Br J Sports Med.* 2008;42:773–778.
7. Finklestein H. Stenosing tendovaginitis at the radial styloid process. *J Bone Joint Surg Am.* 1930;12:509–540.
8. Lindau T, Adlercreutz C, Aspenberg P. Periferal tears of the triangular fibrocartilage complex cause distal radioulnar joint instability after distal radial fracture. *J Hand Surg.* 2000;25(3):464–468.
9. LaStayo PC, Howell J. Clinical provocative tests used in evaluating wrist pain: a descriptive study. *J Hand Ther.* 1995;1:10–17.
10. Weiss AP, Akelman E, Tabatabai M. Treatment of de Quervain's disease. *J Hand Surg [Am].* 1994;19:595–598.
11. Harvey FJ, Harvey PM, Horsley MW. De Quervain's disease: surgical or nonsurgical treatment. *J Hand Surg [Am].* 1990;15:83–87.
12. Lapidus PW, Fenton R. Stenosing tenovaginitis at the wrist and fingers: report of 423 cases in 369 patients with 354 operations. *AMA Arch Surg.* 1952;64:475–487.
13. McMahon MS, Posner MA. Triggering of the thumb due to stenosing tenosynovitis of the extensor pollicis longus: a case report. *J Hand Surg [Am].* 1994;19:623–625.
14. Wood MB, Dobyns JH. Sports-related extraarticular wrist syndromes. *Clin Orthop Relat Res.* 1986;202:93–102.
15. Pantukosit S, Petchkrua W, Stiens SA. Intersection syndrome in Buriram Hospital: a 4-yr prospective study. *Am J Phys Med Rehabil.* 2001;80:656–661.
16. Grundberg AB, Reagan DS. Pathologic anatomy of the fore-arm: intersection syndrome. *J Hand Surg [Am].* 1985;10:299–302.
17. Minami A, Ishikawa J, Suenaga N, et al. Clinical results of treatment of triangular fibrocartilage complex tears by arthroscopic debridement. *J Hand Surg [Am].* 1996;21(3):406–411.
18. Grover R. Clinical assessment of scaphoid injuries and the detection of fractures. *J Hand Surg [Br].* 1996;21:341–343.
19. Trumble TE. Avascular necrosis after scaphoid fracture: a correlation of magnetic resonance imaging and histology. *J Hand Surg [Am].* 1990;15:557–564.
20. Rykman GK, Taleisnik J, Peters G, et al. Treatment of nonunited scaphoid fractures by pulsed electromagnetic field and cast. *J Hand Surg [Am].* 1986;11:344–349.
21. Carter PR, Eaton RG, Littler JW. Ununited fracture of the hook of the hamate. *J Bone Joint Surg Br.* 1977;59:583–588.
22. Andresen R, Radmer S, Sparmann M, et al. Imaging of hamate bone fractures in conventional x-rays and high-resolution computed tomography: an in vitro study. *Invest Radiol.* 1999;34:46–50.
23. Wright TW, Dobyns JH, Linscheid RL, et al. Carpal instability nondissociative. *J Hand Surg [Br].* 1994;19(6):763–773.
24. Albanese SA, Palmer AK, Kerr DR, et al. Wrist pain and distal growth plate closure of the radius in gymnasts. *J Pediatr Orthop.* 1989;9:23–28.
25. Shih C, Chang CY, Penn IW, et al. Chronically stressed wrists in adolescent gymnasts: MR imaging appearance. *Radiology.* 1995;195:855–859.
26. McCue FC, Garroway RY. Sports injuries to the hand and wrist. In: Schneider RC, ed. *Sports Injuries: Mechanisms, Prevention, and Treatment.* Baltimore: Williams & Wilkins; 1985.
27. McMaster PE. Tendons and muscle ruptures: clinical and experimental studies on the causes and location of subcutaneous ruptures. *J Bone Joint Surg.* 1933;15:705–722.
28. Souter WA. The boutonniere deformity: a review of 101 patients with division of the central slip of the extensor expansion of the fingers. *J Bone Joint Surg.* 1967;49B:710.

15

Athlete with Acute Wrist and Hand Injuries

Michelle Mariani

INTRODUCTION

Hand and wrist injuries are common in athletes, making up between 3% and 9% of all athletic injuries. Athletic injuries to the hand and wrist can range from simple sprains to severe fractures. Many injuries of the hand and wrist are obvious, but subtle injuries can be missed and may require a high index of suspicion with a systematic examination and diagnostic imaging. Often injuries to the hand and wrist may be dismissed as trivial; however, delay in diagnosis and treatment may lead to significant and possible permanent disability. Overtreatment or inappropriate treatment can be just as problematic. Swanson appropriately said, "Hand fractures can be complicated by deformity from no treatment, stiffness from over-treatment, and both deformity and stiffness from poor treatment."[1] In this chapter, we will discuss the diagnosis, treatment, and rehabilitation of common hand injuries to the athlete.

FUNCTIONAL ANATOMY

A basic understanding of the complex anatomy of the finger, hand, and wrist is necessary to properly diagnose and treat acute injuries. There are 27 bones that act dynamically to allow oppositional grip: eight carpal bones, five metacarpals, and fourteen phalangeal bones. In general, the radial nerve accounts for wrist and finger extension, the ulnar nerve provides finger flexion on the ulnar side and power grip, and the median nerve provides thumb opposition and circumduction to allow for fine control. Vascularity to the hand is provided by the radial and ulnar arteries, which join together in the palm to make up the deep and superficial palmar arches. Each digit has two neurovascular bundles, which travel volarly on both the radial and ulnar aspects of the digit.

Bony anatomy of the hand includes the five metacarpals, with first, fourth, and fifth metacarpals having increased mobility at their corresponding carpometacarpal (CMC) joints. In contrast, the second and third metacarpals are held rigid at the CMC joint by stout ligaments and congruent articulation with the trapezoid and capitate. The transverse metacarpal ligaments interconnect the second through the

fifth metacarpals adding to their internal support. The thumb metacarpal is positioned on the trapezium in an abducted and pronated position to allow for its prehensile function.

Each finger is an individual skeletal unit made up of a proximal, middle, and distal phalanx (Fig. 15.1A). The proximal and middle phalanges can be divided into the base, shaft, neck, and head, whereas the distal phalanx has a base, shaft, and tuft. There are three ginglymus (hinged) joints in each finger: distal interphalangeal (DIP), proximal interphalangeal (PIP), and metacarpophalangeal (MCP). The interphalangeal (IP) joints in the fingers are bicondylar, providing a great arc of motion as well as bony stability for lateral and rotatory forces. The collateral ligaments, volar plate, and extensor mechanism offer additional stability to the joint, and injury to these structures may compromise function significantly. The thumb CMC joint is unique with its reciprocally biconcave saddle joint allowing for opposition with the other digits.[2] The thumb is made up of the first metacarpal and only two phalanges with a single IP joint.

The most complex anatomy of the hand includes the extensor mechanism of the fingers. The extensor digitorum communis (EDC) splits into four separate tendons, one to each finger. As the extensor tendon passes over the MCP joint, there is some adhesion to the joint capsule, but no formal insertion. The tendon is anchored over the MCP joint by the sagittal bands that arise from the volar plate. In addition to keeping the extensor tendon centralized over the MCP joint, sagittal bands also function to extend the proximal phalanx. At the MCP joint, the extensor tendon splits into three slips. The middle slip, which connects to the proximal phalanx by sagittal bands, inserts on the base of the middle phalanx. The two lateral slips unite more distally on the base of the distal phalanx after receiving contributions from the interossei on both sides and the lumbrical on the radial side (Fig. 15.1B). On the radial side of each digit, the lumbrical unites with the lateral slip to form the lateral band. The interossei also insert into the lateral slips to form the lateral bands in addition to the base of the proximal phalanx and joint capsule.

The flexor tendons on the volar side of the finger include the flexor digitorum superficialis (FDS) and the flexor

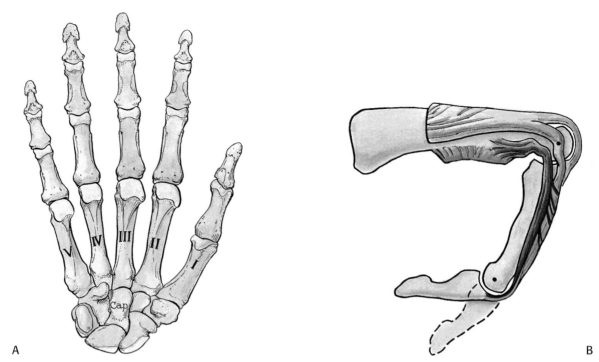

FIG. 15.1. Functional anatomy of the hand and wrist. **A**: Palmar view, bony anatomy of the hand and wrist (metacarpal bones labeled with Roman numerals). **B**: Lateral view of the retinacular ligaments in a flexed digit.

digitorum profundus (FDP). The FDS tendon travels volar to the FDP and splits to form two slips that attach to the base of the middle phalanx and function to flex the PIP joint. The FDP tendon is located dorsal to the FDS and inserts into the base of the distal phalanx and flexes the DIP joint.

The anatomy of the wrist comprises one of the most complex joints in the body. The eight wrist carpal bones articulate with the radius and ulna and allow for a large arc of motion in three degrees of freedom. The proximal row of carpal bones includes the scaphoid, lunate, triquetrum, and pisiform, which are closely approximated to the distal radius. The triangular fibrocartilage complex, an articular disk located between the proximal row of carpals and the ulna, completes the concave surface on which the carpals move. The distal row of carpal bones includes the hamate, capitate, trapezium, and trapezoid, which articulate with the metacarpals. The scaphoid is the common link between the proximal and the distal row of carpals.

EPIDEMIOLOGY

Injuries to the hand and wrist are common in athletes of all levels. The two main types of injuries suffered by athletes include soft-tissue injury (tendon and ligament) or bony injury (fracture and/or dislocation). Thumb injuries should be considered a discrete group of injuries compared with the other digits as the anatomy and function differ significantly.

The hand is usually out in front of the athlete and used to catch a ball in motion, brace any falls, and block opponents. The middle finger is a commonly injured finger because it extends most distally, allowing it to be vulnerable to jamming, catching, and torsion. Thumb injuries are more common in falls to the side or reaching behind to brace a fall, such as during skiing. The small finger can also easily be injured as it gets caught on a jersey. An axial load to a closed fist or a misdirected punch may cause a metacarpal fracture or CMC injury. Any fall on an outstretched hand can cause a hyperextension injury and lead to fracture or ligamentous injury in the wrist.

Injuries to flexor and extensor tendons can occur during athletics, but injuries to the extensor mechanism are more common because they are weaker when compared to the flexors. The common injuries of the extensor mechanism include the mallet finger, acute boutonniere, and sagittal band injuries. The main injury to the flexor tendon suffered during sporting events is an FDP avulsion injury, also known as jersey finger. Whereas most of the extensor injuries seen are easily treated with splinting and observation, all flexor tendon injuries should be referred to a hand surgeon urgently for surgical fixation.

Extensor tendon injuries such as mallet finger and acute boutonniere injuries are common injuries in ball sports such as basketball, when the athlete's fully extended finger is struck by the ball. In a mallet finger, the result is a stretching or disruption of the terminal tendon, which is responsible for active extension of the DIP joint. An acute boutonniere injury ranges from a sprain to complete disruption of the central slip that can result from a volar PIP dislocation. An avulsion fracture is possible with both of these injuries, so x-rays need to be done to evaluate for this variant of injury.

Injury to the sagittal bands can result in pain and extensor tendon subluxation during finger flexion. These injuries may occur from blunt trauma, forced flexion of the MCP joint, or sometimes even minor insults. These injuries usually involve a sagittal hood tear of the radial side of the long finger.

An FDP avulsion/rupture results from a forceful hyperextension of the DIP joint while the FDP is contracting. A classic example is catching the middle finger on a competitor's jersey. The tendon may rupture from its insertion or avulse a small bone fragment from the distal phalanx. The tendon may retract into the finger or palm.

Fractures of the metacarpals and phalanges are the most common fractures of the upper extremity.[3] The thumb and small finger are the most frequently fractured.[4] The majority of these fractures can be managed nonoperatively, but unstable fractures need to be recognized and referred to a hand surgeon for operative management. Regardless of treatment, the goal is to restore hand function and prevent stiffness or deformity.

The most commonly dislocated joint in the body is the PIP joint of the finger. Injury to the PIP joint can range from a jammed finger to a complex irreducible fracture dislocation. The severity of these injuries is often underestimated, and improper treatment may cause long-term disability. The direction of dislocation is usually dorsal, but volar and lateral dislocations may occur.

The DIP and MCP joints are less commonly dislocated. Dorsal dislocations are the more common variant of these IP dislocations. DIP dislocations are usually related to a crushing-type injury and are more prone to open injuries because of the tissue attachments distally. It is important to realize that MCP joint dislocations can be either simple subluxation injuries that can easily be reduced or a complex complete dislocation that usually requires surgery to relocate.

All IP dislocations are associated with some ligamentous injury. The most common soft-tissue injury with joint dislocations is avulsion of the volar plate. Collateral ligament and tendon avulsions are also possible at the time of injury. Intra-articular fractures can occur and range from small, insignificant avulsions to larger triangular or comminuted fractures that make up a significant portion of the joint.

Injuries to the thumb MCP joint are quite common. The most common injury to the MCP joint is an ulnar collateral ligament (UCL) disruption. This injury occurs when an athlete falls on an outstretched hand with the thumb abducted, as might occur when a skier falls while holding a pole.

The wrist is a complex anatomic structure made up of eight carpal bones, the distal radius, distal ulna, and multiple tendons and ligaments. It is beyond the scope of this chapter to discuss every injury that can occur to the intricate wrist, but the more common athletic injuries should be recognized. Appropriate treatment of wrist injuries can prevent future disability. Scaphoid fractures are by far the most common carpal fracture. Other acute sporting injuries to the wrist include hamate fractures and scapholunate ligament tears.

NARROWING THE DIFFERENTIAL DIAGNOSIS

History

A good history and detail of the mechanism of injury may help you focus on a diagnosis prior to the examination and help guide your decision-making. Some injuries are more prevalent in specific sports, such as jersey finger in rugby and football or hook of the hamate fractures in golf and baseball. Also a history of refractory pain in an initial negative assessment should prompt further examination and ·diagnostic imaging as a more subtle diagnosis may be present.

Evidence-based Physical Examination

Start with the basics of inspection, palpation, and a thorough neurovascular examination. Inspect for swelling, deformity, ecchymosis, and possible open injuries. Palpate for point tenderness, stepoffs, and crepitation. The patient should be able to actively extend all of their fingers and thumb. An inability to actively extend a finger should prompt further examination. Examination of finger flexion should include isolating the FDP and the FDS function. The FDP can be tested by holding the PIP straight and asking the patient to flex their DIP joint. Evaluation of rotational deformity may be picked up by observing that the plane of the fingernails lines up. If a rotational deformity is present, there will be finger crossover with flexion. Varus and valgus testing will help determine joint laxity. MCP joints should be stressed with the joint flexed to 90 degrees.

Diagnostic Testing

Imaging

Routine radiographs of the hand or wrist should begin with PA, lateral, and oblique views. If you are suspicious of a specific injury or need better visualization of a fracture, other views should be considered. Individual fingers should have a true lateral of the injured finger. A true AP of the thumb (Roberts view) is obtained by having the patient hyperpronate the hand and rest the dorsum of the thumb on the x-ray cassette. A true lateral of the basal joint is obtained by pronating the hand 20 degrees with the thumb flat on the x-ray cassette and the x-ray tube angled 10 degrees in a distal-to-proximal direction. A 30-degree pronated lateral will help visualize the second and third metacarpals, and a 30-degree supinated lateral will help visualize the fourth and fifth metacarpals. Suspicion of an easily missed CMC fracture dislocation should prompt careful inspection of these oblique views.

MRI may be utilized to better visualize soft-tissue injuries, while CT may be required to assess complex fractures and bony anatomy not visualized on plain radiographs. Musculoskeletal ultrasound is gaining popularity due to its excellent soft-tissue visualization of superficial structures along with the dynamic capabilities. Its relatively low cost and lack of ionizing radiation also make it a good option.

APPROACH TO THE ATHLETE WITH A TENDON INJURY

HISTORY AND PHYSICAL EXAMINATION

A mallet finger and acute boutonniere injuries are both caused by forced flexion of extended DIP and PIP joints, respectively. The history of a mallet injury often involves a ball striking the tip of the finger. The athlete may have only minimal pain and may even continue playing. The patient usually presents after the game or in the office with inability to actively extend the injured finger. Examination will confirm this flexion deformity, but passive extension should be possible.

Central slip injuries are usually from a jamming-type injury to the finger, and the patient will complain of pain at the PIP joint. The examination may demonstrate an acute boutonniere deformity, making the diagnosis easy, but this deformity usually takes several weeks of no treatment to develop. The patient should be tested for active PIP extension. Weak active PIP extension, with intact passive extension, is indicative of an acute central slip injury.

Patients with sagittal band injuries at the MP joint can present with a history of a direct blow or a more mundane activity such as flicking their finger. Boxers can suffer from this injury after repetitive trauma. Symptoms vary from pain and loss of motion at the MP joint to actual extensor tendon snapping during finger flexion. Ulnar deviation of the finger may also be apparent in severe cases. In order of frequency, these injuries are most common in the long, small, index, and ring fingers.

FDP avulsion injuries are an injury not to be missed, as surgical intervention is needed promptly to restore full finger function. The history usually involves catching or jamming the tip of the finger on an opponent or a ball. The DIP joint will be swollen and painful, and a painful fullness may also be appreciated more proximally along the volar aspect of the finger or in the palm. To test the integrity of the FDP, ask the patient to actively flex the DIP joint while immobilizing the PIP joint. Inability to do so should prompt immediate referral to a hand surgeon for surgical repair of the FDP tendon.

DIAGNOSTIC TESTING

Imaging

- AP and lateral x-rays
  - Evaluate for any avulsion fractures of the phalanges
  - Evaluate lateral x-ray for volar subluxation joints (bony mallet or central slip disruption)
  - Large fragment may be an indication for surgery (FDP avulsion)
    - Identify the level of retraction for operative planning.

TREATMENT

Nonoperative

- Most are able to be treated nonoperatively
- Six to eight weeks of continuous extension splinting
- Followed by 2 weeks of splinting at night and sporting activities[5]
- Lightly padded aluminum splint, stack splint, or ring splint
  - Applied to dorsal aspect of the DIP joint
  - Avoid immobilizing the PIP joint
  - Treatment can be initiated up to 6 months after the injury
  - Success rate with splinting approximately 80%[6]
  - Avoid pressure breakdown of skin with splinting
- Acute central slip injuries with a supple joint
  - PIP joint splinting for 6 weeks
  - Followed by night splinting for another 6 weeks
  - DIP and MP joints are left free and DIP flexion encouraged
  - Older patients immobilized for a shorter time to prevent PIP joint stiffness
- Sagittal band injuries not causing extensor tendon subluxation
  - Treated with buddy taping.
- Symptomatic subluxing extensor tendon and is diagnosed less than 3 weeks from injury
  - Hand-based MP extension splint[7,8]
  - Continued for 6 weeks
  - Block MP flexion, and allow for PIP motion.

Operative

- Surgical indications include
  - Open injuries
  - A large avulsion fracture with a volar subluxation of the distal phalanx
  - Closed injuries in patients who may not be able to work with a splint (i.e., surgeon)
- Surgical treatment recommended for
  - Closed boutonniere injuries with a large avulsion fracture[9]

- Repair of the sagittal band in a patient with a symptomatic subluxing extensor tendon
  - Diagnosed more than 3 weeks from injury
  - Or if they failed splint treatment
- All open injuries to tendons and flexor tendon injuries
- FDP tendon avulsion, which is usually repaired primarily
- Protected immobilization of the repair for 6 to 8 weeks

Prognosis/Return to Play

- Prognosis is excellent in a closed mallet or boutonniere injury
- Diligent in continual splinting for 6 to 8 weeks
- If the finger falls into flexion, must start from the beginning
- Return to play varies with the severity
- Most can return with an appropriate splint
- Sagittal band injuries have a good prognosis
- If no tendon subluxation, may return to play with buddy taping
- Surgery may delay return to play until full range of motion and grip strength returns
- Prognosis of flexor tendon injuries prognosis depends on early recognition and treatment
- FDP avulsion injuries require surgical intervention
- May restrict activities for 3 to 4 months

Complications/Indications for Referral

Complications of extensor tendon injuries are not common, but can occur with insufficient treatment or noncompliance. An extensor lag deformity may persist and secondary deformities may develop. A persistent mallet injury will develop into a swan-neck deformity, and the central slip injury will fall into a boutonniere deformity. Complications of sagittal band injuries are rare, but operatively repaired sagittal band injuries may become stiff.

There are specific findings in tendon injuries that should prompt referral to a hand surgeon. Any open tendon injury, unstable joint, lack of passive extension, or avulsion fracture involving greater than 30% are indications for referral and possible surgical intervention. It is also imperative to diagnose the FDP avulsion injury early and refer promptly. A delay of 7 days will make repair difficult and may compromise the outcome of the finger function.

APPROACH TO THE ATHLETE WITH A HAND FRACTURE

HISTORY AND PHYSICAL EXAMINATION

Phalangeal and metacarpal fractures can range from nondisplaced stable fractures to displaced, comminuted fractures. Often the type of fracture is directly related to the mechanism of injury. A direct blow usually causes a transverse fracture. Rotational forces, such as those that occur when an athlete grabs an opponent's jersey, cause spiral fractures. Axial loading to the finger usually causes intra-articular fractures and may be associated with joint dislocation as previously discussed. An axial load on a closed fist is the common mechanism of a fourth or fifth metacarpal neck fracture, commonly referred to as a "boxer's fracture."

Physical examination should include a routine neurovascular examination, range of motion of each joint, inspection of the skin for potential open fractures, and evaluation for any deformity. Every phalangeal and metacarpal fracture should be evaluated specifically for rotational deformity. This can be accomplished by asking the patient to flex all digits and evaluate for any rotation or overlap of the injured finger in comparison with the other digits. All fingers should point toward the scaphoid.

DIAGNOSTIC TESTING

Imaging

- Radiographs – PA, lateral, and oblique views
  - Identify fractures and define the severity of the injury
  - Semipronated view will allow optimal visualization of the index metacarpal
  - Semisupinated view will allow optimal visualization of the ring and small finger metacarpal
  - Individual finger radiographs to assess for phalangeal fractures

TREATMENT

Nonoperative

- Most phalangeal and metacarpal fractures can be managed nonoperatively
- Distal phalanx fractures are divided into tuft and transverse fractures
- Tuft fractures
  - Associated with an open nail bed injury or subungual hematoma
  - If a subungual hematoma that involves greater than 50% of the nail bed is decompressed
  - Dorsal aluminum splint
    - Rarely indicated for more than 3 weeks
    - Should not include the PIP joint[3]
- Nondisplaced and stable middle and proximal phalangeal fractures
  - Buddy taping or splinting
  - Can be reduced to convert to a stable fracture
  - Wrist-based splint, MP joints flexed to 70 degrees and the digits in extension

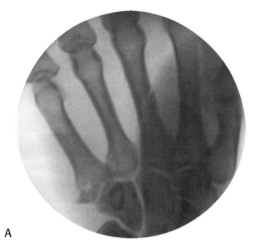 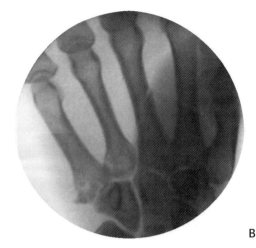

A   B

FIG. 15.2. A: 25-year-old male professional baseball player who sustained a closed carpometacarpal (CMC) fracture dislocation of the left hand after a diving catch. **B:** Note the displaced fracture of the small finger metacarpal base. Reprinted with permission from Strickland JW, Graham TJ. *Master Techniques in Orthopeadic Surgery: The Hand.* 2nd ed. Philadelphia: Lippincott Williams & Wilkins; 2005.

- Follow up radiographs weekly until bony union is evident
- Spiral and oblique fractures have a tendency to redisplace and shorten and often require internal fixation
- Metacarpal fractures
  - Ring and small fingers can tolerate up to 40 degrees of dorsal angulation
  - Index and middle fingers can tolerate only 10 to 15 degrees of dorsal angulation
  - Reduction by flexing the MP joint to 90 degrees and using the proximal phalanx to exert an upward pressure on the flexed metacarpal head[10]
  - Held in place by plaster or fiberglass
  - X-ray is done weekly to confirm satisfactory reduction
  - Nondisplaced metacarpal neck fractures can be treated with simple buddy taping
  - A functional brace is an option in treatment of stable metacarpal fractures
  - Spiral or oblique fractures are more likely to cause a malrotation deformity and need to be corrected to restore normal hand function. If the rotation is not corrected after reduction, surgical intervention may be necessary.

- An intra-articular fracture of the phalangeal condyle
  - Usually requires surgical intervention
  - If nonoperative treatment should be followed very closely
- Phalangeal shaft fractures with angulation, rotation, or shortening that cannot be corrected by reduction and splinting
- Metacarpal neck and shaft fractures
  - Open reduction or percutaneous pinning
  - Ring metacarpal fractures with angulation greater than 20 degrees
  - Small finger metacarpal fractures with angulation greater than 30 degrees[12]
  - Others have accepted much more angulation with no significant disability with up to 70 degrees of angulation[13–15]
- Metacarpal base fracture (Fig. 15.2)
  - Often associated with a CMC dislocation
  - Usually requires closed reduction and percutaneous fixation to maintain the joint reduction
- Other indications for surgical fixation of phalangeal and metacarpal fractures
  - Open fractures, segmental bone loss, and multiple hand and wrist fractures.

Operative

- Unstable fractures that should be recognized and referred for surgical intervention
- Displaced transverse distal phalanx fracture
  - Disruption of the overlying nail matrix
  - Requires internal fixation and debridement of nail matrix
  - Stabilization is accomplished with a longitudinal Kirschner pin or with a small screw[11]

Prognosis/Return to Play

- Intra-articular fractures will have a poorer prognosis than extra-articular fractures[16]
- Fracture patterns associated with poor outcomes
- Extensive comminution, bone loss, and unstable fractures with significant deformity
- Extensive soft-tissue injury and extended splinting are both associated with decreased range of motion and poorer outcomes

- When immobilization exceeded 4 weeks, total active motion declined to 66% of normal[17]
- Metacarpal fractures are inherently stable and may be treated with minimal or no immobilization with good outcomes
- In minimally or nondisplaced fractures in athletes, the average time lost from practice or competition was 14 days[18]
- Displaced metacarpal fractures that require a reduction may return to sports and unrestricted activity as early as 4 to 6 weeks.

Complications/Indications for Referral

Common complications of phalangeal and metacarpal fractures include stiffness and malunions. Nonunions are uncommon, but delayed union may be seen. Malunions can cause angular deformity, rotational deformity, or shortening. These need to be referred for possible corrective osteotomy. Stiffness is fairly common and has a higher likelihood with associated soft-tissue or joint injury. Treatment of this complication should start with an aggressive hand therapy program and may require dynamic splinting. Failure to regain full motion with conservative measures should prompt referral for possible tenolysis. Phalangeal and metacarpal fractures with extensive comminution, bone loss, and unstable fractures with significant deformity are beyond the scope of nonoperative treatment. These fractures are prone to residual disability regardless of the method of treatment, so they should be referred to a hand surgeon early.

APPROACH TO THE ATHLETE WITH AN INTERPHALANGEAL JOINT DISLOCATION

HISTORY AND PHYSICAL EXAMINATION

The usual mechanism of injury in a dorsal PIP dislocation is a hyperextension injury combined with axial compression. This often happens in ball-handling sports such as football. An athlete with a dorsal dislocation will have a fixed deformity, swelling, and tenderness over the volar plate. Volar and rotatory PIP dislocations are rare and are usually the result of a rotatory axial compression force while the PIP joint is flexed. These dislocations will also have diffuse tenderness, swelling, and a fixed deformity, which may have a rotational component.

DIP and MCP joint dislocations are less common but usually present with a fixed deformity at the respective joint. Both usually dislocate dorsally, and flexion of the joint is impossible. MCP joint dislocations occur predominantly in the index and small fingers from a hyperextension-type injury. An MCP joint subluxation (simple dislocation) is usually

locked in about 60 degrees of hyperextension. In contrast, the patient with a complete (complex) MCP joint dislocation presents with the proximal finger held in slight hyperextension with inability to flex the MCP joint, and the metacarpal head is palpable in the palm.

After a reduction, the collateral ligaments should be examined, and active flexion and extension should be evaluated to ensure the integrity of tendons.[19,20] Functional stability of the joint is determined by checking both active and passive stability.[21] Active stability is tested by having the patient move the digit through its normal range of motion. Full active range of motion is an indication of joint stability despite ligament disruption. Passive stability is assessed by applying lateral stress to each collateral ligament at both full extension and 30 degrees of flexion. The dorsovolar stability of the joint is tested by attempting to translate the joint both dorsally and volarly to detect any laxity. Laxity in any plane should be compared to an uninjured joint. The laxity can then be graded I–III, depending on the amount of opening, with I being pain and minimal instability and III being gross instability and complete tearing of the collateral ligament. More than 20 degrees of laxity with lateral testing indicates complete collateral ligament disruption plus injury to at least one other secondary stabilizer.[19]

DIAGNOSTIC TESTING

- Three views (PA, true lateral, oblique) of the are required.
- Hand x-ray or fanned-out four-finger x-ray is not acceptable
  - Subtle dislocations may be missed. The PA and true lateral x-rays should be carefully evaluated for the direction of the dislocation and any associated fractures
- CT is occasionally for complex intra-articular fracture

TREATMENT

Nonoperative

- On-the-field reduction, if suspected IP dislocation
- Splint and follow up x-rays to confirm joint congruity
- Stable PIP dislocation
  - Reduction and splinting
  - Postreduction examination of the joint is key
  - Reduction of a *dorsal* PIP joint by gentle traction and volar-directed pressure to the middle phalanx
  - May need to reproduce the hyperextension injury to unlock the dislocated digit
- *Volar* PIP dislocation
  - The condyle is often buttonholed through the extensor mechanism between the lateral band and the central slip
  - Traction will tighten lateral bands and prevent reduction

- Reduce with flexion of the MP and PIP joint while applying traction
- Splint dorsal PIP dislocation in 30 degrees of flexion
- Splint volar PIP dislocation in extension
- Splint simple dislocations with no ligamentous laxity for 7 to 10 days and then begin protected range of motion with buddy taping
- Ligamentous injury; splinted for 3 weeks
- DIP dislocations reduced with simple traction and direct pressure
  - Uncomplicated DIP splinted for 7 to 10 days
  - Early range of motion
- MCP subluxations treated with closed reduction
  - Reduction by applying distal and volar-directed pressure to the proximal phalanx with the wrist flexed to relax the flexor tendons
  - Hyperextension and traction should be avoided in these injuries because these reduction techniques could convert the injury to a complete (complex) dislocation
  - Early range of motion is encouraged with an extension block
- Complete MCP dislocations require open reduction

Operative

- All irreducible dislocations should be referred
- Unstable fracture/dislocation should also be referred for surgical intervention (Fig. 15.3)
  - Articular fracture greater than 40% of the size of the articular surface
  - Any condylar fracture
  - Incongruency of the joint
- Any complete MCP joint dislocation by definition has some interposed soft tissue and requires an open reduction
- Primary repair of complete collateral ligament tears
  - Decrease the time of disability and provide predictable stability of the joint[20]
  - An option in high-demand athletes
  - Instability is rarely a long-term sequelae of this injury, and stiffness is much more common

- Repair of collateral ligaments reserved for subacute or chronic joint instability

Prognosis/Return to Play

- Most patients with uncomplicated IP dislocations have a good outcome
- Simple dislocations that are reduced and verified to be stable by x-ray and physical examination; the athlete may return to play early
- If any surgical intervention is needed, return to play may be delayed for 4 to 6 weeks.

Complications/Indications for Referral

After joint reduction, you should be able to determine if an IP joint is stable or unstable by physical examination and radiographic evaluation. It is key to identify any residual joint subluxation, joint laxity, and fractures that involve more than 40% of the articular surface. These unstable fractures should be referred to a hand specialist for further treatment. Less common volar PIP dislocations and complete (complex) MCP dislocations should be recognized as more technically difficult injuries. Both are difficult to reduce and often need referral for an open reduction. Most long-term complications are related to stiffness or instability and should be referred to a hand specialist if these arise.

APPROACH TO THE ATHLETE WITH A THUMB INJURY

HISTORY AND PHYSICAL EXAMINATION

The common presentation of an UCL injury is an injury causing forced abduction of the thumb. The athlete will present with tenderness, swelling, and possibly ecchymosis along the ulnar border of the MCP joint. The integrity of the UCL can be assessed for instability by testing for any laxity and an end point to valgus stress in extension and 30 degrees

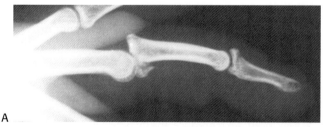

A

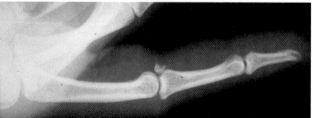

B

FIG. 15.3. Evidence of incongruent reduction ranges from **(A)** the radiographically obvious full subluxation of the major dorsal fragment away from the volar lip to **(B)** extremely subtle evidence of slight dorsal opening and lack of absolute congruence on the lateral view. Reprinted with permission from Bucholz RW, Heckman JD. *Rockwood & Green's Fractures in Adults.* 5th ed. Philadelphia: Lippincott Williams & Wilkins; 2001.

of flexion.[19] A grade I sprain will have pain without laxity. A partially torn ligament (grade II) will have laxity with stressing, but in contrast to a complete UCL tear, it will have an end point. Local anesthesia may be necessary to accurately evaluate for any joint laxity. Occasionally, if the injury is a complete tear, the patient will present with a tender palpable nodule proximal to the MCP joint. This is known as a Stener lesion and is the result of the UCL retracting beyond the adductor aponeurosis.

Injuries of CMC joint are usually caused by axially loading force across a partially flexed thumb. This injury usually results in a two-part intra-articular fracture at the base of the thumb metacarpal known as a Bennett fracture. A Bennett fracture is the most frequent fracture of the thumb and by definition is a fracture dislocation of the thumb CMC joint. The volar–ulnar fragment is held in its anatomic position against the trapezium by the volar beak ligament, but the metacarpal shaft and base displace dorsally and rotate into a supinated position. A Rolando fracture is a comminuted intra-articular fracture of the base of the thumb metacarpal. Rolando fractures can either be a basic three-part Y or T configuration or have further comminution. Patients with an injury of their CMC joint will have localized pain, swelling, and diminished thumb motion.

DIAGNOSTIC TESTING

Imaging

- Radiographs
  - MCP injuries: standard PA, lateral, and oblique radiographs[22]
  - Stress radiographs are rarely needed[23,24]
  - CMC injures: lateral view with hand palm down, pronating the wrist 15 to 35 degrees and directing x-ray tube obliquely 15 degrees[25]
- Alternative modalities
  - Ultrasound
  - CT may be necessary for Rolando fractures
  - MRI angiography

FUNCTIONAL TREATMENT

Nonoperative

- Acute partial UCL injuries
  - Four weeks of immobilization in a thumb spica
  - Followed by 2 weeks of immobilization with active range of motion exercises
  - Strenuous thumb activity avoided for 3 months
- Complete ligament tears are less predictable
  - Exploration and repair of the ligament
  - Immobilization in a thumb spica for complete tears as long as there is no Stener lesion[26]

- Bennett fractures
  - Thumb spica cast immobilization effective with adequate reduction maintained
  - Reduction by traction and metacarpal extension, pronation, and abduction
  - Reduction difficult to maintain due to pull of APL

Operative

- Complete UCL tear/avulsion: operative treatment commonly necessary
  - Stener lesion indicates complete tear
  - Indication for surgery: greater that 30 degrees of laxity or no firm end point
  - Open repair has good results in many studies and complications are infrequent[27–29]
  - Surgical repair should be done early[30]
  - MCP immobilized for approximately 4 to 6 weeks postop
  - Range of motion exercises initiated after 4 weeks
  - By 10 weeks postoperatively, the athlete should have regained nearly full active range of motion and have at least 60% of normal pinch strength.[3]
- CMC fracture surgical indication: 1 mm of articular incongruity or persistent CMC joint subluxation after closed reduction (Fig. 15.4)
  - Closed reduction and casting of Bennett fractures leads to diminished mobility and strength, as well as degenerative arthritis and joint subluxation[31]
  - Closed reduction with percutaneous fixation.
- Immobilized for 4 to 6 weeks before pins are removed
  - Open reduction with internal fixation (ORIF)
- Early active range of motion
  - Rolando fracture: ORIF versus external fixation and bone grafting versus arthrodesis

Prognosis/Return to Play

- If the injury is identified early and treated appropriately, most athletes have an excellent outcome.
- In partial UCL tears (grade I and II) the athlete can return to play early in a well-padded splint or cast to protect the injury during healing.
- In certain sports that require ball handling, the athlete may need to wait for 6 to 8 weeks for complete recovery from this injury.
- Complete UCL tears (grade III) usually require surgery and take 8 to 12 weeks to recover; return sooner is possible with splint or cast protection.[3]

Complications/Indications for Referral

Complications are rare after UCL injury treatment. In nonoperatively treated UCL injuries, the patient may have residual stiffness of the MCP joint, but is likelier to have

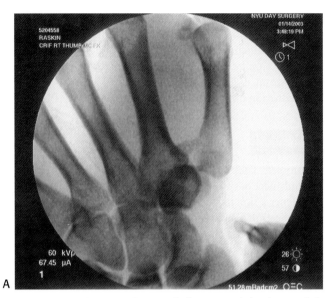
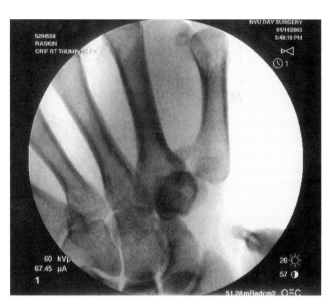

FIG. 15.4. Bennett's fracture of the base of the thumb metacarpal. **A:** Prereduction fluoroscopic image. **B:** Postreduction fluoroscopic image. Reprinted with permission from Strickland JW, Graham TJ. *Master Techniques in Orthopeadic Surgery: The Hand.* 2nd ed. Philadelphia: Lippincott Williams & Wilkins; 2005.

continued laxity or diminished pinch strength in incompletely healed ligaments. Operative complications include injury to the crossing branches of the dorsal sensory branch of the radial nerve or stiffness from over-tightening of the repaired ligament. These two complications can be avoided by careful surgical technique. Patients with complete UCL tear and no Stener lesions are a relative indication for surgery, and complete UCL tear with a Stener lesion is an absolute indication for surgery. Both should be referred to a hand surgeon for consultation.

It is important to recognize fractures of the thumb CMC joint and understand the Bennett fracture is also a dislocation and requires anatomic reduction. Complications of a missed or incorrectly treated thumb CMC fracture can lead to degenerative arthritis and diminished thumb function. All CMC injuries should be referred to a hand surgeon for evaluation.

APPROACH TO THE ATHLETE WITH A WRIST INJURY

HISTORY AND PHYSICAL EXAMINATION

A scaphoid fracture usually occurs from a fall on an outstretched hand but can also occur from a punch. An athlete will usually present with radial-sided wrist pain at the base of the thumb with tenderness over the snuffbox and/or volar scaphoid tubercle. On the dorsum of the wrist, the anatomic snuffbox can be identified easily as the patient abducts and extends the thumb. There is usually no deformity and only minimal swelling. A fall on an outstretched hand can also result in a distal radius fracture, which usually has more swelling and deformity or a scapholunate ligament disruption. A scapholunate ligament tear can be detected on physical examination by tenderness dorsally just distal to Lister's tubercle and provocative maneuvers that cause a painful clunk. If the thumb is placed on the scaphoid tubercle, four fingers can wrap around the distal radius while the wrist is held in ulnar deviation. The patient is then asked to radially deviate his or her wrist. As the patient does this, the scaphoid tubercle will volar flex into the physician's thumb. If pressure is directed dorsally with the thumb, pain may be elicited and an associated clunk may indicate scapholunate instability. This maneuver is termed the Watson or scaphoid shift test.[32]

Scapholunate dissociation (SLD) is the most common carpal instability. An SLD may be easily missed, especially when it is an isolated injury or masked by a more obvious injury such as a fracture. Any history of a fall on an outstretched hand with presenting wrist pain is possibly an SLD injury. Continued radial-sided wrist pain with a negative workup for scaphoid fracture may be an occult or partial SL tear. SLD may also occur in conjunction to distal radius or scaphoid fractures.

A hook of the hamate fracture usually occurs in athletes that use a club, bat, or racquet. This injury can easily be missed because it is not apparent on standard radiographs, so clinical suspicion should prompt further diagnostic imaging. This injury may occur when an athlete falls while holding an object, such as a racquet. A hard hit baseball or a golf club striking the ground may also cause a hamate fracture. The patient will present with pain in the volar and ulnar sides of the wrist. Loss of grip strength may also be another symptom. To locate and palpate the hook of the hamate, place your thumb IP joint over the easily identified pisiform and direct your thumb toward the patient's index finger. With the patient's wrist flexed, the hook of the hamate can be felt with the tip of your thumb. Direct tenderness should raise suspicion of a fracture.

DIAGNOSTIC TESTING

Imaging

- Radiographs (Fig. 15.5)
  - PA, lateral, oblique, and ulnar deviated views
  - PA view is best obtained with a clenched fist
  - Clenched fist view will accentuate scapholunate gap[31]
  - Increased SL joint space of greater than 5 mm is diagnostic of SLD

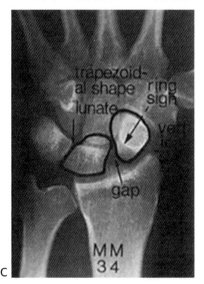
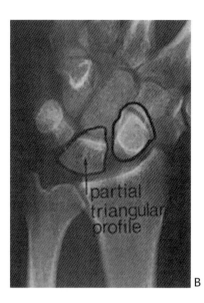
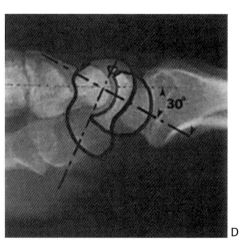

FIG. 15.5. X-ray findings in scapholunate dissociation. **A:** In ulnar deviation, increased scapholunate gap with incomplete radial translation of the lunate. **B:** In radial deviation, the scapholunate gap closes, and the lunate partially rotates and shows a triangular profile. **C:** The gap between scaphoid and lunate exceeds 3 mm; note the trapezoidal shape of the lunate secondary to the volar pole of the lunate rotating under the capitate. Also note foreshortening of the scaphoid due to its palmar flexed position. A ring sign is produced by the cortical outline of the distal pole of the scaphoid. **D:** Lateral view: the scaphoid is palmar flexed and the lunate extended. The capitate is displaced dorsally relative to the radius. Reprinted with permission from Bucholz RW, Heckman JD. *Rockwood & Green's Fractures in Adults*. 5th ed. Philadelphia: Lippincott Williams & Wilkins; 2001.

- Lateral projection of an SLD may demonstrate an increased flexion of the scaphoid or extension of the lunate
- Greater than 60 degrees indicates disruption of the scapholunate ligament
- Ulnar deviated PA view will allow better visualization of scaphoid waist fracture
- Radiographs repeated in 1 to 2 weeks if initial series equivocal
- Hamate fractures difficult to visualize on radiographs
  - Carpal tunnel projection view[33]
  - Oblique radiograph obtained in 45 degrees of supination, slight radial deviation, and dorsiflexion[34]
- MRI if x-ray questionable[35]
- MRA useful for defining SL ligament disruption
- CT if x-ray questionable[36]
  - Sensitivity of 100%, specificity of 94%, and accuracy of 97.2% in detecting hook of the hamate fractures[37]
- Bone scan at 48 to 72 hours following injury
  - Imprecise at localization of the fracture[38]
- Arthroscopy is gold standard for SL disruption

TREATMENT

Nonoperative

- Nondisplaced scaphoid fractures treated with a thumb spica cast
- Usually heals between 8 and 12 weeks but differs based on the location of the fracture
  - Hundred percent of distal scaphoid fractures heal in 6 to 8 weeks
  - Sixty to seventy percent of proximal scaphoid fractures will heal
    - May take up to 24 weeks
  - Ninety percent waist fracture heals by 12 weeks
  - Presentation later than 4 weeks requires longer immobilization to achieve union[39]
- Scapholunate disruption
  - Nonoperative treatment only recommended for dynamic instability
  - Activity modification, wrist splinting, and anti-inflammatory medications
- Hook of the hamate fractures
  - Cast immobilization for 6 weeks
  - Injuries diagnosed late or left untreated will progress to nonunion
  - Displaced and proximal pole scaphoid fractures require surgical intervention
  - The length of cast and duration of treatment are debatable

Operative

- Surgery is recommended for unstable scaphoid fractures and proximal pole fractures[3]
  - Displacement of 1 mm or more

- Fragment angulation
- Abnormal carpal alignment
- Proximal pole scaphoid fractures should be treated operatively[3]
- Other surgical indications for scaphoid fractures include high-demand athletes and scaphoid fractures associated with ligamentous injury or other fractures[40,41]
- Surgical techniques
  - Percutaneous fixation
  - ORIF
- Acute SL ligament tears treated with closed reduction and percutaneous pinning or acute ligament repair and capsulodesis
- The wrist is usually immobilized for 6 to 8 weeks following surgery
- Partial tears of the SL ligament complex are best treated with arthroscopic debridement[3]
- Hook of the hamate fractures diagnosed late, or in those that have progressed to a painful nonunion
  - Excision of the fragment is recommended[42]
  - Osteosynthesis may be considered for delayed union and nonunion in a high-performance athlete such as a professional golfer or baseball player[43]
    - Offers little benefit over excision in terms of functional outcome.

Prognosis / Return To Play

- The vast majority of scaphoid fractures will heal if diagnosed promptly and treated appropriately.
- Early rigid fixation may allow for early active motion and earlier return to sports.[44,45]
- Athletes may be able to return with a cast in some sports, but full unrestricted activities should be restricted until evidence of radiographic healing and return of full range of motion.
- SLD treatment results are more unpredictable and immobilization is needed for at least 8 weeks and athletic restrictions may last 6 to 12 months.
- Hook of the hamate fracture excision has good results.
- Most patients are able to return to full athletic activities shortly after excision with only mild pain and weakness.

Complications/Indications for Referral

Nonunion is the most common complication after scaphoid fracture treatment. Nonunion rates may be as high as 10% of cases despite proper treatment and, if left untreated, will progress to osteoarthritis.[46] All proximal pole fractures and displaced fractures should be referred for a hand surgery consultation as they are at a higher risk of complications and usually require surgical intervention. SLD can lead to changes in the wrist kinematics that increase load concentration across the radioscaphoid joint and progressive degenerative changes. These SLD injuries are often diagnosed weeks to months after the injury but before any evidence of degenerative changes. These injuries are difficult to both diagnose and treat, and all suspected SLD should be referred to a hand surgeon. Hook of the hamate fractures may result in a painful nonunion, but this can be treated by excision of the fragment.

KEY POINTS
• X-rays are needed to evaluate for joint subluxation and avulsion fractures
• Nondisplaced scaphoid waste fractures are best treated in a cast for 12 weeks
• Most phalangeal and metacarpal fractures can be managed nonoperatively
• Splinting for 6 to 8 weeks is appropriate for most extensor tendon injuries
• Indication for surgical referral includes flexor tendon injuries, open tendon injuries, intra-articular fractures, complete MCP dislocations, and CMC fractures

REFERENCES

1. Swanson AB. Fractures involving the digits of the hand. *Orthop Clin North Am.* 1970;1:261–274.
2. Kuczynski K. Carpometacarpal joint of the human thumb. *J Anat.* 1974;118:119–126.
3. Kaplan EB. Anatomy, injuries and treatment of the extensor apparatus of the hand and fingers. *Clin Orthop Relat Res.* 1959;13:24–41.
4. Abouna JM, Brown H. The treatment of mallet finger: the results in a series of 148 consecutive cases and a review of the literature. *Br J Surg.* 1968;55:653–667.
5. Araki S, Ohtani T, Tanaka T. Acute dislocation of the extensor digitorum communis tendon at the metacarpophalangeal joint. *J Bone Joint Surg Am.* 1987;69:616–619.
6. Inoue G, Tamura Y. Dislocation of the extensor tendons over the metacarpophalangeal joints. *J Hand Surg [Am].* 1996;21:464–469.
7. Tubiana R. Surgical repair of the extensor apparatus of the fingers. *Surg Clin North Am.* 1968;48:1015–1031.
8. Green DP, Hotchkiss R. *Green's Operative Hand Surgery.* 5th ed. Philadelphia: JB Lippincott; 2005.
9. Hove LM. Fractures of the hand. *Scand J Plast Reconstr Surg.* 1993;27:317–319.
10. Jahss SA. Fractures of the metacarpals: a new method of reduction and immobilization. *J Bone Joint Surg.* 1938;20:178–186.
11. Richards RR, Khoury G, Young MC. Internal fixation of an unstable open fracture of the distal phalanx with a Herbert screw. *J Hand Surg [Am].* 1988;13:428–432.
12. Amadio PC, Beckenbaugh RD, Bishop AT, et al. Fractures of the hand and wrist. In: Jupiter JB, ed. *Flynn's hand surgery.* Baltimore: Williams & Wilkins; 1991:122–185.
13. Holst-Nielsen F. Subcapital fractures of the four ulnar metacarpal bones. *Hand.* 1976;8:290–293.
14. Hunter JM, Cowen NJ. Fifth metacarpal fractures in a compensation clinic population. *J Bone Joint Surg Am.* 1970;52:1159–1165.
15. Kuokkanen HOM, Mulari-Keranen SK, Niskanen RO, et al. Treatment of subcapital fractures of the fifth metacarpal bone: a prospective randomised comparison between functional treatment and reposition and splinting. *Scand J Plast Reconstr Surg.* 1999;33:315–317.
16. Stark HH. *Troublesome Fractures and Dislocations of the Hand.* St. Louis, AAOS Instructional Course Lectures. Vol. 19. St. Louis: CV Mosby; 1970:130–149.
17. Strickland JW, Steichen JB, Kleinman WB, et al. Phalangeal fractures: factors influencing digital performance. *Orthop Rev.* 1982;11:39–50.
18. Rettig AC, Ryan R, Shelbourne KD, et al. Metacarpal fractures in the athlete. *Am J Sports Med.* 1989;17:567–572.
19. Mintzer CM, Waters PM. Late presentation of a ligamentous ulnar collateral ligament injury in a child. *J Hand Surg [Am].* 1994;19:1048–1049.
20. Bowers WH, Hurst LC. Gamekeeper's thumb: evaluation by arthrography and stress roentgenography. *J Bone Joint Surg Am.* 1977;59:519–524.
21. Downey EF Jr, Curtis DJ. Patient-induced stress test of the first metacarpophalangeal joint: a radiographic assessment of collateral ligament injuries. *Radiology.* 1986;158:679–683.
22. Billing L, Gedda KO. Roentgen examination of Bennett's fracture. *Acta Radiol.* 1952;38:471–476.
23. Abrahamsson SO, Sollerman C, Lundborg G, et al. Diagnosis of displaced ulnar collateral ligament of the metacarpophalangeal joint of the thumb. *J Hand Surg [Am].* 1990;15:457–460.
24. Livesley PJ. The conservative management of Bennett's fracture-dislocation: a 26-year follow-up. *J Hand Surg [Br].* 1990;15:291–294.
25. Bostock S, Morris MA. The range of motion of the MP joint of the thumb following operative repair of the ulnar collateral ligament. *J Hand Surg [Br].* 1993;18:710–711.
26. Gerber C, Senn E, Matter P. Skier's thumb: surgical treatment of recent injuries to the ulnar collateral ligament of the thumb's metacarpophalangeal joint. *Am J Sports Med.* 1981;9:171–177.
27. Jackson M, McQueen MM. Gamekeeper's thumb: a quantitative evaluation of acute surgical repair. *Injury.* 1994;25:21–23.
28. Kiefhaber TR, Stern PJ, Grood ES. Lateral stability of the proximal interphalangeal joint. *J Hand Surg [Am].* 1986;11:661–669.
29. Minamikawa Y, Horii E, Amadio PC, et al. Stability and constraint of the proximal interphalangeal joint. *J Hand Surg [Am].* 1993;18:198–204.
30. Kato H, Minami A, Takahara M, et al. Surgical repair of acute collateral ligament injuries in digits with the Mitek bone suture anchor. *J Hand Surg [Br].* 1999;24(1):70–75.
31. Eaton RG, Littler JW. Joint injuries and their sequelae. *Clin Plast Surg.* 1976;3:85–98.
32. Kiefhaber TR, Stern PJ, Grood ES. Lateral stability of the proximal interphalangeal joint. *J Hand Surg [Am].* 1986;11:661–669.
33. Lewis DM, Osterman AL. Scapholunate instability in athletes. *Clin Sports Med.* 2001;20:131–140.
34. Tiel-van Buul MMC, Bos KE, Dijkstra PF, et al. Carpal instability: the missed diagnosis in patients with clinically suspected scaphoid fracture. *Injury.* 1993;24:257–263.
35. Lepisto J, Mattila K, Nieminen S, et al. Low field MRI and scaphoid fracture. *J Hand Surg.* 1995;20:539–542.
36. Larsen CF, Brandon V, Wienhultz G, et al. An algorithm for acute wrist trauma. *J Hand Surg [Br].* 1995;18:207–212.
37. Murphy D, Eisenhauer M. The utility of a bone scan in the diagnosis of clinical scaphoid fracture. *J Emerg Med.* 1994;12:709–712.
38. Hart VL, Gaynor V. Roentgenographic study of the carpal canal. *J Bone Joint Surg.* 1941;23:382.
39. Nisenfield FG, Neviaser RJ. Fracture of the hook of the hamate: a diagnosis easily missed. *J Trauma.* 1974;14:612–616.
40. Rettig AC, Kollias SC. Internal fixation of acute stable scaphoid fractures in the athlete. *Am J Sports Med.* 1996;24:182–186.
41. Taras J, Sweet S, Shum W, et al. Percutaneous and arthroscopic screw fixation of scaphoid fractures in the athlete. *Hand Clin.* 1999;15:467–473.
42. Andresen R, Radmer S, Sparmann M, et al. Imaging of hamate bone fractures in conventional x-rays and high-resolution computed tomography: an in vitro study. *Invest Radiol.* 1999;34:46–50.
43. Mack GR, Wilckens JH, McPherson SA. Subacute scaphoid fractures: a closer look at closed treatment. *Am J Sports Med.* 1998;26:56–58.
44. Bishop AT, Beckenbaugh RD. Fracture of the hamate hook. *J Hand Surg [Am].* 1988;13:135–139.
45. Watson HK, Rogers WD. Nonunion of the hook of the hamate: an argument for bone grafting the nonunion. *J Hand Surg [Am].* 1989;14:486–490.
46. Mack GR, Bosse MJ, Gelberman RH, et al. The natural history of scaphoid non-union. *J Bone Joint Surg Am.* 1984;66:504–509.

16 Athlete with Back Pain

Peter Hoth and Katherine Riggert

INTRODUCTION

Back pain is a symptom often encountered by athletes of all ages and levels of sports participation. Chronic back pain is the most common reason for missed playing time.[1] Although certain sports such as gymnastics, wrestling, and rowing have a higher prevalence of low back pain due to repetitive mechanical loads placed on the spine, any athlete is at risk. Other factors such as position played, level of training, and gender may also play a role.[1-3] The majority of back pain among active individuals is self-limited and is usually not associated with underlying structural abnormalities; however, back pain may be a symptom of a more serious disease process. An awareness of sport-specific demands, age-related conditions, risk factors, and warning signs can help narrow the wide differential diagnosis, guide the evaluative process, and lead to proper treatment and return-to-play decisions.

FUNCTIONAL ANATOMY

Bony and soft-tissue elements are integral components of the spine that provide strength and stability, and both are vulnerable to injury. Coordinated movement of the spine is highly complex and is governed by neurologic and biomechanical processes. Any disruption in the process can lead to injury, altered function, and may generate a pain response due to mechanical or chemical sources. A fundamental knowledge of the anatomy of the spine and the biomechanical demands of each sport can help to correctly identify the etiology of back pain in active individuals.

The functional unit of the thoracolumbar spine is the vertebrae and intervertebral discs and is located in the anterior column of the thoracolumbar spine. The intervertebral discs separate two vertebrae and are composed of an inner nucleus pulposus and an outer annulus that is attached to the vertebral endplate. The annulus has sensory innervation, while the nucleus pulposus does not. The nucleus pulposus acts as a shock absorber between adjacent vertebrae. Although it is composed primarily of water at birth, age-related desiccation makes the disc increasingly vulnerable to degeneration or failure caused by acute or chronic mechanical forces. The connection between low back pain and degenerative disc disease is somewhat unclear but is believed to be caused by leakage of inflammatory factors within the nucleus pulposus through annular tears where it comes in contact with nociceptive nerve fibers (Fig. 16.1).

Radicular back pain is often generated from the spinal nerves which exit through the intervertebral foramina. While the lumbar spinal nerves increase in size descending down the spine, the intervertebral foramina become smaller. Any process that causes additional narrowing of the intervertebral foramen including loss of disc height and osteoarthritis can lead to symptomatic compression of the spinal nerve roots (Table 16.1).

The posterior column of the thoracolumbar spine consists of the bony vertebral arch, including the pedicles, lamina, pars interarticularis, transverse and spinous processes, and the facet joints (zygapophyseal). The spinal cord is contained within the vertebral arch. The pars interarticularis is particularly vulnerable to injury in young athletes playing sports that involve repetitive trunk rotation and lumbar hyperextension due to the presence of ossification centers in the posterior region of the spine until age 25 and ongoing remodeling and bone growth (Fig. 16.2). A facet joint is

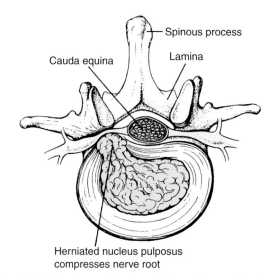

FIG. 16.1. Lumbar disc herniation. From Chaffee EE, Greisheimer EM. *Basic Physiology and Anatomy.* 3rd ed. Philadelphia: J.B. Lippincott; 1974.

TABLE 16.1 **Spinal Nerve Roots**

Root	Motor	Reflex	Sensory
L4	Tibialis anterior/dorsiflexion	Patellar	Lateral thigh, medial leg, and foot
L5	Extensor hallicus longus	None	Lateral leg, dorsum of foot
S1	Peroneus longus and brevis/plantar flexion	Achilles	Posterior thigh and leg, lateral foot

formed by the inferior articular process of the vertebrae above and the superior articular process of the vertebrae below. This region is innervated with proprioceptive and nociceptive fibers.

Supporting soft-tissue structures include paraspinal muscles, ligaments, and thoracolumbar fascia. Maintenance of posture and functional spinal movement depends on the strength and integrity of the intrinsic muscles of the back. The erector spinae muscle group is the predominant extensor of the lumbar spine and includes the spinalis, semispinalis, longissimus, and iliocostalis muscles. The deepest layer includes the multifidus, semispinalis, and the rotatores that act to extend, rotate, and control deceleration of forceful spinal flexion. The intertransversarii and interspinalis intersegmental muscles allow for ipsilateral side bending and extension, respectively.

Other important supporting structures include the anterior longitudinal ligament that covers the anterior aspect of the spine throughout its course and prevents hyperextension. It is twice as strong as its posterior counterpart, the posterior longitudinal ligament, which helps to prevent hyperflexion. The posterior longitudinal ligament narrows as it approaches the lumbar region, providing only central support and an area of relative weakness in the posterolateral aspect overlying the lumbar disc, therefore accounting for the higher prevalence of posterolateral lumbar disc herniations in the lumbar spine. Both the anterior and posterior longitudinal ligaments have nociceptive fibers.

EPIDEMIOLOGY

Although low back pain is a common complaint in the general population with a prevalence of 85% to 95%, comparison studies between athletes and nonathletes indicate that athletes had significantly higher rates.[1] Low back pain, however, was found to be less common among former elite athletes compared to nonathletes, suggesting that sports involvement is not a risk factor for chronic back pain and may even be protective.[4] Muscle strain is the most common

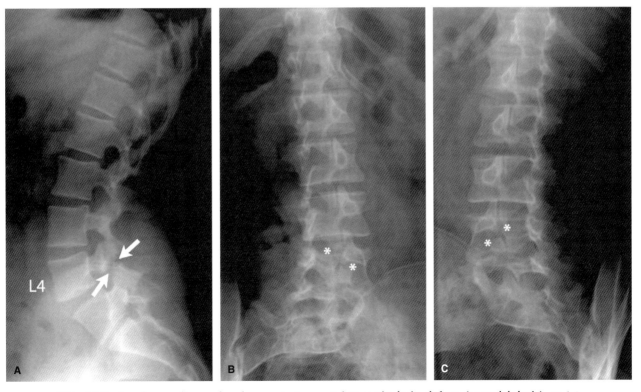

FIG. 16.2. Lumbar radiographs demonstrate pars interarticularis defect (spondylolysis) at L4. **A:** Pars defect (*arrows*). **B and C:** Classic Scotty dog sign (*asterisks*).

TABLE 16.2   **Risk Factors Associated with Low Back Pain/Injury in Athletes**

Risk Factor	Comment
Previous back injury or low back pain	One of the strongest predictors of subsequent low back pain or injury[1,2,9,10]
Training :15 hr/wk	Higher incidence of back injury[5]
Sudden changes in training intensity or duration	Increased risk of low back pain or injury[5]
Overtraining	Increased risk of degenerative changes in weight lifters[1]
Improper technique	Increased risk of degenerative changes in weight lifters[1,5]
Collision sports	Increased risk of low back pain[11]
Warm-up exercises	Little evidence for decreased risk of injury or prevalence of low back pain[1]
Age > 40 years	Increased risk of disc disease in weight lifters[5]
Strength and flexibility imbalances of hamstrings and hip flexors	Increased risk of low back pain[11]
Flexibility	Conflicting evidence regarding relationship with low back pain[1]

cause of back pain among athletes.[1,5] The most common structural etiologies associated with low back pain in athletes are degenerative disc disease and spondylolysis.[1]

The incidence and anatomic location of back pain vary not only with each sport but also with gender, position played, and level of training.[1–3] Divers (63%), wrestlers (54%), gymnasts (32%), and rowers have the highest prevalence of severe low back pain.[1,5] Female rowers (25%) having a higher prevalence of back pain compared to males.[1] Athletes involved in sports requiring repetitive trunk rotation such as golf and racquet sports also frequently experience back pain.[5] Pars interarticularis stress fractures of the spine (spondylolysis) comprise 45% of all stress fractures in female gymnasts.[6] Football lineman have a high prevalence of spondylolysis and spondylolisthesis. Among college and professional players with spondylolisthesis, lineman accounted for nearly 50% in both groups.[5]

The incidence of spondylolysis seems to be bimodal. The first peak is somewhere from age 3 to 7 years. The majority of cases go undetected, are asymptomatic, and are likely due to normal childhood activity. The prevalence in this age group may be as high as 6% to 10% of all children. The second peak of spondylolysis is in early adolescence. It is most frequently seen in athletes participating in sports that involve repetitive lumbar loading in hyperextension and trunk rotation such as gymnastics, diving, wrestling, weight lifting, and rowing, with a prevalence ranging from 23% to 47%.[1,7]

Lumbar disc herniation is a common cause of acute, chronic, or recurrent low back pain, and most frequently occurs at the L5–S1 level.[1] A comparison study of lumbar disc degenerative changes in elite gymnasts versus nonathletes showed a prevalence of 75% and 35%, respectively.[1] Among Olympic athletes studied, 58% had lumbar disc bulging. In contrast, clinically significant thoracic disc herniations comprise less than 1% of all disc ruptures.[8] The prevalence and level of disc degeneration are influenced by the age of the athlete, and type and intensity of the sport.[4,5] Soccer players have degenerative changes almost exclusively at L4 to S1 levels, whereas weight lifters have more severe degenerative changes in the upper lumbar spine.[4] Among weight lifters older than 40 years, 65% of women and 80%

of men demonstrated disc degeneration.[5] The association between radiographic degenerative changes and the prevalence of back pain is unclear.[1] Decreased disc space height was the radiographic finding most strongly associated with low back pain and was more strongly correlated with the greater number of levels involved (Table 16.2).[1]

NARROWING THE DIFFERENTIAL DIAGNOSIS

History

A detailed history should include the acuity of onset, characteristics and location of the pain, aggravating and alleviating factors, as well as history of previous injuries. Pain exacerbated by forward flexion may indicate potential disc pathology or muscle strain, while pain with extension may suggest spondylolysis, spondylolisthesis, or facet arthropathy. Presence of radicular symptoms suggests nerve impingement most commonly from disc bulge/herniation or neuroforaminal narrowing from spondylosis/degenerative disc disease. The athlete's age, gender, sport, level of competition, position played, training patterns, and recent changes in training type, volume, or intensity should be elicited. A nutritional and menstrual history should be obtained in female athletes with a history of low back or sacral pain to assess for stress fracture risk. Table 16.3 highlights common symptoms with potential associated conditions.

Evidence-based Physical Examination

Observation

The examiner should begin by inspecting the spine, shoulders, torso, and abdomen looking for any asymmetry, atrophy, or evidence of traumatic injury, such as ecchymosis or swelling. The shoulder heights should be equal, but in a throwing athlete the dominant shoulder may be slightly lower.[13] Observe for any loss of any of the physiologic spinal curves—cervical lordosis, thoracic kyphosis, and lumbar lordosis that may indicate localized paraspinal muscle spasm.

TABLE 16.3 Key Pain Patterns/History and Associated Conditions

Key Pain Patterns/History	Differential Diagnosis
Low back pain exacerbated by activity, relieved by rest, all age groups	Lumbar strain, myofascial pain, spondylosis
Sharp unilateral radicular pain down posterior or lateral aspect of leg to ankle or foot with associated paresthesias[12]; insidious or acute in onset	Lumbar disc disease
Adolescent athlete, insidious onset axial low back pain exacerbated by sports, improves with rest, may be severe, radiate to buttocks, posterior thighs, exacerbated by extension, often unilateral, involved in sports with repetitive hyperextension	Spondylolysis, spondylolisthesis, facet pain, ring apophyseal injury
Low back or sacral pain, female athlete, low bone mineral density, decreased caloric intake, menstrual irregularity, track or marathon runner	Sacral or pars interarticularis stress fracture Nonspinal diagnoses: ovarian cysts, renal disease
Radicular pain, weakness, low back pain, saddle anesthesia, urinary retention, urinary or bowel incontinence	Cauda equina syndrome
Night pain, unexplained weight loss, fever	Neoplasm, infection (osteomyelitis, epidural abscess, discitis)

Look for asymmetry in scapular appearance, such as scapular winging or scapular height, which may indicate nerve injury or scoliosis. The iliac crest heights should be equal and any differences may indicate a functional leg length discrepancy.

Palpation

The exam is performed in the standing and prone positions. Palpate each spinous and transverse process to ascertain any point tenderness. Point tenderness over one spinous process could indicate an acute bony injury such as vertebral body compression fracture, spinous or transverse process fracture, spondylolysis, or fracture of the posterior bony vertebral arch. Palpate the paraspinal muscles for tenderness and spasm. Note any step-off of the spinous process that may suggest possible spondylolisthesis. Overall, soft-tissue palpation and bony tenderness have poor specificity and reproducibility in determining the etiology of low back pain.[12]

Range of Motion (ROM)

Assess lumbar flexion by having the patient bend forward (normal 40 to 60 degrees), noting whether this maneuver reproduces his/her pain. Assess lumbar extension (normal 20 to 35 degrees), noting whether this reproduces the patient's pain. Flexibility of the hamstrings should also be assessed. ROM is usually normal except for limitations in lumbar spine extension and hamstring flexibility that may occur in pars interarticularis defects.[7] As a general rule, pain with forward flexion is more likely to be anterior column pathology (disc) and pain with extension is most likely posterior column pathology (facets, pars intra-articularis).

Special Tests

Stork test (single-legged hyperextension test): This test is performed by having the patient stand on one leg, followed by flexing the contralateral hip and knee while extending the lumbar spine. The test is then repeated on the opposite leg. The test is positive if it reproduces the athlete's pain. Stork test has a low sensitivity and specificity in detecting spondylolysis and should not be used to exclude the diagnosis (Level B).[14] Stork test may be positive with facet degenerative joint disease (DJD).

Straight leg raising test: This test is performed by slowly raising the leg from the examining table while the patient is supine keeping the knee in full extension. A positive test reproduces the radicular pain and/or paresthesias between 30 and 70 degrees of leg elevation. Ipsilateral straight leg raise (SLR) at 60 degrees is moderately to highly sensitive for herniated lumbar discs but is not specific.[13] Crossed straight leg raising performed on the contralateral leg is less sensitive but highly specific.[13]

Neurologic testing: Muscle strength testing in patients with lumbar radiculopathy should include hip flexors (L1–L3), quadriceps (L2–L4), tibialis anterior (L4–L5), extensor hallucis longus (L5), and gastrocnemius (S1). Decreased strength in ankle dorsiflexion and plantar flexion had a low sensitivity but a moderately high specificity for diagnosis of L4 to S1 disc protrusions.[13] Sensory exam of the lower extremities has a sensitivity ranging from 16% to 66% and specificity 51% to 86% in the diagnosis of lumbar disc herniation.[13]

Reflex testing: Absent ankle reflex had a sensitivity of 0.5 and specificity of 0.6 for L5–S1 disc herniation.[12]

Imaging

Radiographs

Imaging is not warranted in every athlete with back pain but certain signs, symptoms, and mechanisms of injury necessitate further evaluation. Plain radiographs (anteroposterior, lateral, and oblique views) are often the appropriate initial imaging study (Table 16.4). Loss of disc space height is the

TABLE 16.4 Common Radiographic Findings on Plain Radiographs

Finding	Associated Condition
Loss of intervertebral disc space	Disc disease
Vertebral endplate changes	Disc disease
Intervertebral foramina changes	Nerve root impingement
Vertebral wedging/fracture	Compression fracture
Pars defect ("Scotty dog collar sign")	Spondylolysis
Anterior movement of one vertebral body on the one beneath it	Spondylolisthesis
Osteophyte formation	Degenerative disease
Spina bifida occulta	Spondylolysis

most strongly associated radiographic finding with low back pain, and correlation increases with the number of levels involved.[1] If initial radiographs are negative and there is a high clinical suspicion, further imaging studies are warranted (Table 16.5).

Computed Tomography (CT)

To diagnose spondylolysis, some authors recommend a single-photon emission computed tomography (SPECT) bone scan followed by CT if the bone SPECT scan is positive (Level A).[14,15] Because of the relatively large amount of radiation exposure, many will defer a CT unless it would change management.

Magnetic Resonance Imaging (MRI)

The role of MRI in diagnosing pars stress fractures appears to be growing with advances in MRI resolution and the use of fat-saturated image sequences. The advantages include the absence of ionizing radiation and the ability to image lumbar bony as well as disc pathology. These advantages need to be weighed against lower sensitivity and specificity compared with SPECT and CT imaging.[16]

APPROACH TO THE ATHLETE WITH LUMBAR STRAIN

Muscle strain is the most common cause of back pain in athletes and may be acute or chronic in onset.[1,5] Strains are caused by a disruption of muscle fibers. In addition, there may be injury to the ligaments (sprain) or fascia.

HISTORY AND PHYSICAL EXAMINATION

Pain has an insidious onset and becomes worst 24 to 48 hours after inciting activity.[1] The patient may recall a twisting episode or particular activity when pain began, such as weight lifting, which is usually not associated with trauma. The patient may report sudden increase in training intensity, duration, or type.[5] The exam is typically significant for paraspinal muscle spasm and tenderness. It may demonstrate hypertonicity of the entire posterior chain, including the lumbar paraspinal musculature, gluteal musculature, hamstrings, and calves. Radicular pain should be absent in lumbar strain.

DIAGNOSTIC TESTING

Imaging is not necessary for diagnosis but may be used to rule out other potential etiologies including disc space narrowing seen with disc disease, facet DJD, or spondylolysis/spondylolisthesis.

TREATMENT

Nonoperative

- Brief rest (24 to 36 hours) after injury. Prolonged inactivity discouraged.
- Pain control with ice and nonsteroidal anti-inflammatory drugs (NSAIDs).

TABLE 16.5 Circumstances Requiring Further Imaging

Sign/Symptom/Mechanism of Injury	Imaging Study
Acute trauma	Plain radiographs
Hyperextension mechanism injury in adolescent athlete	Plain radiographs to assess for spondylolysis. If nondiagnostic—a single-photon emission computed tomography (SPECT) bone scan is indicated
Neurologic deficit	MRI
Severe pain unresponsive to a trial of appropriate conservative treatment	Plain radiographs, MRI
Night pain and constitutional symptoms	MRI, bone scan, appropriate lab studies

- After acute pain has subsided (usually 48 to 72 hours), begin stretching exercises with emphasis on hamstrings, lumbar flexors, and extensors.
- Core stabilization exercises to improve strength, endurance, and neuromuscular control of spinal and trunk stabilizing muscles are initiated when ROM has improved, usually after 1 to 2 weeks.
- Progression to pain-free sports-specific activities allowed, when full strength and ROM are regained.

Operative

- Usually responds well to conservative therapy.

Prognosis/Return to Play

- Full strength, ROM, and pain free with sport-specific activities.
- Encourage ongoing participation in strength and flexibility exercises.

Complications/Indications for Referral

Pain out of proportion to the injury and persistence of pain despite appropriate conservative treatment warrant further evaluation. Radicular pattern of pain may indicate underlying disc pathology or nerve injury.

APPROACH TO THE ATHLETE WITH LUMBAR DISC DISEASE

Lumbar disc disease involves a spectrum of pathology from disc desiccation (drying of the disc), disc bulging, disc protrusion, to frank disc herniation. The precise relationship between degenerative disc disease and low back pain is unclear, given high rates of radiographic evidence of degenerative discs in asymptomatic athletes.

Repetitive microtrauma or acute trauma can lead to tears in the annulus fibrosis. Circumferential tears occur first, followed by radial tears if the stress continues. The nucleus pulposus may herniate through the annulus leading to radicular pain and paresthesias and low back pain. Disc herniations occur most frequently at the L5–S1, followed by L4–L5.

HISTORY AND PHYSICAL EXAMINATION

Sharp unilateral radicular pain down the posterior or lateral aspect of leg to ankle or foot with associated paresthesias is suggestive of lumbar disc herniation.[12] Pain may be described as burning or shooting. Onset may be insidious or acute. Pain is often exacerbated in lumbar flexion and improved with extension. Periods of prolonged sitting, coughing, and sneezing may also exacerbate the pain. Physical exam may show paraspinal muscle spasm with associated tenderness to palpation, positive straight leg raising test, sensory and motor deficits, and asymmetrical reflexes associated with a lumbar nerve root distribution.

DIAGNOSTIC TESTING

Plain radiographs may show loss of disc space height and vertebral endplate changes. MRI is superior for soft-tissue evaluation. Disc degeneration and herniation, annular tears, and foraminal impingement can be appreciated on an MRI. Electrodiagnostic studies should be considered when clinical findings and imaging studies are inconclusive.

TREATMENT

Nonoperative

- Brief rest (24 to 36 hours) after injury. Prolonged inactivity discouraged.
- Pain control with ice and NSAIDs.
- After acute pain has subsided (usually 48 to 72 hours), begin stretching exercises with emphasis on hamstrings, lumbar flexors, and extensors.
- Core stabilization exercises to improve strength, endurance, and neuromuscular control of spinal and trunk stabilizing muscles are initiated when ROM has improved, usually after 1 to 2 weeks. Extension exercises (McKenzie) may be beneficial.
- Progression to pain-free sports-specific activities permitted, when full strength and ROM are regained.
- Maintenance core stabilization program should be encouraged.

Operative

- There are no randomized controlled trials comparing return to sports using conservative versus surgical treatment of symptomatic lumbar disc herniation in an athletic population.[17]
- A comparison of short-term outcomes of conservative (discontinuing "aggravating activities") versus surgical management of symptomatic lumbar disc herniation demonstrated that nearly 80% of athletes returned to their prior sports activities following conservative treatment in an average time of 4.7 months.[17]
- Athletes with more severe symptoms are less likely to respond to conservative treatment.[17]

- Surgical intervention may be considered in athletes if symptoms persist or worsen after 6 weeks of appropriate conservative care and MRI findings are consistent with physical exam findings.[18]
- Surgery to excise or partially excise the disc may provide symptom relief.[18]
- Percutaneous discectomy has been studied in athletes with return to play 2 months post-procedure.[19]
- A comparison of percutaneous discectomy versus standard discectomy, or discectomy with spinal fusion demonstrated that return to play was significantly shorter (7.5 weeks) with percutaneous discectomy.[18]

Prognosis/Return to Play

- Return to play begins with resolution of symptoms and adequate return of core and lower extremity strength.
- If an athlete is pain free and able to perform all of the activities required to participate in his or her sport, then he or she may safely be returned to participation, even if an underlying disc bulge or other pathology is in place.
- After microdiscectomy, pain-free full ROM is required for return to play, usually 3 months for collision sports and 6 to 8 weeks for noncollision sports.[18]
- After percutaneous discectomy/nucleotomy, 2 to 3 months of rest and rehabilitation are usually required prior to return to play.

Complications/Indications for Referral

Progressively worsening radicular pain, weakness, low back pain, saddle anesthesia, urinary retention, urinary or bowel incontinence are possible signs of Cauda equina syndrome and require prompt referral for neurosurgical evaluation.

APPROACH TO THE ATHLETE WITH SPONDYLOLYSIS AND SPONDYLOLISTHESIS

Low back pain is a common complaint among adolescent athletes, with female gymnasts appearing to be at greater risk for spine stress injuries.[1,7] Stress reaction of the pars interarticularis, spondylolysis, and spondylolisthesis represent a continuum of bone stress injury. Spondylolysis is a term used to refer to a stress fracture, either new or old in the pars interarticularis, most commonly at L5.[1] This condition may be unilateral or bilateral. A stress reaction to the pars interarticularis is a milder form of overuse bone stress injury with a microfracture pattern.

These injuries are caused by repetitive flexion, hyperextension, and rotation of the lumbar spine. The stress injury/fracture itself may be responsible for the low back pain experienced by the athlete, or it may account for abnormal function/wear at the facet joints in the posterior aspect of the spine that may also account for the patient's pain.

Spondylolisthesis refers to vertebral body slippage due to an underlying bilateral pars defect. The direction of slippage is anterior in relation to the underlying vertebral body at the affected level. The fifth lumbar vertebra is the most commonly affected level, followed by L4 and L3, respectively. Spondylolisthesis is graded based on the percentage of slip of one vertebral body over the one below it. Grade 1 is less than 25% slippage, grade 2 is 25% to 50%, grade 3 is 50% to 75%, and grade 4 is greater than 75%.[20]

HISTORY AND PHYSICAL EXAMINATION

Pars interarticularis stress fractures may present as persistent nonradicular low back pain that becomes worse with activity, particularly extension of the lumbar spine. On exam, spinous process point tenderness may be elicited at the affected vertebrae, most commonly L5. ROM may be limited or painful in lumbar extension.[7] A history of pain radiating into the thighs or buttocks or during straight leg raising is usually due to hamstring tightness rather than radiculopathy and does not extend below the knee. Hamstring tightness was found in 80% of patients with spondylolysis.[7] Stork test (single-legged hyperextension test) has low sensitivity and specificity in detecting spondylolysis and should not be used to exclude the diagnosis (Level B).[14]

DIAGNOSTIC TESTING

Plain radiographs (AP, lateral, and oblique views) are the initial imaging study. Positive findings include the Scotty dog sign in spondylolysis and anterior displacement of one vertebral body on the one below it in spondylolisthesis (Fig. 16.3). If initial x-rays are negative and there is a high clinical suspicion, further imaging studies are warranted. Establishing that an identified pars defect is the source of pain can be challenging given that pars defects are evident on plain radiographs in 6% of general adolescent population and in 8% to 14% of elite athletes prior to age 18 years.[21]

CT provides detailed bony anatomy of the lumbar spine; however, it cannot show the chronicity of the lesion (new or old) and exposes the patient to a significant amount of radiation. Some authors recommend a SPECT bone scan followed by CT if the bone SPECT scan is positive (Level A).[14,15] SPECT scan has the highest sensitivity and specificity for diagnosis of acute pars stress injury, particularly a painful pars lesion; however, there is still a significant radiation exposure.[16,21] Bone scans alone are helpful in determining the age of the lesion, but are not overly anatomically specific.

The role of MRI in diagnosing pars stress fractures appears to be growing with advances in MRI resolution and the use of fat-saturated image sequences. The advantages include the absence of ionizing radiation and the ability to image

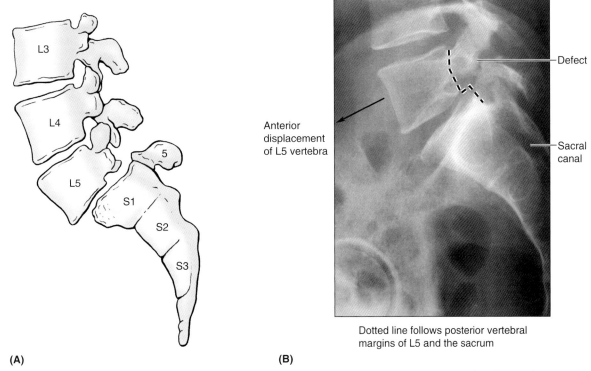

(A)   **(B)**

FIG. 16.3. Anterior spondylolisthesis of L5 on S1 represented by diagram (A) and radiograph (B). From Moore KL, Dalley AF II. *Clinical Oriented Anatomy.* 4th ed. Baltimore: Lippincott Williams & Wilkins; 1999.

lumbar bony as well as disc pathology. These advantages need to be weighed against lower sensitivity and specificity compared with SPECT and CT imaging.[16]

TREATMENT

Nonoperative

- Most athletes, even without bracing, can return to their sport once they have become pain free and have full strength and ROM, even without evidence of healing of the pars defect.[22]
- Treatment involves discontinuation of all painful activities that cause hyperextension and impact loading of the thoracolumbar spine.
- Rehabilitation with emphasis on neutral to flexion-based core strength training; hamstring flexibility should begin within a few weeks with re-evaluation in 4 to 6 weeks, especially to observe for pain-free extension.
- When the athlete is pain free, a gradual increase in activities may begin.
- Reintroduction of hyperextension activities may commence if the athlete remains pain free with activity progression.
- The role of bracing is an area of controversy and debate as good outcomes have been shown to occur with rigid bracing, soft bracing, and no bracing.[21,23] No head-to-head trials of bracing versus nonbracing exist.

Operative

- Surgical stabilization with lumbar fusion is performed in cases of failed conservative therapy with persistent pain with sports and activities of daily living.[7] This is a very rare complication.
- Indications for earlier surgical repair include neurologic deficit, a progressive lesion, or grade 3 or 4 slip.[20]

Prognosis/Return to Play

Return to play allowed after progression to pain free with hyperextension activities. Healing may take as long as 6 months with conservative measures. No sports until 12 months after fusion.[7] Overall prognosis appears to be excellent in long-term studies with incidence of back pain comparable to general population.[24]

Complications/Indications for Referral

Spondylolisthesis and cord compression may present as radicular pain, saddle numbness, and loss of bowel or bladder control with prompt referral recommended. High-grade slips (III–IV) at initial presentation should be referred due to risk of further progression.[20]

<table>
<tr><td colspan="2" align="center">**KEY POINTS**</td></tr>
</table>

- Knowledge of sport-specific demands, age-related conditions, and risk factors can help narrow the differential diagnosis, and guide evaluative, treatment, and return-to-play decisions in athletes with low back pain

- Muscle strain is the most common cause of low back pain in athletes[1,5]

- Athletes who participate in sports involving repetitive lumbar loading and trunk rotation are at risk for par interarticularis stress fractures[1–7]

- Warning signs that may indicate a more serious disease process and require prompt evaluation include progressively worsening radicular pain, weakness, saddle anesthesia, and changes in bladder or bowel function

- Stork test (single-legged hyperextension test) has low sensitivity and specificity in detecting spondylolysis and should not be used to exclude the diagnosis[14]

- When spondylolysis is suspected, the diagnostic imaging modality of choice is bone SPECT scan followed by CT if bone SPECT scan is positive[14,15]

- Core stabilization exercises to improve strength, endurance, and neuromuscular control of spinal and trunk stabilizing muscles are the mainstay of treatment for low back pain

- There are no randomized controlled trials comparing return to sports using conservative versus surgical treatment of symptomatic lumbar disc herniation in an athletic population[17]

- Athletes with more severe symptoms are less likely to respond to conservative treatment[17]

- Surgery may be considered in athletes with persistent symptoms after 6 weeks of appropriate conservative care and if MRI and physical exam findings are congruent[18]

REFERENCES

1. Bono CM. Low back pain in athletes. *J Bone Joint Surg.* 2004;86: 382–396.
2. Tietz CC, O'Kane J, Lind BK, et al. Back pain in intercollegiate rowers. *Am J Sports Med.* 2002;30:674–679.
3. Hickey GJ, Fricker PA, McDonald WA. Injuries to elite rowers over a 10-yr period. *Med Sci Sports Exerc.* 1997;29:1567–1572.
4. Videman T, Sarna S, Battie MC, et al. The long-term effects of physical loading and exercise lifestyles on back related symptoms, disability, and spinal pathology among men. *Spine.* 1995;20:699–709.
5. Trainor TJ, Trainor MA. Etiology of low back pain in athletes. *Curr Sports Med Rep.* 2004;3:41–46.
6. Snyder RA, Koester MC, Dunn WR. Epidemiology of stress fractures. *Clin Sports Med.* 2006;25:37–52.
7. Micheli LJ, Curtis C. Stress fractures in the spine and sacrum. *Clin Sports Med.* 2006;25:75–88.
8. Errico TJ, Stecker S, Kostuik JP. Thoracic pain syndrome. In: Frymoyer JW, ed. *The Adult Spine: Principles and Practice.* 2nd ed. Philadelphia, PA: Lippincott–Raven; 1997:1623–1637.
9. Teitz C, O'Kane JW, Lind BK. Back pain in former intercollegiate rowers: a long-term follow-up study. *Am J Sports Med.* 2003;31: 590–595.
10. Greene HS, Cholewicki J, Galloway MT, et al. A history of low back injury is a risk factor for recurrent back injuries in varsity athletes. *Am J Sports Med.* 2001;29:795–800.
11. Nadler SF, Wu KD, Galski T, et al. Low back pain in college athletes: a prospective study correlating lower extremity overuse or acquired ligamentous laxity with low back pain. *Spine.* 1998;23:828–883.
12. Deyo RA, Rainville J, Kent DL. What can the history and physical examination tell us about low back pain? *JAMA.* 1992;268(6):760–765.
13. Malanga GA, Nadler SF. *Musculoskeletal Physical Examination: An Evidence-based Approach.* Philadelphia, PA: Elsevier; 2006:189–225.
14. Masci L, Pike J, Malara F, et al. Use of one-legged hyperextension test and magnetic resonance imaging in the diagnosis of active spondylolysis. *Br J Sports Med.* 2006;40:940–946.
15. Gregory PL, Batt ME, Kerslake RW, et al. The value of combining photon emission computerized tomography and computerized tomography in the investigation of spondylolysis. *Eur Spine J.* 2004; 13:503–509.
16. Campbell RS, Grainger AJ, Hide IG, et al. Juvenile spondylolysis: a comparative analysis of CT, SPECT and MRI. *Skeletal Radiol.* 2005;34(2):63–73 [Epub November 25, 2004].
17. Iwamoto J, Takeda T, Sato Y, et al. Short-term outcome of conservative treatment in athletes with symptomatic lumbar disc herniation. *Am J Phys Med Rehabil.* 2006;85:667–674.
18. Alsobrook J, Clugston JR. Return to play after surgery of the lumbar spine. *Curr Sports Med Rep.* 2008;7(1):45–48.
19. Sakou T, Masuda A, Yone K, et al. Percutaneous discectomy in athletes. *Spine.* 1993;18:2218–2221.
20. McCleary MD, Congeni JA. Current concepts in the diagnosis and treatment of spondylolysis in young athletes. *Curr Sports Med Rep.* 2007;6:62–66.
21. Standaert CJ, Herring SA. Expert opinion and controversies in sports and musculoskeletal medicine: the diagnosis and treatment of spondylolysis in adolescent athletes. *Arch Phys Med Rehabil.* 2007;88: 537–540.
22. Sys J, Michielsen J, Bracke P, et al. Nonoperative treatment of active spondylolysis in elite athletes with normal X-ray findings: literature review and results of conservative treatment. *Eur Spine J.* 2001;10: 498–504.
23. Steiner ME, Micheli LJ. Treatment of symptomatic spondylolysis and spondylolisthesis with the modified Boston brace. *Spine.* 1985;10: 937–943.
24. Beutler WJ, Fredrickson BE, Murtland A, et al. The natural history of spondylolysis and spondylolisthesis: 45-year follow-up evaluation. *Spine.* 2003;28(10):1027–1035.

CHAPTER 17

Athlete with Hip Pain

Agam Shah and Jonathan Fallon

INTRODUCTION

Athletic hip pain is a common complaint among athletes that historically has been hard to diagnose and treat. The vague nature of hip pain along with the complex anatomy has made it a diagnostic and therapeutic challenge. The advent of magnetic resonance imaging (MRI), improved exam techniques, and better understanding of the pathology surrounding the hip, including the bony, ligamentous, neurovascular, muscular, and intra-articular diseases, have allowed for the diagnosis and treatment of athletic hip pain to become more manageable and an area of active research. This chapter will focus on the overall approach to hip pain in the athlete based on a sound understanding of anatomy and the physical exam. The second half of the chapter will focus on the diagnosis and treatment of common conditions found in athletes that can cause hip pain.

FUNCTIONAL ANATOMY

The hip joint consists of the articulation of the acetabulum with the proximal femur, including the overlying musculature, ligamentous and other soft-tissue structures, and associated neurovascular structures.

The acetabulum serves as the fusion point of the three parts of the innominate bone: the ilium, the ischium, and the pubis. The ilium is located posterior-laterally and articulates with the sacrum at the sacroiliac joint and gives rise to a broad expansion termed "the iliac crest." The ischium is located posterior-inferiorly and is bordered by the ilium superiorly and pubis anteriorly. The pubis forms the third part of the innominate bone and is found in the anterior aspect of the pelvis. All three bones meet at the center of the acetabulum. The acetabulum is a dome-shaped structure that approximates a hemisphere, with the concave portion covered by articular cartilage.

The proximal femur comprises the bony elements of the thigh and articulates with the pelvis at the hip joint. The femur is a diaphyseal structure that broadens proximally to form the trochanteric ridge, greater trochanter, lesser trochanter, and femoral neck. The neck forms an average angle with the shaft of approximately 130 degrees (neck shaft angle) and is found to have an average anteversion angle of 15 degrees. Deviations from normal anatomic geometry can lead to improper mechanics and injury, that is, femoroacetabular impingement (FAI) or stress fracture.[1]

The femoral head forms two thirds of a sphere and is covered with articular cartilage. The ligamentum teres arises from the fovea of the femoral head and attaches to the center of the acetabulum in the pulvinar fossa.

Unlike the shoulder joint, the hip joint is a highly constrained ball-and-socket joint, with motion limited predominantly by its bony configuration. Additionally, the joint is surrounded by three strong ligaments: the pubofemoral ligament inferiorly, the ischiofemoral ligament posteriorly, and the iliofemoral ligament anteriorly (also known as the ligament of Bigalow). These three ligaments integrate to form the hip joint capsule. The capsular attachments are from the intertrochanteric line on the femur to a few millimeters superior to the acetabular rim.

The labrum is a fibrocartilagenous structure that is attached to the acetabular margin. The labrum serves to deepen the hip socket and contributes to the normalization of joint reactive forces across the hip joint. Although the labrum's function remains controversial, studies show that the labrum does not participate in direct load transmission.[2]

The muscles around the hip can be divided into two layers, superficial (Table 17.1) and deep (Table 17.2). Although injury can occur to any of these muscles, there is a general agreement that muscles that cross two joints are more likely to sustain a strain injury than muscles that cross a single joint for two reasons. First, muscles that cross two joints have been found to be less flexible and experience a greater strain per applied force when compared to single-joint muscles.

Second, muscles that cross two joints have a higher ratio of type II fast-twitch fibers, leading to more violent contractions.[3] Special attention should be given to four muscles that are more commonly injured. The gluteus maximus and the tensor fascia lata are superficial posterior lateral structures that combine to form the iliotibial band (ITB), which has been implicated in the etiology of trochanteric bursitis and external snapping hip syndrome. The iliopsoas muscle can be associated with internal snapping hip syndrome and is

TABLE 17.1   **Superficial Muscles Surrounding the Hip Joint**

Name of Muscle	Origin	Insertion	Nerve Supply	Action	Distinguishing Characteristics
Anterior Group Sartorius	Anterior–superior iliac spine	Anteromedial surface of proximal tibia	Femoral nerve	Flexes, abducts, laterally rotates thigh at hip joint	Longest muscle in the body One third of pes anserine
Lateral Group Tensor fascia lata	Iliac crest	Iliotibial band and then Gerdy tubercle	Superior gluteal nerve	Assists in extending the knee joint and abducting the hip	Can be responsible for external snapping hip
Gluteus medius	Outer surface of ilium	Greater trochanter	Superior gluteal nerve	Abducts hip joint	Injury to this muscle leads to trendelenburg gait
Posterior Group Gluteus maximus	Surface of ilium, sacrum, and coccyx	Gluteal tuberosity of femur and iliotibial band	Inferior gluteal nerve	Extends and externally rotates the hip and extends the knee	Termed the "pelvic deltoid" by Henry Largest muscle in the body
Medial Group Gracilus	Inferior ramus	Anteromedial surface of proximal tibia	Obturator nerve	Abducts hip and flexes knee	One third of pes anserinus
Adductor longus	Body of pubis	Linea aspera of femur	Obturator nerve	Adduct hip	—

TABLE 17.2   **Deep Muscles Surrounding the Hip Joint**

Name of Muscle	Origin	Insertion	Nerve Supply	Action	Distinguishing Characteristics
Anterior Group Rectus femoris	Anterior inferior iliac spine and ilium	Quadriceps tendon into patella	Femoral nerve	Flexes hip and extends knee	Only quadriceps muscle that crosses the hip joint
Iliopsoas	Iliac fossa and T12–L5 vertebral bodies	Lesser trochanter	Lumbar plexus	Flexion, adduction, and external rotation of hip joint	Associated with internal "snapping hip syndrome"
Lateral Group Gluteus minimus	Surface of ilium	Greater trochanter	Superior gluteal nerve	Abduction of hip joint	—
Posterior Group Piriformis	Anterior sacrum	Greater trochanter	First and second sacral nerves	Externally rotate the hip joint	Most proximal of the short external rotators
Obturator internus	Obturator membrane and spine of ischium	Greater trochanter	Sacral plexus	Externally rotate the hip joint	—
Quadratus femoris	Ischial tuberosity	Quadrate tubercle of femur	Sacral plexus	Externally rotate the hip joint	Most distal of the short external rotators
Superior gemellus	Spine of ischium	Greater trochanter	Sacral plexus	Externally rotate the hip joint	—
Inferior Gemellus	Ischial tuberosity	Greater trochanter	Sacral plexus	Externally rotate the hip joint	—
Medial Group Adductor brevis	Inferior ramus of pubis	Linea aspera of femur	Obturator nerve	Adduct the hip joint	—
Adductor magnus	Inferior ramus of pubis and ischial tuberosity	Posterior femur and adductor tubercle	Obturator and sciatic nerve	Adduct the hip joint	Muscle has dual innervation

the most common muscle involved with hip flexor strain. Lastly, the adductor longus muscle is the most commonly involved muscle in adductor strains. Free body analysis demonstrates that the adductor longus has the least mechanical advantage on adduction of the hip, making it susceptible to the most strain.

EPIDEMIOLOGY

Muscle strain injuries are fairly common and occur as the result of forceful contraction of a stretched muscle. Eccentric contraction, or muscle contraction during elongation, is the most frequent type of contraction that causes this injury.[4] A strain is the result of partial tearing of a muscle, generally at the myotendinous junction. Repetitive microtrauma can lead to chronic strains. Historically, soccer and hockey players are most prone to adductor strains. Poor adductor strength and conditioning has been found to be a risk factor for adductor strains.[5] Some authors have concluded that decreased preinjury flexibility leads to muscle strain, but recent literature suggests that the two are unrelated.[6] Strains to the iliopsoas muscle are an infrequent cause of hip pain. The mechanism of injury is usually a sudden resistance to hip flexion, that is, a collision while attempting to perform a kick. Patients with suspected strain will exhibit pain in the front of the proximal hip that radiates into the groin. Often, there will be a sharp pain in the groin, which increases with resisted hip flexion or passive external rotation. Patients with iliopsoas strains will not have pain or weakness with resisted knee extension, helping distinguish it from strains of the rectus femoris and gracilis muscles.

Apophyseal injuries and avulsion fractures typically occur in sprinters, jumpers, and soccer and football players. Once thought to be rare, these injuries are more common among the athletic population and comprised greater than 13% of pediatric pelvic fractures in one series.[7] Typically, avulsion injuries are caused by a sudden eccentric contraction of a muscle; however, chronic overuse syndromes can present as apophysitis in the skeletally immature athlete (e.g., Sinding–Larsen dx and Osgood–Schlatter dx).[3]

Osteitis pubis is a painful inflammation of the pubic symphysis. This pathology occurs most commonly in the adolescent and early-adult athletic population. Causative mechanisms are not well understood, but investigators believe that the underlying feature involves overuse of the adductors and gracilis muscles.[8] Alternative causes are hypothesized to include microstrains at the origins of these muscles, avascular necrosis (AVN) of the symphysis, osteochondritis desiccans at the symphysis, or fatigue fracture. Some believe that an imbalance between abdominal wall musculature and hip adductor strength can be a risk factor.[8]

Athletic pubalgia, also termed "Gilmore's groin" or "sports hernia," is a broad spectrum of injuries involving the inguinal ligament, conjoined tendon transversalis fascia,

internal oblique muscle, external oblique muscle, and rectus abdominus insertion. There is thought to be an imbalance between the adductor muscle group of the thigh and the abdominal musculature, leading to a weakening and possible tearing of the structures of the pelvis floor. The pathology is noted to occur more frequently in males versus females.

Coxa sultans, more commonly known as "snapping hip," is a term used to describe several different disease entities. Although these entities can occur in patients of any age, external and internal snapping hip tends to occur in patients in the late teens or early 20s.[9] The common feature of all patients with snapping hip syndrome is that there is a reproducible audible or palpable "snap" with certain hip motion. There are three main categories of coxa sultans: external snapping hip syndrome, internal snapping hip syndrome, and intra-articular snapping hip syndrome. External snapping hip is the most common and is most often caused by thickening of the ITB or gluteus maximus snapping over greater trochanter.[10] In contrast, internal snapping hip, often seen in ballet dancers,[11] is most often caused by the iliopsoas snapping over the iliopectineal eminence of the pelvis or over the femoral head.[10] Intra-articular causes of snapping hip can be labral tears, loose bodies, or osteochondral injuries. Most patients with intra-articular causes have a history of trauma.

Acetabular labral tears have been reported as the most common form of intra-articular pathology in the hip. Increased shear forces in the hip joint have been suggested as a cause for labral tears. Five distinct pathologic entities have recently been linked to this condition: FAI, hip dysplasia, trauma, capsular laxity, and joint degeneration.[12]

FAI in the athletic population is thought to be caused by a combination of subtle morphologic variants in the acetabulum and/or proximal femur and use of the hip through an extreme range of motion.[13] Posttraumatic deformities, deepened acetabulum (protrusion or coxa profunda), and acetabular retroversion are thought to be the most common anatomic variants that cause the femoral neck to repeatedly abut against the rim of the acetabulum. This pathologic impingement, either cam (femoral neck based) or pincer (acetabular based), causes chondral and labral damage that, if left untreated, can lead to early joint degeneration.[14]

AVN of the femoral head in the athletic population is an incompletely understood pathology that frequently affects patients in the third to fifth decade.[15] Interrupted vascular supply secondary to lipid circulation and coagulation pathways are the most commonly cited mechanisms of subchondral bone death. Approximately 80% of cases have a predisposing risk factor, systemic steroid use, hypercoagulable states, and alcoholism, which is the most common. There have also been reports of AVN after traumatic subluxations of the hip in football players.[16]

Degenerative joint disease (DJD) can be the final common pathway of many disease processes that affect the hip, including osteoarthritis, traumatic arthritis, congenital hip dysplasia, systemic inflammatory diseases, and AVN (Table 17.3).

TABLE 17.3   Common Etiologies of Hip Arthritis

Osteoarthritis
Trauma
Rheumatoid arthritis
Infection
Reiter arthropathy
Psoriatic arthropathy
Avascular necrosis
Gout
Pseudogout
Ankylosing spondylitis
Hemophilia
Paget disease
Legg–Calvé–Perthes disease
Slipped capital femoral epiphysis
Developmental dysplasia of the hip

All of these entities result in the destruction of cartilage within the hip joint, increased friction with hip motion, and irritation of the surrounding synovium.

NARROWING THE DIFFERENTIAL DIAGNOSIS

Discerning the cause of hip pain in the athlete can be daunting due to the complex anatomy and large number of potential etiologies. The following is a list of common causes of hip pain in the athlete followed by appropriate history and physical exam findings that can help narrow the differential diagnosis:

- Strain or avulsion injury
- Osteitis pubis
- Athletic pubalgia
- Snapping hip syndrome (external and internal)
- Labral tear
- FAI
- AVN
- DJD
- Stress fracture (femoral neck or pubic ramus – see Chapter 22, "Athlete with Stress Fracture")
- Referred pain from lumbosacral spine or gastrointestinal/gastrourinal process

History

As with any patient, significant diagnostic information can be gained from the injured athlete's history. Physicians should discuss onset, duration, character, intensity, location, exacerbating factors, prior history, and quantification of the athlete's pain. Use of a visual analog scale can provide consistent comparison throughout the treatment process. Information should also be gathered about the athlete's training regimen, noting any recent changes in intensity, frequency, or equipment. Relevant medical and surgical history should

also be gathered, including obstetric, gynecologic, and urologic. Any prior history of hip pain should be thoroughly explored, obtaining old records, films, or test when applicable and available. Finally, prior treatment modalities should be noted along with a measure of their success.

Location of hip pain will often be useful in arriving at an accurate diagnosis. Lateral hip pain associated with snapping or popping may suggest ITB friction syndrome, while painful snapping in the inguinal crease region may indicate iliopsoas tendonitis/bursitis or a labral tear. Diffuse deep groin pain that is gradual onset may suggest a femoral neck stress fracture in the appropriate setting. Diffuse hip pain in the older athlete that improves as the day progresses may indicate underlying hip osteoarthritis.

Pain that radiates past the knee or has any paresthesias or dysthesias may indicate referred pain from the lumbar spine.

Evidence-based Physical Exam

The physical exam of the hip and pelvis should begin with a general inspection of gait, posture, and pelvic and limb alignment. Normal and symmetric anatomic contours should exist when comparing the injured hip to the contralateral hip. In the setting of an acute injury, gross deformity, tenderness, inability to bear weight, ecchymosis, edema, or erythema may be present. Chronic or subacute injuries are more likely to be manifested in altered gait, limited range of motion, or persistent restrictive pain altering the athlete's ability to participate in desired activities. Regions of tenderness, limited range of motion or strength, relevant neurologic findings, and muscle atrophy should all be documented on initial examination. Palpable landmarks that deserve attention include the greater trochanter, the superior and inferior iliac spines, and the femoral pulse.

When evaluating muscle strains and tears, regions of tenderness and rarely identification of palpable defects can isolate involved musculotendinous units. Active and passive range of motion should be tested in all planes. Strength and resistance testing should also be performed focusing on the specific action of the involved muscle. Although strains occur most commonly at the musculotendinous junction, points of origin and insertion should be palpated if an avulsion injury is suspected.[4] Loss of strength in certain planes can be diagnostic in strain injuries, nerve damage, and avulsion injuries. Tenderness in the region of the superior pubic ramus and symphysis is suggestive of ramus stress fractures, osteitis pubis, or athletic pubalgia. Reproduction of this pain with passive abduction and resisted adduction is highly suggestive of osteitis pubis. Athletic pubalgia can have associated tenderness along the conjoined tendon, inguinal ring, or adductor origin. If a hernia is suspected, thorough examination of the abdominal wall, inguinal canal, scrotum, and testicles is indicated. Provocative testing for hernias include pain with resisted sit-ups and with resisted adduction with the hip externally rotated.[17]

The standing sign, the hop test, and the fulcrum test are well-described provocative maneuvers designed to reproduce the pain associated with stress fractures about the hip.[18] A more thorough discussion is provided in the section of this text dedicated to stress fractures.

External and internal snapping hip syndrome can often be delineated by the position of the leg while reproducing the snapping sensation. With internal snapping hip, the symptoms can be reproduced by placing the patient supine, flexing and abducting the hip, followed by an extension and adduction maneuver. Pressure applied over the iliopsoas tendon at the level of the femoral head should block the snapping, thereby corroborating the diagnosis. The snapping sensation associated with external snapping hip can be reproduced by having a supine patient actively flex the affected hip with the examiner's hand over the region of the greater trochanter. As with internal snapping hip, pressure at the point of snapping should block the event. Although there are no scientific data to delineate the specificity or sensitivity of these tests, they are generally considered the most effective test available. Ober's test is helpful in confirming a diagnosis of external snapping hip. The test is performed with the patient in the lateral decubitus position with the affected hip up. With the knee flexed and the hip maximally extended, the hip is brought from a maximally abducted position to an adducted position. If the patient's hip cannot be adducted beyond the midline, then the test is positive, indicating a tight ITB associated with external snapping hip.[9]

The "log roll" is thought to be the most specific indicator of intra-articular pathology. The passive rotation of the leg of a supine patient through maximal internal and external rotation allows for motion of the femoral head relative to the acetabulum and capsule without stressing the surrounding structures.[20]

Physical exam tests suggestive of labral pathology include the flexion abduction external rotation test as well as the anterior–superior impingement test. The FABER test is performed with the patient supine; the involved hip is flexed, abducted, and externally rotated by the examiner while stabilizing the anterior superior iliac spine. The impingement test involves flexing, internally rotating, and adducting the hip of a supine patient. If the original pain is reproduced, these tests are considered positive. These tests are thought to be more sensitive for intra-articular pathology; however, recent studies have questioned their accuracy.[20–22] Both the FABER and impingement tests have demonstrated good interrater reliability and remain the best physical exam tests available to screen for labral pathology.

Diagnostic testing

Laboratory

Routine laboratory analysis is not generally indicated in the athlete with hip pain. If an autoimmune condition including spondyloarthropathy is considered, then appropriate serology would be indicated. If pain is felt secondary to a septic joint, a hip joint aspiration with cell count as well as culture and sensitivities would be indicated.

Imaging

A radiographic pelvis series including anterior–posterior (AP) of the pelvis and lateral of the affected hip is standard when a bony injury is considered. This may allow for immediate diagnosis of an injury such as fracture or avulsion or suggest a diagnosis as in the case of decreased joint space or osteophyte formation in DJD, coxa vara associated with snapping hip, or a crossover sign in FAI.[14,23] Often the radiographic features of a pathology will not be distinguishable immediately (e.g., stress fx, AVN, apophyseal avulsion, osteitis pubis) and may require inlet/outlet views or Judet oblique views of the pelvis. These alternate views are most helpful in characterizing apophyseal avulsion fractures. Single-limb stance flamingo views can be useful in identifying symphysis instability associated with osteitis pubis[24] (Fig. 17.1). Harris and Murray have described three common features of athletic osteitis pubis: bone resorption at the pubis symphysis, widening at symphysis, and rarefaction along the pubic rami.[25]

Computed tomography (CT) scans are a useful adjunct for providing more detail for bony lesions such as avulsion injuries and fractures.

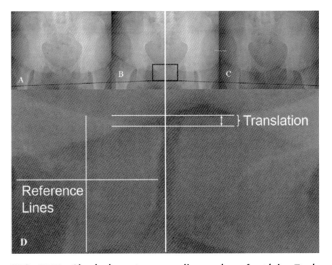

FIG. 17.1. Single-leg stance radiographs of pelvis. Each patient was assessed with three radiographs: one standard anteroposterior view **(A)** with dual-leg stance to show the baseline translation, one flamingo view with weight borne on the left leg **(B)**, and one flamingo view with weight borne on the right leg **(C)**; **(D)** is a magnified view of the pubic symphysis region seen on **(B)**. The total translation is the sum of the translations on the right and left flamingo views or, in this case, 5 mm. Reprinted with permission from Garras DN, Carothers JT, Olson SA. Single-leg-stance (flamingo) radiographs to assess pelvic instability: how much motion is normal? *J Bone Joint Surg.* 2008;90(A):2114–2118.

A technetium bone scan may also provide useful information in narrowing the differential diagnosis, providing a lower cost indicator of bone metabolism. Three-phase bone scan will show a broad area of bone uptake centered on the symphysis in osteitis pubis and possibly in athletic pubalgia.

Recent research and attention has focused on the use of MRI with and without arthrogram for the diagnosis of hip pathology. MRI using 1.5 T magnets allows for soft-tissue definition around the hip and can often diagnose the underlying cause. MRI is excellent for identifying soft-tissue disorders such as an abdominal hernia or adductor tearing; however, it shows limited findings associated with athletic pubalgia.[26] This imaging modality will show a quantifiable area of injury associated with muscle strains and tears, but is not predictive of the level of disability.[3] Regional edema as well as increased signal within the symphysis is suggestive of osteitis pubis.[27] MRI is the current standard for diagnosing AVN, demonstrating a 99% sensitivity and specificity.[28] The presence of an effusion or sublabral cyst has shown to be a good indicator of intra-articular pathology.[20] Unfortunately, the reliability of MRI or MR arthrogram (MRA) to delineate the nature of this pathology is uncertain. Recent studies using a 3 T magnet report greater than 92% sensitivity at discovering labral tears in contrast to a 42% false-negative rate by MRI and a 20% false-positive rate by MRA in a different series.[20,29,30]

The utility of ultrasonography is growing, but it is highly user dependent. The dynamic nature of the test provides for useful information in the diagnosis of snapping hip, allowing the sonographer to delineate between internal and external snapping hip syndromes. Its utility has also been suggested in the diagnosis of apophyseal avulsion injuries.[31]

Other Testing

Diagnostic injections are a highly effective tool in athletic hip pain. Injection of local anesthetic along the external oblique at the point of maximal tenderness can assist in the diagnosis of athletic pubalgia. Intra-articular injections, usually concomitant with MRAs of the hip, are 90% accurate in predicting intra-articular pathology.[20,32] Anesthetic injections in association with bursography can be useful in differentiating internal and intra-articular snapping hip.[13,33]

APPROACH TO THE ATHLETE WITH STRAIN OR AVULSION INJURIES

HISTORY AND PHYSICAL EXAMINATION

Diagnosis of muscle strain injury can be through careful history and physical exam. A history of eccentric muscle injury is usually elicited. Although rare, complete rupture can

result in a palpable musculotendinous defect. Muscle strains are graded upon severity. Grade I strains are classically thought of as "muscle pulls" and generally involve less than 5% of the musculotendinous junction. A strain injury involving greater than 5% and less than 100% is classified as grade II strains. Grade III strains involve complete tear and discontinuity between the muscle origin and insertion.[3] Defects palpable at the bone–tendon interface should alert the clinician to a tendon avulsion injury.

DIAGNOSTIC TESTING

- Plain radiographic evaluation
  - Indicated for suspicion of avulsion injury (Fig. 17.2)
  - Oblique views often helpful
  - May be nondiagnostic if apophysis not ossified
- Adjunct imaging
  - CT scan may better visualize avulsion fragment but not commonly necessary
  - MRI can show a quantifiable area of injury
    - Not predictive of the level of disability
    - Ultrasound rarely used as an alternative to MRI

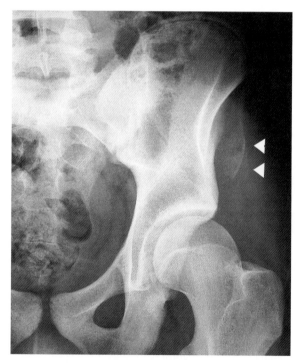

FIG. 17.2. This 14-year-old boy felt a "pop" in his hip while running during a baseball game. The radiograph shows the avulsion fracture (arrowheads) of his anterior inferior iliac spine. Reprinted with permission from Fleisher GR, Ludwig S, Baskin MN. *Atlas of Pediatric Emergency Medicine.* Philadelphia: Lippincott Williams & Wilkins; 2004.

TREATMENT

Nonoperative

- Five-phase protocol for the treatment of muscle strain injuries has been advocated (Table 17.3)[33]
- Modification of Metzmaker and Pappas' descriptive protocol for treating avulsion fractures[34]
  - Emphasizes a reduction in pain and inflammation (24 to 72 hours)
  - Followed by gradual range-of-motion exercises (days 3 to 7)
  - Increases strength, flexibility, and endurance (weeks 1 to 3)
  - Sport-specific training and return to sport (weeks 4 to 6)
- Apophyseal avulsion
  - Rest/protected weight bearing for 3 weeks or until early callus
  - The progress to strain protocol

Operative

- Painful nonunion
- Symptoms greater than 6 months despite appropriate conservative management[35,36]
- Displacement greater than 3 cm
- High-level athlete

Prognosis/Return to Play

- Return to sports is dictated by complete healing of the injury (avulsion or tear)
- Completed rehabilitation is assessed by therapist-supervised isokinetic testing (at least 90% of strength)

Complications/Indications for Referral

Premature return to play can lead to reinjury and further damage.

APPROACH TO THE ATHLETE WITH OSTEITIS PUBIS

HISTORY AND PHYSICAL EXAMINATION

Osteitis pubis presents as pain that has an insidious onset but can be acute in traumatic causes. Although vague, pain begins at the level of the symphysis pubis and may radiate into the groin, medial thigh, or abdomen. History may reveal that the patient is involved in kicking and running-type activities such as soccer, football, and long-distance running.[37]

Physical exam will reveal tenderness along the symphysis. Pain can be elicited by passive abduction and resisted adduction. This disease is easily confused with hernias; therefore, a thorough exam and palpation of the patient's inguinal canal should be performed.

DIAGNOSTIC TESTS

- Radiographic evaluation
  - Negative early
  - Resorbtion, widening, and rarefaction evident late
- Three-phase bone scan
  - Broad area of bone uptake centered around the pubis
- MRI
  - Increased T2 edema at pubic symphysis including surrounding bone edema
  - Advantages include lack of ionizing radiation, better anatomic detail, and ability to assess surrounding soft-tissue structures. Main disadvantage is cost

TREATMENT

Nonoperative

- Ninety percent to 95% success rates[37]
- Activity modification, nonsteroidal anti-inflammatory drugs (NSAIDs), therapeutic modalities
- A progressive rehabilitation program (core strengthening, adductor stretching, and balance control)
- Complete recovery may take *2 to 3 months*
- Corticosteroid injection at the point of maximal tenderness[37]

Operative

- Symptomatic after more than 3 months of nonoperative management
- Surgical debridement, curettage, wide resection, or arthrodesis[17]
- Recovery from these procedures may take up to a year[17,25]

Prognosis/Return to Play

- Patients may return to play once symptoms allow.
- Early return or overly aggressive rehabilitation may exacerbate symptoms.

Complications/Indications for Referral

Continued pain secondary to missed or inappropriate diagnosis is the most likely complication of this condition. Athletic pubalgia or labral tear may mimic symptoms of osteitis pubis.

APPROACH TO THE ATHLETE WITH ATHLETIC PUBALGIA

HISTORY AND PHYSICAL EXAMINATION

The primary complaint with athletic pubalgia is exertional pain in the pubic area. The pain may radiate into the adductor region, inguinal ring, or the testicles. History often reveals the occurrence of a specific aggravating injury. The proposed mechanism of injury is described as a hyperextension injury pivoting around the pubic symphysis, seen frequently in hockey and soccer players.[25] There is an insidious progression of pain, usually only while performing the offending activity. It is not uncommon for these patients to have referrals to multiple specialists in search of a diagnosis.

Meticulous physical exam is necessary because findings for athletic pubalgia are subtle. Inspection and general range-of-motion exam will not reveal any abnormalities, except for decrease motion on hamstring testing. Palpable tenderness along the conjoined tendon or inguinal ring may exist. Patients may also be tender to palpation at the pubic tubercle, symphysis, and adductor origin. Examination of the abdominal wall is essential to rule out abdominal hernia. Neurologic exam will be normal. Provocative testing includes pain with resisted sit-ups and with resisted adduction with the hip externally rotated.[25]

DIAGNOSTIC TESTING

- Radiographic imaging
  - Negative but necessary to rule out other causes of pain
- Three-phase bone scan
  - Results similar to osteitis pubis
- MRI
  - May show abdominal hernia, rectus tear, or symphyseal edema

TREATMENT

Nonoperative

- First-line treatment
- First-time episodes and pre- or midseason athletes
  - Rest, ice, NSAIDs (2 weeks)
  - Corticosteroid injection may facilitate recovery
  - After 2 weeks, progressive physical therapy started
    - Range of motion, modalities, and stretching
  - Strengthening
- Recurrent episodes
  - At least 4 weeks of rest

Operative

- Symptoms lasting greater than 6 weeks, despite conservative management
- Herniorrhaphy[25]
- Ninety-five percent success rate[38]

Prognosis/Return to Play

- Pre- and midseason athletes treated nonoperatively can return to play when pain free and range of motion and strength have fully returned.
- Recovery from the repair takes approximately 4 to 6 weeks.
- Restrictions on strenuous activities continue for 6 weeks total, and patients can usually return to play at 8 weeks.[38]

Complications/Indications for Referral

Major pitfalls associated with this condition can be caused by missed or inappropriate diagnosis causing continued pain and decreased performance level. Osteitis pubis and labral tears may mimic the symptoms of athletic pubalgia in the athlete.

APPROACH TO THE ATHLETE WITH SNAPPING HIP SYNDROME

HISTORY AND PHYSICAL EXAMINATION

Patients with snapping hip often describe a "snap" that may feel as though "the hip is popping in and out." The snap can usually be reproduced by the patient. The history is generally insidious with onset of pain prior to snapping over the region of the snap. Patients with external snapping hip will have pain along the greater trochanter that may radiate distally and proximally. Patients with internal and intra-articular snapping hip generally have pain along the anterior of the hip with radiation into the groin. Physical exam helps confirm the diagnosis and may give insight into the underlying cause. Patients with external snapping hip have the greatest amount of tenderness over the greater trochanter, and the pain can be reproduced with repetitive flexion and extension.[10] The snap can be reproduced when the patient moves from a standing to sitting position. Ober's test is helpful in establishing a diagnosis.

Internal and intra-articular snapping hip causes pain along the anterior thigh, inguinal crease, and medial thigh. In patients with internal snapping hip, the snap can be simply reproduced with patient supine and flexing and extending the hip. The snap can be amplified if the hip is ranged from an abducted, externally rotated, and flexed position to an adducted, internally rotated, and extended position.

Gentle pressure over the femoral head will prohibit the snap from occurring.[10]

Intra-articular injuries should be considered when external and internal causes have been ruled out. Patients present with pain in the groin and a history of trauma. Often patients will have "clicks" on ranging of the hip, but the clicks are not necessarily reproducible. Most likely causes include loose bodies, labral tears, and osteochondral lesions.[39]

DIAGNOSTIC TESTING

- Radiographic imaging
  - Standard AP and frog leg lateral
  - Femoral neck angle should be noted (coxa vara common with internal snapping hip)[40]
- Dynamic ultrasound may differentiate internal or external snapping
  - Technician experience dependent
- Bursography
  - Differentiates between intra-articular and internal causes[9]
  - Therapeutic injection of the bursa (lidocaine and/or steroids) may be useful
- MRA for suspected intra-articular pathology

TREATMENT

Nonoperative

- First-line therapy for internal and external snapping hip
  - NSAIDs, therapy, activity modification
  - Corticosteroid injection into the trochanteric bursa (external)
- Corticosteroid injection into the iliopectineal bursa (internal)
- Requires fluoroscopic or ultrasound guidance
  - Intra-articular snapping hip not amenable to nonoperative therapy

Operative

- Indicated for failed nonoperative treatment (up to 1 year)
- Surgically released tension of the ITB as it crosses over the greater trochanter[4]
- Z-plasty–lengthening techinique[41] or an elliptical incision with bursa removal[42]
- Surgical release of the iliopsoas tendon (open or endoscopically)[43,44]
- See subsequent text on treatment for intra-articular pathology

Prognosis/Return to Play

- A complete return to activity is based on resolution of symptoms.

Complications/Indications for Referral

Postoperatively, patients may complain of continued pain over the incision and return of snapping sensation secondary to scarring. Iliopsoas release requires postoperative limitation on active flexion.

APPROACH TO THE ATHLETE WITH A LABRAL TEAR

HISTORY AND PHYSICAL EXAMINATION

Patients with labral tears complain of pain in the groin with certain motions of the hip. Sudden pivoting or twisting motion often reproduces the pain. They may also have a clicking or catching sensation, known as intra-articular snapping hip. Physical examination may reveal decreased range of motion of the affected hip. Dependent on the location of the labral tear, certain provocative tests can be performed. Ranging the hip from a fully flexed, externally rotated, and abducted position to a position of extension, internal rotation, and adduction will cause pain if an anterior-based labral tear is present.[44] Posterior tears can be painful if the hip is brought from a flexed, adducted, and internally rotated position to one of abduction, external rotation, and extension. Although both of these maneuvers are very sensitive, they have not been found to be specific.[46]

DIAGNOSTIC TESTING

- Radiographic imaging
  - Indirect diagnosis
  - Evidence of hip dysplasia, trauma, joint degeneration, and FAI[23]
- MRI
  - Soft-tissue definition around the hip
  - Questionable accuracy for identification of specific pathology
  - Arthrogram adds to sensitivity but may lead to frequent overreads
- Diagnostic/therapeutic injection
  - Preformed in conjunction with arthrogram
  - Improves diagnosis and potentially treats symptoms

TREATMENT

Nonoperative

- Limited long-term success with labral tear
- Physical therapy, activity modification
- Intra-articular corticosteroid injection
  - Provides temporary relief
  - May allow to continue to play on limited basis

- Indicated if failure of nonoperative modalities[23]
- Arthroscopic repair or debridement highly successful[47–49]

Prognosis/Return to Play

- For simple debridement of labral tears, postoperative recovery usually takes 6 to 8 weeks.
- Poor surgical outcomes if coexisting hip osteoarthritis or significant articular cartilage injury.
- Return to play is allowed once the patient has full motion and full strength.
- Postoperative rehabilitation for arthroscopic labral repair is more protracted and less predictable; however, no long-term data are available.[12]

Complications/Indications for Referral

Debridement of labral tears caused by underlying disorders such as DJD or FAI may provide unpredictable or temporary solution if the causative factors are not completely addressed. Failure to address coexisting FAI, chondral lesions, or loose bodies may result in poor surgical outcome.

APPROACH TO THE ATHLETE WITH FEMOROACETABULAR IMPINGEMENT

HISTORY AND PHYSICAL EXAMINATION

Athletes with FAI typically report a vague intermittent groin pain, brought on by minor trauma and exacerbated with increased demand placed on the hip. Pain may also be present with extended periods of sitting and may be referred to the knee and medial thigh. Examination of the patient often reveals limited internal rotation and reproduction of pain with the impingement test described earlier.[13] If a deep groin pain is produced with forced external rotation, posteroinferior impingement should be suspected.[14]

DIAGNOSTIC TESTING

- Radiographic imaging
  - Slight bony prominence on the anterolateral head and neck junction of the proximal femur suggests "cam impingement"
  - "Crossover sign" suggests acetabular retroversion that can be associated with "pincer-type impingement"

- MRA with diagnostic injection of anesthetic
  - Highly sensitive for intra-articular and labral pathology
  - Important to assess pre- and postanesthetic pain using visual analog scale with provocative exam maneuvers (impingement, FABER, or forced external rotation test)

TREATMENT

Nonoperative

- NSAIDs, activity modification temporarily successful
- Range-of-motion therapy counterproductive

Operative

- Progressive pathology – early surgical intervention warranted
- Arthroscopic and open treatments
- Femoroacetabular osteoplasty to address pathology
- Labral repair/joint debridement

Prognosis/Return to Play

- Return to all activities depends on symptomatic control.
- Analgesia and anti-inflammatories can aid the patients to return to sports quickly.
- Exacerbations are likely to recur until the underlying problem is addressed surgically.
- Studies have demonstrated 75% resolution of pain by 5 months postoperatively and 95% complete resolution by 1 year with arthroscopic intervention.[50]

Complications/Indications for Referral

If left untreated, the chondral and labral damage can propagate, leading to early joint degeneration and osteoarthritis.

APPROACH TO THE ATHLETE WITH AVASCULAR NECROSIS OF THE FEMORAL HEAD

HISTORY AND PHYSICAL EXAMINATION

Athletes with AVN of the femoral head typically present with insidious onset, nonspecific hip or groin pain. Early in the disease process, range of motion and strength should remain within normal limits. There are no provocative signs

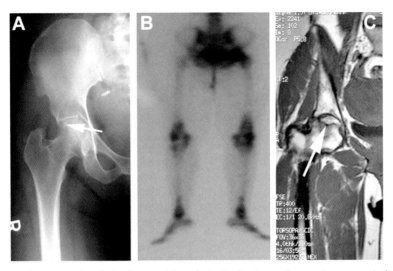

FIG. 17.3. Avascular necrosis of the femoral head. **A:** Early signs of an osteonecrotic lesion *(arrow)* are shown on the plain radiograph. **B:** A normal or "cold" bone scan of both hips. **C:** Evidence of a subchondral osteonecrotic lesion *(arrow)* is seen on the magnetic resonance image. Reprinted with permission from Mont MA, Jones LC, Hungerford DS. Nontraumatic osteonecrosis of the femoral head: ten years later. *J Bone Joint Surg.* 2006;88(A):1117–1132.

specific to this pathology; however; pain elicited with passive internal rotation has been shown to be the most effective predictor.[51]

DIAGNOSTIC TESTING

- Radiographic imaging
  - Standard radiographs are the first step in management
  - Radiographic changes lag 3 months behind symptoms
  - Osteopenia, mottled subchondral bone in femoral head
  - Subchondral collapse indicates advanced disease
- MRI
  - Obtain if radiographs are normal yet suspicion remains high (Fig. 17.3)

TREATMENT

Nonoperative

- Limited weight bearing, symptomatic treatment

Operative

- Immediate referral appropriate
- Core decompression/vascularized fibular graft
  - Provides predictable relief[15,28]
- Joint arthroplasty for advanced disease

Prognosis/Return to Play

- Full weight bearing is resumed at a minimum of 6 weeks after surgical intervention.
- Therapy focuses on range of motion and strength.
- Return to sport is based on radiographic evidence of healing as well as full resolution of symptoms.

Complications/Indications for Referral

Because radiographic evidence is delayed and early surgical intervention is the best chance to preserve the native joint, diagnosis is initially based on a high index of suspicion. Missed diagnosis can lead to advanced degenerative disease. With core decompression, there is the threat of femoral neck fractures with premature weight bearing after surgery.

APPROACH TO THE ATHLETE WITH CHONDRAL DAMAGE OR DEGENERATIVE JOINT DISEASE

HISTORY AND PHYSICAL EXAMINATION

Patients with cartilage disease of the hip present with an insidious onset of pain localized to the groin that may radiate to the buttocks, thigh, and knee. Rarely, patients will present with vague knee pain. History may reveal stiffness that is relieved by activity, that is, "start-up pain." Depending on the severity of the disease, patients will have trouble with activities of daily living such as donning socks, climbing stairs, and walking distances.

Physical exam is essential in ruling out other causes of hip pain. Inspection may reveal muscle atrophy, but is often normal. Tenderness to palpation in the groin or along the lateral aspect of the hip should alert the examiner to possible hernia or trochanteric bursitis, respectively. Because the hip is a deep joint, palpation should not cause pain. With the hip flexed 90 degrees, the external and internal rotations should be checked. Patients with DJD of the hip often have side-to-side differences in internal rotation or pain with the hip internally rotated to maximum. Pain with log rolling or axial load is present in severe forms of the disease.

DIAGNOSTIC TESTING

- Radiographic imaging
  - Plain radiographs are often diagnostic for advanced DJD
  - Joint space narrowing, osteophyte formation, subchondral cysts, and sclerotic bony margins
- MRA
  - Diagnostic anesthetic injection
  - Loose bodies, labral pathology, or AVN may be identified

TREATMENT

Nonoperative

- NSAIDs/analgesics, therapy, activity modification
- Weight loss
- Intra-articular cortisone injection

Operative

- Arthroscopic removal of loose bodies
- Joint arthroplasty—high patient satisfaction rate

Prognosis/Return to Play

- The patient's level of activity will be determined by the adequacy of pain control.

Complications/Indications for Referral

DJD is a progressive condition with no known cure.

KEY POINTS
• There are multiple pathologies that can present as hip pain in the athlete. Consider all possible causes including the bones, joints, muscles, and surrounding soft tissue
• Location of pain can be very helpful in narrowing the differential diagnosis, remembering that intra-articular pathology radiates to the groin
• Careful physical exam is essential to determining the underlying cause of the pain, with special attention to pathology-specific maneuvers and contralateral range of motion
• All patients with hip pain should have plain radiography performed to rule out fracture or malignant causes of hip pain
• If ordering an MRI of the hip to assist in diagnosing the cause of pain, consider MRI with intra-articular contrast as well as concomitant steroid injection, as this will greatly aid in diagnosis and can also be therapeutic
• Treatment should proceed in a stepwise fashion, involving the physician, therapist, trainer, coach, and most importantly the athlete. Premature return to sport could result in more severe or recurrent injury

REFERENCES

1. Nordin M, Frankel VH. Biomechanics of the hip. In: Frankel VH, Burstein AH, eds. *Orthopaedic Biomechanics.* Philadelphia: Lea & Febiger; 1970.
2. Konrath GA, Hamel AJ, Olson SA, et al. The role of the acetabular labrum and the transverse acetabular ligament in load transmission in the hip. *J Bone Joint Surg.* 1998;80(A):1781.
3. Noonan TJ, Garrett WE Jr. Muscle strain injury: diagnosis and treatment. *J Am Acad Orthop Surg.* 1999;7:262–269.
4. Garrett WE, Safran MR, Seaber AV, et al. Biomechanical comparison of stimulated and nonstimulated muscle pulled to failure. *Am J Sports Med.* 1987;15:448.
5. Merrifield HH, Cowan RF. Groin strain injuries in ice hockey. *Am J Sports Med.* 1973;1:41.
6. Tyler TF, Nicholas SJ, Campbell RJ, et al. The association of hip strength and flexibility with the incidence of groin strains in professional ice hockey players. *Am J Sports Med.* 2001;29(2):124–128.
7. Canale ST, King RE. Pelvic and hip fractures. In: Rockwood CA Jr, Wilkins KE, King RE, eds. *Fractures in Children.* Philadelphia: JB Lippincott; 1984.
8. Wiley JJ. Traumatic osteitis pubis: the gracilis syndrome. *Am J Sports Med.* 1983;11:360.
9. Scharberg JE, Harper MC, Allen WC. The snapping hip syndrome. *Am J Sports Med.* 1984;12:361.
10. Allen WC, Cope R. Coxa saltans: the snapping hip syndrome. *J Am Acad Orthop Surg.* 1995;3:303.
11. Howse AJG. Orthopedists and ballet. *Clin Orthop Relat Res.* 1972;89:52–63.
12. Kelly BT, Weiland DE, Schenker ML, et al. Arthroscopic labral repair in the hip: surgical technique and review of the literature. *Arthroscopy.* 2005;21(12):1496–1504.

13. Ganz R, Parvizi J, Beck M, et al. Femoroacetabular impingement: a cause for osteoarthritis of the hip. *Clin Orthop Relat Res.* 2003;417: 112–120.
14. Parvizi J, Leunig M, Ganz R. Femoroacetabular impingement. *J Am Acad Orthop Surg.* 2007;15:561–570.
15. Lieberman JR, Berry DJ, Mont MA, et al. Osteonecrosis of the hip: mangement in the 21st century. In: Vail TP, ed. *AAOS, Instructional Course Lectures: Hip.* Rosemont, IL: AAOS; 2007.
16. Garrick JG. Sports medicine. *Pediatr Clin North Am.* 1986;33:1541–1550.
17. Mehin R, Meek R, O'Brien P, et al. Surgery for osteitis pubis. *Can J Surg.* 2006;49:170–176.
18. Paluska SA. An overview of hip injuries in running. *Sports Med.* 2005;35(1):991–1014.
19. Reider B. *The Orthopaedic Physical Exam.* Philadelphia: WB Saunders; 1999.
20. Byrd JW, Jones KS. Diagnostic accuracy of clinical assessment, MRI, MRA, and intra-articular injection in hip arthroscopy patients. *Am J Sports Med.* 2004;32:1668–1674.
21. Martin RL, Irrgang JJ, Sekiya JK. The diagnostic accuracy of a clinical examination in determining intra-articular hip pain for potential hip arthroscopy candidates. *Arthroscopy.* 2008;24(9):1013–1018.
22. Martin RL, Sekiya JK. The interrater reliability of 4 clinical tests used to assess individuals with musculoskeletal hip pain. *J Orthop Sports Phys Ther.* 2008;38:71–77.
23. Byrd JWT. Labral lesions: an elusive source of hip pain. *Arthroscopy.* 1996;12:603.
24. Siegel J, Templeman DC, Tornetta P III. Single-leg-stance radiographs in the diagnosis of pelvic instability. *J Bone Joint Surg.* 2008;90(A): 2119–2125.
25. Ahumada LA, Ashruf S, Espinosa-de-los-Monteros A, et al. Athletic pubalgia: definition and surgical treatment. *Ann Plast Surg.* 2005;55: 393–396.
26. Mora SA, Mandelbaum BR, Byrd JW. Hip and groin injuries. In: Garrick JG, ed. *Orthopaedic Knowledge Update: Sports Medicine 3.* Rosemont, IL: AAOS; 2004.
27. Long G, Cooper JR, Gibbon WW. MRI of injuries in the child athlete. *Clin Radiol.* 1999;54:781–791.
28. Lieberman JR. Core decompression for osteonecrosis of the hip. *Clin Orthop Relat Res.* 2004;418:29–33.
29. Sundberg TP, Toomayan GA, Major NM. Evaluation of the acetabular labrum at 3.0-T MR imaging compared with 1.5-T MR arthrography: preliminary experience. *Radiology.* 2006;238(2):706–711.
30. Toomayan GA, Holman WR, Major NM, et al. Sensitivity of MR arthrography in the evaluation of acetabular labral tears. *AJR.* 2006; 186(2):449–453.
31. Pisacano RM, Miller TT. Comparing sonography with MRI of apophyseal injuries of the pelvis in four boys. *AJR.* 2003;181(1):223.
32. Crawford RW, Gie GA, Ling RS, et al. Diagnostic value of intra-articular anaesthetic in primary osteoarthritis of the hip. *J Bone Joint Surg Br.* 1998;80:279–281.
33. Nuccion S, Hunter D, Finerman G. Hip and pelvis: adult. In: DeLee JC, Drez D, Miller MD, eds. *Orthopaedic Sports Medicine: Principles and Practice.* Philadelphia: WB Saunders; 2003.
34. Metzmaker JN, Pappas AM. Avulsion fractures of the pelvis. *Am J Sports Med.* 1985;13:349.
35. Akermark C, Johansson C. Tenotomy of the adductor longus tendon in the treatment of chronic groin pain in athletes. *Am J Sports Med.* 1992;20(6):640–643.
36. Tyler TF, Nicholas SJ. Adductor muscle strains in sport. *Sports Med.* 2002;32(5):339–344.
37. Koch R, Jackson D. Pubic symphysitis in runners. *Am J Sports Med.* 1981;9:62.
38. Biedert RM, Warnke K, Meyer S, et al. Symphysis syndrome in athletes: surgical treatment for chronic lower abdominal, groin, and adductor pain in athletes. *Clin J Sports Med.* 2003;13:278–284.
39. McCarthy JC, Busconi B. The role of hip arthroscopy in the diagnosis and treatment of hip disease. *Orthopedics.* 1995;18:753–756.
40. Harper MC, Schaberg JE, Allen WC. Primary iliopsoas bursography in the diagnosis of disorders of the hip. *Clin Orthop Relat Res.* 1987;221: 238–241.
41. Larsen E, Johansen J. Snapping hip. *Acta Orthop Scand.* 1986;57: 168–170.
42. Brignall CG, Stainsby GD. The snapping hip: treatment by Z-plasty. *J Bone Joint Surg.* 1991;73(B):253–254.
43. Zoltan DJ, Clancy WG Jr, Keene JS. A new operative approach to snapping hip and refractory trochanteric bursitis in athletes. *Am J Sports Med.* 1986;14:201–204.
44. Ilizaliturri VM Jr, Viallalobos FE Jr, Chaidez PA, et al. Internal snapping hip syndrome. *Arthroscopy.* 2005;21(11):1375–1380.
45. Taylor GR, Clarke NMP. Surgical release of the "snapping iliopsoas tendon." *J Bone Joint Surg.* 1995;77(6):881–883.
46. McCarthy JC, Mason WB, Wardell SR. Hip arthroscopy for acetabular dysplasia. *Orthopedics.* 1998;21:977.
47. Suenaga E, Noguchi Y, Jingushi S, et al. Relationship between the maximum flexion-internal rotation test and the torn acetabular labrum of a dysplastic hip. *J Orthop Sci.* 2002;7(1):26–32.
48. Santori N, Villar RN. Acetabular labral tears: result of arthroscopic partial limbectomy. *Arthroscopy.* 2000;16:11–15.
49. Farjo LA, Glick JM, Sampson TG. Hip arthroscopy for acetabular labrum tears. *Arthroscopy.* 1999;15:132–137.
50. Byrd JWT, Jones KS. Prospective analysis of hip arthroscopy with two year follow up. *Arthroscopy.* 2000;16:578–587.
51. Sampson TG. Arthroscopic treatment of femoroacetabular impingement. *Tech Orthop.* 2005;20:56–62.
52. Joe GO, Kovacs JA, Miller KD, et al. Diagnosis of avascular necrosis of the hip in asymptomatic HIV-infected patients: clinical correlation of physical examination with magnetic resonance imaging. *J Back Musculoskeletal Rehabil.* 2002;16(4):135–139.

Athlete with Acute Knee Injuries

Nicola DeAngelis and Robert Nascimento

INTRODUCTION

The knee plays a distinct role in a multitude of athletic activities. With the growing participation in competitive and recreational sports, injuries of the knee can affect a broad range of individuals. The general approach to the knee and its associated injuries is best accomplished in a systematic way using a proper history, physical exam, and diagnostic evaluation.

This chapter will review the functional anatomy of the knee as well as the pathophysiology behind various common acute knee injuries in the athlete. With this knowledge, practitioners should have a solid foundation for the diagnosis, initial treatment, and proper reasons for referral, which will best serve and help guide an athlete down the path of a timely recovery.

FUNCTIONAL ANATOMY

The knee is an exceedingly complex hinged (ginglymus) joint, and its anatomy lends to its sophisticated biomechanical function. Bony and ligament balance provide joint stability in a range of knee motions. In the simplest understanding, the bony architecture of the knee consists of three articulations: the patellofemoral, the medial, and the lateral joint space. The medial compartment contains the medial femoral condyle, the medial tibial plateau, and the medial meniscus. The lateral compartment contains the lateral femoral condyle, the lateral tibial plateau, and the lateral meniscus (Fig. 18.1).

The four primary ligamentous stabilizers of the knee include the anterior and posterior cruciates and the medial and lateral collateral ligaments. Combined, these four ligaments give stability in multiple planes of motion (Figs. 18.2 and 18.3).

The medial collateral ligament (MCL) is divided into three distinct layers. The most superficial layer consists of the deep fascia of the patellar tendon anteriorly and the popliteal fascia posteriorly. The second layer is the superficial MCL, and the third layer is the deep MCL or the medial capsular ligament. The medial structures of the knee are the primary stabilizers for valgus force and act as secondary stabilizers to anterior translation. The MCL contributes 78% to the restraining force on the medial side of the knee.[1] It also works in concert with the anterior cruciate ligament (ACL) to allow for external rotation stability. An injury to the MCL increases the stress on the ACL in valgus forces, and thus, ACL-deficient knees rely on the MCL as a secondary stabilizer to anterior translation.[2]

The ACL is the primary restraint to anterior tibial translation throughout the arc of knee motion. The ACL also is a secondary restraint to varus and valgus stress. The tibial insertion of the ACL is along the anterior portion of the lateral tibial plateau—medial to the anterior horn of the lateral meniscus anteriorly and 2 mm anterior to the posterior cruciate ligament (PCL) posteriorly (Fig. 18.4). On the femoral side, it attaches on the posteromedial aspect of the lateral femoral condyle. The ACL contains two bundles—the anteromedial and the posterolateral. The anteromedial bundle is tight in flexion, while the posterolateral bundle is tight in extension.

The PCL originates along the lateral border of the medial femoral condyle and inserts on the posterior cortical surface approximately 1 to 1.5 cm inferior to the articular surface. Along with the PCL are two meniscofemoral ligaments, the ligament of Humphrey and the ligament of Wrisberg (Fig. 18.5). The PCL is the primary restraint to posterior tibial translation.

The lateral structures of the knee include the lateral collateral ligament, the popliteus muscle and tendon, the popliteofibular ligament, the popliteomeniscal attachment, the iliotibial tract, and the arcuate ligament (Fig. 18.1). Combined, these lateral structures comprise the posterolateral corner (PLC) of the knee and are responsible for a variety of knee restraints, namely, posterior, lateral, and rotatory. The lateral collateral ligament is the knee's primary restraint to varus load. Injuries to the lateral collateral ligament in isolation are rare, and therefore, other injuries should be suspected when a lateral knee injury occurs.

The menisci, made of predominantly type I cartilage, are semicircular or C-shaped structures that have multiple functions in the knee. The medial meniscus covers less space over the plateau than its lateral counterpart. Both have attachments to the tibial plateau as well as soft-tissue

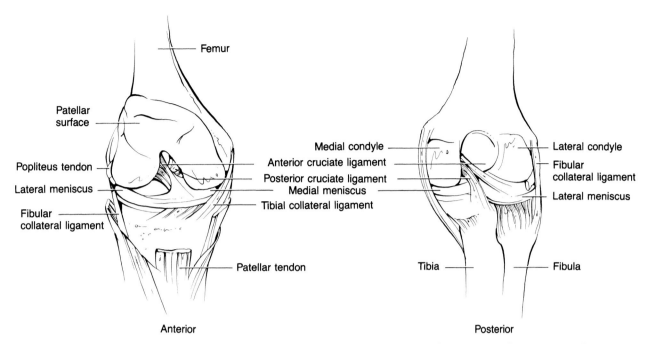

FIG. 18.1. Knee anatomy. Reprinted with permission from Harwood-Nuss A, Wolfson AB, et al. *The Clinical Practice of Emergency Medicine.* 3rd ed. Philadelphia: Lippincott Williams & Wilkins; 2001.

Right Knee
(Anterior)

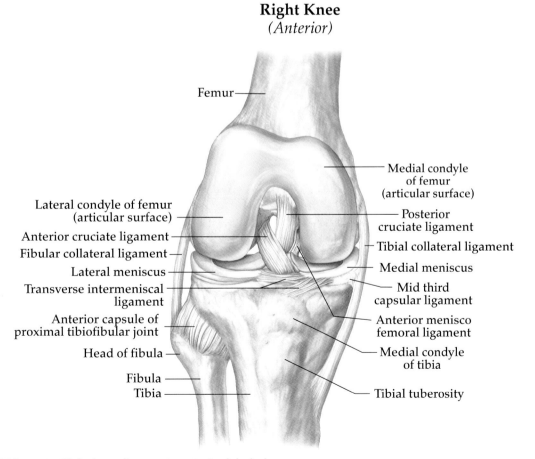

FIG. 18.2. Right-knee ligaments anterior labeled.

Right Knee
(Posterior)

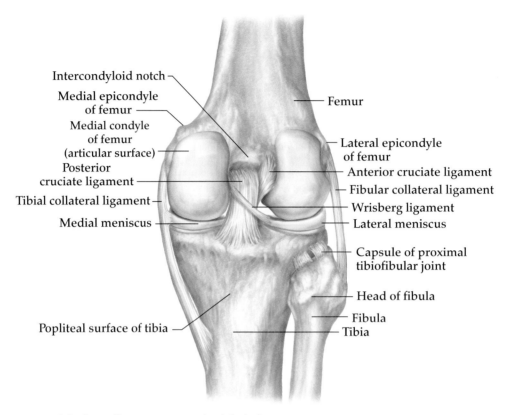

Intercondyloid notch
Medial epicondyle of femur
Medial condyle of femur (articular surface)
Posterior cruciate ligament
Tibial collateral ligament
Medial meniscus
Popliteal surface of tibia

Femur
Lateral epicondyle of femur
Anterior cruciate ligament
Fibular collateral ligament
Wrisberg ligament
Lateral meniscus
Capsule of proximal tibiofibular joint
Head of fibula
Fibula
Tibia

FIG. 18.3. Right-knee ligaments posterior labeled.

Normal Knee Anatomy
(Patella removed)

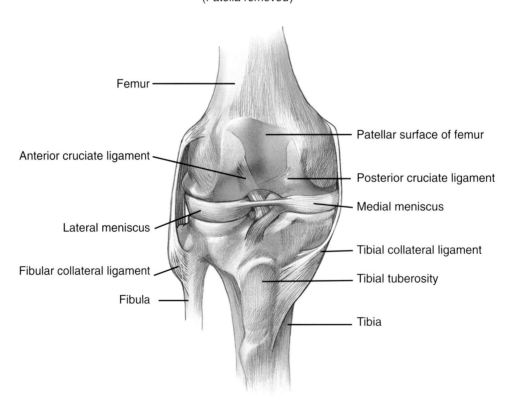

Femur
Anterior cruciate ligament
Lateral meniscus
Fibular collateral ligament
Fibula

Patellar surface of femur
Posterior cruciate ligament
Medial meniscus
Tibial collateral ligament
Tibial tuberosity
Tibia

FIG. 18.4. Knee anatomy anterior view.

Meniscus

The meniscus is a crescent-shaped piece of cartilage that lies between the femur and tibia. Each knee has two menisci, one medial and one lateral. Together, they cushion the joint by distributing downward forces outward and away from the central anchor points of the menisci.

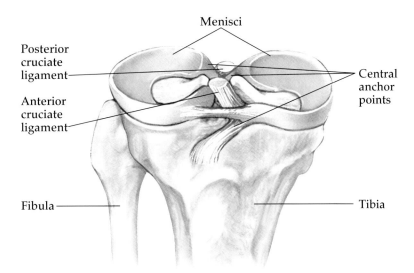

FIG. 18.5. Meniscal Anatomy demonstrating meniscal attachment points and relationship to the cruciate ligaments.

structures within the knee. They derive their blood supply from a perimeniscal capillary plexus as branches from the genicular arteries. Only the outer 10% to 25% of the lateral and 10% to 30% of the medial menisci have direct blood supply; the inner two thirds of the menisci receive nutrition via diffusion. The menisci, in the simplest of senses, function as shock absorbers to the knee. They also participate in load sharing, passive stabilization, reduction in contact stresses within the joint, proprioception, and joint congruity via increased contact surface.

Muscular attachments about the knee also lend to the stability of the joint. The quadriceps musculature anteriorly in conjunction with the patella and patellar tendon, known as the extensor mechanism, is responsible for extension of the knee (ability to straight leg raise). The posterior musculature, and particularly the hamstrings complex, is responsible for flexion of the knee (bending) (Fig. 18.6).

The neurovascular bundle runs along the posterior margin of the knee and can be injured acutely. The blood supply to the knee consists of a network of genicular branches from

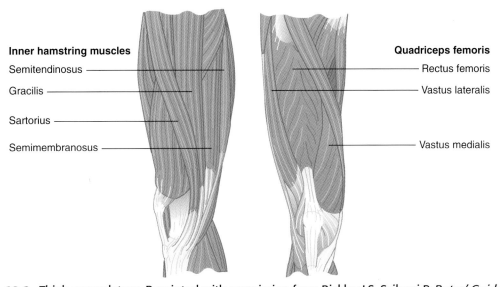

FIG. 18.6. Thigh musculature. Reprinted with permission from Bickley LS, Szilagyi P. *Bates' Guide to Physical Examination and History Taking.* 8th ed. Philadelphia: Lippincott Williams & Wilkins; 2003.

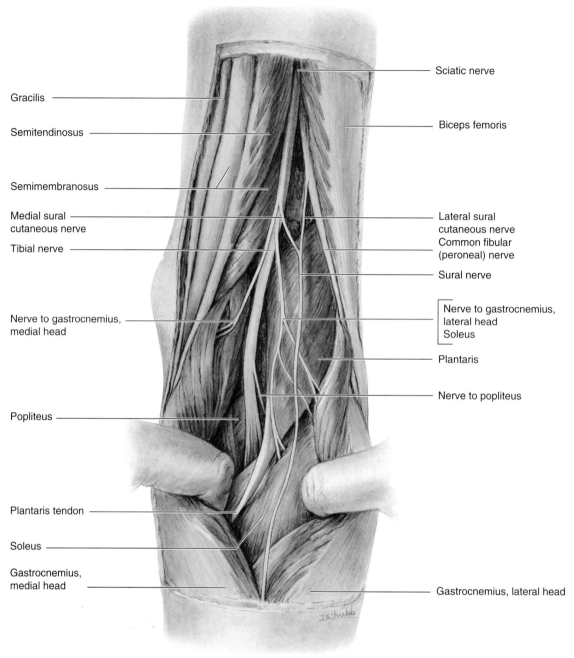

Gracilis

Semitendinosus

Semimembranosus

Medial sural
cutaneous nerve

Tibial nerve

Nerve to gastrocnemius,
medial head

Popliteus

Plantaris tendon

Soleus

Gastrocnemius,
medial head

Sciatic nerve

Biceps femoris

Lateral sural
cutaneous nerve
Common fibular
(peroneal) nerve

Sural nerve

Nerve to gastrocnemius,
lateral head
Soleus

Plantaris

Nerve to popliteus

Gastrocnemius, lateral head

Anterior View

FIG. 18.7. Nerves of the popliteal fossa. Reprinted with permission from Moore KL, Dalley AF II. *Clinical Oriented Anatomy.* 4th ed. Baltimore: Lippincott Williams & Wilkins; 1999.

the popliteal system. The tibial and peroneal nerves, which innervate the lower extremity and foot, also course posterior to the knee and are at risk at the time of initial injury to the knee (Fig. 18.7).

EPIDEMIOLOGY

The potential morbidity of knee injuries has led many physicians, trainers, coaches, and athletes themselves to attempt to identify the factors predisposing to these injuries in the

hope of minimizing risk. Injuries are categorized by bony, ligamentous, or meniscal involvement. The type of injury that is encountered depends, to some extent, on the type of athletic pursuit. The majority of studies on preventing injury have centered around football in the United States and soccer internationally.

The most significant trend in acute knee injuries over the past 20 years has been the rise of ACL tears, with a disproportionately higher rate among female athletes. The incidence of ACL injuries is estimated at approximately 200,000 a year with upward of 100,000 ACL reconstructions a year. Recent studies have shown a difference between the rates of ACL injuries in women compared to men. Speculation as to the reasons for this is unclear. Some authors account for a decreased protective role of dynamic stabilizers (quadriceps and hamstrings) in women, while others note the smaller-diameter ACL and narrower intercondylar notch as reasons for the increased incidence.[3] In any event, an ACL injury can be a devastating injury for the competitive and recreational athletes alike.

PCL injuries have historically been underdiagnosed because these are often asymptomatic. Some studies have shown an incidence of up to 44% of all acute knee injuries.[4]

The overall incidence of posterolateral injuries of the knee is rare and has been reported to be less than 2% of all acute ligament knee injuries.[5] Approximately 40% of all posterolateral knee injuries occur during sports activities.[6]

The annual incidence of meniscal tears is 60 to 70 per 100,000.[7,8] Injuries occur more commonly in men, with the male-to-female ratio of 2.5:1 to 4:1.[9] Meniscal injuries are also highly associated with other injuries within the knee. Lateral meniscal tears are more common acutely with an ACL tear,[10] whereas chronic ACL tears are associated with medial meniscal tears. Meniscal tears also have been reported frequently in the setting of an acute tibial plateau fracture.

The incidence of osteochondritis dissecans (OCD) of the knee has been estimated at between 0.02% and 0.03% based on knee radiographs and 1.2% based on arthroscopy.[11,12] The highest rates are among children aged 10 to 15, and the male-to-female ratio approaches 2:1. Approximately 15% to 30% of cases reported are bilateral.[13] A history of trauma is reported in as many as 40% of OCD lesions, although this has recently been challenged.[14]

NARROWING THE DIFFERENTIAL DIAGNOSIS

History

In the initial approach to the acute knee injury in the athlete, it is imperative to obtain a detailed history. This coupled with a thorough physical exam will significantly narrow the differential and ultimately the diagnosis (Fig. 18.8).

Important questions to ask include a complete description of the mechanism of injury and localizing symptoms. This includes the onset, location, severity, and intensity of the pain as well as the alleviating and modifying factors. Specific questions to ask if not given in the overall description of the mechanism include the following:

1. Position of the knee at the time of injury (i.e., extension vs. flexion)
2. Anterior versus posterior symptoms; medial versus lateral symptoms
3. Twisting/rotational injury versus axial load injury
4. Varus stress/valgus stress
5. Catching or locking of the knee
6. An initial "pop" or later "clicking"
7. Presence of an effusion
8. Ability to range
9. Ability to weight bear
10. Presence of a deformity

Certainly the position of the knee can play a role in the injury process. An extended knee has more inherent stability than a flexed knee but could be subject to axial loading forces with the end result in fracture. These patients will be very uncomfortable with weight bearing. The location of symptoms often helps narrow the differential by assigning a compartment of injury, be it on the medial or the lateral side, where one can have an injury to the collateral ligament, meniscus, or plateau. The presence of an effusion helps to depict between intra-articular and extra-articular pathology, while catching or locking of the knee is often present in meniscal injuries. If the patient complains of a varus or valgus load, meniscal and collateral ligament pathology is brought to the forefront of the differential. Twisting injuries are suspicious for anterior cruciate tears, and the patient can often account for an audible or sensible "pop." Some very common injuries in the athlete will be discussed later in this chapter with keys to the history and physical outlined.

Evidence-based Physical Exam

After a through history has been elicited, physical exam of the knee is an important step to narrow the differential diagnosis. The general exam techniques as well as injury-specific exam techniques described later in this chapter can help to differentiate between the most common diagnoses for each particular compartment, or area, of the knee. Location of tenderness, ligament laxity, presence of an effusion, and range of motion (ROM) are keys to the physical exam that will always be helpful to narrow the differential. It is important to remember that possibly the greatest and most morbid knee injury in an athlete is a frank dislocation. This should be clearly evident by gross deformity, severe pain, an inability to range or weight bear, and sometimes neurovascular compromise. Knee dislocation is an emergency, and failure to recognize a knee dislocation may lead to devastating residual injuries and even amputation. These patients should be evaluated at the nearest emergency department for radiographic confirmation, prompt reduction, and further treatment, as necessary.

Once a proper history is taken, attention can then turn toward the physical exam. A systematic approach to the knee should be preformed with particular attention paid to differences between the affected and unaffected sides. This statement, although true in any athletic extremity injury, is particularly important with the knee exam.

KNEE INJURIES

Anterior View of Normal Knee
(Patella removed)

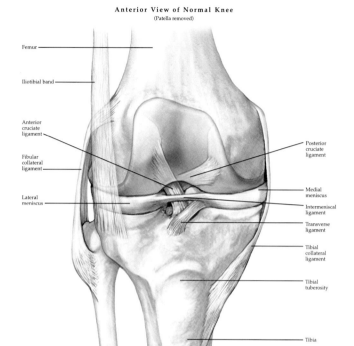

Femur
Iliotibial band
Anterior cruciate ligament
Fibular collateral ligament
Lateral meniscus
Posterior cruciate ligament
Medial meniscus
Intermeniscal ligament
Transverse ligament
Tibial collateral ligament
Tibial tuberosity
Tibia
Fibula

Oblique View

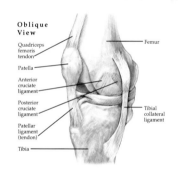

Femur
Quadriceps femoris tendon
Patella
Anterior cruciate ligament
Posterior cruciate ligament
Patellar ligament (tendon)
Tibia
Tibial collateral ligament

Posterior View

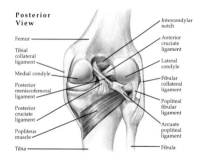

Intercondylar notch
Femur
Tibial collateral ligament
Medial condyle
Posterior meniscofemoral ligament
Posterior cruciate ligament
Popliteus muscle
Tibia
Anterior cruciate ligament
Lateral condyle
Fibular collateral ligament
Popliteal fibular ligament
Arcuate popliteal ligament
Fibula

Traumatic Knee Injuries

Ligament tear   Bone avulsion   Ligament sprain   Patellar dislocation

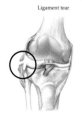 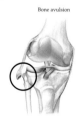 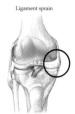 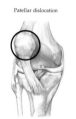

Sports Related Ligament Injuries

 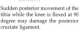   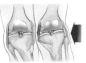

Sudden posterior movement of the tibia while the knee is flexed at 90 degree may damage the posterior cruciate ligament.

Hyperextension of the knee joint can damage the anterior cruciate and tibial collateral ligaments.

Forcible external rotation of the foot in the "whip-kick" causes the lower leg to twist at the knee, putting excessive strain on the tibial collateral ligament. It can also cause plical irritation or exacerbate patellar instability.

A lateral blow to the knees while the feet are firmly planted may cause damage to the tibial and fibular collateral ligaments.

9872   ©1993, 2000, 2003 Anatomical Chart Company, Skokie, Illinois. In consultation with Mark R. Hutchinson, MD, University of Illinois at Chicago.

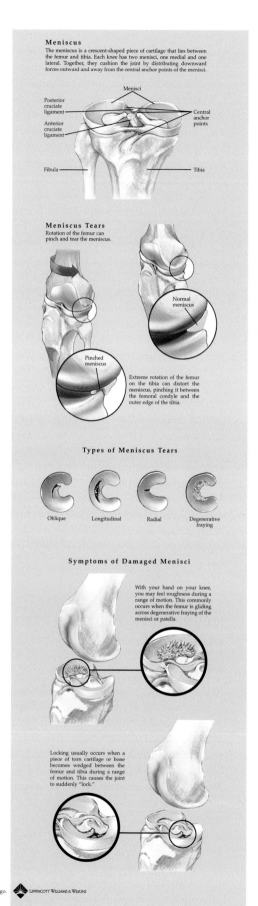

Meniscus
The meniscus is a crescent-shaped piece of cartilage that lies between the femur and tibia. Each knee has two menisci, one medial and one lateral. Together, they cushion the joint by distributing downward forces outward and away from the central anchor points of the menisci.

Menisci
Posterior cruciate ligament
Anterior cruciate ligament
Central anchor points
Fibula
Tibia

Meniscus Tears
Rotation of the femur can pinch and tear the meniscus.

Normal meniscus
Pinched meniscus

Extreme rotation of the femur on the tibia can distort the meniscus, pinching it between the femoral condyle and the outer edge of the tibia.

Types of Meniscus Tears

Oblique   Longitudinal   Radial   Degenerative fraying

Symptoms of Damaged Menisci

With your hand on your knee, you may feel roughness during a range of motion. This commonly occurs when the femur is gliding across degenerative fraying of the menisci or patella.

Locking usually occurs when a piece of torn cartilage or bone becomes wedged between the femur and tibia during a range of motion. This causes the joint to suddenly "lock."

LIPPINCOTT WILLIAMS & WILKINS

FIG. 18.8. Knee injuries.

Inspection

The overall position of the knee can lend some insight into the injury process. Ecchymosis or edema can lead an examiner toward a particular area of injury. Evidence of an effusion helps to differentiate between intra-articular and extra-articular processes. An effusion often presents as swelling about the knee, with the knee held in mild flexion and pain with full extension or moderate flexion. A gross deformity can also be present, and knee dislocation needs to be ruled out immediately because of the associated devastating consequences.

Palpation

Palpation over the three compartments of the knee can help differentiate injuries in each particular location. Anterior or posterior tenderness to palpation may include injuries to the extensor mechanism and/or hamstrings musculature, respectively. Pain along the medial or lateral portions of the knee is suspicious for collateral ligament injuries. Finally, pain along the joint line, especially the medial joint line, is indicative of meniscal pathology.

Evidence of an Effusion

Presence of an effusion in the setting of an acute knee injury signifies an intra-articular injury and is a key part of the knee exam. The effusion is a red flag for a potential significant knee injury that needs to be identified for proper management. A minimal effusion is best tested by milking down any fluid from the suprapatellar area with the knee held in extension. The fluid can then be concentrated into either the medial or the lateral compartment by gentle pressure over the opposite compartment. Once the fluid is concentrated in one area, gentle pressure over that area will force the fluid to traverse the joint, and it will be felt in the opposite compartment. Presence of an effusion in the setting of an acute knee injury signifies an intra-articular injury and generally indicates a more significant knee injury that needs to be identified for proper management.

Range of Motion

The normal ROM of the knee is from 0 degrees (full extension) to approximately 135 degrees of flexion and 10 degrees of internal and external rotation. Acutely, a decreased ROM is a nonspecific sign of knee injury but may be helpful when associated with other exam findings. A mechanical "block" to ROM may be indicative of a bucket-handle tear of the meniscus and should not be forcefully reduced. It is important to note that with many acute knee injuries, it is common to have a limited ROM. This is usually secondary to pain and/or presence of an effusion.

Strength

Strength should be accessed in the acute injury as well. This will often be difficult secondary to pain associated with the injury. The strength both of the hamstrings and of quadriceps should be accessed and documented. The patient should also be asked to perform a *straight leg raise*. This maneuver entails keeping the knee extended and lifting the lower extremity off the bed/ground straight in the air. If the patient is able to straight leg raise, or can at least hold elevation of the leg for a short period of time, the extensor mechanism (quadriceps, patella, patella tendon) is intact.

Ligaments

The most important component to the ligament exam of the knee is the comparison to the opposite (unaffected) knee. This is the best way to gauge an abnormal test. The most basic of approaches to the ligament exam will be discussed here. A more detailed exam will also be outlined with the specific injuries to follow.

Collateral Ligaments

To test the MCL, a valgus stress (knee is stabilized, and pressure is applied on the lateral side of the knee and the medial side of the ankle) is applied with the leg in full extension and in 30 degrees of flexion. To test the lateral collateral ligament, a varus stress is applied with the leg again in full extension and 30 degrees of flexion. Any laxity of these motions with respect to the unaffected side is suspicious for an injury.

Cruciate Ligaments

The Lachmann's examination is the preferred method for assessing the integrity of the ACL. With the femur/thigh stabilized with one hand, take the leg in the opposite hand near the tibial tubercle and attempt to translate the tibia forward with respect to the femur. A positive test will exhibit increased laxity and no firm "end point" in comparison to the unaffected knee.

The posterior cruciate is best tested with the patient lying down with the hip flexed and the knee at 90 degrees. A posterior force is applied to the proximal tibia with respect to the femur. If the subluxation is greater than the other side, and there is no stiff end point, then a PCL injury is suspected. This is called the posterior drawer test.

Diagnostic Testing

In the workup of knee injuries in the athlete, there are many imaging modalities that will aid in the narrowing and, sometimes, confirmation of the diagnosis.

Laboratory

Routine laboratory analysis is generally not required in the setting of an acute knee injury. If infectious or autoimmune etiology is suspected, then appropriate serology and/or cultures should be obtained.

Imaging

Plain radiographs are usually the initial test that can show any associated fractures and dislocations. Any fracture or dislocation should be seen promptly by an orthopedist. X-ray may also show evidence of bony ligament avulsion either on the medial or on the lateral sides. The lateral radiograph lends information about the congruency of the joint as well as evaluation of the patella. A high- or low-riding patella (patella alta or baja) could be an indication of a patellar or quadriceps tendon tear, respectively.

Other Testing

Computerized tomography (CT) is also very useful in the evaluation of the acute knee injury. CT gives very fine definition of the bony structures of the knee and can confirm evidence of an effusion. It is also helpful for the evaluation of an occult fracture.

Magnetic resonance imaging (MRI) has shown to be extremely useful in many acute knee injuries. MRI gives outstanding detail and the precise location of ligament and menisci injuries.

APPROACH TO THE ATHLETE WITH MEDIAL COLLATERAL LIGAMENT INJURIES

HISTORY AND PHYSICAL EXAMINATION

The diagnosis of MCL injuries is related to the mechanism of injury. The typical injury is one of a valgus moment to the knee. Patients typically present with tenderness along the medial portion of the knee from femur to tibia. They sometimes note a sense of instability with weight bearing.

On physical exam the MCL should be tested at both full extension and 30 degrees of flexion. It is imperative for an adequate exam that the patient be completely relaxed. The exam at full extension tests both the MCL as well as the associated capsular and cruciate ligament injuries. Exam at flexion isolates the MCL complex. A difference of only 5 to 8 mm is indicative of significant injury.[1] Palpation along the course of the ligament is helpful in determining the location of the injury. A proximal MCL tear is more common than a distal avulsion. After injury to the MCL is determined, a complete exam of the knee is warranted to rule out concomitant injuries.

MCL injury classification:

- Grade I is a primary sprain and signifies stretching of the fibers with localized tenderness, but no laxity on exam.
- Grade II is more severe injury indicating partial tear with mild to moderate laxity noted on valgus stress at 30 degrees.
- Grade III sprain indicates a complete MCL with gross instability and laxity on exam. There will generally be laxity both with valgus stress at 30 degrees of flexion as well as in full extension.

DIAGNOSTIC TESTING

Plain radiographs may be helpful in the evaluation of an MCL injury by identifying a bony avulsion or associated fractures of the knee. The most useful diagnostic test is MRI, which localizes the area and the extent of injury but may not be indicated in milder cases, particularly in the absence of an effusion. Musculoskeletal ultrasound can also clearly visualize the MCL and assess the extent of the MCL injury.

TREATMENT

Nonoperative

- Grade I– and grade II–isolated MCL injuries usually can be treated successfully in a conservative manner.
- Rest, ice, compression, elevation (RICE)
- Hinged knee brace (to resist valgus stress)
- Weight bearing as tolerated
- ROM exercises
- In one study, collegiate football players with grade I and II injuries showed return to full, unprotected participation at an average of 10.6 and 19.5 days, respectively.[15] Grade III injuries, if present in isolation, can be treated with an aggressive rehab protocol after initial swelling subsides. Protected weight bearing in conjunction with a hinged knee brace has been advocated for these patients.[2]

Operative

- In the past, primary repair of complete MCL injuries was encouraged, but recently the pendulum seems to have swung toward nonoperative treatment.
- Controversy still exists whether MCL repair is needed with combined ACL–MCL injuries.[16]
- Typically, athletes with a grade III injury that is interfering with return to sport or has failed nonoperative management should be considered for operative management.
- Those patients with persistent instability also should be considered for surgery.
- Currently there are no well-defined guidelines or indications for the operative treatment of these injuries.

Prognosis/Return To Play

- Isolated MCL injuries overall hold a good prognosis.
- Athletes with grade I and II injuries typically can return to full activity after 2 to 3 weeks or after participation in practice is not limited.
- For athletes with grade III injury, the return to sport is less predictable. They may benefit from a few more weeks of rest and rehabilitation before returning to activity, usually at 6 to 8 weeks, as long as instability is absent.

Complications/Indications for Referral

In general, athletes who fail conservative treatment, although uncommon, should be referred to an orthopedist for consideration of surgical treatment. Athletes with gross instability or a type III tear should also be evaluated by an orthopedic surgeon. Beware of the patient with a suspected MCL injury and an associated lateral tibial plateau fracture. The latter will exhibit lateral tenderness to palpation as well as significant edema and instability. These patients should be seen immediately by an orthopedist for consideration of surgical management of the fracture.

APPROACH TO THE ATHLETE WITH ANTERIOR CRUCIATE LIGAMENT INJURIES

HISTORY AND PHYSICAL EXAMINATION

An ACL injury is oftentimes a noncontact injury while changing direction or landing from a jump. Patients will give a history of a sudden "pop" with swelling and hemarthrosis within a few hours. Many athletes will feel a sense of instability and often report an inability to weight bear.

The acute evaluation of an athlete with a suspected ACL injury should begin with a general physical exam as for any knee injury. Special tests that can help confirm an ACL injury include the anterior drawer, Lachman, and pivot shift tests.[17] Of these, the Lachman is the most sensitive and specific for ACL injury with rates reportedly as high as 93% and 99%, respectively.[18] This test is preformed with the patient completely relaxed. The leg is held at 30 degrees of flexion, and as the femur is stabilized, an anterior force is applied to the posterior calf attempting to translate the tibia forward with respect to the femur. Displacement should be measured in millimeters and compared to the opposite side. It is also useful to distinguish an end point—firm (normal), marginal, or soft. The pivot shift test is extremely helpful, if present, to rule in ACL injury, but is very difficult to elicit in the acute setting. This test is preformed with the patient supine and the knee extended. The lower extremity is mildly internally rotated at the ankle, and a soft valgus stress is given at the knee as the knee is flexed slowly. In an ACL injury the tibia translates anterior in mild flexion, and as more flexion is obtained, the iliotibial tract reduces the tibia posterior onto the femur. This reduction is the "clunk" that is felt by the examiner and is graded 0 (absent), 1+ (pivot glide), 2+ (pivot shift), and 3+ (momentary locking). The anterior drawer is preformed with the knee at 90 degrees. An anterior force is then applied to the tibia. This test is difficult to perform secondary to spasm and is the most inconsistent of ACL exams in determining injury.[17]

DIAGNOSTIC TESTING

Plain radiographs of the knee can aid in the evaluation of an ACL injury and should be the first imaging study ordered to rule out associated osseous injuries. The lateral knee and tunnel views can show an acute avulsion fracture of the anterior tibia spine suggesting ACL injury. The anterior–posterior (AP) view can show a lateral tibial plateau avulsion fracture (Segond fracture), which has also been associated with ACL injuries.

MRI has also been widely incorporated in the evaluation of ACL injuries. The overall accuracy of MRI in accessing ACL injuries is approximately 95%. The ACL is best seen in the sagittal images through the intercondylar notch. MRI will also sometimes show increased signal intensity (bone bruising) over the lateral femoral condyle and posterior lateral tibial plateau.

TREATMENT

The treatment of an acute ACL injury is reliant on many factors. The goal of treatment is return to play with restoration of normal function. Among the factors to be considered are the presence of concomitant injuries, age of the patient, activity level and type of sport, and degree of instability.[17]

Nonoperative

- Bracing
- Partial weight bearing (crutches)
- ROM exercises
- Closed kinetic chain exercises
- Weight-bearing strengthening (quadriceps/hamstrings)
- Reinjury prevention education
- Knee orthoses

Operative

- The primary candidates for ACL reconstruction are those patients with an active lifestyle in which instability would lead to further knee damage.
- Multiple surgical techniques have been described with no clear consensus as to the best mode of reconstruction.

- Currently, the three major options are bone–patellar tendon–bone autograft, semitendinosus and gracilis bundled autograft, and various allograft choices.
- The initial rehab begins with preoperative ROM exercises with the goal to match the unaffected side (phase I).
- Immediate postoperative ROM from full extension to 90 degrees of flexion as well as complete wound healing is the goal in the first 2 weeks (phase II).
- From weeks 3 to 5, extension should be maintained and gradual increase to full flexion should be reached (phase III).
- Six weeks postop and beyond is considered the safe point for strengthening programs with emphasis on closed-chain weight-bearing exercises.[17]

Prognosis/Return To Play

- The return to play after an ACL tear is less predictable than that after an MCL tear. Most patients will be able to return to some activities, but often at a decreased level as compared to preinjury.
- Patients that elect nonoperative treatment should undergo an extensive rehabilitation protocol and likely could return to sport at around 6 months if return is capable.
- Most high-level athletes elect to have a reconstruction, and this is associated with intensive perireconstructive rehabilitation. Return for such athletes is usually 6 to 9 months, with some requiring up to a year.
- Long-term studies have shown that early arthritic changes are not necessarily prevented by joint stabilization by surgical means. This should be discussed with the patient before surgical intervention.[17]

Complications/Indications for Referral

Athletes that are diagnosed with an acute ACL injury and want to return to their prior activity will likely need referral to an orthopedist. Acute management including the initiation of a comprehensive rehabilitation program can be started by the primary physician, which will help to efficiently manage these athletes. Beware of the patient with associated fractures or multiple ligamentous injuries. Prompt evaluation of these patients is crucial for timing of appropriate surgical procedures.

APPROACH TO THE ATHLETE WITH POSTERIOR CRUCIATE LIGAMENT INJURIES

HISTORY AND PHYSICAL EXAMINATION

The most common cause of PCL injury is via a mechanism in which the tibia is forced posterior with the knee bent. This is frequently the case in a motor vehicle accident when the tibia is struck by the dashboard. In sports, this mechanism can be the result of a direct blow to the proximal tibia anteriorly or with a fall onto the tibial tubercle with the knee bent and the ankle plantarflexed. Acutely, the athlete may describe a sense of instability. Typically there is only minimal pain and effusion. Inspection may reveal abrasion and/or ecchymosis over the anterior proximal tibia. There are many specific exams that may aid in the diagnosis of a PCL injury. The most sensitive exam for an isolated PCL injury is the posterior drawer test. This is preformed with the knee bent at 90 degrees. The examiner then applies a posterior force over the proximal tibia. The amount of laxity is measured against the opposite knee. The posterior sag test is preformed with the patient supine and the hip and knee flexed at 90 degrees. In an injured PCL the tibia will noticeably "sag" as compared to the uninjured knee. The quadriceps active test is preformed with the patient supine and the hip at 45 degrees and knee at 90 degrees. The ankle is stabilized and the patient is asked to fire their quadriceps. With a PCL injury the examiner can observe reduction of the tibia from the original posterior subluxation after quadriceps contraction.

Classification of Acute Injuries

Classification of PCL injuries can be graded during examination and is based on the posterior drawer test. In a grade I injury, the tibial plateau remains proudly anterior to the medial femoral condyle; in a grade II tear, the tibial plateau is palpated flush with the condyles; and in a grade III tear, the tibial plateau is posterior to the femoral condyles.

DIAGNOSTIC TESTING

Plain radiographs can help in the acute evaluation of PCL injuries by ruling out associated osseous injury. The lateral knee view may also show clear evidence of posterior translation of the tibia or acute avulsion fractures. The posterior subluxation can be accentuated by obtaining gravity-assisted stress radiographs. MRI is extremely useful in the evaluation of PCL and associated injuries and is easily seen on sagittal views.

TREATMENT

Nonoperative

- The initial treatment of acute grades I and II PCL tears can be conservative with a brief period of splinting and protected weight bearing.
- Early ROM and quadriceps strengthening can usually be initiated soon after injury, and recovery of strength and ROM generally occurs quickly.
- Most athletes can return to sports within 4 weeks.[19]

- Acute treatment of grade III tears can also be treated successfully nonoperatively, but this is more controversial.
- The current recommendation is to splint the knee in full extension for 2 to 4 weeks followed by early ROM and strengthening.

Operative

- Surgical treatment is indicated for acute bony avulsion fractures and combined PCL injuries with other ligament, meniscal, or bony lesions.[20]
- Patients who fail conservative management should also be considered for surgical treatment. Some orthopedists recommend surgical management of grade III tears as well as combined injuries in the athlete.

Prognosis/Return To Play

- The prognosis for PCL injuries overall is excellent when presenting in isolation.
- *Natural History*: In 1986, Parolie and Bergfeld reported that approximately 2% of college senior football players at the National Football League (NFL) predraft examination were found to have chronic asymptomatic PCL-deficient knees. There have been numerous studies that document good to excellent results for return to play in acute PCL tears.[21]
- Most athletes return to sport between 4 and 6 weeks—those with grade I and II injuries returning earlier than their grade III counterparts.
- If nonsurgical management fails, surgical treatment is considered and may extend the duration away from sport. The athlete should not return to sport with an unstable knee as reinjury can occur.

Complications/Indications for Referral

Patients with an isolated PCL injury are likely to function with minimal disability. Referral should be made when conservative measures fail or instability is significant enough to limit daily activities and sport. Beware of associated ligamentous injuries, especially injuries of the PLC. These injuries are complex and difficult to treat and should be evaluated by an orthopedic specialist.

APPROACH TO THE ATHLETE WITH LATERAL KNEE LIGAMENTOUS INJURIES

HISTORY AND PHYSICAL EXAMINATION

The usual mechanism for posterolateral knee injuries involves knee hyperextension with a varus moment combined with a twisting force. The most common mechanism is a posterolateral-directed blow to the medial tibia, but injury can also occur with sudden deceleration of the upper leg and torso with the lower leg fixed. Patients usually report pain along the lateral and posterolateral knee. Some may have associated motor or sensory changes secondary to peroneal nerve injury/irritation. After the acute swelling resolves, patients typically note instability in extension. They typically have trouble with lateral cutting maneuvers as well as ascending and descending stairs.[22] On examination, patients may exhibit hyperextension of the knee as well as a varus thrust in the stance phase of gait. Examination of the knee may reveal ecchymosis or abrasion over the anteromedial proximal tibia and/or varus alignment of the knee not evident on the opposite side. Few specific physical exam tests are highly sensitive or specific for posterolateral injuries, so a high index of suspicion is needed in the diagnosis of these injuries. In general, the lateral collateral ligament should be examined with a varus stress at full extension and 30 degrees, and laxity should be compared to the unaffected knee. The dial test helps to discern posterolateral injuries from combined posterolateral and PCL injuries. To perform this test the patient should be relaxed and in the prone position on the examination table. The knee is fixed and the tibia is externally rotated at both 30 and 90 degrees of knee flexion. Posterolateral subluxation of the lateral tibial plateau at 30 degrees only suggests PLC injury, whereas subluxation at both 30 and 90 degrees indicates both PLC and PCL injuries.

DIAGNOSTIC TESTING

Plain radiographs of the knee may show acute avulsion fracture of Gerdy's tubercle (indicating iliotibial band injury), fibular tip avulsion, or fibular head fracture. MRI is an excellent diagnostic tool in the evaluation of the PLC and other associated injuries. The soft-tissue detail heavily aids in the diagnosis of these difficult injuries.

TREATMENT

Nonoperative

- It is difficult to predict the natural history of isolated PLC injuries, as significant long-term studies have yet to be published.
- It has been postulated that early degenerative changes can occur as with most other ligament injuries about the knee. Studies have shown that professional and recreational athletes who sustained isolated PLC injuries did not have evidence of impaired function initially.[22,23]
- Initial treatment of the acutely injured athlete with mild instability and minimal to no symptoms or functional limitations should include a period of immobilization (2 to 4 weeks) followed by a rehabilitation program focused on ROM and quadriceps strengthening.[6]

Operative

- Indications for surgical treatment include symptomatic instability with functional limitations.
- In general, surgical repair is recommended within 2 weeks of injury.
- The diagnosis and treatment of combined ligament injury (ACL/PCL + PLC) as well as knee malalignment are important for long-term functional status.
- Knee malalignment is typically treated surgically via a proximal tibial valgus osteotomy or some other bony procedure.

Prognosis/Return To Play

- The effect of the acute PLC injury in the athlete has not yet been clearly defined. Most patients do not exhibit functional disability or impaired function.
- It has been postulated that these injuries predispose the athlete to early degenerative disease.
- Nonoperative treatment of these injuries can be associated with return to full preinjury activities. After the initial 2 to 4 weeks of immobilization, rehabilitation and gradual return to sport-specific drills can typically start at 6 to 8 weeks as strength increases.
- Operative patients typically require a well-supervised rehabilitation program for 9 to 12 months.
- The most severe injuries, especially those with associated ligamentous injuries, typically result in an inability to return to vigorous activities postoperatively.[6]

Complications/Indications for Referral

PLC injuries that are associated with frank instability should be referred to an orthopedic surgeon. It is important to recognize combined injuries, especially those of the ACLs or PCLs, as prompt surgical treatment of these combined injuries has been shown to yield better long-term outcomes.

APPROACH TO THE ATHLETE WITH MENISCAL TEARS OF THE KNEE

HISTORY AND PHYSICAL EXAMINATION

Acute injury to the meniscus can occur both alone and in the setting of other injuries. When isolated, the most common mechanism is a twisting injury or hyperflexion event. Oftentimes, the athlete notes immediate pain and swelling. Pain with squatting is also sometimes a sign of meniscal pathology. Loss of motion with a mechanical block to extension is frequently due to a displaced bucket-handle tear of the meniscus and usually requires surgical management. Examination for meniscal pathology begins like any other acute knee injury. Inspection for an effusion followed by palpation, ROM, and ligament laxity should be initially

accessed. Joint line tenderness has been shown in one study to be the best clinical sign of a meniscal tear with a sensitivity of 74% and positive predictive value of 50%.[24] This was not true in the setting of acute ACL pathology.[25] The McMurray test has been shown not to be as sensitive. This test, though, in combination with history and other physical exam findings may aid in the diagnosis. To perform the McMurray test the patient is positioned supine on the examination table. The knee is flexed, and the medial joint space is palpated with the examiner's thumb. A valgus force is applied to the knee with the lower leg in external rotation, and the leg is extended. If this maneuver causes a palpable or audible "click," there is a probable meniscal tear.[26]

DIAGNOSTIC TESTING

Plain radiographs will be unlikely to show evidence of meniscal injury, but they will help to rule out associated osseous injury. Standard AP, lateral, and weight-bearing views at 30 or 45 degrees should be preformed. These views will allow for the diagnosis of fracture and early joint space narrowing, which may change treatment strategies. In a recent study, MRI was shown to accurately detect meniscal pathology in approximately 95% of cases.[27] The criterion standard for confirmation of meniscal tears is direct visualization through arthroscopy. The types of meniscal tears are beyond the scope of this chapter, but include oblique, transverse (radial), horizontal, vertical–horizontal (can be a displaced bucket-handle tear), or degenerative.

TREATMENT

Nonoperative

- A common misconception is that all meniscal tears need surgical management.
- Short, stable vertical tears (<10 mm); stable partial-thickness tears; and small radial tears (<3 mm) may heal spontaneously or remain asymptomatic.
- It is difficult to know how prevalent these types of tears are since most are likely not reported or imaged.

Operative

- It is rare for an athlete to be treated nonoperatively for an acute meniscal tear, given their symptomatology and activity level.
- The surgical indications for arthroscopic treatment of meniscal tears are given in Table 18.1.

Commonly accepted criteria for meniscal repair include the following:

- A complete, vertical, longitudinal tear greater than 10 mm in length

TABLE 18.1 Indications for Surgical Management of Meniscal Pathology

1. Symptoms of meniscal injury that affect activities of daily living or sports
2. Positive physical findings such as joint line tenderness, joint effusion, limitation of motion, pain with squatting, or positive McMurray test
3. Failure to respond to nonsurgical treatment including activity modification, NSAIDs, and a rehabilitation program
4. Absence of other identifiable causes of knee pain

- A tear within the peripheral 10% to 30% of the meniscus or within 3 to 4 mm of the meniscocapsular junction
- An unstable peripheral tear
- The absence of secondary degenerative changes
- A tear in an active patient
- A tear associated with concurrent ligament stabilization

Prognosis/Return To Play

- Prognosis of meniscal tears depends on the injury type and treatment.
- For stable tears treated nonoperatively or partial menisectomy athletes, there have been no studies to recommend time away from sport.
- The return to play depends on pain, ROM, and strength, when the standard criteria for return to sport are met.
- Following meniscal repair, athletes are typically able to return to all activities three to four months post-operatively.[28]

Complications/Indications for Referral

In general, because successful nonoperative management is rare in athletes, most patients with a confirmed acute meniscal tear should be evaluated by an orthopedist for consideration of operative management. The patient who presents with a displaced bucket-handle tear may be unable to fully extend the lower extremity. It should be recognized that many of these injuries will need acute surgical intervention. Meniscal repair in the setting of ACL reconstruction yields better meniscal healing than repair without ACL reconstruction.

APPROACH TO THE ATHLETE WITH OSTEOCHONDRITIS DISSECANS OF THE KNEE

Numerous theories have been proposed, but the etiology of OCD is unclear. The three major mechanisms are hereditary, vascular, and traumatic. This chapter reviews those lesions precipitated by trauma.

HISTORY AND PHYSICAL EXAMINATION

There is a distinction between adult and juvenile forms of OCD. OCD with open physes is known as the juvenile form. Some authors note that the adult form is likely an unrecognized juvenile form that later becomes apparent on radiographs. Early presentation often consists of poorly defined complaints. Anterior knee pain may be present, as well as intermittent swelling. Periods of increased activity closely relate to pain and increased swelling. In more advanced cases, persistent edema/effusion may be accompanied by catching, locking, or giving way. In late-stage disease the sensation of a loose body is sometimes described.[14]

Exam of the knee begins with a systematic approach, as discussed earlier in this chapter, to identify concurrent pathology. Wilson described an external rotation mechanism of the tibia during the gait cycle signifying compensation for impingement of the tibial eminence on an OCD lesion of the medial femoral condyle.[29] Wilson's test involves reproduction of pain on exam with internal rotation of the tibia during extension of the knee from 90 to 30 degrees. Once pain is elicited, external rotation usually alleviates the pain. This test has a poor predictive valve but may be helpful in following the disease for resolution.

DIAGNOSTIC TESTING

Plain radiographs are the primary tools in initial diagnosis of an OCD lesion. Standard anterior/posterior, lateral, axial, notch, and weight-bearing views should be obtained. Occasionally OCD lesions can be missed on standard anterior/posterior views in full extension because of its location—flexion views may allow visualization. The classic location for an OCD lesion is the lateral aspect of the medial femoral condyle. Plain radiographs provide insight into lesion size, location, and sclerosis.

MRI has also been shown to aid in the workup by attempting to characterize stability. Typically, lesions are identified as fluid behind the cartilage, as shown on T2-weighted images. This is indicative of a partial or total breech of the cartilage. Criteria for fragment instability include (1) an area of increased homogenous signal 5 mm or greater in diameter beneath the lesion, (2) a focal defect 5 mm or greater in the articular surface, and (3) a high-signal line traversing the subchondral plate into the lesion. The criterion standard for diagnosing stability is direct visualization—as with arthroscopy.

Classification

The classification system described by Cahill and Berg[30] is the one most commonly used. In this system, anteroposterior and lateral radiographic views are divided into multiple regions. Anteroposterior zones are signified by numerical values ranging from 1 to 5 (1 medial to 5 lateral). The lateral radiograph is divided by lettered zones A through C (Blumensaat's line anteriorly and the posterior cortical line posteriorly).

TREATMENT

Nonoperative

- The goal of treatment is to promote healing of the lesion and prevent further displacement or propagation.
- Stable lesions on radiographs and MRI can usually be treated nonsurgically with activity modification and restricted weight bearing for a 3-month period with re-evaluation following that course.
- Nonsteroidal anti-inflammatory drugs (NSAIDs) can be used.
- ROM exercises can be performed to maintain flexibility.
- In some cases in which a patient cannot be compliant with non–weight bearing, a brace or cast can be used.

Operative

- Transchondral drilling
- Chondrocyte transplantation
- Osteochondral grafts[14]

Prognosis/Return to Play

- The approach to return to play of an athlete with an OCD lesion sometimes can be a difficult task. Oftentimes it is unclear as to the healing stage of the lesion.
- Conservative management entails observation with no weight bearing for 3 months, and depending on symptoms and radiographs, return to sport-specific activities can usually commence shortly thereafter.
- Return to play after surgical treatment is dependent on the type of procedure preformed. Return after microfracture, periosteal grafting, and osteochondral autogenous transfer typically begins at 3 to 6 months postoperatively.
- Some advocate repeat MRI to evaluate the amount of incorporation for osteochondral transfers.
- Recommendations for return to play following osteochondral allografts and autologous chondrocyte implantation approach 6 months and 14 to 16 months, respectively.[28]

Complications/Indications for Referral

Osteochondral lesions that are unstable or become unstable need prompt referral to an orthopedist for consideration of surgical management. Stable lesions that do not respond to conservative management can also be referred, or if other injuries are suspected to contribute to the clinical picture.

APPROACH TO THE ATHLETE WITH A TIBIAL PLATEAU FRACTURE

Tibial plateau fractures are injuries associated with a high-energy mechanism. The majority of tibial plateau fractures are secondary to high-speed motor vehicle accidents and falls from heights. They are typically axial compressive injuries with either a valgus (more common) or a varus moment. When a single plateau is involved, it is usually the lateral plateau. Although it is uncommon for these injuries to occur in the athlete, it is essential to diagnose and treat them appropriately, as a delay in diagnosis can lead to a devastating long-term outcome.

Tibial plateau injuries are associated with a variety of ligamentous injuries, which include (1) collateral ligament injuries (7% to 43%), (2) ACL tear (23%), and (3) meniscal injuries (50%). These injuries may be difficult to diagnose acutely secondary to the pain and swelling associated with plateau fractures. In the case of a bicondylar tibial plateau fracture, frank knee dislocation must also be suspected and evaluated.[31]

HISTORY AND PHYSICAL EXAMINATION

The typical patient with a tibial plateau fracture complains of moderate to severe pain in the knee. The knee is often visually swollen, with the most severe injuries at risk for compartment syndrome secondary to the swelling. Pain out of proportion to injury and pain with passive flexion or extension of the ankle and toes are the most sensitive history and physical exam findings indicative of compartment syndrome. This, if present, is a surgical emergency. Most patients will be unable to weight bear secondary to pain and/or instability.

A complete physical exam of the knee is warranted as outlined earlier in this chapter. A comprehensive ligamentous examination may be exceedingly difficult with a very painful and swollen knee and may be misleading if gross displacement of a tibial plateau fracture is present. A careful neurovascular exam should also be preformed. The peroneal nerve is in proximity to the lateral tibial plateau and thus can be injured acutely.

DIAGNOSTIC TESTING

Plain radiographs are the initial diagnostic test that will aid in the diagnosis of a tibial plateau fracture. Anteroposterior, lateral, and oblique views should be obtained in the acute setting. Injuries can include stress, nondisplaced, displaced, and impacted fractures. For the highly displaced fracture, a traction view may be helpful to delineate fracture pattern. Classification of these injuries is based on plain radiographs and has been described by Schatzker.

CT has highly increased the diagnostic accuracy in the evaluation of tibial plateau fractures and is useful in preoperative planning. CT with sagittal and coronal reconstructions should be obtained in the majority of these injuries.

TREATMENT

Nonoperative

- Completely nondisplaced or very minimally displaced fractures can usually be managed successfully without surgery.
- These patients are placed in either a knee immobilizer or a hinged knee brace and made non–weight bearing for a period of 8 to 12 weeks.
- During this time, fracture displacement is an indication for operative management.
- Early knee ROM to prevent stiffness is essential and encouraged as soon as acute swelling subsides.

Operative

- High-energy traumatic tibial plateau fractures are serious injuries and will require surgical management.
- Varus or valgus instability greater than 10 degrees in full extension is usually an indication for operative treatment.[32]
- A displaced or unstable fracture is usually best treated acutely with external fixation to stabilize the fracture and allow for an adequate soft-tissue envelope for delayed open reduction and internal fixation.
- The main goals of surgical treatment are reconstruction of the articular surface and re-establishment of tibial alignment.[32,33]

Prognosis/Return To Play

- The athlete with a tibial plateau stress fracture has a relatively good prognosis.
- The guideline for return to activity is reliant on the healing of the fracture. This can be accessed by plain films, CT scan, or MRI—MRI being the most sensitive in assessing occult fractures.
- Once healing has occurred, weight bearing can be advanced, and a slow return to sport-specific activities is begun with the emphasis that bony architecture is weakened secondary to disuse.
- Weight bearing is usually advanced to as tolerated at the 6- to 8-week point. If there is no pain associated with normal gait, the slow progression into sport is initiated. Please refer to Appendix C, "Interval Running Program," for details on a graduated return to running program.
- Those athletes with more severe bony injuries that warrant surgery should expect to be away from sport for at least 6 months to a year.

Complications/Indications for Referral

In general, any patient with an acute tibial plateau fracture should be referred to an orthopedic surgeon. Beware of any knee injury that incurs large amounts of swelling or deformity, as this may be a sign of a displaced tibial plateau fracture or dislocation. These injuries can be surgical emergencies if compartment syndrome ensues or a dislocation is found. The amount of long-term bony, chondral, and soft-tissue damage of a dislocation or gross deformity is directly related to the time from initial injury to the time of reduction or stabilization.

KEY POINTS
• Knee injuries are common in the athlete, can lead to major disability, and can decrease the athlete's ability to return to prior level of play
• Medial collateral ligament (MCL) injuries, in general, can be treated nonoperatively with great success
• Most athletes who engage in pivoting sports and want to return to such activities will benefit from surgical reconstruction of anterior cruciate ligament tears
• The majority of posterior cruciate ligament injuries can be treated conservatively
• OCD lesions are difficult to diagnose and treat, but there are well-defined surgical indications
• Tibial plateau fractures, when associated with a high-energy mechanism of injury, should be evaluated and treated by an orthopedic specialist for consideration of operative management

REFERENCES

1. Grood ES, Noyes FR, Butler DL, et al. Ligamentous and capsular restraints preventing straight medial and lateral laxity in intact human cadaver knees. *J Bone Joint Surg Am*. 1981;63:1257–1269.
2. Indelicato PA. Non-operative treatment of complete tears of the medial collateral ligament of the knee. *J Bone Joint Surg Am*. 1983;65:323–329.
3. Anderson AF, Dome DC, Gautam S, et al. Correlation of anthropometric measurements, strength, anterior cruciate ligament size, and intercondylar notch characteristics to sex differences in anterior cruciate ligament tear rates. *Am J Sports Med*. 2001;29:58–66.
4. Shelbourne KD, Davis TJ, Patel DV. The natural history of acute, isolated, nonoperatively treated posterior cruciate ligament injuries: a prospective study. *Am J Sports Med*. 1999;27:276–283.
5. Houghston JC, Andrews JR, Cross MJ, et al. Classification of knee ligament instabilities: part II. The lateral compartment. *J Bone Joint Surg Am*. 1976;58:173–179.
6. Chen FS, Rokito AS, Pitman MI. Acute and chronic posterolateral rotatory instability of the knee. *J Am Acad Orthop Surg*. 2000;8:97–110.
7. Hede A, Jensen DB, Blyme P, et al. Epidemiology of meniscal lesions in the knee: 1,215 open operations in Copenhagen 1982-84. *Acta Orthop Scand*. 1990;61:435–437.
8. Nielson AB, Yde J. Epidemiology of acute knee injuries: a prospective hospital investigation. *J Trauma*. 1991;31:1644–1648.
9. Greis PE, Bardana DD, Holmstrom MC, et al. Meniscal injury: I. Basic science and evaluation. *J Am Acad Orthop Surg*. 2002;10:168–176.

10. Duncan JB, Hunter R, Purnell M, et al. Meniscal injuries associated with acute anterior cruciate ligament tears in alpine skiers. *Am J Sports Med.* 1995;23:170–172.

11. Linden B. The incidence of osteochondritis dissecans in the condyles of the femur. *Acta Orthop Scand.* 1976;47:664–667.

12. Bradley J, Dandy DJ. Osteochondritis dissecans and other lesions of the femoral condyles. *J Bone Joint Surg Br.* 1989;71:518–522.

13. Hefti F, Beguiristain J, Krauspe R, et al. Osteochondritis dissecans: a multicenter study of the European Pediatric Orthopedic Society. *J Pediatr Orthop B.* 1999;8:231–245.

14. Crawford DC, Safran MR. Osteochondritis dissecans of the knee. *J Am Acad Orthop Surg.* 2006;14:90–100.

15. Derschied GL, Garrick JG. Medial collateral ligament injuries in football: nonoperative management of grade I and grade II sprains. *Am J Sports Med.* 1981;9:365–368.

16. Indelicato PA. Isolated medial collateral ligament injuries in the knee. *J Am Acad Orthop Surg.* 1995;3:9–14.

17. Larson RL, Taillon M. Anterior cruciate ligament insufficiency: principles of treatment. *J Am Acad Orthop Surg.* 1994;2:26–35.

18. Scholten RJPM, Opstelten W, van der Plas CG, et al. Accuracy of physical diagnostic tests for assessing ruptures of the anterior cruciate ligament: a meta-analysis. *J Fam Pract.* 2003;52:689–694.

19. Harner CD, Hoher J. Evaluation and treatment of posterior cruciate ligament injuries. *Am J Sports Med.* 1998;26:471–482.

20. Cosgarea AJ, Jay PR. Posterior cruciate ligament injuries: evaluation and management. *J Am Acad Orthop Surg.* 2001;9:297–307.

21. Parolie JM, Bergfeld JA. Long-term results of nonoperative treatment of isolated posterior cruciate ligament injuries in the athlete. *Am J Sports Med.* 1986;14:35–38.

22. Jakob RP, Warner JP. Lateral and posterolateral rotatory instability of the knee. In: DeLee JC, Drez D Jr, eds. *Orthopaedic Sports Medicine: Principles and Practice.* Vol 2. Philadelphia: WB Saunders; 1974: 1275–1312.

23. Baker CL Jr, Norwood LA, Hughston JC. Acute posterolateral rotatory instability of the knee. *J Bone Joint Surg Am.* 1983;65:614–618.

24. Weinstabl R, Muellner T, Vecsei V, et al.. Economic considerations for the diagnosis and therapy of meniscal lesions: can magnetic resonance imaging help reduce the expense? *World J Surg.* 1997;21:363–368.

25. Shelbourne KD, Martini DJ, McCarroll JR, et al. Correlation of joint line tenderness and meniscal lesions in patients with acute anterior cruciate ligament tears. *Am J Sports Med.* 1995;23:166–169.

26. Hoppenfeld S. *Physical Exam of the Spine & Extremities.* New Jersey: Prentice Hall; 1976:171–196.

27. Muellner T, Weinstabl R, Schabus R, et al. The diagnosis of meniscal tears in athletes: a comparison of clinical and magnetic resonance imaging investigations. *Am J Sports Med.* 1997;25:7–12.

28. Bowen TR, Feldmann DD, Miller MD. Return to play following surgical treatment of meniscal and chondral injuries to the knee. *Clin Sports Med.* 2004;23:381–393.

29. Wilson JN. A diagnostic sign in osteochondritis dissecans of the knee. *J Bone Joint Surg Am.* 1967;49:477–480.

30. Cahill BR, Berg BC. 99m-Technetium phosphate compound scintigraphy in the management of juvenile osteochondritis dissecans of the femoral condyles. *Am J Sports Med.* 1983;11:329–335.

31. Egol KA, Koval KJ. Fractures of the proximal tibia. In: Bucholz RW, Heckman JD, Court-Brown C, eds. *Rockwood and Green's Fractures in Adults.* Vol 2. 6th ed. New York: Lippincott Williams & Wilkins; 2006: 1999–2029.

32. Koval KJ, Helfet MD. Tibial plateau fractures: evaluation and treatment. *J Am Acad Orthop Surg.* 1995;3:86–94.

33. Berkson EM, Virkus WW. High energy tibial plateau fractures. *J Am Acad Orthop Surg.* 2006;14:20–31.

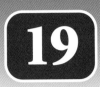

CHAPTER 19

Athlete with Knee Pain

Carolyn Saluti

INTRODUCTION

Running is an excellent activity to keep a person healthy. Many people choose to run because of its convenience and affordability. It has many health benefits, but along with the benefits, there are also injuries. Knee pain is a common symptom seen in runners with up to 50% of running injuries occurring at the knee.[1] There are many etiologies of knee pain, but a good history and physical exam can differentiate between the causes.

FUNCTIONAL ANATOMY

The tibiofemoral joint is the largest joint in the body (see Figs. 18.1 and 18.2). The femur sits on the articular surface of the tibia with the meniscus acting as a cushion between the two bones. The menisci are essential parts of the knee joint for weight bearing, stabilization, energy absorption, and joint lubrication. The capsule of the tibiofemoral joint is continuous with the capsule of the patellofemoral joint. The patellofemoral joint is comprised of the femoral trochlea in which the patella glides. The patella lies within the quadriceps tendon. The quadriceps tendon becomes the patellar tendon distal to the patella, which inserts onto the tibial tuberosity. Smooth hyaline cartilage covers the undersurface of the patella, which protects the patella during weight bearing. This is actually the thickest articular cartilage in the body. The iliotibial band (ITB) originates in the lateral hip region, crosses the knee joint, and attaches on the lateral tibia at Gerdy's tubercle. The pes anserinus lies just medial to the tibial tuberosity and is the insertion site of the semitendinosus, sartorius, and gracilis tendons. There is a bursa located at this area known as the pes anserine bursa.

EPIDEMIOLOGY

The knee is the most common site for injury in a runner. Studies have shown that the predominant site of lower extremity injury in runners is the knee, with the incidence ranging from 7.2% to 50%.[1] Females have a greater incidence of lower extremity injuries compared to males.[1]

Greater training distance per week (more than 64 km/wk) is a risk factor for lower extremity injury in men, while an increase in training distance per week is a protective factor against knee injuries in both men and women.[1] History of previous injuries is a risk factor for future injuries while running. High endurance strength in adolescence is a predictor of knee injury in men.[2]

NARROWING THE DIFFERENTIAL DIAGNOSIS

History

A thorough history may give enough information for the diagnosis. Important questions to ask are if the athlete has had any changes in training surface, intensity of exercise, mileage, or footwear. Inquire if the athlete has had an injury in the knee before, how long they have had pain, what the pain inhibits them from doing, and if they have done any rehabilitation. Find out if they have any joint swelling, locking or giving out of the knee, any night pain, systemic symptoms, or pain in joints other than their knee.

The location of the pain can help focus the differential to particular conditions (see Fig. 18.9).

Anterior knee pain may be caused by patellofemoral pain syndrome (PFPS), patella subluxation, chondromalacia patellae, osteochondral defect, patellar tendinopathy, Osgood–Schlatter disease (OSD), Sinding-Larsen–Johansson syndrome, prepatellar bursitis, quadriceps tendinopathy, fat pad syndrome, or degenerative joint disease (DJD). Lateral knee pain may be due to ITB friction syndrome, lateral meniscus tear, or lateral collateral ligament sprain. Medial knee pain may be secondary to plica, medial collateral ligament (MCL) sprain, medial mensical injury, or pes anserine bursitis. Posterior knee pain can be from popliteal cyst, hamstring strain, or posterior horn meniscal cyst.

Evidence-based Physical Exam

It is important to examine the asymptomatic knee so that a comparison can be made between the two. While examining the knee, keep in mind that knee pain can be referred from other areas, such as the hip, particularly with young children. Description of specific knee exam maneuvers as related to overuse knee injuries is listed later in the chapter. Examination of acute injuries is reviewed in Chapter 18, *Athlete with Acute Knee Injuries*. Key point to remember is that the presence of an effusion in overuse knee pain strongly suggests intra-articular pathology including a degenerative meniscal tear, osteoarthritis (OA), osteochondritis dissecans (OCD), articular cartilage injury, or occult intra-articular fracture. Majority of overuse knee injuries, however, do not result in knee effusion as the structures are extra-articular (patella tendon, ITB) or are functional in nature (patellofemoral syndrome). Pain that radiates down the leg, dysthesias, or paresthesias is typically secondary to lumbar spine etiology. The following is a systematic approach to the knee exam with focus on overuse etiologies.

Inspection

The exam can begin with observation of the patient standing. Focus should be on any evidence of genu valgum or varum (Fig. 19.1). Genu valgum can be associated with patellofemoral syndrome, while genu varum is most often associated with medial compartment knee OA. While standing, observe for any quadriceps atrophy by having the patient contract their quadriceps. Note the position of the patellae, whether they face in or out. Patellae that face in are a sign of femoral anteversion or increased medial femoral torsion and can be seen in patients with PFPS. The examiner should also observe the patient's gait for signs of a painful or antalgic gait. Once supine, observe the knee for any swelling, erythema, or ecchymosis of the knee.

Palpation

After observing the knee, the examiner should palpate it for signs of an effusion, warmth, or tenderness. An effusion tends to signify an intra-articular injury such as anterior cruciate ligament, posterior cruciate ligament, or mensical injury, none of which are common in straightforward activities such as running.

Tenderness at the distal pole of the patella is found in patellar tendinopathy and also in Sinding-Larsen–Johansson syndrome. Tenderness in the patellar tendon itself can also be found in patellar tendinopathy. OSD will exhibit tenderness and prominence at the tibial tuberosity. Palpate the medial and lateral patella facets by displacing the patella medially and laterally to feel the undersurface of the patella. Tenderness is seen in PFPS, chondromalacia, plica syndrome, and patella joint OA. Palpate for the pes anserinus, which is located medial and slightly distal to the tibial tubercle. Tenderness is seen in pes anserine tendonitis and bursitis. Moving lateral from the tibial tubercle, the insertion of the ITB can be felt at Gerdy's tubercle. Palpate along the entire ITB. Tenderness may indicate ITB friction syndrome.

Palpate the medial and lateral joint lines with the knee flexed to 90 degrees. Athletes with mensical injuries will have tenderness along the joint line. Tenderness at the medial or lateral tibial plateau or along the distal femur could indicate a stress fracture.

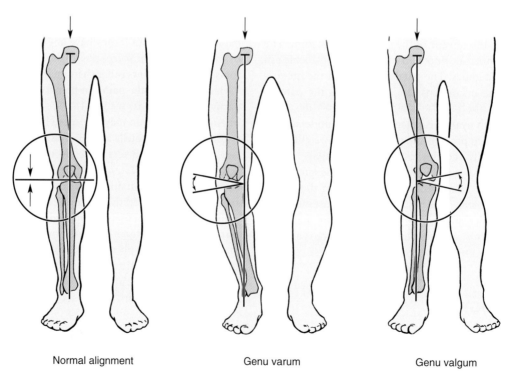

Normal alignment   Genu varum   Genu valgum

FIG. 19.1. Knee alignment: normal, genu varum, genu valgus. From Moore KL, Dalley AF II. *Clinical Oriented Anatomy*. 4th ed. Baltimore: Lippincott Williams & Wilkins; 1999.

Range of Motion

Normal range of motion is 0 to 140 degrees. It is common to be able to extend into 3 to 5 degrees of hyperextension. Loss of passive range of motion may be due to effusion, loose body, or mensical injury.

Strength

Having the patient perform a single leg squat is another method to look for quadriceps atrophy and weakness. Patients with PFPS tend to have quadriceps atrophy and weakness especially of the vastus medialis oblique.[3]

Special Tests

Examine the mobility of the patella. It should move about half of its width medially and laterally with the knee in extension. A tight ITB may cause the patella to track laterally. Assessment of the ligaments and menisci can be done via joint line palpation and McMurray's test. Meniscal tears and their exam are fully reviewed in Chapter 18, *Athlete with Acute Knee Injuries.*

Special tests found to be helpful in the assessment of knee pain in the runner include the patella grind test, the patella apprehension test, Ober's test, and Noble's test. The sensitivity and specificity of these tests have not been documented in the literature.

The patellar grind test assesses for patellofemoral dysfunction. It is performed by pressing on the area just proximal to the upper pole of the patella and having the patient contract their quadriceps. If they have pain with this maneuver, it is a positive patella grind test.

The Ober's test examines the flexibility of the ITB. The patient should lie on their side with the affected leg facing up. The lower hip and knee should be straight. Standing behind the patient, place one hand on the hip to stabilize it and the other hand on the patient's knee of the upper leg. The hip of the upper leg is then passively abducted and extended to about 40 degrees while the knee is in a flexed position. Finally, lower the leg into adduction as far as gravity will allow. If the ITB is tight, the leg will remain abducted, or not fall below horizontal, which results in a positive Ober's test.

The Noble's test assesses for ITB friction syndrome. While the patient is in the supine position, flex the knee to 90 degrees. The examiner should place their thumb on the lateral femoral epicondyle and move the leg into extension. Pain with this maneuver (a positive Noble's test) is caused by the ITB rolling over the lateral femoral epicondyle.

Diagnostic Testing

Laboratory

Laboratory work is usually not required when diagnosing the etiology of knee pain. If the patient has systemic or infectious symptoms, then there may be a need for appropriate serology or cultures. A knee effusion without history of trauma should raise suspicion for possible autoimmune or infectious etiology and prompt serologic evaluation including lyme titers in endemic regions.

Imaging

X-rays should be the initial study when attempting to diagnose knee pain. Anteroposterior (AP) and lateral views should be obtained. AP weight bearing of the knees in 30 degrees of flexion (tunnel view) should be assessed for joint space narrowing if concerned about OA; this will also show evidence of an osteochondral defect if one is present. The lateral view should be obtained to evaluate for OSD. An axial view (also known as sunrise, skyline, or merchant view) will show the position of the patella in relation to the femur. It is common to see laterally displaced patellae in patients with patellofemoral syndrome.

Magnetic resonance imaging (MRI), computed tomography (CT), and bone scintigraphy may be needed if patient requires further evaluation. MRI is the preferred study for soft-tissue structures, while a CT can delineate bony structures including cortical defects not appreciated on plain radiographs. Due to the relatively high radiation exposure with CT, its use should be limited to cases where imaging results would significantly alter management. Bone scintigraphy (bone scans) may be utilized to rule out metabolically active bone lesions or bone stress injuries.

Other Testing

Other diagnostic testing is generally not required in the routine evaluation of overuse knee injuries.

APPROACH TO THE ATHLETE WITH PATELLOFEMORAL PAIN SYNDROME (RUNNER'S KNEE)

PFPS, also called "runner's knee," is the most common cause of overuse anterior knee pain in athletes, and studies have shown it to be the most common cause of knee pain in runners.[4,5] PFPS is pain localized to the patellofemoral joint with unaffected articular cartilage. Among adolescents and young adults, patella disorders are the most common knee problems seen.[6] Incidence has been reported to be as high as one in four in athletes. PFPS is typically an overuse injury, but can be a traumatic injury as well. PFPS affects 15% to 33% of adults and 21% to 45% of adolescents, being more common in female adolescents. The exact etiology of pain is unknown, but the syndrome is felt to be secondary to abnormal tracking of the patella in the femoral groove. Contact stresses on the patellofemoral joint are higher than any other weight-bearing joint. Predisposing factors have been suggested to be a lateral tracking patella,[7] tight lateral retinaculum, tight

ITB, hip musculature weakness, abnormal vastus medialis oblique/vastus lateralis reflex timing, or an excessive Q angle (>20 degrees).[8] PFPS should be differentiated from other causes of anterior knee pain including chondromalacia, patellar tendinopathy, and patellofemoral joint OA.

HISTORY AND PHYSICAL EXAM

Patients will complain of anterior knee pain, or pain behind the patella. They may isolate the pain to the medial or lateral aspect of the patella. When asked where the pain is, patients often draw a circle around the patella with their finger. Running, jumping, and walking up- and downstairs tend to exacerbate PFPS. They may also have pain after prolonged periods of sitting (theater sign), getting up from a chair, and squatting. The onset of pain is insidious and will often stop the athlete from participating in activity when severe.

On physical exam, conditions such as femoral anteversion and external tibial torsion should be noted as they may lead to patellofemoral joint pain. Increased patella mobility may play a role in PFPS.[6] A tight ITB or lateral retinaculum may cause a lateral tracking patella and create pain. Palpate the medial and lateral patella facets for tenderness by medially and laterally deviating the patella and palpating its undersurface. Patella grind test will generally recreate patients' pain with PFPS. Check the flexibility of the quadriceps and gastrocnemius muscles because decreased flexibility has been shown to be a risk factor for PFPS.[6] A single leg squat performed by the patient enables the examiner to evaluate the quadriceps strength, in particular the vastus medialis oblique. Also, patients with PFPS tend to have pain with squats. Studies have shown that runners with higher knee abduction impulses are at increased risk for PFPS.[9]

DIAGNOSTIC TESTING

For athletes with chronic knee pain or history of trauma, imaging helps to rule out more serious conditions. Radiographs, especially the sunrise or merchant view, of the knees may show lateral tracking of the patella. The presence of patella spurring indicates patellofemoral OA rather than PFPS. If symptoms persist, consider an MRI to look for osteochondral defects, chondromalacia, or occult intra-articular pathology.

TREATMENT

Nonoperative

- Nonoperative treatment is the mainstay of therapy.
- Activity modification involves limiting bending, kneeling, squatting, or excessive stairs.

- Physical therapy (PT) to increase strength of quadriceps, especially the vastus medialis oblique, and the gluteus muscles.
- One study showed that by strengthening hip flexors, stretching the ITB, and improving iliopsoas flexibility, patients were able to decrease their knee pain.[10]
- A randomized placebo-controlled study found a 6-week, once weekly program significantly reduced PFPS symptoms compared with a sham PT program.[11] The program consisted of quadriceps muscle retraining, patellofemoral joint mobilization, patellar taping, and daily home exercises.
- Nonsteroidal anti-inflammatory drugs (NSAIDs) help alleviate the pain of PFPS on a short-term basis, but have not been proven to help in the long term.[12]

Operative

- Surgery is rarely required and reserved for recalcitrant cases that have not responded to a prolonged course of conservative treatment.
- The type of surgical procedure depends on the characteristics of patellar maltracking.
- Patients with a tight lateral retinaculum associated with a rotational tilt of the patella may benefit from a lateral release surgery, usually done by arthroscopy. Side effect of the surgery is medial patellar subluxation.
- Arthroscopic patellar debridement alone may be enough for some patients to decrease their pain.
- Other surgeries are proximal realignment or distal realignment: both procedures are often done with anteromedialization of the tibial tubercle.[13]
- One study of patients with chronic PFPS concluded that when arthroscopy was used in addition to a home exercise program, there was no better outcome compared to when a home exercise program was used alone.[14]

Prognosis/Return to Play

- Patients generally have a good prognosis and respond well to conservative treatment.
- Athletes may return to play on an as-tolerated basis as pain improves.

Complications/Indications for Referral

Prolonged symptoms, progressively worsening symptoms, or failure of conservative measures are indications for referral to a sports medicine physician. Consider surgery when the athlete has completed a thorough rehabilitation program for 6 to 12 months, yet pain persists. Indications for surgery include inability to perform activities of daily living. Complications are rare, but include patella dislocation if PFPS is associated with patella instability. A large knee effusion or signs of infection are red flags warranting immediate attention.

APPROACH TO THE ATHLETE WITH ILIOTIBIAL BAND FRICTION SYNDROME

ITB friction syndrome is an overuse injury and is the second most common overuse injury in runners.[5,9] It is the most common running injury of the lateral knee and has an incidence of 1.6% to 12%.[15] The ITB originates in the lateral hip region, crosses the knee joint, and attaches on the lateral tibia at Gerdy's tubercle (Fig. 19.2).

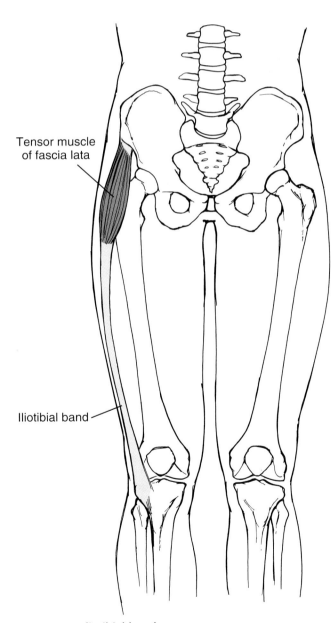

Tensor muscle of fascia lata

Iliotibial band

FIG. 19.2. Iliotibial band.

Pain is caused by friction between the ITB and the lateral femoral epicondyle; friction is maximized when the knee is flexed to 30 degrees. Contact with the epicondyle occurs near foot strike, and in runners, the repetitive contact may cause inflammation of the ITB, which then leads to degenerative changes or bursitis.

HISTORY AND PHYSICAL EXAM

ITB friction syndrome causes pain in the lateral aspect of the knee. Pain is often worse with running downhill. The pain will tend to resolve once the athlete stops running; however, chronic ITB friction syndrome may cause pain with activities of daily living. The pain may stop them from running when severe. A history of an increase in running distance or weakly mileage is a risk factor but should also raise concern for potential stress fracture.

On physical exam, patients will exhibit tenderness over the lateral femoral epicondyle, 3 cm proximal from the lateral joint line. The runner will often have a positive Ober's test indicating a tight ITB. Noble's test is considered diagnostic of the condition, but may be absent in milder cases.

DIAGNOSTIC TESTING

Imaging is not necessary for diagnosis but may rule out coexisting pathology. Plain radiographs will be normal. An MRI will show thickening of the ITB over the lateral femoral epicondyle and occasionally a small bursa inferior to the ITB in chronic conditions; however, MRI is generally not needed for diagnosis.

TREATMENT

Nonoperative

- The athlete needs to rest from running.
- Cross-training by swimming using arms only is a good way to remain active.
- PT should be initiated with emphasis placed on stretching the ITB, in particular with a foam roller. Additional focus is on core, hip, and knee strengthening.
- PT helps reduce daily pain and treadmill running pain.[15]
- Deep transverse friction massage (DTFM) is a technique used to break up myofascial tissue restrictions in ITB friction syndrome. DTFM combined with other physiotherapy modalities has not shown consistent benefit over PT alone.[15,16]
- Running modification should also be a part of the treatment:
  - Decrease mileage
  - Refrain from hills
  - Alternate which side of the street they run on to avoid a sloped surface

- The athlete may return to running when they can perform strengthening and stretching exercises without pain; up to 6 weeks is common.
- The athlete should start with running every other day and then slowly increasing their distance (about 10% per week) until they are able to run their previous routine without pain.
- Corticosteroid injection just under the ITB at the lateral femoral epicondyle can be very effective, especially in the acute phase of ITB friction syndrome.[15] Patients occasionally need more than one injection. Allow 4 to 6 weeks to see improvement prior to reinjecting.
- NSAIDs can help alleviate the pain and reduce inflammation, especially if used while participating in PT.

Operative

- Surgery may be an option if the patient is having pain after 6 months of conservative treatment.
- The surgery entails resecting a triangular piece of the posterior half of the ITB at the lateral femoral epicondyle.

Prognosis/Return to Play

- Overall prognosis is excellent with conservative treatment.
- Graduated return to running as symptoms resolve will reduce risk of reinjury.

Complications/Indications for Referral

Prolonged symptoms, progressive worsening of symptoms, and failure of conservative measures are indications for referral to sports medicine physician. Complications are rare but may include occult stress fracture. Large knee effusion, locking, or signs of infection are red flags warranting attention.

APPROACH TO THE ATHLETE WITH PATELLAR TENDINOPATHY (JUMPER'S KNEE)

Patella tendinopathy is an overuse tendon injury caused by repetitive overloading of the extensor mechanism. Previously, it was believed to be an inflammatory process and called tendinitis; however, it is now believed to be mostly a degenerative condition (tendinosis). The term tendinopathy encompasses both tendinosis and tendinitis and better describes the underlying pathology.[17] The tendon changes are most commonly at the proximal insertion of the patellar tendon; however, they can also occur at the distal portion or within the tendon itself (Fig. 19.3).

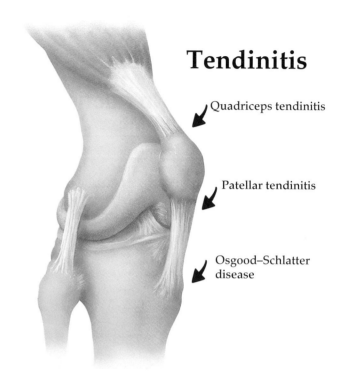

FIG. 19.3. Patellar tendinopathy.

Patella tendinopathy is also known as "jumper's knee" because it occurs more commonly in athletes who participate in sports that involve explosive jumping, such as basketball and volleyball. Estimated incidence is between 13% and 20% in athletes.[18] As many as 40% to 50% of athletes who participate in volleyball, basketball, and soccer have patellar tendinopathy.[19] Predisposing factors are felt to include OSD, patella alta, chondromalacia, leg length discrepancy, or abnormal tracking of the patella. Sinding-Larsen–Johansson syndrome is a traction apophysitis at the distal pole of the patella that may present similarly and is found in the skeletally immature runner (see Chapter 24, *Pediatric Athlete*).

HISTORY AND PHYSICAL EXAM

The patient will complain of pain in the anterior knee, specifically at the proximal end of the patellar tendon. The pain is described as a dull ache during or after activity. The pain may exist with walking up- and downstairs or after sitting for long periods of time (theater sign). If they have had pain for some time, it may start to interfere with their running. It is often an insidious onset and can occur after an increase in activity.

On palpation, they will be tender at the inferior pole of the patella and may exhibit swelling in that same area. There may be bogginess in the tendon. The runner may have pain in the main body of the tendon with the knee in extension. Resisted knee extension and squatting tend to cause pain in the patient.

DIAGNOSTIC TESTING

A diagnosis of patella tendinopathy can be made clinically. Occasionally, plain radiographs display osteopenia at the distal pole of the patella, calcification of the tendon, or a traction osteophyte. MRI and ultrasound, although not needed for diagnosis, will show thickening of the tendon. Structural tendon changes seen on ultrasound and revascularization seen on power Doppler are associated with a clinical diagnosis of patellar tendinopathy and may also indicate a risk for developing tendinopathy when seen in asymptomatic athletes.[20]

TREATMENT

Nonoperative

- Resting or minimizing running/jumping should be the initial treatment.
- Apply ice after exercise.
- PT should focus on strengthening and stretching of quadriceps, hamstrings, and calf muscles.
- Eccentric strengthening has been shown to be 50% to 70% successful in improving knee function and pain.[20] A decline board should be involved in the eccentric training program, and the program should be performed with some level of discomfort.[19]
- An eccentric drop squat program and a concentric leg extension/curl program have been shown to be effective strengthening techniques.[21]
- Other modalities that may help are taping, massage, electrotherapy, and ultrasound, though outcome studies are lacking.
- Some athletes' pain is alleviated with an infrapatellar strap or band.
- NSAIDs help to reduce the pain, but have not been shown to enhance healing.
- Other new techniques such as prolotherapy, autologous blood, and platelet-rich plasma injections are currently being studied for efficacy.
- Corticosteroid injections are contraindicated due to high risk of tendon rupture associated with injection of a weight-bearing tendon.

Operative

- Patients with chronic tendinopathy who have not responded to conservative methods after 3 to 6 months may benefit from surgery.
- The objective of surgery is to excise the degenerative area and then promote tendon restoration. Different techniques to promote tendon repair include:
  - Drilling of the inferior pole of the patella
  - Removing the inferior pole of the patella and suturing of the paratenon.

- Success rate of surgery has been found to be 70.9% to 91.5% depending on the surgical method used; however, there is not enough evidence in the literature to assure a full return to activity after surgery[22] (level of evidence (LOE) = 4).

Prognosis/Return to Play

- Overall prognosis is good; however, some athletes may have prolonged mild symptoms. In one study, patients had mild pain 15 years after the initiation of the study.[23]
- Return to running should be done in a graduated and progressive manner as pain improves.
- Recovery is slower if patients run while performing rehabilitation.

Complications/Indications for Referral

Prolonged symptoms, progressive worsening of symptoms, and failure of conservative measures are indications for referral to sports medicine physician. Complications are rare but may include potential tendon rupture in chronic severe cases. Knee swelling, effusion, or signs of infection are red flags warranting immediate attention.

APPROACH TO THE ATHLETE WITH CHONDROMALACIA PATELLAE

Chondromalacia is an overuse condition causing anterior knee pain secondary to softening and fissuring of the patella femoral joint articular cartilage. Chondromalacia has been used in the past to describe all causes of anterior knee pain, but its current usage should be applied only to softening and fissuring of the articular cartilage noted either on MRI or on arthroscopy. It is not known whether chondromalacia is progressive or a predisposing risk factor for OA. Etiologies include trauma, malalignment, biomechanical, or metabolic. It is seen in young adults and more commonly in females.

HISTORY AND PHYSICAL EXAM

On history, the runner may state that they have pain with walking up- and downstairs, squatting, sitting for prolonged periods of time (theater sign), or rising from a chair. It is usually an insidious onset and presents as a dull ache in the anterior knee.

On exam, observe for femoral anteversion, external tibial torsion, foot pronation, and genu varum or valgum, as these conditions may predispose patients to chondromalacia patella. Palpate the medial and lateral patella facets for tenderness. The athlete may also have a positive patellar grind test (pain with contraction of the quadriceps as pressure is held on the patella).

DIAGNOSTIC TESTING

MRI will show the articular cartilage thinning and fissuring.

TREATMENT

Nonoperative

- Initial treatment is activity modification.
- Rehabilitation includes stretching of the hamstrings and strengthening of the quadriceps and gluteus muscles along with single-leg proprioception exercises.
- NSAIDs may be used to decrease the pain and inflammation.
- Corticosteroid injection may temporarily decrease pain and inflammation.

Operative

- Occasionally, surgery is needed to correct malalignment in patients that do not respond to conservative treatment.

Prognosis/Return to Play

- Overall prognosis is good with conservative measures.
- Running may need to be modified to limit hills.
- Athletes may run on an as-tolerated basis.

Complications/Indications for Referral

Prolonged symptoms, progressive worsening of symptoms, or failure of conservative measures are indications for referral to a sports medicine physician. Complications are rare but may include loose body formation from articular cartilage degeneration. Knee swelling, effusion, or signs of infection are red flags warranting immediate attention.

APPROACH TO THE ATHLETE WITH OSGOOD–SCHLATTER DISEASE

OSD is a traction apophysitis of the tibial tuberosity caused by repetitive stress. It is a common cause of knee pain secondary to running in females of ages 11 to 13 and males of ages 13 to 15. The full description of the evaluation and treatment of OSD can be found in Chapter 24, *Pediatric Athlete.*

APPROACH TO THE ATHLETE WITH KNEE OSTEOARTHRITIS

Knee OA is a progressive degenerative condition affecting the articular cartilage and meniscus of the knee (Fig. 19.4).

Knee OA may affect the medial or lateral femorotibial compartment and/or the patellofemoral compartment of the knee. It can vary from mild to severe and can be associated with a degenerative mensical tear. Knee OA incidence rates rise over the age of 30 or with a history of trauma. Knee OA is the most common cause of overuse knee pain in the running athlete over the age of 40.

The beneficial or detrimental effects of running on knee OA have been an area of active debate and research. The beneficial effects include an increase in articular cartilage thickness and a decreased risk of obesity.[24,25] Additionally, physical activity has been shown to increase diffusion of nourishing substances from joint fluid through the avascular articular cartilage matrix.[26] One study found running did not accelerate OA in the hands, knees, or lumbar spine over a 5-year period.[27]

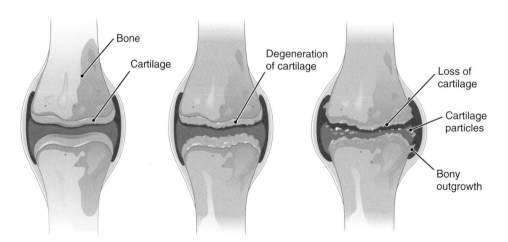

FIG. 19.4. Osteoarthritis: normal joint, early stages of OA, late stages of OA. From Cohen BJ. *Medical Terminology.* 4th ed. Philadelphia: Lippincott Williams & Wilkins; 2003.

The main risk factors for OA are age, family history, developmental conditions that affect joint growth or shape, injuries to the joint, certain occupations, muscle weakness, and obesity.[28] High levels of physical activity may be a risk factor for symptomatic OA among men under age 50, but it has not been shown to be a risk factor for women or men over the age of 50.[26] There may be a correlation with anterior knee pain as an adolescent and patellofemoral arthritis because a significant number of athletes with patellofemoral arthritis have a history of anterior knee pain in their adolescence and early adult years.[29]

HISTORY AND PHYSICAL EXAM

Activity-related knee pain, stiffness, and/or swelling are common complaints in an athlete with knee OA. Walking up- and downstairs will often exacerbate their symptoms, particularly if the patellofemoral joint is involved. Runners may present with pain on the medial, lateral, or anterior aspect of the knee depending on where the degeneration is. Unlike a mensical tear, significant locking should not be present.

Exam may reveal decreased range of motion of the knee, crepitus, or mild joint effusion. Joint line tenderness or patellofemoral joint tenderness is commonly found depending on the compartments affected. The pes anserinus will often be tender to palpation if an associated pes anserine bursitis/tendonitis is present. Moderate or severe knee OA will often exhibit a varus or valgus deformity. Varus deformity is associated with medial compartment OA, while a valgus deformity is associated with lateral compartment OA. Pain with compression of the patella against the femur during quadriceps contraction (patella grind test) may be a sign of patellofemoral compartment OA. If McMurray's test is significantly painful or causes a painful click, consider an associated mensical tear.

DIAGNOSTIC TESTING

Radiographs are the preferred imaging modality as they can play an important role in identifying the location and severity of knee OA. The views should include *weight-bearing* AP and tunnel views along with lateral and merchant views. Weight-bearing views allow an accurate assessment of joint space narrowing (Fig. 19.5). The images will also commonly show subchondral bony sclerosis and hypertrophic osteophyte formation. The merchant and lateral views best assess the patellofemoral joint and will often show decreased joint space and bone spur formation. MRI is rarely required and reserved for atypical symptoms or mechanical symptoms unresponsive to conservative treatments.

Laboratory studies are rarely required unless symptoms of infection or systemic symptoms are present.

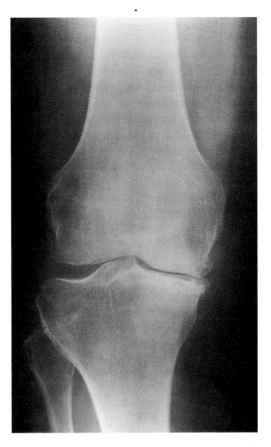

FIG. 19.5. Osteoarthritis: weight-bearing AP x-ray demonstrating decreased joint space. From Koval KJ, Zuckerman JD. *Atlas of Orthopaedic Surgery: A Multimedia Reference.* Philadelphia: Lippincott Williams & Wilkins; 2004.

TREATMENT

Nonoperative

- Relative rest and activity modification are first-line treatments in knee OA.
- Cross-training with biking, elliptical training, or swimming helps maintain cardiovascular activity until the patient is able to return to running.
- PT may be initiated to strengthen the musculature around the knee, including the gluteus, quadriceps, and hamstring muscles.
- A Cochrane review for transcutaneous electrical nerve stimulation (TENS) for knee OA revealed that pain relief from TENS treatment was significantly better than placebo. TENS also decreases the amount of knee stiffness.[30]
- Both acetaminophen and NSAIDs have been proven to be effective in the treatment of OA[31] (LOE 1A).
- The short-term benefit of intra-articular corticosteroid injections is well established for the treatment of knee OA, and they have few side effects; however, long-term benefits have not been confirmed.[32]

- Viscosupplementation can be used for OA if corticosteroid injections have failed or no longer provide relief. Level I evidence demonstrates that the use of hyluronic acid in patients with OA results in modest improvement.[33] Hyluronic acid treatments have been shown to have better long-term effects compared to corticosteroid injections.[32]
- Glucosamine supplementation is an effective and safe treatment for OA of the knee. It delays the progression and improves the symptoms of OA.[34] In one particular study, high doses (2,000 mg/day) over an extended period of time (at least 12 weeks) showed an improvement in knee pain.[35]
- Studies on chondroitin sulfate have shown it to have a slight-to-moderate efficacy in the symptomatic treatment of OA, and it has an excellent safety profile.[36]

Operative

- Operative management can range from surgical debridement to joint replacement.
- Degenerative meniscal tears that cause continued pain or mechanical symptoms despite conservative treatment may require partial meniscectomy.

Prognosis/Return to Play

- Overall prognosis for mild-to-moderate OA is good.
- The athlete may need to decrease their mileage and/or run every other day to minimize the pain from DJD.
- In severe cases, changing to less impact or nonimpact exercise, such as biking, elliptical, and swimming, may be necessary.
- Return to play is as symptoms allow.

Complications/Indications for Referral

Prolonged symptoms, progressive worsening of symptoms, or failure of conservative measures are indications for referral to a sports medicine or orthopedic physician. Complications are rare but may include loose body formation from articular cartilage degeneration or degenerative mensical tears unresponsive to conservative treatment. Signs of infection are red flags warranting immediate attention.

APPROACH TO THE ATHLETE WITH PES ANSERINE TENDINITIS

The pes anserine bursa lies on the medial aspect of the proximal tibia, just medial to the tibial tuberosity. The pes anserinus is where the semitendinosus, sartorius, and gracilis tendons attach (Fig. 19.6). The bursa can become inflamed from overuse, direct trauma, or coexisting knee OA. This can be a commonly overlooked source of knee pain in runners.

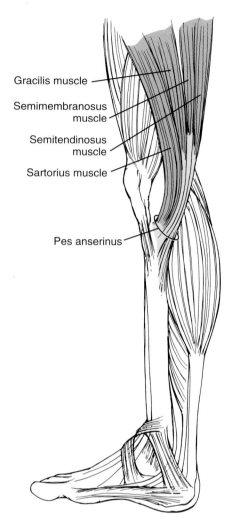

FIG. 19.6. Pes anserinus.

HISTORY AND PHYSICAL EXAM

The patient will report pain along the proximal tibial metaphysis. They may report a history of pain with running hills. The pes anserinus will be tender to palpation, and swelling may be evident. Flexion of the knee against resistance may exacerbate the pain.

DIAGNOSTIC TESTING

Plain radiographs will be normal. MRI generally not required unless there is concern for a tibia plateau stress fracture.

TREATMENT

Nonoperative

- Icing the area may help.
- Elastic bandage wrapped over the area can decrease and prevent swelling.

- The runner should rest from painful activity.
- Corticosteroid injection into the bursa decreases the inflammation and pain.
- PT includes hamstring stretching, strengthening, and knee proprioception along with core strengthening.
- NSAIDs may help alleviate the pain and swelling.

Operative

- Pes anserine tendonitis generally responds well to conservative treatment with no need for surgical intervention.

Prognosis/Return to Play

- Overall prognosis is excellent.
- The athlete may gradually return to running as pain allows.

Complications/Indications for Referral

If patients are not improving, an MRI may be necessary to evaluate for a stress fracture of the medial tibial plateau.

APPROACH TO THE ATHLETE WITH A STRESS FRACTURE OF THE KNEE

Stress fractures involving the knee can be an overlooked source of knee pain in the running athlete. They can occur within the distal femur, proximal tibia, or patella. A high suspicion for stress fracture should occur in running athletes with a recent increase in running mileage or intensity, history of prior stress fracture, underlying osteopenia/osteoporosis, or presence of the female athletic triad (disordered eating, amenorrhea, and osteopenia/osteoporosis). Most lower extremity stress fractures will occur in the running athlete. A history of OSD can be a risk factor for tibial tuberosity stress fractures. Patellar stress fractures are more common in young athletes. A complete description of the evaluation and treatment of stress fractures can be found in Chapter 22, *Athlete with Stress Fracture.*

APPROACH TO THE ATHLETE WITH OSTEOCHONDRITIS DISSECANS

OCD describes a focal area of subchondral bone avascular necrosis. This can lead to varying degrees of articular cartilage separation from the subchondral bone. OCD is of unknown etiology, possibly due to ischemia, infection, genetics, or trauma. Most commonly, OCD is found in the femoral condyles, in particular the lateral aspect of the medial condyle (70% of incidences), and less likely in the patella. OCD occurs in active children and adolescents. A thorough review of OCD can be found in Chapter 24, *Pediatric Athlete.*

HISTORY AND PHYSICAL EXAM

Patients may have swelling with activity. There is usually no history of trauma; however, some patients do recall a significant trauma to their knee in the past. They may describe vague knee pain worse with activity and complain of morning stiffness. If there is a loose body, they may complain of their knee locking or catching. On physical exam, there may be an effusion and quadriceps atrophy secondary to the effusion. Decreased range of motion may be present if there is a loose body. Palpate the flexed knee along the femoral condyles for tenderness. Pain may also be elicited with patellar compression.

DIAGNOSTIC TESTING

Radiographs may show a lesion on the femoral condyle. The best view to obtain is the posteroanterior tunnel view, which shows the articular surface (Fig. 19.7). If plain films are negative and clinical suspicion remains, an MRI should be obtained to further evaluate for OCD. MRIs are highly sensitive in detecting OCD lesions. They are essential in grading stage of the OCD lesions, which will help in treatment decisions.

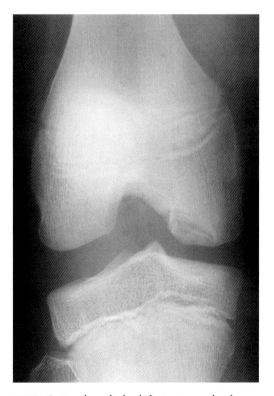

FIG. 19.7. Osteochondral defect: tunnel view x-rays demonstrating lesion on lateral aspect of medial femoral condyle. Reprinted with permission from Fleisher GR, Ludwig S, Baskin MN. *Atlas of Pediatric Emergency Medicine.* Philadelphia: Lippincott Williams & Wilkins; 2004.

FUNCTIONAL TREATMENT

Nonoperative

- For stable lesions in athletes with open growth plates, rest followed by a graduated asymptomatic return to sport is acceptable as long as lesion demonstrates signs of healing.
- The patient may need to be made non–weight bearing and immobilized.
- Rehabilitation should start with non–weight-bearing activities and progress to weight bearing as symptoms allow.
- Healing may take anywhere from 6 to 18 months.
- Athletes with open physes have a higher rate of healing.

Operative

- Operative treatment should be considered in patients with detached or unstable lesions and in those with lesions that are unresponsive to nonoperative management after 6 to 18 months.
- Goals of surgery include maintenance of joint congruity, fixation of unstable lesions, and repair of osteochondral defects. This is accomplished by drilling, fixation, bone grafting, fragment removal, and/or chondral resurfacing.
- Following surgery, the athlete will be partial weight bearing from 3 to 8 weeks, depending on the method of the procedure.

Prognosis/Return to Play

- Gradual return to play is necessary to allow proper healing.
- If the athlete returns too soon, there is risk of prolonging the healing process or making a stable lesion unstable.
- Radiographs should be obtained every 3 months to monitor for healing.

Complications/Indications for Referral

If the athlete does not show improvement within 8 to 10 weeks, surgery may be needed. Depending on the grading of the OCD lesion, surgery is occasionally the first line of treatment. In skeletally immature patients with an unstable lesion, surgery should be considered. Surgical options include debridement, drilling of the defect, open reduction internal fixation (ORIF), osteoarticular transplant technique (OATS), and autologous chondrocyte transplantation.

KEY POINTS

- Patellofemoral pain syndrome is the most common cause of knee pain in runners[4,5]
- Physical therapy for patellofemoral syndrome can significantly reduce pain and improve function[10,11]
- Iliotibial band friction syndrome is the second most common overuse injury in runners[5,9]
- Both acetaminophen and NSAIDs have been proven to be effective in the treatment of osteoarthritis[31]
- The short-term benefit of corticosteroid injections is well established for the treatment of knee OA; however, long-term benefits have not been confirmed[32]
- While examining the knee, keep in mind that 5% of knee pain is referred from other areas, such as the hip, particularly with young children

REFERENCES

1. van Gent RN, Siem D, van Middelkoop M, et al. Incidence and determinants of lower extremity running injuries in long distance runners: a systematic review. *Br J Sports Med.* 2007;41:469–480.
2. Mikkelsson LO, Nupponen H, Kaprio J, et al. Adolescent flexibility, endurance strength, and physical activity as predictors of adult tension neck, low back pain and knee injury: a 25 year follow up study. *Br J Sports Med.* 2006;40:107–113.
3. Callaghan MJ, Oldham JA. Quadriceps atrophy: to what extent does it exist in patellofemoral pain syndrome? *Br J Sports Med.* 2004;38: 295–299.
4. Lun V, Meeuwisse WH, Stergiou P, et al. Relation between running injury and static lower limb alignment in recreational runners. *Br J Sports Med.* 2004;38:576–580.
5. Taunton JE, Ryan MB, Clement DB, et al. A retrospective case-control analysis of 2002 running injuries. *Br J Sports Med.* 2002;36:95–101.
6. Witvrouw E, Lysens R, Bellemans J, et al. Intrinsic risk factors for the development of anterior knee pain in an athletic population: a two-year prospective study. *Am J Sports Med.* 2000;28:480–489.
7. Cown S, Bennell K, Hodges P, et al. Delayed onset of electromyographic activity of vastus medialis oblique relative to vastus lateralis in patients with patellofemoral pain syndrome. *Arch Phys Med Rehabil.* 2001;82: 183–189.
8. Waryasz G. Patellofemoral pain syndrome (PFPS): a systematic review of anatomy and risk factors. *Dyn Med.* 2008;7:9.
9. Stefanyshyn D, Stergiou P, Lun V, et al. Knee angular impulse as a predictor of patellofemoral pain in runners. *Am J Sports Med.* 2006; 34(11):1844–1851.
10. Tyler T, Nicholas S, Mullaney M, et al. The role of hip function in the treatment of patellofemoral pain syndrome. *Am J Sports Med.* 2006; 34(4):630–636.
11. Crossley K, Bennell K, Green S, et al. Physical therapy for patellofemoral pain: a randomized, double-blinded, placebo-controlled trial. *Am J Sports Med.* 2002;30:857–865.
12. Heintjes EM, Berger M, Bierma-Zeinstra SMA, et al. Pharmacotherapy for patellofemoral pain syndrome. *Cochrane Database of Systematic Rev.* 2004, Issue 3. Art. No.:CD003470. DOI: 10.1002/14651858.CD003470.pub2.
13. Fulkerson JP. Diagnosis and treatment of patients with patellofemoral pain. *Am J Sports Med.* 2002;30:447–456.
14. Kettunen J, Harilainen A, Sandelin J, et al. Knee arthroscopy and exercise versus exercise alone for chronic patellofemoral pain syndrome: a randomized controlled trial. *BMC Med.* 2007;5:38.
15. Ellis R, Hing W, Reid D. Iliotibial band friction syndrome—a systematic review. *Man Ther.* 2007;12:200–208.

16. Brosseau L, Casimiro L, Milne S, et al. Deep transverse friction massage for treating tendinitis. *Cochrane Database of Systematic Rev.* 2002, Issue 4. Art. No.:CD003528. DOI: 10.1002/14651858.CD003528.

17. Panni A, Biedert R, Maffulli N, et al. Overuse injuries of the extensor mechanism in athletes. *Clin Sports Med.* 2002;21:483–498.

18. James S, Ali K, Pocock C, et al. Ultrasound guided dry needling and autologous blood injection for patellar tendinosis. *Br J Sports Med.* 2007;41:518–522.

19. Visnes H, Bahr R. The evolution of eccentric training as treatment for patellar tendinopathy (jumper's knee): a critical review of exercise programmes. *Br J Sports Med.* 2007;41:217–223.

20. Gisslen K, Alfredson H. Neovascularisation and pain in jumper's knee: a prospective clinical and sonographic study in elite junior volleyball players. *Br J Sports Med.* 2005;39:423–428.

21. Cannell L, Taunton J, Clement D, et al. A randomized clinical trial of the efficacy of drop squats or leg extension/leg curl exercises to treat clinically diagnosed jumper's knee in athletes: pilot study. *Br J Sports Med.* 2001;35:60–64.

22. Kaeding C, Pedroza A, Powers B. Surgical treatment of chronic patellar tendinosis: a systematic review. *Clin Orthop Relat Res.* 2007;455:102–106.

23. Kettunen J, Kvist M, Alanen E, et al. Long-term prognosis for jumper's knee in male athletes: a prospective follow-up study. *Am J Sports Med.* 2002;30:689–692.

24. Hanna F, Teichtahl A, Bell R, et al. The cross-sectional relationship between fortnightly exercise and knee cartilage properties in healthy adult women in midlife. *Menopause.* 2007;14(5):830–834.

25. Racunica T, Teichtahl A, Wang Y, et al. Effect of physical activity on articular knee joint structures in community-based adults. *Arthritis Rheum.* 2007;57(7):1261–1268.

26. Cheng Y, Macera C, Davis D, et al. Physical activity and self-reported, physician-diagnosed osteoarthritis: is physical activity a risk factor? *J Clin Epidemiol.* 2000;53(3):315–322.

27. Lane N, Michel B, Bjorkengren A, et al. The risk of osteoarthritis with running and aging: a 5-year longitudinal study. *J Rheumatol.* 1993;20(3):461–468.

28. Lohmander LS, Englund PM, Dahl LL, et al. The long-term consequence of anterior cruciate ligament and meniscus injuries: osteoarthritis. *Am J Sports Med.* 2007;35:1756.

29. Utting MR, Davies G, Newman JH. Is anterior knee pain a predisposing factor to patellofemoral osteoarthritis? *Knee.* 2005;12(5):362–365.

30. Osiri M, Welch V, Brosseau L, et al. Transcutaneous electrical nerve stimulation for knee osteoarthritis. *Cochrane Database of Systematic Rev.* 2000, Issue 4. Art. No.:CD002823. DOI: 10.1002/14651858.CD002823.

31. Zhang W, Moskowitz RW, Nuki G, et al. OARSI Recommendations for the management of hip and knee osteoarthritis, part I: critical appraisal of existing treatment guidelines and systematic review of current research evidence. *Osteoarthritis Cartilage.* 2007;15(9):981–1000.

32. Bellamy N, Campbell J, Robinson V, et al. Intraarticular corticosteroid for treatment of osteoarthritis of the Knee. The Cochrane Library (Oxford) 2005;4 (ID #CD005328).

33. Divine JG, Zazulak BT, Hewett TE. Viscosupplementation for knee osteoarthritis: a systematic review. *Clin Orthop Relat Res.* 2007;459:283.

34. Poolsup N, Suthisisang C, Channark P, et al. Glucosamine long-term treatment and the progression of knee osteoarthritis: systematic review of randomized controlled trials. *Ann Pharmacother.* 2005;39(6):1080–1087.

35. Braham R, Dawson B, Goodman C. The effect of glucosamine supplementation on people experiencing regular knee pain. *Br J Sports Med.* 2003;37:45–49.

36. Monfort J, Martel-Pelletier J, Pelletier J. Chondroitin sulfate for symptomatic osteoarthritis: critical appraisal of meta-analyses. *Curr Med Res Opin.* 2008;24(5):1303–1308.

Athlete with Overuse Foot and Ankle Injuries

Jeremy McCormick

INTRODUCTION

With increasing participation in athletics, foot and ankle injuries are becoming more prevalent. While many injuries occur with an acute incident, others are the product of repetitive stress or overuse. With these types of injuries, patients develop symptoms slowly over a period of several weeks or months. In some situations, the athlete cannot recall a specific incident, but presents because of dull pain or discomfort that has lingered for some time without improvement. The duty of the physician is to assess, diagnose, and treat these injuries as expeditiously as possible so that the athlete can return to play quickly, without compromising the healing or recovery process.

This chapter reviews some of the more common overuse foot and ankle injuries. Patients can fully recover from all of these injuries if they are properly diagnosed and treated in the early stages of their disease process. It is our hope that by reviewing these injuries with their classic signs, symptoms, and treatment regimens, an athlete will be well served with early intervention and a path toward recovery that enables full participation in return to their sport.

FUNCTIONAL ANATOMY

The anatomy of the foot and ankle can be very involved, and a whole chapter might be dedicated to its finest detail. However, a working knowledge of the anatomy of this region of the body is critical to proper examination and diagnosis of chronic injuries. The bony structures of the foot are divided into regions called the forefoot (phalanges, metatarsals), midfoot (cuneiforms, cuboid, navicular), and hindfoot (calcaneus, talus), and there are named joints between all of these bones (Fig. 20.1).

Additionally, there are numerous muscular structures intrinsic to the foot and tendons that pass across the ankle, with origin in the lower leg. Crossing on the lateral aspect of the ankle are the peroneal tendons and crossing on the medial aspect are the posterior tibialis, flexor digitorum longus, and flexor hallucis longus tendons (Fig. 20.2).

The primary nerve supply for intrinsic function in the foot comes from the tibial nerve, which passes medially and

branches just beyond the ankle. There are also the deep and superficial branches of the peroneal nerve, the sural nerve, and the saphenous nerve, which all cross the ankle and enter the foot. The main vascular supply to the foot comes from the dorsalis pedis and posterior tibialis arteries (Fig. 20.3).

Within each section of this chapter, the anatomy, as it pertains to a specific chronic foot and ankle injury, is explained in greater detail.

EPIDEMIOLOGY

Millions of people play football, soccer, basketball, and baseball, and some studies have shown that up to 40% of athletes may suffer some type of foot or ankle injury during their participation in these sports.[1] With that in mind, it is important to be aware of the different injuries that can exist, particularly when patients present with chronic complaints. These can be more challenging in that the complaints might be vague and there may not be a discrete source of pain. The differential diagnosis for any presenting complaint of foot or ankle pain can be broad, but with a careful history and physical examination, the list can be narrowed. The subsequent sections on specific etiologies of chronic foot and ankle injuries will help in their diagnosis and subsequent treatment and help sports physicians accurately and expeditiously treat their patients.

NARROWING THE DIFFERENTIAL DIAGNOSIS

History

A careful history should include questions characterizing the complaint. Information such as the mechanism of injury can be extremely useful. One should also determine the severity of pain, quality of pain, location of pain, timing of pain, onset of pain, and the alleviating or exacerbating factors. It is also important to determine if a patient has ever experienced or been treated for the pain in the past. While in some measure, patients of certain age groups or activity profiles are more

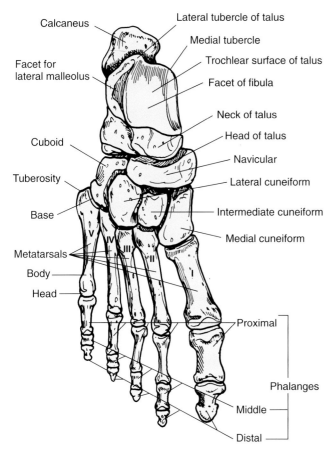

Calcaneus
Lateral tubercle of talus
Medial tubercle
Facet for lateral malleolus
Trochlear surface of talus
Facet of fibula
Neck of talus
Head of talus
Cuboid
Navicular
Tuberosity
Lateral cuneiform
Base
Intermediate cuneiform
Medial cuneiform
Metatarsals
Body
Head
Proximal
Phalanges
Middle
Distal

FIG. 20.1. Foot anatomy. Reprinted with permission from Anderson M, Hall SJ. *Sports Injury Management.* 2nd ed. Baltimore: Lippincott Williams & Wilkins; 2000.

predisposed to an injury, a physician should not limit themselves when investigating a patient's complaints.

The subsequent sections discussing the approach to patients with specific foot and ankle complaints will help guide one down a path from a large list of possible diagnoses to the correct one. There are also classic descriptions for some disease processes, such as pain worse with the first few steps of the day in plantar fasciitis, which will be discussed.

Evidence-based Physical Examination

While gathering a detailed history regarding a patient's complaint can provide valuable information in localizing symptoms, one should always approach the foot and ankle examination with a systematic approach so as to not miss any important detail. Using the opposite, noninjured side as a reference is always helpful as a control. As problems are presented in this chapter, we will discuss specific details of the physical examination important to diagnosing that specific problem. In general, however, the examination should proceed as follows.

Inspection

Observe for evidence of swelling, ecchymosis, or skin injury, which might be indicative of trauma. Observe for erythema, which might be indicative of infection or inflammation. Be aware of skin changes or ulcerations that could suggest vascular problems or diabetes, particularly between the toes. Areas of thickened skin could point to bony prominences. Note any foot or toe deformity, particularly in stance, which could hint at the underlying cause of a chronic foot and ankle complaint (i.e., hindfoot varus in chronic ankle instability).

Palpation

Attempt to find areas of tenderness to localize symptoms. This might be over a bony prominence in the case of a stress fracture or over a tendon sheath as in posterior tibialis dysfunction. Also, determine if malalignment or deformities are flexible or fixed as this may influence treatment options. Check for intact sensation through all distributions in the foot. This includes superficial peroneal nerve, deep peroneal nerve, sural nerve, saphenous nerve, and tibial nerve, which divides into lateral plantar and medial plantar nerves.

Range of Motion

Test both active and passive ranges of motion to assure there is no restriction. Joints that should be assessed are the ankle joint, subtalar joint, midfoot, metatarsophalangeal (MTP) joints, and interphalangeal joints. Any restriction or pain with range of motion should be noted, again helping to localize the etiology of a patient's presenting complaint.

Strength Testing

The basic function of all muscle groups crossing the ankle and within the foot should be tested. This includes ankle dorsiflexion and plantarflexion as well as foot inversion and eversion and toe flexion and extension. In addition to proper function, their strength should be examined. Asking a patient to walk on their heels and on their tiptoes is a simple way to assure all muscle groups are functioning, and at full strength. Specific tests such as a single heel rise to look for posterior tibialis dysfunction can be helpful in localizing pathology.

Laxity Tests

Examining the joints of the foot and ankle for stability is valuable in attempting to determine a source of discomfort. When testing for laxity, comparison to the uninjured side gives a valuable frame of reference. For instance, a test such as the anterior drawer test at the ankle is helpful in trying to discern between ankle joint instability and peroneal tendon degeneration.

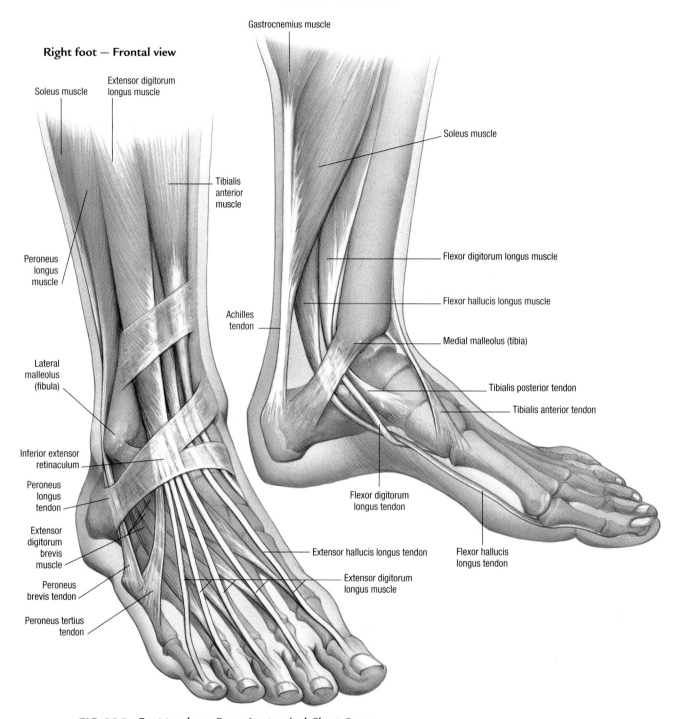

Left foot — Medial view

Gastrocnemius muscle

Soleus muscle

Flexor digitorum longus muscle

Flexor hallucis longus muscle

Medial malleolus (tibia)

Tibialis posterior tendon

Tibialis anterior tendon

Flexor digitorum longus tendon

Flexor hallucis longus tendon

Right foot — Frontal view

Soleus muscle

Extensor digitorum longus muscle

Tibialis anterior muscle

Peroneus longus muscle

Achilles tendon

Lateral malleolus (fibula)

Inferior extensor retinaculum

Peroneus longus tendon

Extensor digitorum brevis muscle

Peroneus brevis tendon

Peroneus tertius tendon

Extensor hallucis longus tendon

Extensor digitorum longus muscle

FIG. 20.2. Foot tendons. From Anatomical Chart Company.

As with a careful history, a detailed and systematic physical examination is critical to narrowing a broad list of differential diagnoses. The examination techniques discussed earlier and those discussed in the following approaches to disease sections are all an important part of the diagnosis puzzle. As one becomes more facile with the foot and ankle and the presenting complaints and physical findings, navigat- ing the list of possible diagnoses will become much easier. It is important, however, especially when one is unsure of the diagnosis, to be as thorough as possible so as not to bypass any critical finding. For instance, numbness and tingling of the medial foot could represent a tarsal tunnel syndrome, if accompanied by a positive nerve compression test or Tinel's sign at the ankle. If, however, one has not attempted a straight

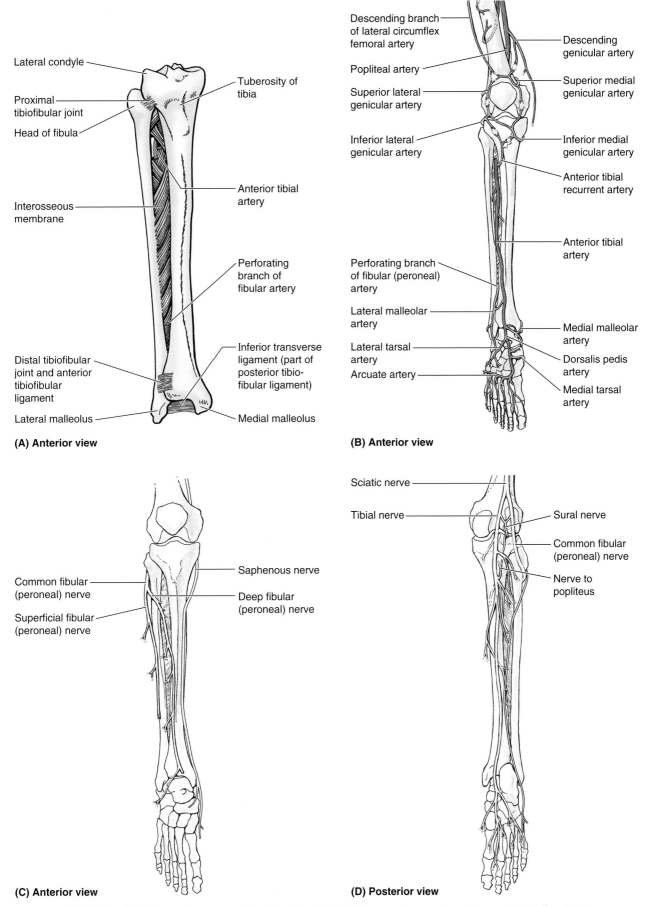

Lateral condyle

Proximal tibiofibular joint

Head of fibula

Interosseous membrane

Tuberosity of tibia

Anterior tibial artery

Perforating branch of fibular artery

Distal tibiofibular joint and anterior tibiofibular ligament

Lateral malleolus

Inferior transverse ligament (part of posterior tibio-fibular ligament)

Medial malleolus

(A) Anterior view

Descending branch of lateral circumflex femoral artery

Popliteal artery

Superior lateral genicular artery

Inferior lateral genicular artery

Perforating branch of fibular (peroneal) artery

Lateral malleolar artery

Lateral tarsal artery

Arcuate artery

Descending genicular artery

Superior medial genicular artery

Inferior medial genicular artery

Anterior tibial recurrent artery

Anterior tibial artery

Medial malleolar artery

Dorsalis pedis artery

Medial tarsal artery

(B) Anterior view

Common fibular (peroneal) nerve

Superficial fibular (peroneal) nerve

Saphenous nerve

Deep fibular (peroneal) nerve

(C) Anterior view

Sciatic nerve

Tibial nerve

Sural nerve

Common fibular (peroneal) nerve

Nerve to popliteus

(D) Posterior view

FIG. 20.3. Arteries and nerves of the leg. Reprinted with permission from Moore KL, Dalley AF II. *Clinical Oriented Anatomy.* 4th ed. Baltimore: Lippincott Williams & Wilkins; 1999.

leg raise or found similar symptoms in a stocking pattern on the other foot, one may not be able to discern a patient's tarsal tunnel syndrome from another etiology for foot pain such as disk herniation in the spine or diabetic neuropathy.

Diagnostic Testing

Diagnostic tests acquired in investigating complaints of the foot and ankle should be ordered with a purpose. That is to say, any test that is obtained should help in delineating a diagnosis from a list of possibilities.

Laboratory

Laboratory tests are helpful when it is thought that a chronic foot and ankle injury stems from an underlying medical disease. Lab values are helpful in investigating rheumatoid arthritis or inflammatory disease as a possible cause of joint pain or inflammation. Also, if there is a concern for infection, inflammatory markers are helpful.

Imaging

Imaging studies are the most commonly ordered and most useful studies available for investigating chronic injuries of the foot and ankle. X-rays are always the first line of imaging, where anteroposterior (AP), oblique, and lateral views of the foot and AP, mortise, and lateral views of the ankle should be obtained (Figs. 20.4–20.6). The subsequent sections on specific diagnoses discuss specific x-ray findings, but in general one should look for obvious fractures, dislocations, or malalignment.

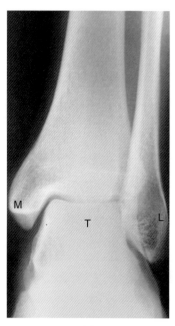
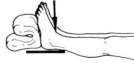

FIG. 20.4. Ankle XR, AP. From Drs. P. Bobechko and E. Becker, Department of Medical Imaging, University of Toronto, Ontario, Canada. M, medial malleolus; T, talus; L, lateral malleolus.

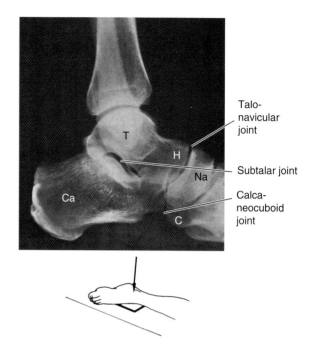

FIG. 20.5. Ankle XR, lateral. Reprinted with permission from Moore KL, Dalley AF II. *Clinical Oriented Anatomy.* 4th ed. Baltimore: Lippincott Williams & Wilkins; 1999. Ca, calcaneus; C, cuboid; Na, navicular; T, talus.

In addition to x-rays, computerized tomography (CT) and magnetic resonance imaging (MRI) are helpful for additional detail. CT is most helpful for bony injury, namely, stress fracture. They can be obtained with coronal, sagittal, and axial cuts to create the geometry of a bony injury. The advantage of MRI is the ability to evaluate soft-tissue structures such as tendons and ligaments. These studies are extremely helpful in diagnosis such as for peroneal tendon subluxation where it is important to evaluate the integrity of the superficial peroneal retinaculum and determine if there is any midsubstance tendon degeneration.

Ultrasound is another imaging modality that can be used to investigate tendinous degeneration or soft-tissue lesions. It has also been helpful in investigating and diagnosing Morton's neuromas.

Lastly, a bone scan is used in the instance where bone pathology cannot be properly seen on plain x-ray. This arises mostly in the instance of Freiberg's infraction or stress fractures. In these circumstances, the bone scan shows increased uptake in the area of question, aiding in the diagnosis of injury with normal radiographs.

Other Testing

In cases of concern for nerve injury or compression, electromyography (EMG) can be obtained to verify the diagnosis. Problems such as tarsal tunnel syndrome can be diagnosed with history and physical examination. The added information of the EMG can help not only in reassuring proper diagnosis but also in documenting preoperative function for a means of comparison to postoperative result.

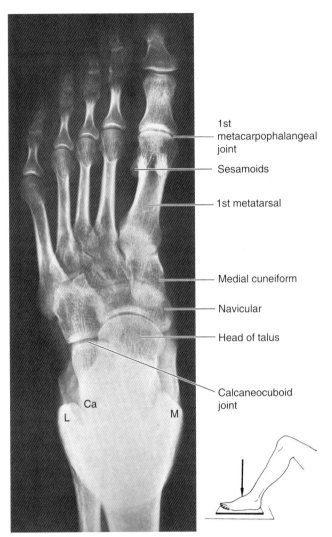

FIG. 20.6. Foot XR, AP. Reprinted with permission from Moore KL, Dalley AF II. *Clinical Oriented Anatomy.* 4th ed. Baltimore: Lippincott Williams & Wilkins; 1999. L, lateral malleolus; M, medial malleolus; Ca, calcaneus.

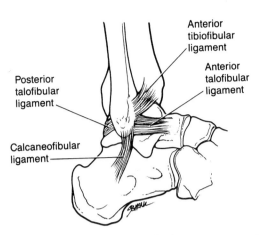

FIG. 20.7. Lateral collateral ankle ligaments. Reprinted with permission from Buchholz RW, Heckman JD. *Rockwood & Green's Fractures in Adults.* 5th ed. Philadelphia, PA: Lippincott Williams & Wilkins; 2001.

APPROACH TO THE ATHLETE WITH FUNCTIONAL ANKLE INSTABILITY

Ankle injuries are very common, accounting for 40% of all sports injuries.[2] The injury often occurs on the lateral aspect of the ankle where three separate ligaments function to stabilize the joint—the anterior talofibular ligament (ATFL), the calcaneofibular ligament (CFL), and the posterior talofibular ligament (PFL) (Fig. 20.7). Also contributing to stability at the ankle through dynamic restraint are the peroneal muscles. Bony structures add a last element of stability to the ankle, particularly in dorsiflexion where the wider anterior aspect of the talus rests within the mortise.

Only about half of the patients presenting with ankle injury develop long-term sequelae, most notably chronic ankle instability. Chronic ankle instability can be mechanical, where the patient does not have any symptoms of instability, but the lateral ankle feels lax on examination, or functional, where the patient describes a history of instability.

HISTORY AND PHYSICAL EXAMINATION

Patients primarily complain of their ankle "giving way" or "rolling over," demonstrating motion at the ankle beyond their control. One might also describe a snap or pop sound with the instability episodes that might be followed by pain and swelling. It is important, however, to determine if the pain lasts between sprains. This might suggest another source of pathology other than lateral ankle instability such as osteochondral injury to the talus, peroneal tendon instability, or synovitis.

On physical examination, one might find a varus position to the hindfoot, perhaps predisposing the ankle to lateral ankle sprains. Patients might have tenderness to palpation at the lateral ankle. The most common test is the anterior drawer test, which is performed with the leg hanging off a table at 90 degrees. With one hand stabilizing the tibia, the other attempts to translate the foot forward at the ankle, with the foot about 25 degrees plantarflexed while allowing for internal rotation of the foot with translation. If the motion is greater than 9 to 10 mm or more than 5 mm greater than the opposite side, then it is considered a positive test. Another examination is the varus instability test, where the foot is stressed to inversion to examine lateral-sided laxity. One should remember, however, to examine the entire foot and ankle as other problems such as peroneal tendon pathology can create similar symptoms.

DIAGNOSTIC TESTING

Overall, the diagnosis of chronic functional ankle instability is generally made by patient history and physical examination. X-rays should be ordered to help eliminate bony lesions such as tarsal coalition as a source of pathology for ankle instability. There has been investigation into stress radiographs to examine the excursion of the talus with anterior drawer maneuver, but this method has been shown to not have much clinical relevance[3]; thus, it is not routinely used.

Another helpful study is an MRI, which can help evaluate the ligaments of the ankle. One might find an attenuated or ruptured ATFL. Perhaps just as important is the ability of the MRI to evaluate the peroneal tendons, the dome of the talus for osteochondral lesions, and the joint space for loose bodies, all of which could cause symptoms simulating ankle instability.

TREATMENT

Nonoperative

- Rest
- Ice
- Elevation
- NSAIDs
- Physical therapy (stretching, strengthening, proprioception)
- Orthotics (lateral heel wedge/post)
- Taping (if continuing sports)
- Reusable ankle bracing

Operative

- Operative treatment should only be considered when nonoperative measures fail.
- Many different types of procedures exist with the Brostrom procedure (lateral ligament repair/reconstruction) being very common.
- Arthroscopy can be performed to evaluate intra-articular pathology.[4]
- Postoperatively, patients will be casted and non–weight bearing for 2 to 3 weeks followed by a weight-bearing cast or boot and gentle range of motion
- At 4 to 6 weeks, patients will begin active range of motion and peroneal strengthening exercises.
- By 10 to 12 weeks, patients should be nearing full recovery, and if they are not able to return to their preoperative level of function, physical therapy should resume.

Prognosis/Return to Play

- The prognosis for functional ankle instability is very good.
- Nonoperative intervention works well, and patients can return to play when symptoms subside, using taping or bracing as needed.
- Should nonoperative management not be successful, the operative options are many and very successful. Whether an anatomic or nonanatomic repair, patients recover from surgery to near preinjury status.
- Assuming postoperative management proceeds without complication, athletes can start returning to their sport by

12 weeks, with return to competition when there is no limitation to function.
- Athletes may tape their ankles or brace postoperatively. Patients who may not do as well with functional ankle instability are those with long-standing instability, those with generalized ligament laxity, and those with underlying osteoarthritis in the ankle.

Complications/Indications for Referral

With functional ankle instability, patients should be referred to a surgeon when they have failed conservative measures and are still experiencing episodes of instability. Even patients with severe ankle sprains do well with late stabilization surgery,[5] so nonoperative measures should be exhausted. Postoperative complications include sural nerve or superficial peroneal nerve irritation. In addition, those patients who have had a stabilization procedure and present with a new instability episode should be sent to see their surgeon. Other indications for referral to a surgeon include patients whose workup for ankle instability revealed another pathology that needs more timely intervention, such as a fracture.

APPROACH TO THE ATHLETE WITH PERONEAL TENDON STRAIN/SUBLUXATION

The peroneal tendons function as the main everters of the foot. They are located on the lateral aspect of the ankle, posterior to the fibula. The peroneus brevis (PB) and peroneus longus (PL) run within the posterior fibular groove and are contained by the superior peroneal retinaculum (SPR), which runs from the fibula to the calcaneus.

Acute injury can cause strain of the tendons or injury to the SPR, which over time could lead to chronic subluxation or degeneration of the peroneal tendons. Generally, the mechanism of injury is sudden dorsiflexion of a plantarflexed, inverted foot. An attenuation or rupture of the SPR in this setting would allow the peroneal tendons to sublux out of the fibular groove and slowly cause tendinosis or tearing of the tendon over time. Additionally, stenosis within the peroneal tendon sheath can lead to development of pathology within the tendons themselves. A peroneus quartus tendon (a normal variant) can cause injury to the PB tendon by compressing it within a narrower space.

HISTORY AND PHYSICAL EXAMINATION

In an acute setting, patients will complain of lateral ankle swelling and ecchymosis, occasionally after hearing or feeling a "pop" (SPR rupture or avulsion) with sudden dorsiflexion of the foot. With chronic peroneal tendon injury, patients will most commonly present with complaint of pain at the lateral ankle often accompanied by the uncomfortable snapping of subluxing tendons across the fibula. The patient may also complain of ankle instability or a sensation of the ankle giving way. There is not always a discrete event that led to the symptoms, and in some cases, an SPR avulsion or rupture that was previously undiagnosed will be found.

On examination, patients will have tenderness with manual pressure over the peroneal tendons. The peroneal tunnel compression test is performed with the knee flexed and the thumb applying pressure over the SPR. Pain as the foot dorsiflexes and everts from a plantarflexed and inverted position is considered positive. Further, patients may be able to voluntarily sublux the tendons with a similar maneuver of eversion and dorsiflexion, which demonstrates instability of the tendons or incompetence of the SPR. Strength examination of the tendons is most often normal; however, it may be uncomfortable for the patient.

DIAGNOSTIC TESTING

X-rays may not be helpful in diagnosing chronic peroneal tendon pathology. However, these images should be obtained, particularly in a patient who had a previous foot or ankle trauma. In an acute setting, one may see a tiny bone fragment signifying an SPR avulsion. In the chronic patient, one might be able to identify a fibular or calcaneal malunion that might have predisposed a patient to developing peroneal tendonitis.

MRI is a helpful diagnostic study as one can see longitudinal split tears of the PB tendon and other tendon irregularities.[6] Additionally, one can see fluid in the peroneal tendon sheath or a peroneus quartus that might be creating stenosis. Lastly, MRI can help evaluate the depth of the posterior fibular groove.

TREATMENT

Nonoperative

- Rest
- NSAIDs
- Immobilization
- Activity modification
- Physical therapy

Operative

- Techniques for operative repair include debridement or repair of the peroneal tendons with repair or reconstruction of the SPR.
- Postoperatively, patients will be non-weight bearing in a splint for 2 weeks and then weight bearing in a cast for 4 to 6 weeks.

- Following this, they will wear a walking boot with gradual progression of range of motion and weight bearing.

Prognosis/Return to Play

- Patients generally have a favorable outcome with peroneal tendon injury, particularly if there is a clear etiology to their problem.
- Patients managed successfully nonoperatively may require 4 to 6 weeks of decreased activity or immobilization prior to return to full function.
- Those undergoing surgery will begin strengthening exercises at 8 weeks and, by 3 months, return to normal activities. Return to competition is usually about 4 to 6 months.

Complications/Indications for Referral

Nonoperative management tends not to have many complications. In the case of an acute injury, one should rule out SPR injury. If an SPR injury occurred acutely, patients should be referred for surgical intervention as it may help expedite return to play. Those who have chronic injury or subluxation should be referred for surgical management after failing conservative measures if they are candidates for the procedure.

APPROACH TO THE ATHLETE WITH POSTERIOR TIBIALIS DYSFUNCTION

Posterior tibial tendon dysfunction is also known as acquired flatfoot deformity or posterior tibial tendon insufficiency. It is the most common cause of adult flatfoot deformity. The posterior tibialis muscle originates proximally from the tibia, fibula, and interosseous membrane and passes distally, posterior to the medial malleolus, before inserting primarily on the navicular of the medial foot. The muscle has a short excursion, so even a small degree of attenuation can gradually worsen and cause deformity. One theory on tendon degenerating is increased susceptibility to injury or degradation in a zone of decreased blood supply between the medial malleolus and the navicular.

HISTORY AND PHYSICAL EXAMINATION

Patients will generally present with medial-based ankle pain that radiates to the medial foot. This discomfort is worse with activity and improves with rest. The patient may have memory of an injury, but this is not a consistent finding. One may have noticed his foot becoming more flat over time and falling into a hindfoot valgus position. With this, patients may actually complain of lateral-sided hindfoot pain where the fibula begins to abut on the calcaneus. Interestingly, as the disease progresses, the early inflammation of the tendon may resolve, leading to less pain through the tendon with greater degeneration.

Physical examination will demonstrate tenderness to palpation along the posterior tibial tendon, often just proximal to its insertion on the navicular. There may be swelling at the medial ankle. The patient should be examined standing, with careful observation of the hindfoot. One will find a valgus heel position, decreased arch height, and difficulty with single heel rise. A classic examination finding is the "too many toes" sign, where the valgus hindfoot, fallen arch, and abducted forefoot allow one to see multiple toes of the foot lateral to the ankle when looking from behind. As the disease progresses, not only patients will have increasing difficulty with single heel rise, but their foot will also become less mobile, eventually developing a rigid hindfoot and progressive attenuation of the deltoid ligament.

DIAGNOSTIC TESTING

Standing AP, lateral, and oblique x-rays should be obtained on all patients. Aside from examining for other sources of foot pain, suspicion for posterior tibial tendon pathology would lead you to examine the height of the midfoot arch and assess any talonavicular subluxation. One can consider obtaining similar views of the contralateral side for comparison.

Other studies such as CT, MRI, or bone scan can be ordered, but are generally not as helpful as x-rays. Of the choices, MRI is a good second study to obtain to evaluate the integrity and quality of the tendon. One might see tendinosis, a longitudinal split, or in extreme cases, a complete rupture of the posterior tibialis tendon. Also, one can determine from the MRI that the inflammation is limited to the synovium or involves the tendon.

TREATMENT

Management of posterior tibialis dysfunction is aided by classifying the stage of disease process. Stage I is degeneration or inflammation of the tendon with no foot deformity. Stage II is tendon degeneration with the beginnings of foot deformity that remains flexible. Stage III is tendon degeneration and foot deformity that becomes fixed. Stage IV is tendon degeneration with fixed foot deformity that involves the ankle joint as well.

Nonoperative

- NSAIDs.
- Medial wedge orthotic with arch support.
- Immobilization (cast vs. walking boot).
- Nonoperative modalities for at least 6 weeks.
- Likelihood for success decreases with progressive stages of posterior tibialis dysfunction

Operative

- Patients should be referred to a surgeon if 6 weeks of non-operative management has failed for stage I disease or if a patient has presented with or progressed to foot deformity.
- Presentation with foot deformity (stage II or greater) should be considered for operative referral sooner than a patient with only medial ankle pain and tenderness over the posterior tibialis tendon (stage I).
- Development of hindfoot valgus with collapse of the medial arch is an indication to proceed with surgery.
- As is the case with most disease processes, surgical options for posterior tibialis dysfunction become more difficult in the late stages of progression. Surgical options are as follows:
  - Posterior tibial tendon debridement/tenosynovectomy
  - Posterior tibial tendon end-to-end repair
  - Reattachment or advancement of the tendon to its primary site of insertion on the navicular bone
  - Tendon reconstruction with transfer (typically flexor digitorum longus)
  - Triple arthrodesis (subtalar/talonavicular/calcaneocuboid)
- With all surgeries, the post-op management involves a 6- to 8-week period of non–weight bearing and immobilization with a cast or boot.
- Weight bearing may progress starting between 6 and 12 weeks postoperatively (earlier with less complex surgery).
- At 12 weeks, patients who underwent tenosynovectomy should begin normal shoe wear with an orthotic.
- Those who had fusion procedures for late-stage disease will still need a walking boot and may not be able to weight bear until there is x-ray evidence of bone healing.

Prognosis/Return to Play

- Prognosis for surgery depends on the degree of disease present preoperatively.
- Stage I patients will be able to return to near-normal function; however, they may not be able to participate in competitive running or jumping sports.
- Patients with stage II disease will have some return of strength and will be able to have normal gait, but running or sports participation may be difficult.
- With stage III and IV disease, patients will likely not be able to run and may even have trouble with walking, particularly those having undergone pantalar fusion.

Complications/Indications for Referral

Patients with posterior tibialis tendon dysfunction should be referred to a surgeon when foot deformity is noted, whether that is on presentation or after initiation of nonoperative treatment. Red flags, therefore, would be valgus deformity of the ankle and flattening of the midfoot arch. While stage I posterior tibial tendonitis can be treated well nonoperatively, a patient should be referred if doubt surrounds the progression of disease. The hope would be that earlier intervention would prevent the need for fusion procedures and allow the patient a more functional foot and ankle after treatment.

APPROACH TO THE ATHLETE WITH TARSAL TUNNEL SYNDROME

Tarsal tunnel syndrome is an entrapment neuropathy of the tibial nerve or its medial and/or lateral plantar branches. The tarsal tunnel, which is on the medial side of the ankle, contains the tibial nerve, the tibial artery and vein, the posterior tibialis tendon, the flexor hallucis longus tendon, and the flexor digitorum longus tendon. Overlying the tunnel is the flexor retinaculum that traverses from the medial malleolus anteriorly to the calcaneus posteriorly.

Anything that decreases space within the tunnel for the tibial nerve to pass could lead to a tarsal tunnel syndrome. Trauma, such as a sprained deltoid ligament or displaced fracture, and tenosynovitis of tendons within the tunnel are etiologies that can cause compression or irritation of the tibial nerve. Additionally, a patient may have a ganglion, lipoma, or other mass within the tunnel. The impingement can occur proximally, where the entire nerve is involved and symptoms are noted throughout the foot, or distally, where the medial or lateral plantar branch may be involved and contribute only medial or lateral symptoms, respectively. There is an entity known as "jogger's foot" where a distance runner develops burning pain through the medial arch and first through third toes. This is due to compression or irritation of the medial plantar nerve. Other athletes who may be predisposed to developing tarsal tunnel syndrome are those who place a heavy load on their ankles such as sprinters and jumpers.[7]

HISTORY AND PHYSICAL EXAMINATION

A patient will present with complaint of diffuse burning, tingling, or numbing pain through the plantar aspect of the foot. The pain is exacerbated with activity and improved with rest, can be intermittent or consistent, localized or global, distal or proximal. The poorly localized quality of the discomfort helps differentiate a tarsal tunnel syndrome from the more directed discomfort of a tendonitis within the tunnel. In collecting a patient history, it is also important to determine any other causes of distal neuropathy such as diabetes, vitamin deficiency, lower back pathology, or rheumatologic disease.

In examining the patient, one should perform a Tinel's sign by percussion over the tibial nerve as it passes through the flexor retinaculum in an attempt to reproduce symptoms. If symptoms are elicited, this is considered a positive test and is indicative of nerve pathology. Also, maintaining direct pressure over the nerve at the tarsal tunnel for about 30 seconds can reproduce symptoms. This is called the nerve compression test. Interestingly, a peripheral sensory examination may be normal in this patient, but decreased two-point discrimination is an early clue to the disease process. A last test would be positioning the foot with eversion and dorsiflexion to stretch the tibial nerve in an attempt to create symptoms and indicate tibial tunnel syndrome.[8]

More long-standing tibial nerve compression will slowly cause atrophy of the foot intrinsic muscles and development of a cavus deformity to the foot. A patient might also have a planovalgus foot or forefoot abduction, which might contribute to the disease by stretching the tibial nerve as it passes into the foot.

DIAGNOSTIC TESTING

A diagnosis can be reached with the combination of the history and physical examination, as well as evidence of a compressive lesion. An x-ray or CT scan would evaluate for a bony lesion on the medial side of the ankle that may contribute to tibial nerve compression. Beyond that, an MRI can be important in locating a space-occupying soft-tissue lesion (i.e., ganglion) that may exist within the tibial tunnel.

In addition to imaging, electrodiagnostic studies can be performed to look for diagnostic clues such as slowed conduction or fibrillation potentials of intrinsic muscles. EMG can also help discern between nerve compression, peripheral neuropathy, and double crush syndrome, where there might be a proximal nerve compression such as a herniated lumbar disk. Ultimately, the correct diagnosis will be reached with the combination of the patient's report of pain and paresthesias, positive physical examination findings, and an EMG report showing delayed sensory nerve conduction.

TREATMENT

Nonoperative

- NSAIDs
- Immobilization
- Steroid injection (beware of the risk of tendon injury)
- Medial wedge orthotic with arch support
- Ankle-foot orthosis

Operative

- Operative intervention is indicated for patients who have failed conservative management or those who clearly have a lesion that is causing the nerve compression as determined by MRI or other imaging study.

- Surgical procedure consists of release of the flexor retinaculum with complete decompression of the tibial nerve and plantar branches.
- Postoperative management consists of splinting and non-weight bearing for 2 weeks followed by weight bearing in a boot for 2 to 4 weeks.

Prognosis/Return to Play

- Patients with the best prognosis are those who have a space-occupying lesion that can be surgically removed. A review of literature finds studies that quote from 40% to 90% success, but almost universally find that if the source of compression can be clearly identified and eliminated, the patient does more predictably well.
- Assuming there is no residual nerve dysfunction from long-standing compression, patients should be able to begin gradual return to play at 6 to 8 weeks of recovery.

Complications/Indications for Referral

Indications for more expeditious referral for tibial tunnel syndrome would be evidence of intrinsic muscle weakness or wasting, suggesting more severe disease. Also, if the workup shows a discrete mass or lesion that directs surgical attention, an earlier referral might be warranted.

The main complication to be aware of would be recurrence of symptoms. If a patient had a surgical decompression performed and had resolution of symptoms, only to have them recur, it is possible that scar tissue has recreated compression on the nerve. In this situation, the patient should return to their surgeon for re-evaluation.

APPROACH TO THE ATHLETE WITH STRESS FRACTURE OF THE FOOT

Stress fractures of the bony structures in the foot arise from repetitive injury. The metatarsals, navicular, and calcaneus are common sites for fractures that occur as a result of overuse or sudden increase in activity. In cases such as the proximal fifth metatarsal and navicular, the bone has areas of tenuous blood supply, which render it susceptible to stress injury. An injury to the fifth metatarsal through the proximal diaphyseal/metaphyseal junction is known as a Jones fracture and can be difficult to manage (Figs. 20.8–20.10). Fractures in zone 1 and zone 2 typically heal uneventfully, but special attention should be paid to zone 3 injuries as they may be more difficult to heal. Decreased bone density or factors such as steroids or endocrine dysfunction that predispose one to osteoporosis can also predispose a patient to stress fractures.

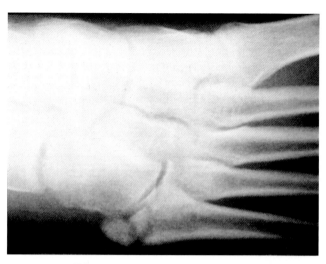

FIG. 20.8. Fifth metatarsal zone 1 injury. Reprinted with permission from Buchholz RW, Heckman JD. *Rockwood & Green's Fractures in Adults.* 5th ed. Philadelphia, PA: Lippincott Williams & Wilkins; 2001.

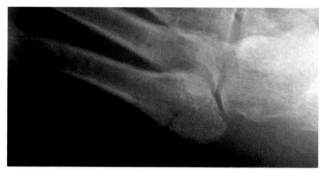

FIG. 20.9. Fifth metatarsal zone 2 injury. Reprinted with permission from Buchholz RW, Heckman JD. *Rockwood & Green's Fractures in Adults.* 5th ed. Philadelphia, PA: Lippincott Williams & Wilkins; 2001.

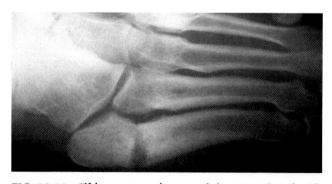

FIG. 20.10. Fifth metatarsal zone 3 injury. Reprinted with permission from Buchholz RW, Heckman JD. *Rockwood & Green's Fractures in Adults.* 5th ed. Philadelphia, PA: Lippincott Williams & Wilkins; 2001.

HISTORY AND PHYSICAL EXAMINATION

Patients will present with pain on weight bearing, localized to the area of injury. Often, they are athletes involved in activities with repetitive loading such as football or ballet. The discomfort increases with activity and becomes more intense over time as the stress fracture propagates. A patient may have difficulty with training or running, with symptoms developing over 2 to 6 weeks without acute injury or incident. Because of the indolent nature of symptoms, physicians must have a high index of suspicion when investigating these injuries so as not to misdiagnose a patient's foot pain.

On physical examination, point tenderness to palpation helps localize the injury and focus further study. There may be swelling as well, which can be important in differentiating plantar fasciitis from a calcaneus stress fracture. Classically, ballet dancers will develop pain over the metatarsals, most frequently the second metatarsal base. Patients with fifth metatarsal stress fractures will have lateral foot pain and frequently underlying cavovarus deformity that increases lateral weight bearing in the foot. Navicular stress fractures will present with dorsal midfoot pain. Discomfort in the posterior–superior aspect of the calcaneus along with pain on medial/lateral compression of the calcaneus suggests stress fracture in that bone.

DIAGNOSTIC TESTING

Diagnostic testing should always begin with x-rays of the foot. If there is a fracture visible, then the diagnosis is easy. Unfortunately, stress fractures are not always easily visible. If there is no fracture clearly seen on x-ray, one should look carefully in areas that were tender on physical examination for periosteal reaction and sclerosis that can diagnose the stress fracture.

If the x-rays are negative, and there is a high index of suspicion, then a bone scan is a helpful follow-up study. The bone scan will be positive in areas of fracture within 48 to 72 hours of initial injury. In most cases, patients present with stress fractures after several weeks of symptoms and thus the bone scans should be positive. An MRI is an additional test that frequently gives helpful information. Stress fractures appear as areas of bony edema and help localize the injury. One can also rule out other soft-tissue injuries as sources of pain. Lastly, a CT scan can help characterize a fracture line more clearly, particularly in the navicular stress fractures where the bone is not as easily seen on plain x-rays.

TREATMENT

Nonoperative

- Immobilization.
- Non–weight bearing.
- Hard-soled shoe.

- Walking boot/cast.
- Nonoperative management should heal about 75% of Jones fractures, but may take as long as 5 or 6 months of treatment.[9]
- Navicular stress fractures should be treated similarly to Jones fractures with immobilization in a non–weight-bearing cast for at least 6 weeks followed by at least 6 weeks of progressive weight bearing out of the cast.[10]

Operative

- Indications for referral for operative management would be displaced fractures or those that fail nonoperative management by having persisting pain even after prolonged immobilization and restricted weight bearing.
- Elite or high-level competitive athletes with Jones fractures, Navicular stress fractures, or other stress fractures should immediately be referred for operative intervention as it frequently allows for earlier return to play.[11]
- Postoperative management for foot fractures involves non–weight bearing and immobilization postoperatively.
- For metatarsal and Jones fractures, this period may be as short as 2 weeks, whereas for navicular fractures it might be as long as 6 weeks, depending on the severity of the fracture and fixation necessary in surgery.
- After this period, patients can progress weight bearing gradually, and when there is motion and weight bearing without any pain, the patient can return to their regular activities and progress to return to play.

Prognosis/Return to Play

- Nonoperative management will be successful in the majority of cases, but can take several months of healing.
- A key for allowing athletes to return to play is healing of the fracture (as seen on x-ray) with no evidence of tenderness on palpation, weight bearing, or other stress. Most frequently, this takes about 6 to 8 weeks.
- Once pain is completely gone, patients can begin training again and can return to play once cutting and running can be performed without discomfort.
- The patient may be aided by an orthotic support to help decrease load through the injured bone.
- Return too soon, without complete healing of the fracture, can lead to refracture of the bone and restart of the healing process.

Complications/Indications for Referral

The main complication in managing stress fractures is that they may not heal. In cases of delayed union or nonunion, patients should be referred for operative intervention. Additionally, elite or professional athletes can be referred for earlier intervention. Lastly, patients with recurrent stress fractures should be considered for investigation of underlying metabolic or endocrine dysfunction that may contribute to decreased bone density. Also, recurrent stress fractures may be a sign of an underlying problem with the posture of the foot or hindfoot and should be referred for further investigation.

APPROACH TO THE ATHLETE WITH PLANTAR FASCIITIS

The plantar fascia is a thick, fibrous layer of tissue that originates on the medial aspect of the calcaneus and inserts at the bases of the five proximal phalanges. Inflammation of this fascia is known as plantar fasciitis, which stems from degeneration and microtears within the fascia, usually near its calcaneal origin. It is regarded as the most common cause of heel pain in athletes.

HISTORY AND PHYSICAL EXAMINATION

The patient with plantar fasciitis is generally a middle-aged, overweight person who will present with complaint of heel pain that is at the plantar, medial heel without radiation. It is gradual in onset without antecedent trauma. Classically, the patient will describe pain when taking the first steps of the day after arising from bed. These patients will improve through the day as the plantar fascia is able to stretch with walking. The pain generally subsides with rest and will increase with overuse. As the fasciitis becomes more chronic, it can alter gait and illicit pain with every step.

On physical examination, the patient will often localize pain to the medial calcaneal tuberosity (plantar fascia insertion). Palpation there or stretching the fascia should reproduce the patient's symptoms. Be sure to palpate the medial border of the fascia itself with the toes dorsiflexed, as laxity or incompetence of the fascia by comparison to the unaffected foot may indicate a plantar fascial rupture. It is important to remember that one should examine the entire foot and ankle to determine if there is any malalignment, swelling, warmth, or neuropathic symptoms that may point toward another diagnosis, even if the history may be very convincing for plantar fasciitis.

DIAGNOSTIC TESTING

Diagnosis of plantar fasciitis is most often made by obtaining a thorough history and physical examination. Obtaining weight-bearing x-rays would be helpful to evaluate foot and ankle position and alignment. Also, one could determine if a plantar heel spur exists that could be contributing to the fasciitis symptoms. Other imaging might include an MRI that could show a thickened fascia and edema through the fascial insertion. Lastly, a bone scan would show increased uptake at the calcaneus, and an ultrasound would show a thickened fascia, but generally, these tests are unnecessary to make the diagnosis.

If one is trying to rule out tarsal tunnel syndrome or other nerve compression as the etiology for heel pain, one could consider an anesthetic injection. If the anesthetic injection decreases the pain, it is likely not plantar fasciitis.

TREATMENT

Nonoperative

- Nonoperative management of plantar fasciitis successful in almost 100% of patients[13]
- Ice
- Stretching the plantar fascia and achilles
- NSAIDs
- Minimize overuse
- Night splints
- Orthotics (over the counter vs. custom)[12]
- Casting/immobilization particularly with fascial rupture
- Injection (anesthetic vs. corticosteroid)[13]
- Extracorporeal shock-wave therapy (ESWT)[14]
- A combination of any or all of the nonoperative options employed for as long as 6 to 12 months before considering surgery

Operative

- An operation for plantar fasciitis is controversial, and as such, the American Orthopaedic Foot and Ankle Society has issued a position statement as a guide to open heel surgery.
- The goal of the statement is to emphasize the importance of nonoperative management and assure careful consideration and discussion before intervention.
- One study showed only about 50% of patients with complete satisfaction after operative intervention.[15]
- Should one work through up to 1 year of nonoperative management and still have symptoms, then referral may be needed.
- If surgery is decided upon, it usually involves release of the fascia through an incision on the medial side of the calcaneus.
- Postoperatively, patients can expect to be non–weight bearing for about 3 weeks followed by weight bearing in a cast for an additional 4 weeks.
- Overall, activity will begin to increase toward normal at about 12 weeks.

Prognosis/Return to Play

- A patient will have difficulty returning to full activity until symptoms resolve completely.
- It may be that an athlete can return for short periods of time as symptoms improve, but this may prove detrimental

as the fasciitis may not have completely resolved and symptoms may return.

- The problem may not be eliminated until a prolonged period of rest and nonoperative intervention.
- For those who elect surgery, a patient may gradually return to play starting at about 3 months after surgery. It may be, however, that it takes a patient as long as 12 months postoperatively to return to full strength.

Complications/Indications for Referral

Unfortunately, plantar fasciitis can be a difficult problem to resolve. Patients should be referred if there is no progress with nonoperative intervention or if there is a question about another etiology for the heel pain that may warrant surgical intervention.

APPROACH TO THE ATHLETE WITH METATARSALGIA

Metatarsalgia is a nonspecific term used to describe pain on the plantar aspect of the foot in the region of the MTP joints. The symptoms can occur for a wide variety of reasons, but the majority seem to stem from improper footwear. Athletes involved in high-impact sports, where overuse injury to the forefoot is more likely, can develop symptoms as well.

The position of the toes is controlled by the intrinsic and extrinsic forces of muscles, tendons, and static stabilizers such as ligamentous and capsular structures that act at the MTP, proximal interphalangeal (PIP), and distal interphalangeal (DIP) joints. A disruption to the balance of this system can lead to pathology in the toe that eventually causes the metatarsalgia symptom of plantar foot pain. The causes are numerous and include the following:

1. Claw toe – hyperextension at the MTP with flexion at the PIP and DIP joints
2. Hammer toe – hyperextension of the MTP and DIP with flexion at the PIP joint
3. Mallet toe – flexion of the DIP joint
4. Synovitis – inflammation of an isolated MTP joint synovium and capsule causing pain
5. Systemic inflammatory disease – systemic illness leading to inflammation of the MTP joints, causing pain, subluxation, and dislocation
6. Intractable plantar keratosis – development of localized, discrete thickening of skin under metatarsal heads
7. Freiberg's infraction – osteochondrosis of the metatarsal head, most often the second metatarsal

In general, these deformities or pathologies lead to altered mechanics at the MTP joints, which causes plantar displacement of the metatarsal heads. Over time, this causes increasing pain and may lead to the plantar fat pad migrating distally. This leaves the metatarsal heads uncovered, furthering symptoms in this area of the foot.

HISTORY AND PHYSICAL EXAMINATION

The goal of the history and physical examination is to begin to discern what the source of the metatarsalgia is, as this is key to the proper treatment of the disease. The presenting complaint involves pain on the plantar aspect of the foot, in the area of the MTP joints. Patients will have the most discomfort with the push-off phase of gait, as the MTP becomes dorsiflexed. The pain might be difficult to localize, having developed over several weeks or months.

On physical examination, one should note the position of the toes in stance as normal, claw, hammer, or mallet toes and identify any corresponding callosities or plantar keratosis. If a patient describes relief of pain with walking barefoot, this might suggest that shoe wear is contributing to their disease process. Conversely, they may describe relief of pain with shoe wear, hinting at uncovered metatarsal heads due to displacement of the plantar fat pad as the source of discomfort. The anterior drawer test can be performed at the MTP joints by stabilizing the metatarsal and attempting to dorsally displace the proximal phalanx of the corresponding toe. Joint displacement and pain suggest instability at the MTP joint. If there is a toe deformity, it should be manipulated to see if it is corectable (flexible) or not (fixed), as this will influence treatment options, particularly at the time of surgery. Lastly, the gastrocnemius/soleus complex and Achilles tendon should be examined for tightness or contracture which can lead to forefoot overload and pain at the plantar aspect of the MTP joints.

Further findings might include a swollen, erythematous, or boggy toe that suggest synovitis or a systemic inflammatory process. Warmth and swelling with decreased range of motion at the MTP joint might suggest Freiberg's infraction, so this should be considered carefully as well.

Because there are so many causes for forefoot pain, one must be sure to also consider diabetic neuropathy, radicular pathology from low-back problems, and vascular disease among other more systemic causes for metatarsalgia-type symptoms.

DIAGNOSTIC TESTING

With all metatarsalgia complaints, weight-bearing x-rays of the foot should be obtained. A widened MTP joint space suggests a synovitic or inflammatory process, whereas a narrowed MTP joint space suggests MTP hyperextension or subluxation. In extreme subluxation or dislocation, one might find a "gun-barrel" sign on the AP x-ray, where the proximal phalanx is seen on end, as the projection looks down the shaft of the phalanx. One might find erosions of the MTP joint in rheumatoid disease or sclerosis and collapse of the metatarsal head in the later stages of Freiberg's infraction. In addition to the joint and joint space, one should look carefully for bony prominences that might contribute to pain or development of keratoses. Lastly, the x-rays are important for ruling out other midfoot or hindfoot problems such as cavovarus deformity that might be contributing to the metatarsalgia.

If there does not seem to be a reason for the forefoot pain that is evident by history, physical examination, and x-rays, then one should consider early Freiberg's infraction or stress fracture as the source of pathology. In this circumstance, a bone scan or an MRI would be helpful for further investigation to identify bony edema or other evidence of osteonecrosis. The MRI would also be helpful in further evaluating the joint capsule, ligamentous structures, and tendinous structures around the MTP joint and toes.

TREATMENT

Nonoperative

- Shoe modification
  - Wide toe box
  - Extra-depth shoes
  - Metatarsal bar/pad
  - Steel plate/stiff sole
- NSAIDs
- Steroid injection[16]
- Plantar keratosis shaving
- Immobilization

Operative

- Soft-tissue release
- Tendon transfer
- Osteotomy
- Combination of the above

Prognosis/Return to Play

- Patients do well if the source of metatarsalgia can be properly identified and treated.
- Return to play for athletes will be dictated by the nature of the injury and the nature of treatment they receive.
- For nonoperative interventions, athletes can return to sport gradually once their metatarsalgia symptoms have subsided.
- For surgical intervention, return to athletics can occur once the toe range of motion and function has returned and the patient is free of pain. In both scenarios, this can take several months.

Complications/Indications for Referral

In general, patients should be referred to an orthopedic surgeon when nonoperative intervention has failed or when the deformity causing the metatarsalgia seems fixed and nonflexible. Further, if a patient has had a foot and ankle procedure in the past and presents with new onset or recurrence of metatarsalgia, the patient should be referred back to their surgeon. An entity called transfer metatarsalgia can occur where a procedure such as a metatarsal osteotomy alters the weight-bearing mechanics of the foot and creates increased pressure at the other MTP joints.

APPROACH TO THE ATHLETE WITH MORTON'S NEUROMA

A Morton's neuroma is a painful entrapment neuropathy of a digital nerve in the foot. The interdigital nerve courses beneath the transverse intermetatarsal ligament and becomes compressed at this point, often because of thickening of the ligament or direct trauma. The vast majority of neuromas occur in the third webspace of the foot, with the second webspace being next most common. Rarely do they occur in the first or fourth webspaces.

HISTORY AND PHYSICAL EXAMINATION

A patient with a Morton's neuroma will present with pain at the plantar aspect of the foot in a webspace, at or just distal to the metatarsal heads. This pain burns and radiates to the toes. Often, patients will describe that they feel as if they are walking on a marble or wrinkle in their sock. Typically, the patient wears narrow-toed shoes or high heels frequently, as dorsiflexion and compression of the toes over time can lead to increased irritation of the digital nerve. Pain is relieved by resting the feet or removing the offending footwear.

Physical examination will find tenderness to palpation in a webspace. A neuroma as the source of pain may be difficult to discern from other structures or causes of pain in that region such as MTP joint synovitis. Careful examination is therefore warranted. One can attempt to reproduce the patient's pain by directing dorsal pressure on the plantar interspace over the digital nerve in question. With this directed force, the foot should then be squeezed in a medial to lateral direction. The digital nerve will then be pushed in the plantar direction. If a clicking occurs and reproduces the patient's pain, this is called Mulder's sign, suggesting an interdigital neuroma is present.

DIAGNOSTIC TESTING

In the large majority of cases, the diagnosis can be made with a thorough history and physical examination. Most patients do not need diagnostic studies to be performed. If the diagnosis is in doubt, however, ultrasound has been shown to correlate closely to clinical findings at the time of surgery and can be used for diagnosis.[17] MRI has also been suggested, but has not been shown to have the same association to findings.

Alternatively, one can consider an injection of anesthetic into the webspace to help with the diagnosis. If a patient has relief of symptoms from this injection, it can support a neuroma as the cause of pain. One must be careful, however, that other local pathology (i.e., synovitis) may also be relieved by an injection of anesthetic.

TREATMENT

Nonoperative

- Shoe modification
  - Wide toe box
  - Lower heel
  - Stiffer sole
  - Metatarsal pad
- Steroid injection[18]

Operative

- If conservative measures have failed, then operative intervention would be indicated.
- Importantly, as with any operation, one should do one's best to be sure of the diagnosis.
- The procedure itself is customarily done as an outpatient and involves a dorsal or plantar incision to resect the diseased portion of nerve.
- Postoperatively, with a dorsal approach, the patient will customarily walk as tolerated in a post-op shoe until the wound is healed. With a plantar approach, the patient will heel-weight bear until the wound is completely healed.
- When the wound is completely healed, the patient can resume wearing a regular shoe and working with active and passive range of motion as tolerated, resuming their normal activity.

Prognosis/Return to Play

- At 5 years after surgery, the satisfaction rate with operative intervention was found to be 85%.[19]
- Patients can expect to have numbness through the webspace and a portion of their toes that remains after surgery.
- As they move from their postoperative period and the surgical wound heals, patients should be able to return to play as tolerated.

Complications/Indications for Referral

Patients should be referred to a surgeon if nonoperative measures fail. Also, if a patient returns with persisting complaints that have not improved postoperatively, it is possible that they were initially misdiagnosed and there is a source of pain other than a neuroma. Also, if the patient's symptoms resolve and then slowly return, it is possible that a neuroma at the stump of the resected digital nerve has formed. In either of these situations, one should consider a referral to a specialist for further intervention.

APPROACH TO THE ATHLETE WITH SESAMOIDITIS

The sesamoid bones of the great toe lie within the flexor hallucis brevis tendon, plantar to the distal aspect of the first metatarsal. They function to absorb and transmit weight to the foot while increasing mechanical advantage in flexion of the great toe. The sesamoids can cause pain in the foot for reasons such as fracture, subluxation, arthritis, and osteonecrosis. If there does not appear to be a clear etiology for sesamoidal pain, then one is diagnosed with sesamoiditis as a diagnosis of exclusion.

Sesamoiditis is pain that occurs from the sesamoids of the great toe without known trauma. It can be disabling and has increased in incidence with participation in athletics and use of artificial surfaces for competition. Sesamoid cartilage is thought to be abnormal as sesamoiditis develops with repetitive injury or stress.

HISTORY AND PHYSICAL EXAMINATION

A patient will present with pain on the plantar aspect of the first metatarsal head that is worse with push-off in gait or running and relieved by rest. The onset of pain seems to be insidious, with a gradual progression of discomfort and no clear evidence of trauma.

An examination will reveal a maximal area of tenderness overlying the sesamoid bones on the plantar foot. It may be possible to distinguish medial from lateral sesamoid pathology, with the medial being a classically bigger bone with greater weight bearing and thus more common injury. A callus might be noted in this area of the foot and occasionally swelling as well. Hyperextension of the great toe will exacerbate symptoms as tension is exerted through the flexor tendons with this maneuver.

Lastly, the position of the foot should be examined, as a cavus foot may be predisposed to developing sesamoiditis. These patients often have a plantarflexed first ray that could proportionally increase the weight-bearing load of the sesamoid bones and lead to pain.

DIAGNOSTIC TESTING

AP and lateral x-rays should be taken to rule out fracture in the foot and examine overall foot position. Additionally, an axial view of the sesamoids (similar to a sunrise view of the patella) should be taken to examine for joint space narrowing or subluxation that might be leading to pathology. Medial and lateral oblique x-rays of the sesamoids can also be performed to help more clearly evaluate the bones without obstruction from overlying metatarsals. In reviewing x-rays, consideration should be given to fracture, dislocation, and arthritis of the bones. Also, if the sesamoids appear to have migrated proximally, consideration should be given to a plantar plate injury or turf toe. It should be noted that occasionally the sesamoid can be bipartite (medial more than lateral), which should not be mistaken for a fracture.

Other studies can be helpful such as a bone scan. It can help discern between an acute fracture and a bipartite sesamoid or between osteonecrosis and sesamoiditis. Bone scans should be interpreted carefully, however, as there can be false-positive results.

MRI is another imaging study that can be ordered to gather information. It might be helpful in diagnosing a plantar plate injury or stress fracture.

TREATMENT

Nonoperative

- Activity modification
- NSAIDs
- Metatarsal bar/pad
- Taping of the great toe in neutral or plantarflexed position
- Short leg cast for 6 to 8 weeks
- Steroid injection

Operative

- Surgical intervention should be considered only after exhausting conservative measures for 6 to 12 months or in the case of a complete plantar plate disruption.
- If the sesamoids are still causing pain, then one can consider excision of the bone.
- Generally, only one of the two sesamoids is excised so as not to predispose the great toe to a hyperdorsiflexion deformity or clawing.
- Most procedures are performed on the plantar aspect of the foot.
- Postoperatively, the patient will be in a soft dressing for about 7 to 10 days and then heel-weight bearing in a postoperative shoe until the wound is completely healed.
- One might tape the great toe in neutral or slight plantarflexion to decrease the extension stresses across the surgical site.
- Full weight bearing and return to normal activities would begin as tolerated gradually after 8 weeks.

Prognosis/Return to Play

- Patients with sesamoiditis can return to play as tolerated, understanding that their symptoms may never completely resolve until a prolonged period of decreased activity or immobilization.
- If the point of surgery is reached, a patient can often return gradually after 8 weeks of recovery.

Complications/Indications for Referral

Indications for referral would include acute fracture, plantar plate avulsion, flexor tendon injury, severe bunion deformity, or other great toe pathology that has specific etiology in need of surgical attention. If the diagnosis of sesamoiditis is reached by exclusion, one should be aware that it can take up to a year to resolve completely.

KEY POINTS
• A working knowledge of foot and ankle anatomy and function is critical to proper examination and diagnosis of chronic injuries
• Functional ankle instability can be successfully treated with surgery after a course of nonoperative modalities
• Patients with foot deformity in posterior tibialis dysfunction should be referred to a surgeon
• Evidence of muscle weakness or wasting in tarsal tunnel syndrome should be documented with EMG and referred to a surgeon
• One must maintain a high index of suspicion for stress fractures so as not to miss a diagnosis
• Surgery for plantar fasciitis is controversial and should be considered only after exhaustive attempts at nonoperative management
• It is critical to determine the cause of metatarsalgia to properly direct management

REFERENCES

1. Messina DF, Farney WC, DeLee JC. The incidence of injury in Texas high school basketball. A prospective study among male and female athletes. *Am J Sports Med.* 1999;27:294–299.
2. Thordarson DB, ed. *Orthopaedic Surgery Essentials: Foot and Ankle.* New York, NY: Lippincott Williams & Wilkins; 2004.
3. Frost SC, Amendola A. Is stress radiography necessary in the diagnosis of acute or chronic ankle instability? *Clin J Sports Med.* 1999;9: 40–45.
4. Komenda GA, Ferkel RD. Arthroscopic findings associated with the unstable ankle. *Foot Ankle Int.* 1999;20(11):708–713.
5. Kitaoka HB, Lee MD, Morrey BF, et al. Acute repair and delayed reconstruction for lateral instability: twenty-year follow-up study. *J Orthop Trauma.* 1997;11:530–535.
6. Rosenberg ZS, Beltran J, Cheung YY, et al. MR features of longitudinal tears of the peroneus brevis tendon. *Am J Roentgenol.* 1997;168: 141–147.
7. Kinoshita M, Okuda R, Yasuda T, et al. Tarsal tunnel syndrome in athletes. *Am J Sports Med.* 2006;34(8):1307–1312.
8. Kinoshita M, Okuda R, Morikawa J, et al. The dorsiflexion-eversion test for diagnosis of tarsal tunnel syndrome. *J Bone Joint Surg Am.* 2001;83:1835–1839.
9. Clapper M, O'Brien TJ, Lyons PM. Fractures of the fifth metatarsal. Analysis of fracture registry. *Clin Orthop Relat Res.* 1995;315: 238–241.
10. Khan K, Brukner PD, Kearney C, et al. Tarsal navicular stress fracture in athletes. *Sports Med.* 1994;17:65–76.
11. DeLee J, Evans JP, Julian J. Stress fractures of the fifth metatarsal. *Am J Sports Med.* 1983;5:349–353.

12. Pfeffer G, Bacchetti P, Deland J, et al. Comparison of custom and pre-fabricated orthoses in the initial treatment of proximal plantar fasciitis. *Foot Ankle Int.* 1999;20:214–221.

13. Crawford F, Atkins D, Young P, et al. Steroid injection for heel pain: evidence of short-term effectiveness. A randomized controlled trial. *Rheumatology.* 1999;38:974–977.

14. Ogden JA, Alvarez R, Levitt R, et al. Shock wave therapy for chronic proximal plantar fasciitis. *Clin Orthop Relat Res.* 2001;387:47–59.

15. Davies MS, Weiss GA, Saxby TS. Plantar fasciitis: how successful is surgical intervention? *Foot Ankle Int.* 1999;20:803–807.

16. Mizel MS, Trepman ET. Non-operative treatment of metatarsophalangeal joint synovitis. *Foot Ankle.* 1993;14:305.

17. Quinn TJ, Jacobson JA, Craig JG, et al. Sonography of Morton's neuromas. *Am J Roentgenol.* 2000;174:1723–1728.

18. Rasmussen MR, Kitaoka HB, Patzer GL. Nonoperative treatment of plantar interdigital neuroma with a single corticosteroid injection. *Clin Orthop Relat Res.* 1996;326:188–193.

19. Coughlin MJ, Pinsonneault T. Operative treatment of interdigital neuroma: a long-term follow-up study. *J Bone Joint Surg Am.* 2001;83: 1321–1328.

Athlete with Acute Foot and Ankle Injuries

Daniel Osuch and Nicola DeAngelis

INTRODUCTION

The ankle is a complex joint composed of three bones, stabilized by several ligaments, and traversed by a number of tendons. It is a relatively constrained joint that is subject to complex forces and stresses. As such, it is the most commonly injured joint in the body and prone to a number of acute and chronic conditions that can lead to significant disability if not recognized or treated properly. To that end, this chapter aims to provide a relatively concise understanding of ankle joint anatomy and several commonly encountered injuries. A thorough understanding of these concepts will serve to minimize disability and help to efficiently return athletes to their sports-related activities.

FUNCTIONAL ANATOMY

When considering the anatomy of the ankle, it is useful to break the ankle down into its three main components: bony, ligamentous, and musculotendinous. Understanding each of these individually is essential to understanding the ankle as a whole. In its simplest form, the ankle is a hinge joint composed of three bones, the tibia, fibula, and talus, and three ligamentous complexes, the medial, lateral, and syndesmotic. Its anatomic features leave the tibiotalar articulation more rigid medially than laterally, more stable in dorsiflexion than in plantar flexion, and sensitive to minor changes in biomechanical stability. Since the tibiotalar articulation is subjected to more load per unit area than any other joint in the body, understanding these relationships is paramount.[1] Three bones compose the ankle joint: the tibia, fibula, and talus. The tibia and fibula form the mortise around the talus (Fig. 21.1). It is important to note that the talus also articulates with the navicular and calcaneus in the foot.

The tibia provides most of the proximal articular surface (plafond) and medial bony constraint (medial malleolus) to the ankle joint. The tibia is the larger of the long bones of the leg and flares distally, where it contributes to the tibiotalar articulation. The plafond is concave when viewed laterally, which accommodates the talar dome. The plafond is also wider medially than laterally and extends further distally

posteriorly (the posterior malleolus) than anteriorly. Because of this complex shape, a minimal subluxation of the talus under the tibia can lead to significantly increased contact stresses and predispose to osteoarthritis.[2,3] The medial malleolus is found anteromedially in the ankle joint and serves as the attachment site for the deltoid ligaments, an important medial stabilizer. It has two subtle prominences called colliculi: the anterior colliculus, which serves as the attachment point for the superficial deltoid ligament, and the posterior colliculus, which anchors the deep deltoid ligament.

The fibula provides lateral bony stability to the ankle joint. It is the smaller of the long bones of the leg and flares distally to form the lateral malleolus. The lateral malleolus extends more posteriorly and distally than the medial malleolus. It also slopes laterally as it comes to its tip. The medial fibula serves as the attachment point of the syndesmotic ligaments and some of the lateral ankle ligaments. The fibula must also externally rotate and migrate proximally to accommodate the talus in ankle dorsiflexion.

The talus is found distal to the tibia and fibula and within the bony confines of the medial and lateral malleoli. It is composed of three main parts: the body (or dome), neck, and head. Sixty percent to 70% of the talar surface is covered by articular cartilage. The talar body articulates with the tibial plafond and is convex in shape. It is also wider anteriorly than posteriorly, which contributes stability to the ankle in dorsiflexion. Many ligamentous attachments from the malleoli and the subtalar joint serve to anchor the talus in place. Also, since its surface is mostly articular, its blood supply is relatively sparse, leaving the talus prone to avascular necrosis, particularly when the neck is fractured.

The ankle is supported by three sets of ligaments: the medial deltoid ligaments, the lateral ligaments, and the syndesmotic ligaments (Fig. 21.1). Three ligaments make up the lateral ankle ligamentous complex, the anterior talofibular ligament (ATFL), the calcaneofibular ligament (CFL), and the posterior talofibular ligament (PTFL). Since each of these ligaments is under varied tension throughout ankle range of motion, the lateral tibiotalar articulation is somewhat flexible.

Each of these ligaments is also confluent with the ankle joint capsule. The ATFL originates from the anterior lateral

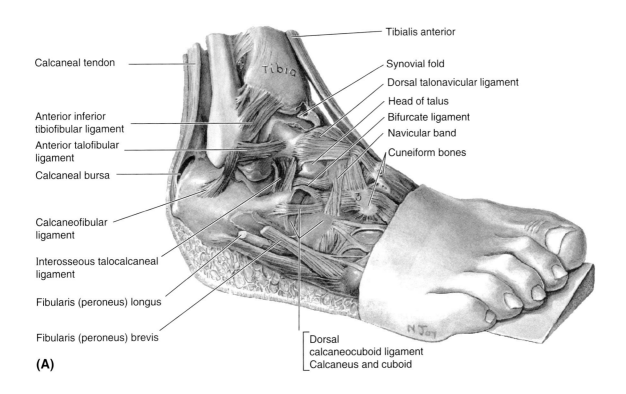

Tibialis anterior

Calcaneal tendon

Synovial fold

Dorsal talonavicular ligament

Head of talus

Bifurcate ligament

Anterior inferior
tibiofibular ligament

Navicular band

Anterior talofibular
ligament

Cuneiform bones

Calcaneal bursa

Calcaneofibular
ligament

Interosseous talocalcaneal
ligament

Fibularis (peroneus) longus

Fibularis (peroneus) brevis

Dorsal
calcaneocuboid ligament
Calcaneus and cuboid

(A)

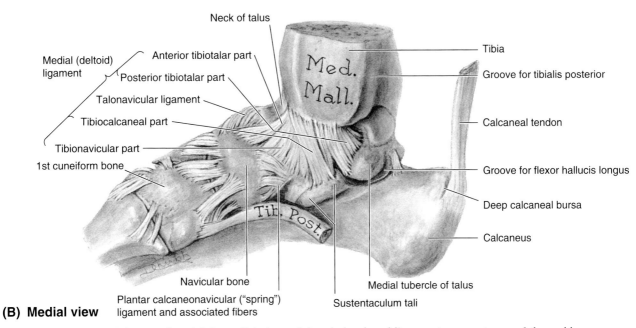

Neck of talus

Tibia

Medial (deltoid)
ligament

Anterior tibiotalar part

Groove for tibialis posterior

Posterior tibiotalar part

Talonavicular ligament

Tibiocalcaneal part

Calcaneal tendon

Tibionavicular part

Groove for flexor hallucis longus

1st cuneiform bone

Deep calcaneal bursa

Calcaneus

Navicular bone

Medial tubercle of talus

(B) Medial view   Plantar calcaneonavicular ("spring")
ligament and associated fibers

Sustentaculum tali

FIG. 21.1. (A) Lateral and **(B)** medial view of the skeletal and ligamentous anatomy of the ankle
and hindfoot. Reprinted with permission from Moore KL, Dalley AF II. *Clinically Oriented Anatomy.*
4th ed. Baltimore: Lippincott Williams & Wilkins; 1999.

malleolus and inserts on the anterior articular facet of the
talus. It provides stability to the ankle when it is plantar
flexed and inverted. With the ankle in neutral, the ATFL
limits rotation and anterior talar translation. Since it is the
weakest of the lateral ankle ligaments, the ATFL is most
commonly injured in an ankle sprain. The CFL originates

just distal and posterior to the ATFL on the lateral malleolus
and inserts posteriorly on the posterior–superior tubercle
of the calcaneus. The CFL is taut in neutral and tightens
with ankle dorsiflexion. It is susceptible to injury with ankle
dorsiflexion and inversion. It also serves to help stabilize the
subtalar joint. The PTFL originates on the posterior–medial

lateral malleolus and inserts broadly on the posterior talus. It is very stout, limits dorsiflexion, and is rarely injured. However, with an injured ATFL, the PTFL assumes a larger role in limiting talar internal rotation.

The deltoid ligament confers stability to the medial ankle. It is composed of two portions: the thinner superficial layer, which originates on the anterior colliculus and inserts on the sustentaculum tali and spring ligaments, and the thicker deep layer, which originates on the posterior colliculus and inserts on the medial talus. The deep deltoid ligament is also intra-articular and confluent with the ankle capsule. Both parts of the deltoid ligament limit ankle eversion, but the deep layer is the primary medial stabilizer.[4] With lateral ligament injury, the deltoid ligament helps to stabilize anterior and lateral migration of the talus.

There are four syndesmotic ligaments which run between the tibia and fibula, and they are essential to the structural integrity of the ankle. They are the interosseous ligament, anterior–inferior tibiofibular ligament (AITFL), the posterior–inferior tibiofibular ligament (PITFL), and the transverse tibiofibular ligament. The syndesmotic ligaments maintain the relationship between the tibia and fibula throughout the arc of ankle motion and also help prevent excessive external rotation of the fibula when the lateral ankle ligaments are torn and the ankle is dorsiflexed. The most commonly injured syndesmotic ligament is the AITFL. The PITFL serves to deepen the ankle joint. The interosseous ligament is the primary connection between the tibia and fibula and is confluent proximally with the interosseous membrane. Injury to the syndesmotic ligaments generally takes a good degree of force, typically with external rotation. This injury is commonly referred to as a "high ankle sprain" and is considered serious.

A number of tendons cross the ankle joint; several of these contribute to ankle stability (Fig. 21.1). The primary dynamic stabilizers of the ankle are the peroneus longus and brevis, the tendons of which course posterior and inferior to the lateral malleolus below the superior peroneal retinaculum. Both are innervated by the deep peroneal nerve and originate on the lateral fibula. The peroneus brevis inserts on the base of the fifth metatarsal and the peroneus longus courses across the plantar aspect of the foot where it inserts on the base of the first metatarsal and medial cuneiform. They both serve to evert and stabilize the ankle and are important to ankle proprioception (an essential aspect of recovery from ankle injury).

There are a number of other important tendons about the ankle joint. The Achilles tendon runs posteriorly and inserts on the calcaneal tuberosity. It is the primary ankle plantar flexor. The tibialis posterior, flexor digitorum longus, and flexor hallucis longus are found posterior medially and are secondary ankle plantar flexors and inverters. Anteriorly, the tibialis anterior (the primary ankle dorsiflexor), extensor digitorum longus, and extensor hallucis longus also cross the ankle joint.

EPIDEMIOLOGY

Inversion ankle sprains are the most common athletic injury to the ankle. They account for up to 75% of ankle injuries.[5] Occurrence rates have been quoted anywhere from 0.68 to 3.85 sprains per 1,000 person-days of exposure.[6–10] Though traditionally considered minor, ankle sprains can lead to significant disability in the athlete.[11] These injuries are classified according to severity from grade I through grade III. A grade I injury is consistent with ligament stretching or partial tear. It typically leads to mild tenderness and swelling, minimal functional loss, and no mechanical instability. A grade II injury involves an incomplete ligament tear, leading to moderate pain and swelling with ecchymoses, tenderness to palpation, loss of motion and function, and mild to moderate instability. A grade III injury involves a complete tear and loss of integrity of a ligament, leading to more severe swelling and ecchymoses, loss of function and motion, and mechanical instability on stress testing.[12]

Though less common than conventional ankle sprains, syndesmotic injuries or high ankle sprains represent a significant injury to the ankle that can result in prolonged disability. These injuries represent approximately 1% of all ankle "sprains."[13] Syndesmotic injuries have gained increasing attention in recent years, because they are often difficult to diagnose and are associated with prolonged recovery compared to conventional ankle sprains, and optimal management is controversial. High ankle sprains occur by an external rotation stress to the ankle that stretches/tears the syndesmotic ligaments, often in the absence of an associated fracture. They can be classified into three categories: sprain without diastasis, sprain with latent diastasis (present on stress x-rays only), and sprain with frank diastasis (present on initial x-rays).[14]

Ankle fractures are one of the most common skeletal injuries and are increasing in incidence, especially with an aging population.[15,16] The incidence of ankle fractures is estimated at approximately 175 per 100,000 persons.[17] Risk factors for ankle fractures include increased body mass index and a history of smoking.[18] Though most work on ankle fractures has focused on the general population, they are also quite common in athletes. Surgical fixation of ankle fractures is the fifth most common procedure performed on prospective National Football League (NFL) players and the most common form of fracture fixation in this population.[19] Improperly managed ankle fractures can lead to significant disability such as posttraumatic arthritis, especially in a young athlete.

Osteochondral lesions of the talus are relatively rare, but since the talus has a tenuous blood supply and limited capacity for healing, these can be devastating injuries to the ankle. These lesions affect the articular cartilage and subchondral bone of the talus and can lead to significant degenerative changes and loss of range of motion.[20] They typically arise from previous ankle trauma and should be suspected in patients with chronic ankle pain, especially with previous injury.[21] Fractures of the talar body compose approximately 1% of all fractures and are often unrecognized because they are associated with other more obvious injuries.[22] For example, 28% of these lesions have been shown to be associated with other fractures, and some authors estimate that osteochondral lesions accompany up to 6.5% of ankle sprains.[23,24] Lesions are generally thought to be split nearly evenly between the medial and lateral talar dome.

Achilles tendon problems represent a spectrum of overuse injuries that are multifactorial in origin and commonly related to poor training practices and advancing age. They represent common ailments, affecting up to 10% of serious runners per year, especially those who have recently stepped up a training program.[25,26] The Achilles tendon is the largest tendon in the body and connects the gastrocnemius and soleus muscles to the calcaneal tuberosity. As such, it crosses the knee, ankle, and subtalar joints. During running, forces up to 10 times body weight are imparted on the Achilles tendon. It lacks a synovial sheath and instead has a paratenon, which helps with gliding. The blood supply to the Achilles tendon leaves a relative watershed region approximately 4 cm proximal to its insertion.[27] With normal aging, the Achilles tendon undergoes morphologic changes that may leave it susceptible to injury.[28] However, a healthy tendon possesses a strong ability to adapt to mechanical stimuli and gradual changes in athletic training. Achilles tendon injuries can be classified according to severity from paratenonitis to paratenonitis with tendinosis to tendinosis to frank rupture.[29,30] In paratenonitis, the inflammation is limited to the paratenon and is accompanied by inflammatory signs over the tendon. In paratenonitis with tendinosis, one encounters the beginnings of intratendinous degeneration usually indicated by a palpable nodule in the tendon accompanied by inflammation. Tendinosis involves further intratendinous degeneration indicated by atrophy and palpable tendon nodule without inflammation. Tendinosis typically occurs 2 to 6 cm proximal to the tendon's insertion and is consistently found in regions of frank tendon rupture.[29,30]

Lisfranc injuries are a relatively rare, but potentially devastating, athletic injury. The Lisfranc joint is formed by the base of the first and second metatarsal and their articulations with the medial and middle cuneiforms. A stout plantar ligament and less stout dorsal ligament between the medial cuneiform and base of the second metatarsal serve as key supporting elements to the transverse arch of the midfoot. Loss of integrity of this ligament can lead to significant distortion of the architecture of the foot, arthritis, and chronic disability. Injuries to the Lisfranc joint include damage to this ligament, fractures of the bones that comprise this joint, dislocations, or combined injuries. The mechanisms of injury commonly associated with a Lisfranc sprain are axial loading of the midfoot, twisting of the midfoot, and landing on a plantar-flexed forefoot. Lisfranc injuries can occur with most sporting activities, but are particularly common in football, especially with pileups.

Turf toe represents an injury to the forefoot at the base of the first toe. It has become more common in recent years due to the increased use of artificial turf and other relatively hard playing surfaces. Hard surfaces combined with flexible footwear that provides less forefoot stability when running and jumping have been thought to be the prime contributors to turf toe. This injury represents damage to the plantar capsule of the first-toe metatarsal–phalangeal joint. Capsular damage can be quite painful and can even lead to joint instability. Patients typically complain of pain at the base of the first toe, stiffness, and swelling. Turf toe is particularly common in sports that require running and jumping on artificial turf such as football, soccer, and lacrosse.

NARROWING THE DIFFERENTIAL DIAGNOSIS

History

One of the most useful tools in evaluating a complaint of ankle pain is the patient's history. Factors to consider include the patient's age, mechanism of injury, location of pain, exacerbating and alleviating factors, associated symptoms, and past medical history.

The patient's age is a key factor when evaluating ankle pain. Children often have ankle pain as a result of trauma. Children are also more likely to suffer avulsion fractures, as their apophyses are relatively weaker than their tendons and ligaments. A history of chronic ankle sprains in a child aged 10 to 15 years should raise the concern for a tarsal coalition. Children can also develop primary bone or soft-tissue tumors. Acute trauma is the most likely cause of ankle pain in young adults. This includes sprains, fractures, tendon injuries, and osteochondral lesions of the talus. Middle-aged adults, especially the "weekend warrior" types, commonly suffer Achilles tendon injuries, sprains, and fractures. Fractures are becoming increasingly common in osteoporotic elderly individuals. Chronic conditions such as osteoarthritis, inflammatory arthritis, posterior tibial tendon dysfunction, and metastatic neoplasms must be considered in the elderly population as well.

Another key feature of the patient's history with ankle pain is the mechanism of injury. Typically, an inversion injury to the ankle results in a sprain. An external rotation injury commonly results in fracture and/or syndesmotic injury. A sudden eccentric contraction of the Achilles tendon accompanied by a pop is common in rupture of this tendon. Fall from a height is commonly associated with hindfoot fractures or fractures of the tibial plafond. More insidious mechanisms and gradual onset of pain suggest chronic conditions such as osteoarthritis, inflammatory arthritis, or neoplasm. The relatively sudden onset of pain in the setting of a fever or other infectious process is concerning for septic arthritis, a surgical emergency. Pain that occurs with discrete periods of exacerbations and remissions is common with chronic ankle instability and osteochondral lesions of the talus. Night pain is especially concerning for a neoplastic process.

The location of ankle pain can also help narrow the differential diagnosis. Pain along the dorsum of the foot, especially if lateral, is typical with ankle sprains. Pain directly over one or both malleoli is associated with fracture and/or ligament injury. Posterior ankle pain is commonly seen with Achilles tendon or hindfoot injury. Diffuse, deep-seated ankle pain is common with the different forms of arthritis. Pain distal to the lateral malleolus or along the lateral border of the foot is common with peroneal tendon instability.

Many ankle conditions have exacerbating and alleviating factors. Pain with weight bearing is common in acute trauma. Typically, there is more difficulty with weight bearing in the setting of a fracture than in the setting of a sprain. The pain associated with inflammatory arthritis is commonly worse early in the day and relieved by anti-inflammatory medications. The pain with osteoarthritis is typically worse with weight bearing, worsens as the day progresses, and responds to anti-inflammatory medications. Pain that does not respond to ice and elevation is concerning for an infectious process. Although pain with range of motion is typical with most ankle processes, the pain with a septic joint is usually markedly worse than that seen with osteoarthritis or inflammatory arthritis.

The patient's past medical history is especially important to consider when evaluating ankle pain. A history of multiple sprains can lead to chronic ankle instability. Multiple sprains are also concerning for a tarsal coalition, particularly in a teenager or young adult. A history of trauma makes posttraumatic osteoarthritis a concern. A previous ankle infection or a history of bacteremia makes a septic joint more likely. Metastatic disease should be considered if the patient has a history of neoplasm. One should consider gout or another inflammatory arthritis if the patient has had previous exacerbations. Diabetics or patients with neuropathy are particularly prone to developing a Charcot joint, as their lack of protective sensation predisposes them to repeat injury.

Evidence-based Physical Examination

Inspection

The examination of the ankle begins with visual inspection. Compare the symptomatic ankle with the unaffected contralateral ankle, as this can give a nice approximation of the baseline appearance of the symptomatic ankle. Observe the affected ankle from midtibia down to the foot. Be sure to look at the bony and tendinous prominences for evidence of cutaneous trauma and/or swelling. Localized swelling serves to help determine the area(s) of maximal injury. Examples of common areas of localized swelling include the anterior/lateral ankle and proximal dorsal foot for ankle sprains, the

malleoli for fractures, and just proximal to the ankle for syndesmotic injuries. Generalized foot/ankle swelling suggests more severe trauma. Bruising and other color changes can help to assess the chronicity of the injury as well. It is also useful to assess the patient's gait and weight-bearing ability to help narrow the potential area(s) of injury/pain. Assessment of overall alignment, especially compared to the contralateral ankle, is also important.

Palpation

Palpate the ankle to assess the various areas of bony anatomy and ligament and tendon origin and insertion. A consistent systematic approach is advised. Palpate the prominent medial malleolus and distal tibia medially. Moving toward the plantar aspect of the foot, palpate the medial talus as well as the prominent sustentaculum tali of the calcaneus. The medial tubercle of the talus is also palpable just posterior to the medial malleolus. The deltoid ligament is palpable as a firm band just inferior to the medial malleolus. Posterior to the deltoid ligament in a soft spot anterior to the Achilles tendon lay the tibialis posterior tendon, flexor digitorum longus tendon, posterior tibial artery and nerve, and flexor hallucis longus tendon. Moving posteriorly, palpate the Achilles tendon down to its insertion on the calcaneus. Laterally, start with bony palpation of the lateral malleolus. Palpation of the proximal/lateral foot includes the prominence of the base of the fifth metatarsal. The peroneal tendons are palpable, tracing back proximally from the base of the fifth metatarsal inferior and lateral to the distal fibula. The lateral ligamentous structures are more difficult to palpate, but tenderness anterior/distal to the lateral malleolus suggests ATFL injury. Similarly, tenderness posterior/medial to the lateral malleolus suggests PTFL or CFL injury. Anterior and medial to the lateral malleolus is a soft area often referred to as the sinus tarsi. In addition to the ATFL, it is also possible to palpate the tibiofibular articulation and dome of the talus in this area. Further anteriorly, palpate the prominent tibialis anterior tendon. Just lateral to this tendon on the dorsum of the foot is the dorsalis pedis artery.

Range of Motion

Range of motion of the ankle can be simplified to plantar flexion and dorsiflexion (which primarily occur through the tibiotalar joint) and inversion and eversion (which primarily occur through the subtalar joint). Passive range of motion is most easily assessed with the patient sitting with the legs dangling over the side of the table. Assess ankle range of motion with the knees bent because the gastrocnemius crosses both the ankle and knee joints. It is important to stabilize the subtalar joint by holding the calcaneus when assessing plantar flexion and dorsiflexion. While grasping the midfoot/forefoot with the other hand, one can assess plantar flexion and dorsiflexion, which averages 50 and 20 degrees, respectively. The shape of the talus leaves the ankle with more medial and lateral motion in plantar flexion than in dorsiflexion. A decrease in range of motion can be caused by prolonged immobilization (e.g., casting), intra- or extra-articular swelling, joint fusion, joint capsule contracture, or impingement due to osteophyte formation seen with osteoarthritis. A loss of dorsiflexion is particularly debilitating because it can lead to difficulty clearing the floor with the toes during the swing phase of gait, which can cause frequent stumbles and/or falls. Assessing subtalar motion through inversion and eversion requires stabilizing the tibia with one hand and using the contralateral hand to hold the calcaneus and hindfoot. There is usually 5 degrees each of subtalar inversion or eversion. Decreased inversion and eversion is seen in conditions such as osteoarthritis, joint fusion, and tarsal coalition. A loss of inversion and eversion makes it particularly difficult to walk on uneven surfaces. Active range of motion can be assessed with the patient sitting as above or standing. Asking the patient to stand/walk on the toes, heels, lateral foot, or medial foot assesses ankle plantar flexion, dorsiflexion, and subtalar inversion and eversion, respectively.

Strength Testing

Strength testing about the ankle involves assessing the function of the main ankle dorsiflexor and inverter (tibialis anterior), plantar flexors (gastrocsoleus complex), and everters (peroneus longus and brevis). Strength testing is a nonspecific test that examines musculotendinous integrity, intact neurologic function, and the ability to move a joint. It is important in assisting the evaluation of the cause of a patient's complaint. To assess the tibialis anterior, observe the patient walking on his/her heels and resist dorsiflexion/inversion by stabilizing the tibia and pushing the foot into plantar flexion/eversion by pressing on the first metatarsal. As mentioned earlier, a weak tibialis anterior and loss of ankle dorsiflexion make it difficult to clear the floor with the toes during swing phase of gait and can contribute to a steppage or drop foot gait. To assess the gastrocsoleus complex, observe the patient walking on his/her toes, hopping up and down on one foot, and resisting plantar flexion by stabilizing the tibia with one hand and pressing up on the dorsum of the foot with the contralateral hand. Weakness with plantar flexion may suggest Achilles tendon injury/inflammation. To assess the peroneus longus and brevis, observe the patient walking on the medial border of the foot and resisting eversion by stabilizing the calcaneus with one hand and providing an inversion/plantar flexion force with the other hand pressing along the fifth metatarsal. Pain with resisted eversion or inability to evert the foot suggests derangement of the peroneal tendons such as tendonitis, sprain, or subluxation. There are also a number of tests to assess the other musculotendinous structures that cross the ankle joint, but these perform a secondary function with ankle joint motion and are not covered in this chapter.

Laxity Tests

A number of different maneuvers are designed to assess the various structural elements of the ankle for stability.[31] One such test is the talar tilt test, which assesses the integrity of the ATFL and CFL. It is performed with the patient seated and the foot unsupported. With the foot in 10 to 20 degrees of plantar flexion (which tests the ATFL primarily), stabilize the leg just above the medial malleolus and supply an inversion force to the hindfoot with the contralateral hand. Normally an angle of approximately 5 degrees is achieved between the tibial plafond and talar dome. An increase in this tilt is suggestive of injury to both the ATFL and CFL. However, there is a lack of consensus on just how much talar tilt is indicative of injury to both ligaments. Comparison to the contralateral ankle is useful in this circumstance.[32–34]

Another test useful for assessing the integrity of the ATFL is the anterior drawer test. This test can be performed with the patient either sitting or supine. In the sitting position, have the knee flexed over the side of the table and let the ankle fall into plantar flexion. Stabilize the distal tibia with one hand and provide an anteriorly directed force on the calcaneus with the other. If the patient is supine, hyperflex the knee, place the ankle in plantar flexion, fix the foot in one hand (or against the table), and apply a posteriorly directed force to the anterior aspect of the distal tibia. This is often called the modified anterior drawer test.[35] A positive test involves pain and/or translation of 8 mm or greater compared to the contralateral side. In a study comparing physical examination to surgical and arthrography findings, the anterior drawer test was found to have a positive predictive value of 91% and a negative predictive value of 51%, with a sensitivity of 80% and specificity of 74%.[36]

Special Tests

Two tests are commonly cited for assessment of injury to the syndesmosis. The first of these is often called the squeeze test, which is performed by squeezing the fibula against the tibia at the midcalf level. A positive test produces pain distally at the level of the syndesmosis just proximal to the ankle joint and indicates severe syndesmotic injury. This test has shown moderate interrater reliability.[13,37] The second test is the external rotation test. In this test, the tibia is stabilized and the foot externally rotated through the ankle joint, thereby stressing the syndesmosis. A positive test causes pain at the level of the syndesmosis in the setting of syndesmotic ligament injury. This test has demonstrated high interrater reliability and significant association with ankle pathology.[37,38]

If the patient has lateral ankle pain, especially with a sensation of popping, it is important to test for peroneal tendon subluxation. This occurs with loss of superior peroneal retinaculum integrity. To perform this test, have the patient further dorsiflex the ankle from a position of slight dorsiflexion and eversion. A positive test recreates the popping sensation and may allow visual observation or palpation of the tendons actively subluxing.

Another test to consider when evaluating ankle pain is the Thompson test for a ruptured Achilles tendon. This test is performed with the patient prone and both feet extending past the end of the table. Squeezing the calf muscles should produce plantar flexion of the ankle if the tendon is intact. The foot should not plantar flex if the tendon is ruptured. This test was found to have a positive predictive value of 98%, with a 96% sensitivity and 93% specificity.[39] False positives may be present if the secondary ankle plantar flexors remain intact.

Diagnostic Testing

Laboratory

Laboratory studies are not commonly obtained in the setting of acute ankle injury. If there are concerns for infectious or inflammatory arthritis, obtaining a white blood cell count, erythrocyte sedimentation rate (ESR), C-reactive protein (CRP), and uric acid level is suggested. Specific markers for inflammatory disease such as rheumatoid factor or antinuclear antibody should also be considered. A Lyme titer should also be considered, given the appropriate history and demographic considerations.

Imaging

One of the best-studied areas in evaluating ankle pain surrounds whether or not to obtain plain x-rays. In the setting of acute injury, the Ottawa ankle rules have proven to be nearly 100% sensitive for detecting clinically significant ankle fractures while reducing the need for x-ray by 30% to 40%.[40,41] The Ottawa ankle rules suggest that ankle x-rays are indicated if there is tenderness over the inferior or posterior pole of either malleolus, including the distal 6 cm, or if there is the inability to bear weight (four steps taken independently, even if limping) at the time of injury and at the time of evaluation. If there is tenderness over the base of the fifth metatarsal or navicular bone, foot x-rays are indicated. X-rays should also be considered in the setting of more chronic ankle pain to evaluate for degenerative changes, osteochondral lesions, or the possibility of neoplasm.

A typical x-ray series of the ankle involves three views: the anteroposterior (AP), mortise, and lateral. On each view, a systematic approach should be employed, looking at all visualized bone and spaces between bones, especially sites of ligament/tendon attachment and joint surfaces. The AP radiograph is taken in the long axis of the foot. Areas of particular importance on the AP radiograph include the tibiofibular clear space and tibiofibular overlap. A clear space of less than 5 mm and an overlap of greater than 10 mm indicate a normal syndesmotic relationship. The mortise radiograph is taken with the foot in 15 to 20 degrees

of internal rotation so that the x-ray beam is perpendicular to the intermalleolar line. On a well-taken mortise x-ray, there should be a universal amount of clear space around the talus and minimal overlap of the tibia and fibula. An increase in the clear space, especially greater than 4 mm medially, suggests lateral talar shift and either medial ligamentous or syndesmotic injury. Talar tilt can be assessed on the mortise x-ray by drawing lines parallel to the tibial plafond and talar articular surface. These lines should be parallel, and greater than 2 degrees of angulation indicates talar tilt. Another important aspect of the mortise view is the talocrural angle. This angle is formed by a line drawn from the tip of one malleolus to the other and a line drawn parallel to the tibial plafond and usually measures 8 to 15 degrees. A smaller angle suggests fibular shortening. Lastly, less than 1 cm of tibiofibular overlap and greater than 1 mm of talar shift are considered abnormal on the mortise view. The final view in an ankle series is the lateral view. On this view, the dome of the talus should be centered under the tibia and congruous with the tibial plafond.[16]

Computed tomography (CT) scans are useful in the 3-dimensional evaluation of bony structures. The use of CT scan is fairly limited in the evaluation of acute ankle pain. CT scan may reveal a tarsal coalition or an osteochondral lesion of the talus that is not appreciated on plain x-ray. CT is also useful to delineate complex fracture patterns or complex bony anatomy for preoperative planning purposes.

Magnetic resonance imaging (MRI) scans are another means of obtaining 3-dimensional information about the ankle. MRI is useful in assessing soft-tissue injury or bony edema about the ankle. MRI is often indicated in the setting of pain or disorders refractory to conservative therapy. MRI has traditionally been used in the evaluation of chronic conditions, but has become increasingly more common in the setting of acute injury. Indications for MRI in acute ankle injury are still being worked out. MRI should be considered when working up suspected Achilles tendon injury, chronic ankle instability, osteochondral lesions of the talus, stress fractures, or peroneal tendon subluxation as outlined in the sections that follow. MRI is also useful in the evaluation of infectious processes. An MRI may also be considered in the evaluation of a potential neoplastic process.

Other Testing

An aspiration of the ankle joint may be considered to help distinguish inflammatory from infectious arthritis. The aspirate should be sent for cell count, Gram stain, culture and sensitivity, and crystal analysis. An ankle aspiration is most easily performed by directing a needle posterior laterally in the soft spot found just lateral to the medial malleolus and medial to the tibialis anterior tendon.

Ultrasound is also of limited utility in evaluating ankle pain. The main indication for ultrasound exists in the dynamic evaluation of a suspected Achilles tendon rupture to assess if the tendon ends reapproximate or not with ankle plantar flexion. Ultrasound is relatively quick and inexpensive, but carries a steep learning curve for those performing and interpreting the test.

APPROACH TO THE ATHLETE WITH AN ANKLE SPRAIN

HISTORY AND PHYSICAL EXAMINATION

Inversion ankle sprains represent injury to the lateral ligamentous complex of the ankle. Patients will typically report an inversion twisting injury, usually with the foot plantar flexed. An ankle sprain will typically produce immediate lateral ankle pain and swelling. It will also commonly produce dorsal–lateral foot pain and swelling in the region of the sinus tarsi, which represent injury to the ATFL. In ankle sprains, the injury typically progresses in an anterior-to-posterior direction, with the ATFL injured first (and most commonly), followed by the CFL, and rarely the PTFL. Patients may experience pain with weight bearing, but will typically be able to ambulate with only mild to moderate difficulty. Patients may also report the sensation of the talus subluxating from under the tibia. The ankle is usually tender and focally swollen in the region of the distal tip of the fibula as well as the course of the ATFL to the talus in the sinus tarsi. Diffuse ankle swelling is less common. The talar tilt and/or anterior drawer tests typically exacerbate the patient's pain. Active and passive range of motion of the ankle should be recorded as well, but typically produce pain, and are not particularly useful when making a diagnosis.

DIAGNOSTIC TESTING

If the Ottawa ankle rules are followed, x-rays are typically not indicated when working up an ankle sprain. X-rays are important when the Ottawa ankle rules are positive to rule out a clinically significant fracture. Inversion stress radiographs are not typically necessary, but can be useful when assessing the integrity of the CFL. A side-to-side difference of greater than 3 mm of anterior subluxation on a lateral stress radiograph while performing the anterior drawer test signifies a rupture of the ATFL. A side-to-side difference of 10 degrees or more on an AP stress radiograph while performing the talar tilt test indicates rupture of both the ATFL and CFL.[42–44] As with plain x-rays, MRI is not typically obtained in the setting of an acute ankle sprain. When obtained, it is useful to investigate the integrity of the ligaments and can also help to grade the severity of injury. MRI should be considered if an ankle sprain does not improve after 6 weeks of conservative treatment.

TREATMENT

Nonoperative

- First-line treatment
- RICE (rest, ice, compression, and elevation)
  - Early management focuses on decreasing swelling while preserving range of motion[45]
  - Weight bearing typically can occur as tolerated
  - An air-filled stirrup brace is useful to restrict inversion/eversion but still allow plantar flexion and dorsiflexion[46]
  - An ankle foot orthosis or well-molded posterior splint can be considered in the setting of significant swelling and stiffness in plantar flexion[12]
  - Prolonged immobilization should be avoided and has been shown to be detrimental[47,48]
- Start a functional rehabilitation program immediately (grade I and II sprains)[6]
- Functional rehabilitation is typically delayed in the setting of a grade III sprain
  - Until swelling and pain have subsided
- Components of this rehabilitation program:
  - Range of motion, muscle strengthening, proprioceptive training, and training for return to activity
  - Achilles tendon stretching is a key component to preserving range of motion
  - Strengthening the peroneal muscles is essential in preventing chronic instability[49,50]
  - Proprioceptive training typically commences after resumption of full weight bearing without pain
  - Proprioceptive training is essential to returning patients to a high functional level[51,52]
  - The final step in functional rehabilitation can begin when walking is no longer limited by pain
  - The patient can begin increasing activity gradually with jogging and sport-specific activities.

Operative

- Can be considered in the setting of grade III injuries with gross instability, especially in high-performance athletes
- Consider operative intervention with chronic instability[53]
- Indicated with concomitant osteochondral lesion of the talus
- Operative options include reconstruction of the lateral ligamentous support to the ankle
  - Requires a significant recovery period of 6 or more months before return to play

Prognosis/Return to Play

- Useful general return-to-play criteria for ankle injuries in general and sprains in specific include the following: normal ankle joint range of motion, no pain or tenderness, negative clinical examination, strength of ankle muscles 90% of the unaffected side, and ability to complete a functional examination.[54]

- Clinical tests such as the anterior drawer or talar tilt tests can be used to assure that the athlete's ankle is stable clinically.
- In general, an athlete is safe for return to play if he or she can perform sport-related activities pain free and feel fully recovered.
- Ankle taping and/or bracing are useful in prophylaxis against reinjury and important during the recovery and initial return-to-play periods.

Complications/Indications for Referral

Complications of ankle sprains typically include associated injuries and warrant referral to an emergency department or orthopaedist. These include fracture or dislocation, osteochondral injury of the talus, neurovascular compromise, tendon rupture or subluxation, traumatic arthrotomy, mechanical locking of the joint, or syndesmotic injury. A referral should be considered if the diagnosis is uncertain or if the patient has pain out of proportion to the degree of trauma.[12] Recurrent ankle sprains should raise the concern for a tarsal coalition or chronic instability and warrant further workup, imaging (MRI or CT), and/or referral.

APPROACH TO THE ATHLETE WITH A SYNDESMOTIC INJURY (HIGH ANKLE SPRAIN)

HISTORY AND PHYSICAL EXAMINATION

Patients with a syndesmotic injury typically report an external rotation injury to the ankle. They often complain of pain and tenderness anteriorly over the syndesmosis somewhat proximal to the ankle joint itself. Syndesmotic injuries often lack the ankle and foot swelling typically associated with an ankle sprain. Since the medial and lateral ligaments are not typically injured, patients usually do not demonstrate tenderness over either malleoli or the course of these ligaments. Tenderness is usually located anterior to the syndesmosis, and pain is usually exacerbated by the squeeze test or external rotation test, as outlined previously.[13,55]

DIAGNOSTIC TESTING

Radiographic examination of the ankle is particularly useful in the setting of a suspected syndesmotic injury. An AP and lateral view of the entire tibia and fibula should also be obtained, as syndesmotic injuries are associated with proximal fibula fractures (also known as Maisonneuve fractures).

On the ankle films, an increased tibiofibular clear space, decreased tibiofibular overlap, and increased medial clear space indicate a syndesmotic injury[56–58](Fig. 21.2). If a syndesmotic injury is highly suspected but x-rays are nondiagnostic, an external rotation stress radiograph (typically the mortise) can be used to help establish the diagnosis. MRIs, or less frequently CTs, can also be used in the suspected occult syndesmotic injury, but are not the usual first-line studies.

TREATMENT

Nonoperative

- Nonoperative treatment is reserved for injuries without syndesmotic diastasis or instability.
- Treatment begins with RICE and a non–weight-bearing cast for 2 to 3 weeks.
- Following casting, the patient is allowed to progressively increase to weight bearing as tolerated in a walking boot.
- Syndesmotic sprains with latent instability:
  - Some authors advocate nonsurgical treatment with a non–weight-bearing cast for 4 to 6 weeks with serial x-rays to assure anatomic tibiofibular relationships during healing.[59]
  - Proceed to progressive weight bearing in a walking boot.
- A functional rehabilitation program as outlined in the ankle sprain section is typically employed with nonoperative treatment of syndesmotic injuries.

Operative

- Operative treatment is indicated for patients with sprain and frank diastasis and most patients with sprain and latent diastasis.
- Operative treatment is also indicated in patients with associated ankle and/or proximal fibula fractures (Fig. 21.2).
- Operative treatment typically consists of two screws placed from the fibula into the tibia with the syndesmosis held in a reduced position.
- Postoperative weight-bearing regimens differ.
  - Most patients are maintained non–weight bearing for 10 to 12 weeks.
  - General consensus is that syndesmotic screws should be removed 3 to 6 months after surgery.
  - If left in, syndesmotic screws will inevitably break due to metal fatigue.

Prognosis/Return to Play

- These sprains typically take longer than conventional ankle sprains for full recovery and return to play.
- Return to play is generally allowed after completion of a functional rehabilitation program when range of motion

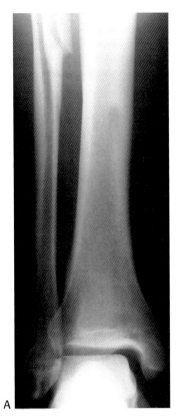

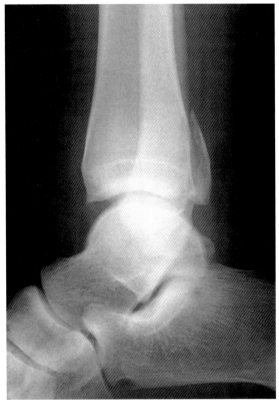

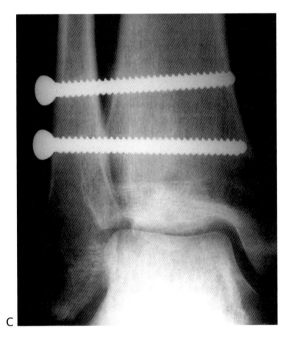

FIG. 21.2. A 22-year-old man sustained an external rotation injury to the right ankle. The initial anteroposterior radiograph **(A)** of the distal tibia and fibula shows a midshaft fibula fracture and a lateral shift of the talus with a wide medial clear space. The lateral radiograph **(B)** shows a small posterior malleolar fracture, indicating a posterior syndesmosis injury. The patient was treated with closed reduction and fixation with two 4.5-mm syndesmosis screws. The postoperative anteroposterior **(C)** and lateral radiographs show the position of the screws and the reduction of the mortise. These screws were removed in the outpatient clinic 4 months after the injury. Reprinted with permission from Bucholz RW, Heckman JD. *Rockwood & Green's Fractures in Adults.* 5th ed. Baltimore: Lippincott Williams & Wilkins; 2001.

has been restored and local tenderness and swelling have resolved.

- The criteria outlined in the ankle sprain section are generally applicable to syndesmotic injuries as well.
- An ankle stirrup brace and/or ankle taping is particularly useful in the final recovery and return-to-play period.[54]

The most common and significant complication following a syndesmotic injury is prolonged ankle stiffness. Delayed or failed diagnoses can lead to adverse outcomes and prolonged disability.[60–64] Referral should be considered in all syndesmotic injuries, especially displaced syndesmotic injuries whether latent or frank. A syndesmotic injury in the setting of an ankle fracture is also an indication for referral.

APPROACH TO THE ATHLETE WITH A ROTATIONAL ANKLE FRACTURE

HISTORY AND PHYSICAL EXAMINATION

Ankle fractures are usually the result of an external rotation injury. The patient typically reports immediate pain in the region of one or both of the ankle malleoli and inability to bear weight. The ankle typically swells quickly, and ecchymoses are common, especially around and inferior to the malleoli. The patient is tender to palpation over the malleoli, and crepitus may be appreciated with attempted ankle motion or stress testing. Evaluating both malleoli is critical to determining the degree of ankle injury, as bimalleolar ankle fractures are typically unstable. It is important to assess skin integrity, the neurovascular status of the foot, and the degree of swelling associated with an ankle fracture, as these factors can alter the treatment algorithm and timing of surgery.

DIAGNOSTIC TESTING

As mentioned previously, the use of the Ottawa ankle rules is paramount in the evaluation of ankle injuries. Since fractures typically involve tenderness over the malleoli and difficulty weight bearing, a three-view ankle x-ray is obtained. When evaluating an ankle fracture, it is also important to image the hindfoot and full extent of the tibia and fibula. Evaluation of ankle films involves looking for fractures to the medial malleolus, lateral malleolus, and posterior tibial plafond (or posterior malleolus) and noting the tibiofibular clear space, medial clear space, and tibiofibular overlap as outlined earlier (Fig. 21.3). External rotation stress mortise radiographs can help to evaluate occult medial ligamentous or syndesmotic injury and should be considered in the setting of an isolated lateral malleolar fracture with medial symptoms/signs on history and physical examination.[65]

A number of classification schemes have been described for ankle fractures, the simplest of which being the Weber classification[66] (Fig. 21.4). Weber A injuries involve the tip of the fibula distal to the tibial plafond, Weber B injuries describe a fibular fracture at the level of the tibial plafond, and Weber C injuries involve a fibula fracture proximal to the level of the tibial plafond. Fractures that involve both the lateral and medial malleoli or demonstrate disruption of the radiographic spaces/parameters represent unstable injuries that are usually treated operatively. As mentioned earlier, stress radiographs have particular utility with a high suspicion of medial or syndesmotic ligament injury.

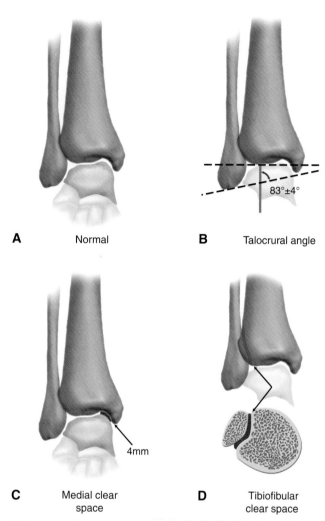

A Normal   **B** Talocrural angle   83°±4°

C Medial clear space   4mm   **D** Tibiofibular clear space

FIG. 21.3. X-ray appearance of the normal ankle on mortise view. **A:** The condensed subchondral bone should form a continuous line around the talus. **B:** The talocrural angle should be approximately 83 degrees. When the opposite side can be used as a control, the talocrural angle of the injured side should be within a few degrees of the noninjured side. **C:** The medial clear space should be equal to the superior clear space between the talus and the distal tibia and less than or equal to 4 mm on standard x-rays. **D:** The distance between the medial wall of the fibula and the incisural surface of the tibia, the tibiofibular clear space, should be less than 6 mm. Adapted from Browner B, Jupiter J, Levine A, eds. *Skeletal Trauma: Fractures, Dislocations, and Ligamentous Injuries.* 2nd ed. Philadelphia: WB Saunders; 1997.

CT scan is not usually necessary in the setting of an acute ankle fracture, but can be useful in the evaluation of injuries to the articular surface of the tibia (also known as pilon injuries). These represent higher-energy injuries of a different spectrum than rotational ankle fractures and are not discussed further here. MRI can be useful to evaluate for occult or stress fractures, but is typically not needed in the setting of an acute fracture.

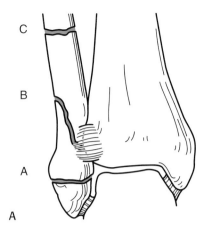

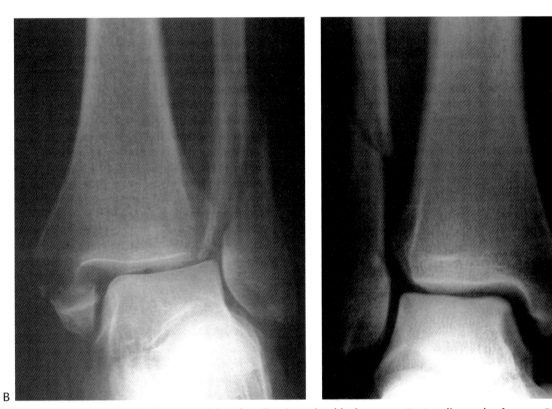

FIG. 21.4. A: Schematic diagram of the classification of ankle fractures. **B:** A radiograph of a type B ankle fracture in which the fibula fracture begins anteriorly at the level of the distal tibiofibular syndesmosis. **C:** A mortise radiograph of a type C injury with disruption of the syndesmosis up to the level of the fibula fracture, which is completely above the distal syndesmotic ligament complex. There is a medial deltoid ligament injury. Reprinted with permission from Bucholz RW, Heckman JD. *Rockwood & Green's Fractures in Adults.* 5th ed. Baltimore: Lippincott Williams & Wilkins; 2001.

TREATMENT

Nonoperative

- Isolated lateral fractures are considered stable injuries and can be treated effectively nonoperatively.[67–69]
- Weber A distal fibular fractures can be treated in a fashion similar to a type 3 lateral ankle sprain with RICE, a removable stirrup brace, weight bearing as tolerated, and functional rehabilitation.
- Weber type B and C injuries require some critical analysis before opting for nonoperative treatment.
  - A lateral malleolus fracture is considered isolated if there is no evidence of medial malleolar injury or disruption of the mortise clinically and radiographically.[70]
- The keys to effective nonoperative treatment of an isolated lateral ankle fracture involve immobilization designed to protect the ankle from further injury.
  - This is typically in the form of a well-molded short-leg walking cast or prefabricated cast boot for 4 to 6 weeks.[16,70]
- Weight bearing can occur as tolerated, as symptoms allow.
- Patients can come out of a removable boot at night to work on gentle range of motion.
- Follow-up x-rays usually at 1 week after injury and at varying periods thereafter are important to assess healing and to assure displacement has not occurred.
- After the immobilization period, with evidence of sufficient healing (improved symptoms, radiologic evidence of healing), a functional rehabilitation program can be instituted.
- It is important to note that nonoperative treatment may also be chosen in patients with significant medical comorbidities and diabetics, though these situations are not typical of an athletic population.

Operative

- Unstable ankle fractures are usually treated operatively.[15,16]
- Unstable ankle fractures include bimalleolar ankle fractures, bimalleolar equivalent ankle fractures with deltoid ligament disruption, trimalleolar ankle fractures, and fractures with syndesmotic disruption.
- Other surgical indications include open fractures, fractures with vascular compromise, or impending compartment syndrome.
- Ankle fractures are typically treated with open reduction and internal fixation.
- Postoperatively, patients are typically placed in a splint or cast and undergo a period of 2 to 4 weeks of strict non–weight bearing.
- The patient is typically progressed to a removable boot or walking cast for a period of 6 to 12 weeks with gradual resumption of full weight bearing.

- With evidence of sufficient healing, a functional rehabilitation program can be instituted.

Prognosis/Return to Play

- Return to play is typically delayed for 3 or more months.[16]
- Fractures treated nonoperatively usually return to play sooner than operatively treated fractures.
- A general guideline for safe return to play is clinical and radiographic evidence of healing, completion of a functional rehabilitation program, and assessment of the patient's strength, agility, and confidence in the ankle.
- As with other ankle injuries, bracing and/or taping is typically useful in the rehabilitation and early return-to-play period.

Complications/Indications for Referral

Complications surrounding ankle fractures typically involve misdiagnosis or delayed diagnosis. Ankle fractures deemed stable that are in fact unstable are prone to failure/disability. Axial load fractures such as pilon fractures require a different treatment algorithm than a rotational ankle fracture. Patient factors such as diabetes, neuropathy, and other medical comorbidities may also compromise outcome. Surgical complications also include soft-tissue compromise, infection, hardware failure, or neurovascular injury.

Referral should be considered for all ankle fractures, whether stable or unstable. The exception to this rule is the Weber A fracture in an adult. This injury represents lateral ligamentous avulsion of the distal fibula and can be treated like a moderate to severe ankle sprain. Weber A–appearing fractures in children typically represent injuries to the growth plate and warrant referral as well.

APPROACH TO THE ATHLETE WITH AN OSTEOCHONDRAL LESION OF THE TALUS

HISTORY AND PHYSICAL EXAMINATION

Osteochondral injuries of the talus should be considered in all traumatic ankle injuries. They commonly present in the setting of chronic ankle pain with or without an obvious preceding traumatic event. A number of possible mechanisms for osteochondral injury have been proposed. These include a shearing impaction force between the talar dome and tibial plafond. This shearing can be caused by a compressive injury to an ankle positioned in dorsiflexion and inversion, a plantar-flexed ankle subjected to inversion and external rotation, or impaction of the lateral dome against the lateral malleolus.[71,72]

As with the history, the physical examination for osteochondral injuries is somewhat nonspecific. It should include palpation of the joint line for discrete regions of tenderness, instability testing if possible (including inversion and eversion stress testing), evaluation of range of motion, and careful neurovascular assessment.[21] In the acute setting, the ankle is typically swollen, and another associated diagnosis is usually more obvious. In the chronic setting, decreased range of motion and pain with range of motion may be the only indicators of an osteochondral injury.

DIAGNOSTIC TESTING

Traditionally, a standard three-view x-ray series of the ankle has been used to assist in the diagnosis of an osteochondral lesion. Some authors have suggested other views that may help to better visualize the talus. These include a view taken with the foot pronated 15 degrees and the x-ray tube angled 75 degrees cephalad and a mortise view taken with the ankle in plantar flexion. However, since plain x-rays do not visualize nonosseous structures, they may not demonstrate an osteochondral lesion.[73] Similarly, CT scans are also limited in their ability to visualize some osteochondral lesions. However, CT remains useful in the 3-dimensional assessment of the subchondral bone and for preoperative planning purposes.[73,74] Bone scans have also been suggested in the evaluation of posttraumatic ankle pain and disability. They have been shown to be 94% sensitive and 96% specific, but authors recommend a positive bone scan be followed by an MRI.[75,76] Currently, MRI is probably the most useful study in assessing a suspected osteochondral lesion. MRI affords multiplanar evaluation, visualizes both the articular cartilage and subchondral bone, demonstrates bone edema, has been shown to detect early/minor osteochondral injuries, and correlates well with arthroscopic findings.[77]

Stone has proposed the following algorithm for evaluating osteochondral lesions of the talus; Plain x-rays should be employed in the setting of acute ankle injury with tenderness at the bony landmarks or hemarthrosis. If an osteochondral lesion is noted on plain x-ray, a CT scan is used to further evaluate the 3-dimensional characteristics of the lesion. If plain x-rays are normal and pain persists, an MRI (and, less commonly, a bone scan) can be used for further evaluation and to identify other associated injuries.

TREATMENT

Nonoperative

- The treatment of osteochondral lesions of the talus is based on the severity and stability of the lesion.
- Lesions are classified based on MRI and arthroscopic evaluation (Table 21.1).

TABLE 21.1 **Staging Guidelines for Osteochondral Lesions of the Talus[71]**

Stage I—localized impaction and an area of bone bruising without violation of the cortex

Stage II—osteochondral fracture that is only partially detached

Stage III—osteochondral fractures that are detached but nondisplaced

Stage IV—displaced osteochondral fracture fragments

- Osteochondral lesions are also classified as stable or loose by the lack or presence of underlying bony edema on MRI.
- Acute stage I and II lesions can be managed nonoperatively.
- Initial period of non–weight bearing and cast immobilization is followed by progressive weight bearing and mobilization by 12 to 16 weeks.[78,79]
- Authors have quoted lower success rates with nonoperative treatment in recent years, especially in the setting of a chronic lesion.[80]
- As with other ankle injuries, once pain has begun to resolve and after the initial period of immobilization, a functional rehabilitation program can be initiated.

Operative

- This typically been reserved for stage I and II lesions that have failed conservative treatment for 1 year and for most stage III and IV lesions.
- Surgical options include both open and arthroscopic techniques.
- Excision of the lesion followed by curettage of the bed of the lesion and drilling the underlying subchondral bone to form vascular channels is typically performed.
- Success rate for this procedure is 78% to 88%.[80]
- If a lesion is acute and comprises one third of the talar dome, internal fixation is preferred.[81]
- Newer trends include osteochondral allografts and autografts, especially for unstable and larger lesions.[82,83]

Prognosis/Return to Play

- Prognosis surrounding osteochondral lesions of the talus is related to the stage of lesion and treatment modality chosen.
- Lower-stage lesions carry a more favorable prognosis.
- Surgical treatment has shown relatively high success rates as well.
- Return-to-play guidelines have not been as strictly defined for these lesions as for other injuries to the ankle, but the same general rules apply.

- An athlete is usually ready to return to play with resolution of symptoms, confidence in the ankle, the ability to perform sports-related activities, and the completion of a functional rehabilitation program.

Complications/Indications for Referral

Complications of osteochondral lesions of the talus are mainly related to delayed diagnosis. The key to avoiding this is considering these lesions in chronic ankle pain and in association with other forms of ankle trauma. Referral should be considered for stage I and II injuries that have failed an initial period of conservative treatment and for all stage III and IV injuries. Referral is also indicated in osteochondral lesions associated with other injuries such as fractures.

APPROACH TO THE ATHLETE WITH ACHILLES TENDON INJURY

HISTORY AND PHYSICAL EXAMINATION

Evaluating a patient with an Achilles tendon injury starts with a thorough history and physical examination. History should focus on athletic training history and participation patterns. Achilles injuries have been associated with recent increases in training and with "weekend warrior"–type activities, especially those that require jumping. In paratenonitis, patients report localized pain with burning during or after engaging in athletic activities. On the other hand, tendinosis is often painless. These two modalities are not exclusive. Partial and complete tendon ruptures involve sharp pain, and patients typically report feeling as if they have been "kicked in the leg."

The physical examination should be performed with the patient prone, feet hanging off the table. Palpation of the entire gastrocnemius–soleus myotendinous complex should be performed at rest and with both passive and active ankle motion. Calf atrophy, tenderness to palpation, warmth, swelling, nodularity, and tendinous defects should all be noted. Abnormal forefoot position should also be noticed, as this is often easily correctable with an orthotic. With paratenonitis, patients have well-localized tenderness and signs of inflammation. Tendinosis involves a palpable nodule in the tendon. A partial rupture demonstrates a focally tender and swollen area with a subtle defect. A complete rupture typically has a palpable defect or depression in the tendon and a positive Thompson test, and patients cannot perform a single heel raise. A complete rupture can occasionally be masked by a hematoma and intact accessory ankle flexors.

DIAGNOSTIC TESTING

There are basically two modalities commonly used to evaluate the integrity of the Achilles tendon: ultrasound and MRI. Ultrasound is inexpensive and fast, allows dynamic examination, and is useful at determining tendon thickness and evaluating the size of the tendon gap after a rupture. On the other hand, it requires experience to both perform and interpret the examination. MRI is more expensive and does not allow dynamic examination. It is far superior in the detection of incomplete ruptures and chronic degenerative changes. It is also useful in following tendon healing. If reliable sonography is available, some authors prefer this as a first-line study. If sonography is unreliable or the results of the test are equivocal, MRI becomes the study of choice.[84]

TREATMENT

Nonoperative

- Paratenonitis is typically treated conservatively.
  - An acute exacerbation is managed by rest.
  - Ice and nonsteroidal anti-inflammatory drugs (NSAIDs) further serve to decrease inflammation.
  - A custom orthotic designed to absorb shock or a small heel lift can also be employed.
- With a chronic presentation, a period of complete rest followed by gradual structured return to activities is recommended.
- Modification of an athlete's training program focusing on lower-impact cross-training is often warranted.[85]
- Stretching of the heel cord can be assisted by the use of a 5-degree dorsiflexion ankle foot orthosis worn at night for 3 months.[26]
- Corticosteroid injection is *not* recommended due to a lack of proven efficacy and risk of adverse effects to the mechanical properties of the tendon.
- Brisement has been demonstrated to be a useful modality.
  - A dilute local anesthetic is injected directly into the paratenon sheath under ultrasound guidance to break up adhesions.
- Tendinosis is typically asymptomatic.
  - If activity-related pain develops, the patient can be managed conservatively, as outlined earlier.
- Nonoperative treatment for an acute Achilles tendon rupture is as follows:
  - Initial period of immobilization is performed.
  - If ultrasound demonstrates tendon apposition at 20 degrees or less of plantar flexion, nonoperative treatment can persist.
  - The leg is initially placed in a splint in plantar flexion for 2 weeks.

- A short-leg cast or a removable boot with an elevated heel is typically worn for 6 to 8 weeks.
- The patient is then progressively weaned and gentle range of motion begins.
- When transitioning to shoes, a 2-cm heel lift is used for 1 month.
- After this, a 1-cm heel lift can be worn for an additional 2 months.
- Strengthening can begin at 8 to 10 weeks with return to running at 4 to 6 months, though maximal strength may not be achieved for 12 months, and residual weakness may remain.[26]

Operative

- Chronic recalcitrant paratenonitis that has failed conservative therapy is occasionally treated with surgery.
  - This involves excising the thickened paratenon.
  - Postoperatively, motion is initiated immediately, weight bearing begins at 7 to 10 days, and progressive strengthening is employed.
  - When the patient can walk without pain, rehabilitation can be expanded.
  - Running is typically reintroduced at 6 to 10 weeks and return to competition at 3 to 6 months.[26]
- The acute onset of pain in the setting of tendinosis is suggestive of a partial tendon rupture.
- If such pain fails conservative treatment, surgery can be performed.
  - Surgical treatment consists of excising the diseased tendon with a side-to-side repair of healthy tendon tissue and repair of the paratenon.
  - Postoperatively, the tendon is protected with weight bearing as tolerated in a walking boot for 2 to 4 weeks.
  - Range of motion is allowed several times a day, and gradual return to sports is allowed after resolution of symptoms and the completion of a strength rehabilitation program.[26]
- Surgical treatment is a valid option in the setting of an acute Achilles tendon rupture.
  - This is recommended for younger and more athletic patients.
  - Surgery is also indicated when a tendon apposition cannot be achieved with 20 degrees of plantar flexion.
  - The tendon ends are reapproximated using suture and the paratenon is repaired.
  - Postoperative regimens differ, with some authors advocating a more aggressive rehabilitation for elite athletes.
  - Range of motion consisting of active dorsiflexion to 20 degrees and passive plantar flexion may begin 3 to 7 days after surgery.
  - Patients wear a walking boot for 6 weeks with progression to sport thereafter, as outlined for nonoperative treatment.

- More typically, a short-leg cast is typically worn for 6 to 8 weeks followed by shoe wear with a 1-cm lift for 1 month.
- Resistance exercises begin at 8 to 10 weeks with return to running at 4 to 6 months.[26]
- Chronic Achilles tendon ruptures result in significant plantar flexion weakness and invariably require surgery. Repair of these ruptures is beyond the scope of this chapter.

Prognosis/Return to Play

- Return to play generally occurs after the time periods outlined in the above-mentioned functional treatment sections.
- With paratenonitis, it is reasonable to resume sports-related activity with the resolution of symptoms.
- The patients must be counseled on the importance of gradually increasing training regimens to allow the tendon to fully accommodate to its workload.
- Both nonoperative and operative means of treating acute Achilles tendon ruptures have been shown to have satisfactory outcomes.
- Return to play may occur slightly sooner with operatively repaired tendons than with nonoperatively treated tendons.
- In either case, return to play typically occurs 4 to 6 months after the injury after completion of a sport-specific rehabilitation program.

Complications/Indications for Referral

The major complication of paratenonitis and tendinosis is rupture of the Achilles tendon. That is why effective treatment of these conditions emphasizes modifying the factors that contributed to the conditions in the first place. As alluded to earlier, a controversy exists surrounding nonoperative and operative treatment for acute Achilles tendon ruptures. Nonoperative treatment avoids surgical risk and has rerupture rates quoted at 8% to 39%. Surgical repair carries the surgical risks of wound infection, skin necrosis, and nerve injury, but is quoted to have a rerupture rate of only approximately 2% and slightly superior strength.[86] Referral is indicated in the setting of chronic, recalcitrant paratenonitis and with partial and acute tendon ruptures.

APPROACH TO THE ATHLETE WITH A LISFRANC SPRAIN

HISTORY AND PHYSICAL EXAMINATION

When evaluating a patient with forefoot/midfoot pain, it is important to understand the mechanism of injury. Patients with a Lisfranc injury typically report immediate midfoot pain after an axial load or twisting injury to the foot. They often have significant difficulty with immediate weight bearing. Since the deep peroneal nerve runs almost directly over the Lisfranc joint, they may also report paresthesias in the first dorsal webspace. A less severe injury may mask itself as pain in the midfoot exacerbated by cutting or pushing off.

The physical examination of a suspected Lisfranc injury is an important part of the evaluation. Patients usually demonstrate difficulty with weight bearing, if they are able to weight bear at all. Swelling is common to just about all Lisfranc injuries. In fact, ligamentous rupture and/or fracture to the Lisfranc joint typically produce significant swelling in the midfoot. It is important to palpate all of the midfoot joints, and tenderness at the base of the first and/or second metatarsal is common with Lisfranc injuries. Two provocative tests are useful in the evaluation of these injuries: the metatarsal squeeze and Lisfranc stress tests.[87] In the metatarsal squeeze test, compression of the metatarsal necks may produce pain and/or abnormal motion at the metatarsal bases. With the Lisfranc stress test, anterior or posterior translation of the first metatarsal head may demonstrate increased or painful motion. Since the dorsalis pedis artery and deep peroneal nerve run in the vicinity of the Lisfranc joint, a careful neurovascular examination is also imperative when evaluating these injuries.

DIAGNOSTIC TESTING

Suspected injuries of the Lisfranc joint should be evaluated with AP, oblique, and lateral x-rays of the foot. If possible, weight-bearing x-rays are preferred, as they serve to help make more subtle injuries easier to identify (Fig. 21.5). These films should be evaluated for fractures and dislocations of the bones of the Lisfranc joints. Subtle avulsion/chip fractures can be indicative of avulsion injuries of the ligaments. Joint spaces may be widened between the metatarsals and cuneiforms, neighboring metatarsal bases, and/or neighboring cuneiforms. The first or second metatarsal base may be displaced dorsally or plantarly on lateral imaging.

Advanced imaging, such as CT or MRI scans, is also useful with the evaluation of Lisfranc injuries. These scans often serve to augment plain imaging. CT scans are best to show the bony anatomy of the Lisfranc joint and can help identify subtle avulsion fractures. MRI scans are particularly useful in evaluating more subtle soft tissue injuries such as ligament sprains and tears not evident on normal plain x-rays. MRI should be considered in patients with normal x-ray or CT studies but persistent pain and a compelling physical examination.

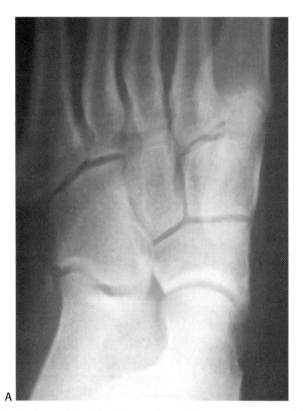

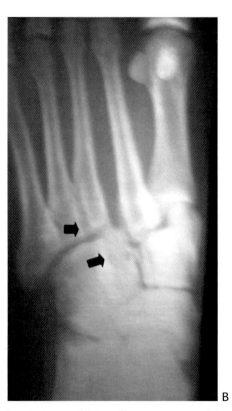

A   B

FIG. 21.5. Medial oblique view of the tarsometatarsal joint. **A:** Normal joint alignment on weight bearing. **B:** View of tarsometatarsal injury with lateral displacement of the fourth metatarsal in relation to the medial border of the cuboid *(arrows)*. Reprinted with permission from Bucholz RW, Heckman JD. *Rockwood & Green's Fractures in Adults.* 5th ed. Baltimore: Lippincott Williams & Wilkins; 2001.

TREATMENT

Nonoperative

- Nonoperative treatment for Lisfranc injuries is reserved for sprains and nondisplaced injuries.
  - Patients are treated with a period of protected weight bearing and measures to decrease inflammation such as ice and elevation.
  - Patients will also usually benefit from orthotic support to the arch of the midfoot.
  - Patients with grade I or II sprains can usually advance their activities, as symptoms permit.
  - Repeat x-rays are an important part of the treatment plan for these patients to rule out displacement of the Lisfranc joint.
- Avulsion fractures with good bony alignment can also be treated nonoperatively.
  - These patients should be kept non–weight bearing in a cast or cast boot for 6 to 8 weeks.
  - Serial x-rays should be obtained to rule out displacement.
  - After this period, weight bearing and activity should be advanced slowly, as symptoms allow.
  - Nondisplaced fractures and/or ligamentous injuries can be treated in a similar fashion, provided there is close vigilance for potential displacement.

Operative

- Operative treatment is indicated for all displaced Lisfranc injuries.
- Surgery for Lisfranc injuries involves reestablishing anatomic alignment of the midfoot via open or closed manipulation and fixation in the form of screws, plates, or pins.
- Postoperatively, patients are treated with immobilization and a period of non–weight bearing for 10 to 12 weeks.
- At this point, the patient can begin progressive weight bearing and a functional rehabilitation program, as outlined previously.

Prognosis/Return to Play

- It is critically important to ease back into weight-bearing activities and functional rehabilitation before return to play can occur.
- Patients with residual pain should not be allowed to return to play until symptoms have resolved.
- During the treatment period, it is also important to perform periodic x-rays, as mentioned earlier, to assure normal anatomic relationships in the midfoot.

Complications/Indications for Referral

As mentioned previously, Lisfranc injuries can lead to significant disability if treated inappropriately. Missed injuries or initially nondisplaced injuries that go on to undetected displacement are particularly important to avoid. Therefore, serial weight-bearing x-rays are important. Grade I or II sprains can be treated successfully nonoperatively and do not necessarily warrant referral, just close observation. Any patient with a complete ligamentous disruption, fracture, or displaced injury should be referred to an orthopaedist for further evaluation and treatment.

APPROACH TO THE ATHLETE WITH TURF TOE

HISTORY AND PHYSICAL EXAMINATION

When evaluating a patient with forefoot pain or suspected turf toe, it is important to gather information around the sport(s) played. Such information includes frequency of play, the types of playing surfaces involved, and footwear. Patients with turf toe typically play frequently on hard surfaces (artificial turf, hard court, hard dry ground, etc.). As mentioned earlier, modern athletic footwear is often quite flexible and may contribute to the injury. Patients will usually complain of pain in the base of the first toe, usually on the plantar surface, which is exacerbated by athletic activities such as running, cutting, and jumping, particularly on artificial turf.

The physical examination of a suspected turf toe injury is a very important part of the diagnosis. These patients may exhibit some degree of edema about the first metatarsal phalangeal joint. Passive and active range of motion of this joint is usually painful and may even be restricted compared to the opposite side. A stiff first toe is often referred to as hallux rigidus. In some instances, instability of the first metatarsal phalangeal joint may even be evident.

DIAGNOSTIC TESTING

The diagnosis of turf toe is made primarily on the basis of history and physical examination. However, it is important to rule out more serious injuries such as fractures and dislocations. It is therefore recommended to obtain AP, oblique, and lateral x-rays of the foot. Patients with turf toe usually have normal x-rays, but may show subluxation of the first metatarsal phalangeal joint if there is loss of capsular integrity and/or significant joint effusion. With longstanding turf toe/hallux rigidus with joint instability, patients may develop degenerative changes such as osteophyte formation on x-ray as well. MRI or CT scan is typically not indicated in evaluation of a suspected turf toe injury.

TREATMENT

Nonoperative

- Treatment focuses around limiting inflammation.
- Activity modification for at least 3 weeks to allow the joint capsule to heal.
- Other modalities include ice, elevation, and NSAIDs.
- Other conservative treatment measures include taping the first toe, stiffer footwear, and turf toe shoe inserts, which are both designed to limit first-toe motion and recurrent injury.
- These are typically employed during the return-to-play period.

Operative

- Operative treatment for turf toe is rarely necessary and is usually the last treatment option.
- Patients who develop degenerative changes and/or hallux rigidus may benefit from surgery.
- Patients with prominent osteophytes may benefit from osteophyte removal or cheilectomy.
- Significant degeneration of the first metatarsal phalangeal joint may be an indication for fusion of this joint to limit pain.

Prognosis/Return to Play

- Athletes diagnosed with turf toe should take at least a 3-week hiatus from athletic activity.
- They should be considered for return to play when symptoms and evidence of inflammation have subsided.
- Upon return to play, they often benefit from measures to restrict reinjury such as taping the first toe, shoe inserts designed to support the first toe, and stiffer foot wear.
- Despite adequate treatment and prevention strategies, turf toe can be a recurrent problem; therefore, vigilance for early symptoms is necessary.

Complications/Indications for Referral

It is important to rule out more serious problems such as fracture or stress fracture in a patient with suspected turf toe. Patients with a fracture or stress fracture should be referred to a sports medicine physician and/or surgeon for further management. Another complication with turf toe is recurrence, which is common in athletes who return to play too soon. Patients with recurrent, refractory turf toe should be considered for referral, as should those with evidence of significant degenerative disease of the first metatarsal phalangeal joint.

KEY POINTS

- The Ottawa ankle rules should be applied while deciding when to obtain x-rays of the foot and ankle
- Ankle sprains are common and can usually be treated by conservative means and functional rehabilitation
- Syndesmotic injuries represent a more serious injury to the ankle and may require operative treatment
- Isolated lateral malleolus fractures can be treated conservatively, whereas unstable ankle fractures require operative treatment
- Osteochondral lesions of the talus are difficult to diagnose and warrant referral to a surgeon
- Achilles tendon ruptures can be treated successfully either conservatively or operatively, with operative treatment favored for athletes
- Injuries to the Lisfranc joint are potentially seriously debilitating and warrant close observation and/or early referral
- Athletes with turf toe should refrain from sporting activities for at least 3 weeks, longer if symptoms have not subsided

REFERENCES

1. Boyd HS, Knight RA. Fractures of the astralgus. *South Med J.* 1942;35:160–167.
2. Burns WC, Prakash K, Adelaar R, et al. Tibiotalar joint dynamics: indications for the syndesmotic screw, a cadaver study. *Foot Ankle.* 1993;14:153–158.
3. Hartford JM, Gorczyca JT, McNamara JL, et al. Tibiotalar contact area. Contribution of posterior malleolus and deltoid ligament. *Clin Orthop Relat Res.* 1995;320:182–187.
4. Vinton CV, DeAngelis N, Lahey P, et al. Diagnosing deltoid ligament injury in supination-external rotation ankle fractures: the external rotation stress test. Podium Presentation, OTA Annual Meeting; October 2006; Phoenix, AZ.
5. Barker HB, Beynnon BD, Renstron PA. Ankle injury risk factors in sports. *Sports Med.* 1997;23:69–74.
6. Jones MH, Amendola AS. Acute treatment of inversion ankle sprains. *Clin Orthop Relat Res.* 2007;455:169–172.
7. Beynnon BD, Renstrom PA, Alosa DM, et al. Ankle ligament injury risk factors: a prospective study of college athletes. *J Orthop Res.* 2001;19:213–220.
8. Beynnon BD, Webb G, Huber BM, et al. Radiographic measurement of anterior talar translation in the ankle: determination of the most reliable method. *Clin Biomech.* 2005;20:301–306.
9. McGuine TA, Greene JJ, Best T, et al. Balance as a predictor of ankle injuries in high school basketball players. *Clin J Sport Med.* 2000;10:239–244.
10. McKay GD, Goldie PA, Payne WR, et al. A prospective study of injuries in basketball: a total profile and comparison by gender and standard of competition. *J Sci Med Sport.* 2001;4:196–211.
11. Gerber JP, Williams GN, Scoville CR, et al. Persistent disability associated with ankle sprains: a prospective examination of an athletic population. *Foot Ankle Int.* 1998;19:653–660.
12. Wolfe MW, Uhl TL, Mattacola CG, et al. Management of ankle sprains. *Am Fam Physician.* 2001;63:93–104.
13. Hopkinson WJ, St Pierre P, Ryan JB, et al. Syndesmosis sprains of the ankle. *Foot Ankle.* 1990;10:325–330.

14. Edwards GS Jr, DeLee JC. Ankle diastasis without fracture. *Foot Ankle.* 1984;4:305–312.
15. Michelson JD. Ankle fractures resulting from rotational injuries. *J Am Acad Orthop Surg.* 2003;11:403–412.
16. Bucholz RW, Heckman JD, Court-Brown C, eds. *Rockwood and Green's Fractures in Adults.* 6th ed. Philadelphia, PA: Lippincott Williams & Wilkins; 2006.
17. Kannus P, Palvanen M, Niemi S, et al. Increasing number and incidence of low-trauma ankle fractures in elderly people: Finnish statistics during 1970–2000 and projections for the future. *Bone.* 2002;31: 430–433.
18. Honkanen R, Tuppurainen M, Kroger H, et al. Relationships between risk factors and fractures differ by type of fracture: a population-based study of 12,192 perimenopausal women. *Osteoporos Int.* 1998;8: 25–31.
19. Brophy RH, Barnes R, Rodeo SA, et al. Prevalence of musculoskeletal disorders at the NFL combine—trends from 1987–2000. *Med Sci Sports Exerc.* 2007;39:22–27.
20. Saunders R. Fractures and fracture dislocations of the talus. In: Mann RA, Coughlin MJ, eds. *Surgery of the Foot and Ankle.* Vol 2. 7th ed. St. Louis, MO: Mosby; 1991:1465–1518.
21. Schacter AK, Chen AL, Reddy PD, et al. Osteochondral lesions of the talus. *J Am Acad Orthop Surg.* 2005;13:152–158.
22. Sneppen O, Christensen SB, Krogsoe O, et al. Fracture of the body of the talus. *Acta Orthop Scand.* 1977;48:317–324.
23. Alexander AH, Lictman DM. Surgical treatment of transchondral talar-dome fractures (osteochondritis dessicans): long-term follow-up. *J Bone Joint Surg Am.* 1980;62:646–652.
24. Van Buecken K, Barrack RL, Alexander AH, et al. Arthroscopic treatment of trancshondral talar dome fractures. *Am J Sports Med.* 1989;17: 350–356.
25. Lysholm J, Wiklander J. Injuries in runners. *Am J Sports Med.* 1987;15: 168–171.
26. Saltzman CL, Tearse DS. Achilles tendon injuries. *J Am Acad Orthop Surg.* 1998;6:316–325.
27. Carr AJ, Norris SH. The blood supply of the calcaneal tendon. *J Bone Joint Surg Br.* 1989;71:100–101.
28. Strocchi R, DePasquale V, Guizzardi S, et al. Human Achilles tendon: morphological and morphometric variations as a function of age. *Foot Ankle.* 1991;12:100–104.
29. Puddu G, Ippolito E, Postacchini F. A classification of Achilles tendon disease. *Am J Sports Med.* 1976;4:145–150.
30. Leadbetter WB. The pathohistology of overuse tendon injury in sports (poster exhibit). Presented at the 59th Annual Meeting of the American Academy of Orthopaedic Surgeons; February 20, 1992; Washington, DC.
31. Marder R. Current methods for the evaluation of ankle ligament injuries. *J Bone Joint Surg Am.* 1993;76:1103–1111.
32. Rasmussen O. Stability of the ankle joint. Analysis of the function and traumatology of the ankle ligaments. *Acta Orthop Scand Suppl.* 1985; 211:1–75.
33. Rubin G, Witten M. The talar-tilt angle and the fibular collateral ligaments. A method for the determination of talar tilt. *J Bone Joint Surg Am.* 1960;42:311–326.
34. Cox JS, Hewes TF. "Normal" talar tilt angle. *Clin Orthop Relat Res.* 1979; 140:37–41.
35. Nyska M, Amir H, Porath A, et al. Radiological assessment of a modified anterior drawer test of the ankle. *Foot Ankle.* 1992;13:400–403.
36. van Dijk CN, Lim LS, Bossuyt PM, et al. Physical examination is sufficient for the diagnosis of sprained ankles. *J Bone Joint Surg Br.* 1996; 78(6):958–962.
37. Alonso A, Khoury L, Adams R. Clinical test for the ankle syndesmosis injury: reliability and prediction of return of function. *J Orthop Sports Phys Ther.* 1998;27:276–284.
38. Stricker PR, Spindler KP, Gauter KB. Prospective evaluation of history and physical examination: variables to determine radiography in acute ankle injuries. *Clin J Sport Med.* 1998;8:209–214.
39. Maffulli N. The clinical diagnosis of subcutaneous tear of the Achilles tendon: a prospective study in 174 patients. *Am J Sports Med.* 1998;26: 266–270.
40. Stiell IG, Greenberg GH, McKnight RD, et al. Decision rules for the use of radiography in acute ankle injuries. Refinement and prospective validation. *JAMA.* 1993;269:1127–1132.
41. Nugent PJ. Ottawa ankle rules accurately assess injuries and reduce reliance on radiographs. *J Fam Pract.* 2004;53:785–788.

42. Cass JR, Borrey BF. Ankle instability: current concepts, diagnosis, and treatment. *Mayo Clin Proc.* 1984;59:165–170.
43. Cox JS. Surgical and nonsurgical treatment of acute ankle sprains. *Clin Orthop Relat Res.* 1985;198:118–126.
44. Ryan JB, Hopkinson WJ, Wheeler JH, et al. Office management of the acute ankle sprain. *Clin Sports Med.* 1989;8:477–495.
45. Knight KL. Initial care of acute injuries: the RICES technique. In: *Cryotherapy in Sport Injury Management.* Champaign, Ill: Human Kinetics; 1995:209–215.
46. Wexler RK. The injured ankle. *Am Fam Physician.* 1998;57:474–480.
47. Karlsson J, Lundin O, Lind K, et al. Early mobilization versus immobilization after ankle ligament stabilization. *Scand J Med Sci Sports.* 1999; 9:299–303.
48. Dettori JR, Pearson BD, Basmania CJ, et al. Early ankle mobilization. Part I: the immediate effect on acute, lateral ankle sprains (a randomized clinical trial). *Mil Med.* 1994;159:5–20.
49. Thacker SB, Stroup DF, Branche CM, et al. The prevention of ankle sprains in sports. a systematic review of the literature. *Am J Sports Med.* 1999;27:753–760.
50. Hartsell HD, Spaulding SJ. Eccentric/concentric ratios at selected velocities for the inverter and evertor muscles of the chronically unstable ankle. *Br J Sports Med.* 1999;33:255–258.
51. Bahr R, Lian O, Bahr IA. A twofold reduction in the incidence of acute ankle sprains in volleyball after the introduction of an injury prevention program: a prospective cohort study. *Scand J Med Sci Sports.* 1997; 7:172–177.
52. Mattacola CG, Lloyd JW. Effects of a 6 week strength and proprioception training program on measures of dynamic balance: a single-case design. *J Athl Train.* 1997;32:127–135.
53. Safran MR, Zachazewski JE, Benedetti RS, et al. Lateral ankle sprains: a comprehensive review. Part 2: treatment and rehabilitation with an emphasis on the athlete. *Med Sci Sports Exerc.* 1999;31(suppl):S438–S447.
54. DeLee JC, Drez D, Miller MD, eds. *Orthopaedic Sports Medicine: Principles and Practice.* Foot and Ankle. Vol 2. Philadelphia, PA: WB Saunders; 2003.
55. Teitz CC, Harrington RM. A biochemical analysis of the squeeze test for sprains of the syndesmotic ligaments of the ankle. *Foot Ankle Int.* 1998; 19:489–492.
56. Harper MC, Keller TS. A radiographic evaluation of the tibiofibular syndesmosis. *Foot Ankle.* 1989;10:156–160.
57. Pneumaticos SG, Noble PC, Chatziioannou SN, et al. The effects of rotation on radiographic evaluation of the tibiofibular syndesmosis. *Foot Ankle Int.* 2002;23:107–111.
58. Beumer A, van Hemert WL, Niesing R, et al. Radiographic measurement of the distal tibiofibular syndesmosis has limited use. *Clin Orthop Relat Res.* 2004;423:227–234.
59. Clanton TO, Paul P. Syndesmosis injuries in athletes. *Foot Ankle Clin.* 2002;7:529–549.
60. Weening B, Bhandari M. Predictors of functional outcome following trans-syndesmotic screw fixation of ankle fractures. *J Orthop Trauma.* 2005;19:102–108.
61. Joy G, Patzakis MJ, Harvey JP Jr. Precise evaluation of the reduction of severe ankle fractures. *J Bone Joint Surg Am.* 1974;56:979–993.
62. Leeds HC, Erlich MG. Instability of the distal tibiofibular syndesmosis after bimalleolar and trimalleolar ankle fractures. *J Bone Joint Surg Am.* 1984;66:490–503.
63. Pettrone FA, Gail M, Pee D, et al. Quantitative criteria for prediction of the results after displaced fracture of the ankle. *J Bone Joint Surg Am.* 1983;65:667–677.
64. Chissell HR, Jones J. The influence of a diastasis screw on the outcome of Weber type-c ankle fractures. *J Bone Joint Surg Br.* 1995;77:435–438.
65. DeAngelis NA, Eskander MS, French BG. Does medial tenderness predict deep deltoid ligament incompetence in supination-external rotation type ankle fractures? *J Orthop Trauma.* 2007;21(4):244–247.
66. Muller ME, Allgower M, Schneider R, eds. *Manual of Internal Fixation: Techniques Recommended by the AO Group.* 2nd ed. Berlin, Germany: Springer-Verlag; 1979:282–299.
67. Kristensen KD, Hansen T. Closed treatment of ankle fractures: stage II supination-eversion fractures followed for 20 years. *Acta Orthop Scand.* 1985;56:107–109.
68. Yde J, Kristensen KD. Ankle fractures: supination-eversion fractures stage II. Primary and late results of operative and non-operative treatment. *Acta Orthop Scand.* 1980;51:695–702.
69. Bauer M, Jonsson K, Nilsson B. Thirty year follow-up of ankle fractures. *Acta Orthop Scand.* 1985;56:103–106.

70. Michelson JD. Fractures about the ankle. *J Bone Joint Surg Am.* 1995;77: 142–152.

71. Berndt AL, Harty M. Transchondral fractures (osteochondritis dessicans) of the talus. *J Bone Joint Surg Am.* 1959;41:988–1020.

72. Davidson AM, Steele HD, MacKenzie DA, et al. A review of twenty-one cases of transchondral fractures of the talus. *J Trauma.* 1967;7: 378–415.

73. Canale ST, Kelly FB Jr. Fractures of the neck of the talus: long-term evaluation of seventy-one cases. *J Bone Joint Surg Am.* 1978;60:143–156.

74. Reis ND, Zinman C, Besser MIB, et al. High-resolution computerized tomography in clinical orthopaedics. *J Bone Joint Surg Br.* 1982;64: 20–24.

75. Anderson IF, Crichton KJ, Grattan-Smith T, et al. Osteochondral fractures of the dome of the talus. *J Bone Joint Surg Am.* 1989;71: 1143–1152.

76. Urman M, Ammann W, Sisler J, et al. The role of bone scintigraphy in the evaluation of talar dome fractures. *J Nucl Med.* 1991;32: 2241–2244.

77. Dipaolo JD, Nelson DW, Colville MR. Characterizing osteochondral lesions by magnetic resonance imaging. *Arthroscopy.* 1991;7: 101–104.

78. Schacter AK, Chen AL, Reddy PD, et al. Osteochondral lesions of the talus. *J Am Acad Orthop Surg.* 2005;13:152–158.

79. Saunders R. Fractures and fracture dislocations of the talus. In: Mann RA, Coughlin MJ, eds. *Surgery of the Foot and Ankle.* Vol 2. 7th ed. St. Louis, MO: Mosby; 1991:1465–1518.

80. Tol JL, Struijs PAA, Bossuyt PMM, et al. Treatment strategies in osteochondral defects of the talar dome: a systematic review. *Foot Ankle Int.* 2000;21:119–126.

81. DeLee JC. Fractures and dislocations of the foot. In: Mann RA, Couglin MJ, eds. *Surgery of the Foot and Ankle.* 6th ed. St. Louis, MO: Mosby; 1991:1465–1518.

82. Gross AE, Agnidis Z, Hutchison CR. Osteochondritis defects of the talus treated with fresh osteochondral allograft transplantation. *Foot Ankle Int.* 2001;22:385–391.

83. Assenmacher JA, Kelikian AS, Gottlob C, et al. Arthorscopically assisted autologous osteochondral transplantation for osteochondral lesions of the talar dome: an MRI and clinical follow-up study. *Foot Ankle Int.* 2001;22:544–587.

84. Neuhold A, Stiskal M, Kainberger F, et al. Degenerative Achilles tendon disease: assessment by magnetic resonance and ultrasonography. *Eur J Radiol.* 1992;14:213–220.

85. Clement DB, Taunton JE, Smart GW. Achilles tendinits and peritendinitis: etiology and treatment. *Am J Sports Med.* 1981;12:179–184.

86. Cetti R, Christensen SE, Ejsted R, et al. Operative versus nonoperative treatment of Achilles tendon rupture: a prospective randomized study and review of the literature. *Am J Sports Med.* 1993;21:791–799.

87. Arntz T, Veith RG, Hansen ST. Fractures and fracture-dislocations of the tarsometatarsal joint. *J Bone Joint Dis.* 1988;70A:173–181.

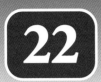

22 Athlete with Stress Fracture

Katherine M. Riggert

INTRODUCTION

Stress fractures are common injuries that occur in both competitive and recreational athletes. Although the majority of stress fractures are diagnosed in runners, any athlete participating in activities that involve repetitive loading is at risk, including swimmers, rowers, and baseball players.[1–3] The most common sites in runners are the tibia and metatarsals; however, the ribs, olecranon, and spine are recognized as frequent sites among rowers, baseball pitchers, and gymnasts, respectively.[1,2,4,5] Stress fractures can be a diagnostic challenge due to the insidious onset of symptoms. They can mimic other common musculoskeletal injuries such as muscle strains and tendinopathies. Having a high index of clinical suspicion and an awareness of the risk factors and sport-specific demands can narrow the time to the correct diagnosis and treatment. Clinical knowledge of high-risk sites is important because management differs from that of low-risk sites and early treatment may prevent catastrophic outcomes.

FUNCTIONAL ANATOMY

Proper bone health is dependent on the equilibrium of bone resorption by osteoclasts with bone rebuilding and remodeling by osteoblasts (Fig. 22.1). Bone injury occurs on a continuum and begins when normal bone reparation and remodeling is disrupted. In this state, osteoclastic bone resorption outpaces osteoblastic bone building. In the earliest phases, cumulative microdamage occurs due to repetitive loading and may progress to microscopic crack initiation.[6,7] If this imbalance between bone stress and reparation continues, crack propagation occurs, with the final stage being a nondisplaced or displaced fracture.[6]

Fatigue stress reaction or fracture is the most common type of bone stress injury in athletes and occurs when repetitive mechanical bone stress overloads the bone's ability to repair and rebuild. This often occurs when there is insufficient rest between exercise bouts or rapid increases in training demands. The majority of fatigue fractures occur in cortical (compact) bone, which is found at the diaphysis of long bones and the outer layer of short bones such as the tarsals and vertebral bodies.[3,6]

A second type of bone stress injury called an insufficiency reaction or fracture occurs when normal strains are placed on histologically abnormal bone as seen in osteopenia and osteoporosis. Athletes in a negative energy balance and hypoestrogenic state associated with the female athlete triad, osteoporosis, amenorrhea, and disordered eating, are at risk for this type of bone injury.[3,6] Among female distance runners, 10% had osteoporosis, while 50% were osteopenic.[8] A negative energy balance with associated amenorrhea places an athlete at risk for low bone density, particularly cancellous bone.[8] Cancellous stress fractures in female athletes have been associated with osteopenia.[9] Cancellous bone is found at the metaphysis and epiphysis of long bones and in the interior of short bones.

Stress fractures are grouped into low-risk and high-risk sites. Low-risk sites are more likely to heal through conservative management, whereas high-risk sites tend to have delayed union or nonunion, progression to complete fracture, and recurrence and often require operative management. Common low-risk sites are ribs, ulna shaft, femoral shaft, posteromedial tibia, and the first four metatarsals.[10] Low-risk sites are loaded with compressive forces. High-risk sites include the femoral neck, patella, anterior tibial diaphysis, medial malleolus, talus, navicular, first metatarsal sesamoids, and the proximal fifth metatarsal.[10] High-risk sites tend to be loaded with tensile forces, increasing the risk of adverse outcomes (Table 22.1).

EPIDEMIOLOGY

The incidence and anatomic location of stress injuries vary not only with each sport but also with regional and national sporting trends.[1,5] In track and field athletes, the incidence is 8.7% to 21.1% in males and females combined, although one study reported an incidence of greater than 30% in collegiate female track and field athletes alone.[1,8,11] The majority of studies cite the lower extremities as the most frequently affected anatomic region, with the tibia, fibula, metatarsals, and tarsals reported as the most common sites, with bilateral stress fractures occurring in 16.6% of cases.[1,2,8] More recently, the tibia and ribs were reported as the most common sites when greater representation of overhead

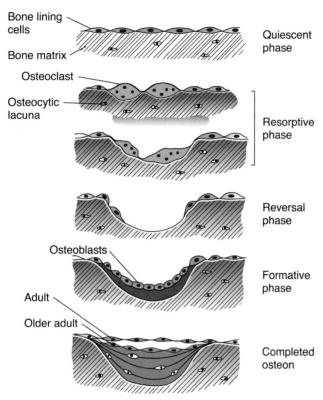

Bone lining cells

Bone matrix

Quiescent phase

Osteoclast

Osteocytic lacuna

Resorptive phase

Reversal phase

Osteoblasts

Formative phase

Adult

Older adult

Completed osteon

FIG. 22.1. Bone remodeling phases. Increased osteoclast activity during resorptive phase. Osteoblasts deposit new bone. Reprinted with permission from Rubin E, Farber JL. *Pathology.* 3rd ed. Philadelphia: Lippincott Williams & Wilkins; 1999.

throwing and rowing athletes was included than in previous studies.[5]

Among track and field athletes, distance runners were more likely to sustain stress fractures of the tibia, femur, fibula, and pelvis. Jumpers, sprinters, hurdlers, and those participating in multiple events had more foot fractures. Jumping and sprinting events were associated with navicular stress fractures.[3] Upper-extremity stress fractures occur in overhead throwing and racquet sports. Rib stress fractures

TABLE 22.1 High-risk versus Low-risk Stress Fracture Sites

High Risk	Low Risk
Femoral neck	Ribs
Patella	Ulna shaft
Anterior tibial diaphysis	Femoral shaft
Medial malleolus	Posteromedial tibia
Talus	First four metatarsals
Navicular	
First metatarsal sesamoids	
Proximal fifth metatarsal	

Data adapted from Boden BP, Osbahr DC, Jimenez C. Low risk stress fractures. *Am J Sports Med.* 2001;29:100–111.

have been associated with overhead throwing athletes and rowers and ulnar stress fractures with baseball pitchers.[5] Pars interarticularis stress fractures of the spine (spondylolysis) comprise 45% of all stress fractures in female gymnasts.[1]

Bone health in athletes is influenced by multiple factors, but the lack of well-designed, large prospective studies has resulted in a paucity of epidemiologic data regarding risk factors for stress fractures.[1] Intrinsic factors include nutritional status, gender, hormonal status, fitness levels, and biomechanical factors.[6,12] Extrinsic factors include training errors associated with changes in intensity, frequency, and duration of activities.[2,6] The effect of oral contraceptives on bone mineral density is unclear.[6,8,13] Oral contraceptive pills normalize menses in athletes with hypothalamic amenorrhea through estrogen replacement, but may mask underlying nutritional insufficiencies.[8]

Limited data identify disordered eating and menstrual dysfunction as significant risk factors for stress fractures among female athletes.[1] Amenorrheic and oligomenorrheic girls had an incidence of 15% versus 4% among eumenorrheic girls.[1] Osteopenia and amenorrhea in female athletes have been associated with cancellous stress fractures.[8,9] Limited comparative data suggest that there is no difference in the incidence of stress fractures between female and male athletes. However, adjustment of training hours for stress fracture rates has been suggested as a more definitive method to demonstrate that women are at higher risk.[1] With regard to age and race, there are no consistent or significant findings in the literature among athletes.[1] Hard training surfaces have not been associated with an increased risk for stress fractures.[8] Training errors were associated with 22.4% of all stress fractures in one study.[2]

NARROWING THE DIFFERENTIAL DIAGNOSIS

History

The earliest symptom of bone stress injury is insidious onset of lower-extremity pain during weight-bearing or sport-specific activities, which is relieved with rest. If the condition goes unrecognized and the athlete ignores the pain without activity modification, the pain may begin earlier in each exercise session and with greater severity. The pain may transition to a sharp, severe localized pain that occurs with all weight-bearing or inciting activities, with progression to resting pain.[3]

The patient will usually deny any specific trauma or injury prior to the onset of pain. An exception may be the tarsal bones, where a history of trauma was found to be associated with this type of stress fracture.[2] A specific episode of direct trauma or injury to a joint associated with torsional or hyperextension forces followed by swelling or joint instability should be investigated for ligamentous or cartilaginous pathology. Severe localized pain with fever as an initial symptom in the absence of trauma may be indicative of an acute infectious or inflammatory process. Night sweats and weight loss should raise concern for malignancy.

Activity and nutrition patterns often provide significant clues in the diagnosis of bone stress injuries. Any alteration in the training routine can place both experienced and novice athletes at risk for stress fractures. Competitive athletes may reveal a change in the type, intensity, or duration of their training. Recreational athletes may report beginning a new activity or embarking on an ambitious training program. Nutrition and training patterns should be assessed in all male and female athletes with a suspected eating disorder. A thorough menstrual history should be obtained in females since amenorrhea is a risk factor for stress fractures.[8] Even subtle menstrual irregularities may put the athlete at risk for poor bone health.[14] A direct correlation exists between the number of stress fractures and the length of amenorrhea.[8]

The underlying pathophysiology of menstrual dysfunction in female athletes relates to an energy imbalance that causes hypothalamic dysfunction.[8,13] A state of undernutrition leads to the loss of pulsatile hypothalamic hormone release.[8,13] This may occur when the athlete fails to meet his or her caloric needs either intentionally through excessive exercise and restrictive eating or through a combination of both. It may also occur unknowingly when minor alterations in a training program result in higher energy demands.[13]

Stress fractures often mimic other conditions. Thorough history taking and knowledge of particular pain patterns may help to narrow the differential (Table 22.2).

Evidence-based Physical Examination

Observation

Varus alignment (forefoot 72.6%, subtalar 71.9%, genu 29%, and tibial 18.9%) has been identified as a frequent finding among athletes with stress fractures.[2] No association was found between the severity of varus alignment and the stress fracture site.[2] Foot overpronation was associated with tarsal, fibular, and tibial stress fractures. Rigid pes cavus was observed most often in metatarsal and femoral stress fractures.[2]

Palpation

Localized bony tenderness is a common finding.[2,20] Palpable deformities and swelling may occur at the fracture site.[20] Swelling was found most commonly in the metatarsal and tarsal bones (Table 22.3).[2]

Range of Motion (ROM)

ROM is usually normal except for limitations in lumbar spine extension and hamstring flexibility that may occur in pars interarticularis defects.[16] Strength testing is usually normal.[12]

Special Tests

Hop Test

This test is used to assist in the clinical diagnosis of lower-extremity stress fractures, especially of the femoral neck and tibia. The test is positive when the patient is single-leg hopping and experiences pain in the area of concern for a stress fracture. A positive hop test has been associated with femoral stress fractures.[2,3,14]

Fulcrum Test

This test is used to assist in the clinical diagnosis of femoral shaft stress fractures. The athlete is seated on the edge of the examination table. The examiner's arm acts as a fulcrum under the patient's thigh and is moved from the distal to

TABLE 22.2	Pain Patterns and Associated Conditions
Location of Pain	**Differential Diagnosis**
Rib or thoracic	Rib stress fracture, scapulothoracic bursitis, slipped rib syndrome, disc pathology, intercostal muscle strain, pleuritis[15]
Low back or buttock	Sacral stress fracture, pars interarticularis stress fracture, disc pathology, sciatica, sacroiliac joint pathology, hip labral tear, iliopsoas pathology[3,16,17]
Proximal femur	Femoral neck stress fracture, avascular necrosis, bursitis, tendonitis, synovitis, neoplasm, muscle or tendon injuries[12]
Distal femur	Femoral shaft stress fracture, knee joint ligamentous or cartilaginous pathology, femoral condyle avascular necrosis, infection, neoplasm.[12] Older athletes—evaluate for spontaneous osteonecrosis of the femoral condyle[12]
Lower leg	Tibial stress fracture, exertional or chronic compartment syndrome, tendinopathy, muscle strain, ligamentous or cartilaginous injuries, myositis, nerve entrapment, neoplasm[18,19]

TABLE 22.3   **Common Localized Findings on Physical Examination**

Injury Site	Physical Examination
Foot	
Sesamoids	Tenderness over the plantar aspect of the first metatarsophalangeal joint, exacerbated by passive doriflexion and plantar flexion of the great toe[3]
Metatarsals	Tenderness directly over involved metatarsal Well-circumscribed swelling limited to dorsum of forefoot[21]
Navicular	Dorsal midfoot tenderness radiating to the medial arch in navicular stress fracture[3]
Leg	
Tibia	Medial or anterior tibial tenderness, swelling, palpable callus[3,19] Compartment swelling, tenderness, and neurovascular changes may help to distinguish between compartment syndrome and a bone stress injury[19]
Distal tibia	Chronic medial malleolar tenderness[3]
Fibula	Proximal or distal fibula tenderness[3]
Thigh	
Femoral shaft	Deep thigh tenderness, antalgic gait, positive hop test, positive fulcrum test[2,3,14,22]
Hip	
Femoral neck	Pain with end-range passive internal and external rotation of the hip with thigh flexed to 90 degrees, palpation of the groin, logrolling of the thigh[3,12,14]
Spine	Pain during extension, positive stork test (single-leg lumbar extension with pain on ipsilateral side), paravertebral tenderness at affected vertebrae[16]

proximal thigh while pressure is applied to the dorsum of the knee with the other hand. The test is positive if the patient experiences sharp pain localized to an area on the thigh that is being compressed by the examiner's arm that is an area of concern for a stress fracture.[22]

Tuning Fork Test

This test is used to assist in the clinical diagnosis of tibial stress fractures. A 128-Hz tuning fork is applied to the anterior surface of the tibia. The test is considered positive if the patient reports a marked exacerbation or reproduction of shin pain in a focal area of the tibia.[23]

Diagnostic Testing

The clinical presentation of bone injuries frequently mimics other musculoskeletal problems; therefore, laboratory testing and imaging studies can expedite the diagnostic process. Imaging studies vary in their specificity and sensitivity and therefore utility in making a diagnosis, grading the injury and guiding treatment, and return-to-play decisions. Common imaging studies include plain radiographs, magnetic resonance imaging (MRI), computed tomography (CT), and bone scan. Laboratory testing is not required to diagnose a stress fracture, but it can be valuable in the evaluation of multiple stress fractures and insufficiency fractures and in suspected cases of spondyloarthropathy or an eating disorder.

Laboratory Studies

Laboratory studies are not necessary for the diagnosis of stress fractures but may be useful to determine underlying causes and rule out other conditions (Table 22.4).

Imaging

Radiographs

- Plain radiographs are the first step in the evaluation of a suspected stress injury, even though within the first few

TABLE 22.4   **Laboratory Evaluation**

Conditions	Laboratory Studies
Female athlete triad/menstrual irregularities	CBC, chemistry panel, TSH, LH, estrodiol, urine pregnancy, testosterone, serum prolactin dexamethasone-suppression testing[8,14]
Insufficiency fracture/multiple stress fractures	CBC, ESR, TSH, PTH, alkaline phosphatase, calcium, phosphorus, 25-hydroxyvitamin D[8,12]
Spondyloarthropathies	HLA-B27, ANA, RF, ESR

CBC, complete blood count; TSH, thyroid-stimulating hormone; LH, luteinizing hormone; ESR, erythrocyte sedimentation rate; PTH, parathyroid hormone; HLA, human leukocyte antigen; ANA, antinuclear antibody; RF, rheumatoid factor.

weeks of the injury they are normal in up to two thirds of patients with stress fractures.[4,17,20]

- Because of the delay between the onset of clinical symptoms and radiographic findings, cortical fracture and periosteal reaction identified on radiography indicate progression to an advanced stage.[3,4]
- If radiographs are negative, but there is a high clinical suspicion for stress fracture, then either an MRI or bone scan should be performed.

MRI   MRI has emerged as the leading diagnostic modality for stress fractures, because it is highly specific in determining the site and grade of the injury and, as a result, treatment options.[3,4,17,24]

- MRI has a higher specificity than bone scan and a high sensitivity to bone marrow edema, an early indication of stress injury to bone.[17] Other benefits include absence of radiation exposure, less time consuming than bone scan, and cost may be equal to or less than bone scan at some institutions.
- A stress reaction appears on MRI as periosteal edema and bone marrow edema without a detectable fracture line. Stress fractures are represented by a low-signal cortical fracture line.
- MRI is particularly useful for sacral and femoral neck stress fractures because radiographic detection may lag behind clinical symptoms by weeks to months.[17]
- MRI was found to be the most sensitive and specific imaging modality for the detection of early tibial stress injuries in a comparison study between MRI, CT, and bone scan. The sensitivity of MRI, CT, and bone scan was 88%, 42%, and 74%, respectively. MRI and CT each had a specificity of 100%. MRI had a positive predictive value of 100% and a negative predictive value of 62%, whereas these values for CT were 100% and 26%, respectively.[18]

A radiographic grading system is used to determine the extent of injury, which can guide treatment and return-to-play decisions.[4,24]

- Grade 1—early stress phenomenon is exhibited by increased activity on bone scan and bone marrow edema on fat-suppressed or short T1 inversion recovery (STIR) sequence images.
- Grade 2—stress phenomenon is characterized by bone marrow edema on T2-weighted images.
- Grade 3—stress reaction is characterized by bone marrow edema on T1- and T2-weighted images but without evidence of a true stress fracture on plain radiographs.
- Grade 4—true stress fracture is exhibited by findings of cortical failure on MRI and radiography.[24]

Treatment is based on a progressive four-phase treatment plan that involves activity modification to a pain-free level.[4] Patients should be placed on crutches if they are symptomatic with weight-bearing activities. Using this standardized

TABLE 22.5	Four-phase Return-to-play Protocol[4]
Phase I	Pain control with ice and physical therapy modalities
	Swimming, aqua running, and cycling allowed if pain free
	Begin a trial of walking every second day
	If any discomfort with activities, regress back to a lower phase of the program or NWB if in phase 1
Phase II	Commence when there is pain-free ambulation for 3–5 days
	Allowed activities: low-impact aerobic conditioning equipment
	Initiate sport-specific muscle rehabilitation
Phase III	Progress from sport-specific drills every other day to limited, brief sports play, then gradual increase in sports play
	Stop activities if pain occurs at the original site of injury
Phase IV	Athlete permitted to return to full unrestricted activity

NWB, non–weight bearing.

protocol, average time to return to full sports activities was found to be 3.3 weeks for a grade 1 stress injury, 5.5 weeks for grade 2, 11.4 weeks for grade 3, and 14.3 weeks for grade 4.[4] The majority of bone stress injuries to the feet were grades 3 or 4 (Table 22.5).[4]

Bone Scan   Triple-phase bone scintigraphy is highly sensitive (84% to 100%) for detecting early bone stress remodeling and stress fractures and allows for detection of injury within 72 hours.[12] The specificity of the bone scan is reduced because increased tracer uptake is demonstrated in all areas of bone remodeling, including areas of inflammation, infection, neoplasm, and trauma.[3,17] Bone scan is also time consuming for patients and is not useful in grading injury, guiding treatment options, or evaluating healing progress.[20] The leading diagnostic modality for pars interarticularis stress fractures is bone scan using a single-photon emission CT scan (SPECT scan), followed by CT if the SPECT scan is positive.[25,26]

CT   This is useful for detection of pars interarticularis stress fractures when combined with SPECT bone scan.[25,26] Useful for detection of stress fractures when MRI is contraindicated. Limitations are that it cannot determine the acuity of bone lesions because it cannot effectively detect bone edema or early stress reactions.[17]

Ultrasound   This has a limited role for the detection of bone stress injuries: 43% sensitivity and 49% specificity.[27]

Dual-Energy X-ray Absorptiometry (DEXA) Scan   Bone mineral density testing with DEXA scan is recommended in athletes with cancellous stress fractures.[9]

APPROACH TO THE ATHLETE WITH A SESAMOID STRESS FRACTURE

Nearly 1% of running injuries involve the sesamoids, with 40% due to stress fractures and 30% due to sesamoiditis.[3] Other conditions with similar presentations include avascular necrosis, traumatic fractures, osteomyelitis, and bursitis.[3]

HISTORY AND PHYSICAL EXAMINATION

Insidious onset of medial forefoot pain with weight-bearing and toe-off activities suggests a sesamoid stress injury. Physical examination shows tenderness over the plantar aspect of the first metatarsophalangeal joint, exacerbated by passive dorsiflexion and plantar flexion of the great toe.[3] Athletes who engage in activities involving jumping, running, and repetitive forced dorsiflexion are at greatest risk.[3]

DIAGNOSTIC TESTING

Plain radiographs may show a transverse fracture of the sesamoid, but it may be difficult to differentiate between a fracture and a bipartite sesamoid, with bipartite sesamoid found in up to 15% of population.[28] Bone scintigraphy may show focal uptake and assist in the diagnosis. MRI demonstrating increased STIR signal intensity, and low T1 signal helps to differentiate a stress injury from sesamoiditis.[3]

TREATMENT

- High-risk sites such as the first metatarsal sesamoids tend to result in delayed union or nonunion, may require operative management, and are more likely to recur.[10]
- Treatment of high-risk stress fractures should be aggressively managed, aimed at fracture healing and prevention of fracture progression and recurrence.
- Treatment involves non–weight-bearing status and operative fixation.

Nonoperative

- Treatment involves a non–weight-bearing cast for 6 to 8 weeks.[20]
- Identification of risk factors is important to prevent recurrence.
- Menstrual history, nutritional assessment, and a review of the training regimen may provide important clues.
- Cross-training with cycling, aqua running, swimming are acceptable forms of low- and nonimpact activities that may be used to maintain cardiovascular fitness.

- After pain-free activity has been achieved, gradual progression of activities may begin (refer to Appendix C "Interval Running Program").

Operative

- Operative treatment is recommended in recalcitrant cases and with refracture.[20]
- Operative management involves sesamoid resection.

Prognosis/Return to Play

Gradual return to play when pain free with activities, often in 6 to 12 weeks.[20] Pain-free interval running program (Appendix C) should be initiated once there is clinical and radiographic evidence of healing.

Complications/Indications for Referral

Delayed union, nonunion, and refracture should be referred for operative consultation.[20]

APPROACH TO THE ATHLETE WITH A PROXIMAL FIFTH METATARSAL STRESS FRACTURE (JONES)

Proximal fifth metatarsal stress fractures, especially at the metaphyseal–diaphyseal junction, called a Jones fracture, are high risk due to the propensity for nonunion owing to poor blood supply (Fig. 22.2).

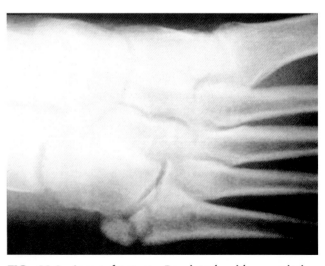

FIG. 22.2. Jones fracture. Reprinted with permission from Bucholz RW, Heckman JD. *Rockwood & Green's Fractures in Adults.* 5th ed. Philadelphia: Lippincott Williams & Wilkins; 2001.

HISTORY AND PHYSICAL EXAMINATION

The usual course is insidious onset of pain with activity; however, the athlete may present with an acute fracture without prior symptoms.[7] Tenderness is elicited over the proximal fifth metatarsal with possible swelling. Pain may be exacerbated with foot inversion.[7]

DIAGNOSTIC TESTING

Early radiographs are often negative. Chronic cases and nonunions will generally be evident on x-ray. MRI is useful for localizing stress injuries at this site.[3]

TREATMENT

High risk sites such as the proximal fifth metatarsal at the metaphyseal-diaphyseal junction tend to result in delayed union or non-union, may require operative management and are more likely to recur.[10] Treatment of high-risk stress fractures should be aggressively managed, aimed at fracture healing and prevention of fracture progression and recurrence.

Nonoperative

- Acute nondisplaced Jones fracture and an acute diaphyseal stress fracture are treated with non–weight-bearing status and immobilization in a short-leg cast for 4 to 6 weeks, followed by a weight-bearing cast until healing has occurred (10 to 12 weeks on average).[20,21]
- CT scan can be used to monitor healing.[20]

Operative

- Operative treatment is recommended in patients with acute displaced fractures, failed nonoperative management, and delayed union, nonunion, or recurrent symptoms.[21]
- Surgical screw fixation with a 4.5-mm cannulated screw demonstrated 100% healing with a mean return to sports in 7.5 weeks (level C).[29]
- Some advocate surgical fixation for Jones fractures in high-level athletes due to faster healing and lower rates of complication compared with nonoperative treatment.[29]

Prognosis/Return to Play

Return to play ranges from 6 to 12 weeks and is based on nontender examination and pain free with activities.[20,21] Jones fractures tend to have longer healing time. Pain-free

interval running program (Appendix C) should be initiated once there is clinical and radiographic evidence of healing.

Complications/Indications for Referral

Nonunion, delayed union, and refracture should be referred for consultation.

APPROACH TO THE ATHLETE WITH A METATARSAL SHAFT STRESS FRACTURE

Metatarsal stress fractures are one of the most common sites of stress fractures.[2,4,5] Overall metatarsal stress fractures carry a good prognosis, with the exception of proximal fifth metatarsal fractures. Management of these fractures is detailed in a separate section.

HISTORY AND PHYSICAL EXAMINATION

Patients often present with a history of rapid increases in training duration, frequency, or intensity, with ballet dancers and runners at highest risk.[21] The most common symptom is pain exacerbated by weight bearing.[21] On examination there is generally tenderness directly over the metatarsal and well-circumscribed swelling limited to the dorsum of the forefoot.[21]

DIAGNOSTIC TESTING

Initial radiographs are often negative, but weight-bearing anteroposterior (AP), oblique, and lateral views should be obtained to rule out acute fractures and to observe for joint subluxation or dislocation.[21] Serial x-rays may show evidence of healing even if initial x-rays are negative. MRI is useful for localizing stress injuries of the metatarsals, but may not be necessary if there is high clinical suspicion.[3] Clinical correlation is important because neoplasm and infection may have a similar appearance. Bone scan is less specific than MRI in elucidating the location of injury in bones of the foot.[3]

TREATMENT

Treatment is based on whether the stress fracture is at a high-risk (Jones, head of the second metatarsal) versus a low-risk site and the grade of the injury based on imaging studies.[4,8,24] Low-risk sites, including the first four metatarsals, are more likely to heal through conservative management with activity modification and are less likely to recur or lead to the complications associated with high-risk stress fractures.[10]

Nonoperative

- Treatment of minimally displaced, isolated metatarsal stress fractures includes activity modification, progressive weight bearing, and wearing a rigid-bottom postsurgical shoe, a walking boot, or a short-leg cast for 3 to 4 weeks, transitioning to a stiff-soled shoe for another 3 to 4 weeks.[21]
- Isolated minimally displaced first metatarsal stress fractures should be non–weight bearing in a short-leg cast for 4 to 6 weeks.[21]
- Treatment of low-risk stress fractures requires sufficient activity modification to allow for healing while at the same time avoiding unnecessary activity restrictions that lead to deconditioning and loss of sport-specific skills.
- No prospective, randomized studies have demonstrated the relationship between weight-bearing status and healing rates.[21]
- Treatment protocols range from non–weight-bearing status to pain-free activities only.
- Cross-training with cycling, aqua running, and swimming is an acceptable form of low- and nonimpact activities that may be used to maintain cardiovascular fitness. The interval running program outlined in Appendix C is an example of a graduated return-to-run program.

Operative

- Complications include displacement with subsequent malunion, delayed union, or nonunion, requiring surgical repair.[21]
- First metatarsal stress fractures with instability or significant displacement require operative treatment.

Prognosis/Return to Play

After pain-free activity has been achieved, gradual progression of activities may begin. Typical return to play is 6 to 12 weeks. Pain-free interval running program (see Appendix C) should be initiated once there is clinical and radiographic evidence of healing.

Complications/Indications for Referral

Malunion, delayed union, nonunion, first metatarsal stress fractures with instability, or significant displacement should be referred for operative consultation.

APPROACH TO THE ATHLETE WITH A TARSAL STRESS FRACTURE

The tarsals are the second most common stress fracture site in the foot, with the navicular being the most commonly involved tarsal bone.[2,4] Runners, particularly track athletes, who complain of insidious onset of midfoot pain should be evaluated for a stress fracture. Jumping and sprinting events were associated with navicular stress fractures.[3] Because of the poor blood supply, navicular stress fractures have a high propensity for nonunion and are frequently diagnosed late.[7] Early diagnosis and treatment are keys to a successful outcome.

HISTORY AND PHYSICAL EXAMINATION

Midfoot pain and tenderness may be indicative of a tarsal stress fracture. Dorsal midfoot pain radiating to the medial arch may be a sign of a tarsal stress fracture, most commonly the navicular.[3,7,30] Matheson found a frequent history of trauma in tarsal bone stress fractures.

DIAGNOSTIC TESTING

MRI is useful for diagnosis and grading the injury, while CT is useful for staging and following healing.[3,7,30]

TREATMENT

Nonoperative

- Treatment of navicular stress fractures involves non–weight-bearing cast immobilization for at least 6 weeks with subsequent 6 weeks of progressive rehabilitation (level B and level C).[31,32]
- If tenderness has resolved after casting, then weight-bearing rehabilitation may begin.
- There is no evidence of the effectiveness of ultrasound or electric bone stimulator in the treatment of navicular stress fractures.[30]

Operative

- Surgical intervention should be considered for high-risk stress fractures (1) to prevent completion of fractures associated with a high level of morbidity and (2) to prevent fracture recurrence to accelerate healing and return to play.[20]
- Surgical intervention is indicated in displaced, comminuted fractures and in failure of nonoperative treatment.
- Operative procedures include bone grafting and screw fixation.[3,7]

Return to play in 3 to 6 months depending on severity.[30] Pain-free interval running program (see Appendix C) should be initiated once there is clinical and radiographic evidence of healing.

Complications/Indications for Referral

This is a high-risk site due to avascularity, making complications of delayed union, nonunion, and chronic pain more likely.

APPROACH TO THE ATHLETE WITH A TIBIAL STRESS FRACTURE

Tibia pain is a common complaint in runners and is the most common site of stress fracture in the running athlete.[2,4,5] The major challenge for the provider is differentiating medial tibia stress syndrome (MTSS, also known as shin splints) from a tibial stress reaction or stress fracture. MTSS is a relatively benign condition that can mimic a stress fracture with medial tibia pain. MTSS is a syndrome that can include the diagnosis of periostitis and/or pain along the fascial insertion of the soleus. It is not known whether MTSS is the earliest presentation of bone stress injury along a continuum, leading to stress reaction/fracture or an entity unto itself. Once a stress fracture is considered or diagnosed, the next question is whether it is a posteromedial cortex versus anterior cortex stress fracture. The main distinction is that posteromedial tibia stress fractures occur on the concave surface of the tibia, are due to compressive forces, and are low risk. Anterior tibia stress fractures are caused by tensile forces on the convex surface of the tibia and are high risk due to increased rates of delayed union and nonunion (Fig. 22.3).

HISTORY AND PHYSICAL EXAMINATION

Athletes often complain of lower leg pain exacerbated by weight-bearing exercise that is relieved with rest.[3] It is common to have tenderness to palpation and percussion at the junction between the middle and distal thirds of the medial tibial shaft.[3] Swelling and a palpable callus may be present.[7,19] Clinically it can be difficult to discern a stress fracture from MTSS. Compartment swelling, tenderness, and neurovascular changes may help to distinguish between exertional compartment syndrome and a bone stress injury.[19] Proximal tibial stress fractures at the medial tibial condyle may mimic intra-articular and ligamentous pathology of the knee. Conditions to consider in athletes presenting with exercise-associated leg pain are noted in Table 22.6 along with pearls to diagnosis.

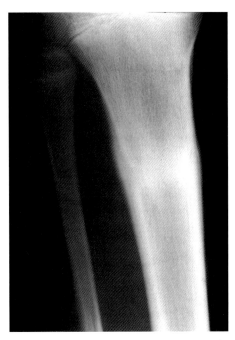

FIG. 22.3. Stress fracture in a young male athlete. Note sclerosis and widened cortices associated with bone healing. Reprinted with permission from Bucholz RW, Heckman JD. *Rockwood & Green's Fractures in Adults.* 5th ed. Philadelphia: Lippincott Williams & Wilkins; 2001.

DIAGNOSTIC TESTING

Plain radiographs are usually negative early in the course of injury but may demonstrate periosteal thickening or frank fracture after several weeks. Lateral radiographs may show the *dreaded black line* representing a fracture line in the anterior cortex consistent with delayed or nonunion. MRI is the best imaging study to detect early tibial stress injuries (Fig. 22.4).[18]

TREATMENT

Treatment is based on whether the stress fracture is at a high-risk versus a low-risk site and the grade of the injury based on imaging studies.[4,8,24] The posterior medial tibia is a low-risk site and is more likely to heal through conservative management with activity modification. The anterior tibia is a high-risk site due to the propensity for delayed union or nonunion, requiring operative management.[10]

Nonoperative

• Low-risk stress fractures require sufficient activity modification to allow for healing while at the same time avoiding unnecessary activity restrictions that lead to deconditioning and loss of sport-specific skills.

TABLE 22.6   **Diagnosis of Exercise-associated Leg Pain**

Common Conditions	Keys to Diagnosis
Medial tibia stress syndrome	Pain posterior medial tibia distal one third Improves quickly with running cessation
Tibia stress reaction or fracture	Pain takes longer to resolve with running cessation Escalating pain Pain with ambulation Anterior tibial cortex pain
Exertional compartment syndrome	Exercise-related pain that quickly resolves with rest Calf tightness Numbness, tingling, or weakness associated with pain
Radiculopathy from LS spine	Pain, paresthesia, or dysthesia May radiate from LS spine in dermatomal distribution Classically posterior calf/thigh pain
Peripheral nerve entrapment	Numbness, tingling, weakness along peripheral nerve innervation
Popliteal artery entrapment	Exercise-related calf pain that improves with rest Often congenital
Claudication	Exercise-related calf pain that improves with rest Found in older athletes or athletes with PVD risk factors

LS, lumbosacral; PVD, peripheral vascular disease.

- Conversely, undertreatment of high-risk stress fractures may result in progression or recurrence of the fracture, leading to prolonged periods of time away from sport.
- No prospective, randomized studies have demonstrated the relationship between weight-bearing status and healing rates.[8]
- Treatment of MTSS, anterior, and posterior–medial stress fractures involves activity modification to pain-free activities only.
- In medial tibial stress fractures, non–weight-bearing status should be initiated when ambulatory pain is present, otherwise a cam walker boot is sufficient.
- Treatment of anterior tibial stress fractures involves *non–weight bearing* until pain-free ambulation is achieved due to risk of nonunion or propagation of fracture.[20]
- A graduated exercise program beginning with 50% of preinjury levels and increasing 10% to 15% each week over 3 to 6 weeks may begin when pain-free ambulation is achieved.
- Cross-training with cycling, aqua running, and swimming is an acceptable form of low- and nonimpact activities that may be used to maintain cardiovascular fitness.[4]
- Pain should be used as a guide and activity levels kept below the threshold of pain when attempting to advance activity levels.[24,33] An alternative is the interval running program outlined in Appendix C.
- There is limited evidence that in tibial stress fractures, early mobilization with a pneumatic brace may accelerate return to athletic activity.[34]
- Electrical stimulation has not been demonstrated to accelerate tibial stress fracture healing.[35]

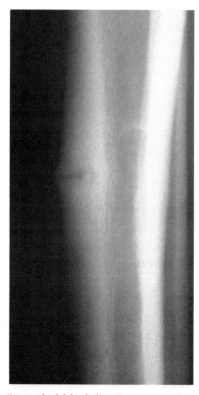

FIG. 22.4. "Dreaded black line" representing stress fracture in anterior cortex of the tibial diaphysis. Reprinted with permission from Schepsis AA, Busconi BD. *Sports Medicine.* Baltimore: Lippincott Williams & Wilkins; 2006.

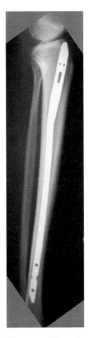

FIG. 22.5. Intramedullary nailing for anterior tibia stress fracture due to nonunion. Reprinted with permission from Schepsis AA, Busconi BD. *Sports Medicine.* Baltimore: Lippincott Williams & Wilkins; 2006.

Operative

- Surgical intervention should be considered for high-risk stress fractures such as the anterior tibia.[20]
- Intramedullary nailing of the tibia in cases of failed non-operative treatment, delayed union, or nonunion is an effective treatment and allowed for return to sports in a mean of 4 months after surgery (Fig. 22.5).[36]

Medications

Bisphosphonates

One small study on collegiate athletes using intravenous pamidronate demonstrated a possible benefit in the treatment of tibial stress fracture, resulting in rapid return to competition (level C).[37] No large, prospective randomized trials on the role of bisphosphonates in stress fracture treatment and prevention have been conducted. Because of the long half-life of bisphosphonates and potential teratogenic effects, future use in young females will likely remain controversial.[38]

Nonsteroidal Anti-inflammatory Drugs (NSAIDs)

The use of NSAIDs for pain control in stress fractures is controversial due to mixed findings in the literature regarding the potential for impaired bone healing. Among the limited number of prospective randomized, controlled trials in humans, no impairment of fracture healing was seen with COX-2 inhibitors.[38] Nonspecific NSAID use has been associated with impaired fracture healing in animal models.[38]

Prognosis/Return to Play

Return to play when pain free during activity, usually in 4 to 6 weeks for mild stress reaction and up to 12 weeks for stress fracture. Pain-free interval running program (Appendix C) should be initiated once there is clinical and radiographic evidence of healing.

Complications/Indications for Referral

Delayed union or nonunion are indications for surgical referral.

APPROACH TO THE ATHLETE WITH A FEMORAL STRESS FRACTURE

Femoral stress fractures are the fourth most common type of stress fracture.[2] Fracture sites include the femoral shaft, neck, and trochanteric and subtrochanteric regions. Femoral neck stress fractures have an incidence of 11% to 20% among athletes and are considered a high-risk site due to potential for long-term complications including displaced fracture and increased risk of avascular necrosis of the femoral head.[3,7,12]

HISTORY AND PHYSICAL EXAMINATION

Depending on the site, the most common symptoms are anterior thigh pain, hip pain, and groin pain.[3,22,39] Ipsilateral knee pain was the most common symptom in one study.[12] Vague groin pain is a common complaint in femoral neck stress fractures, but the athlete may present with pain in the low back, anterior thigh, lateral hip, or knee.[3,12,14,17]

Patients may complain of worsening hip pain with activity and night pain.[12] The history may reveal abrupt increases in training mileage or changes in terrain with symptoms occurring as early as 2 weeks.[12] Older athletes with distal femoral pain should be evaluated for spontaneous osteonecrosis of the femoral condyle.[12]

On physical examination, the hop test and fulcrum test are used to elicit pain and identify the site of a femoral stress fracture.[2,22,39] Pain may be elicited with end-range passive internal and external rotation of the hip with thigh flexed to 90 degrees, with palpation of the groin and logrolling of the thigh.[3,12,14] Bilateral femoral neck stress fractures may occur.

DIAGNOSTIC TESTING

Plain radiographs are positive in 30% to 70% of cases at symptom onset and should be the first imaging study ordered.[39] If the radiograph does not reveal a stress injury, an

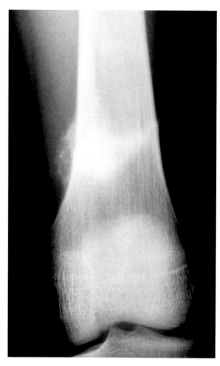

FIG. 22.6. Femoral shaft stress fracture in a runner with worsening thigh pain after increased training mileage over previous months. AP radiograph of distal femur shows increased density and periosteal reaction. Reprinted with permission from Bucholz RW, Heckman JD. *Rockwood & Green's Fractures in Adults.* 5th ed. Philadelphia: Lippincott Williams & Wilkins; 2001.

MRI or bone scan should be obtained to ensure prompt diagnosis.[3,12,39] MRI has the advantage of localizing the stress fracture more accurately. If femoral neck stress fracture is suspected, patient should be made non–weight bearing till results of imaging studies are reviewed.

TREATMENT

- Treatment is based on whether the stress fracture is at a high-risk versus a low-risk site and the grade of the injury based on imaging studies.[4,8,24] Low-risk sites, including the femoral shaft, are more likely to heal through conservative management with activity modification (Figs. 22.6 and 22.7).[10]
- High-risk sites including the femoral neck tend to result in delayed union or nonunion, may require operative management, and are more likely to recur.[10]

Nonoperative

- Femoral shaft stress fractures are managed conservatively with non–weight bearing on the affected leg.
- Progression is made to pain-free ambulation and non–weight-bearing exercises. The next phase allows for some weight-bearing activities, with initiation of a graduated

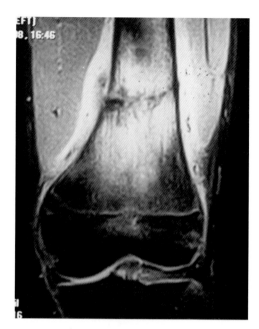

FIG. 22.7. MRI shows fracture line and bright signal of surrounding bone edema. Reprinted with permission from Bucholz RW, Heckman JD. *Rockwood & Green's Fractures in Adults.* 5th ed. Philadelphia: Lippincott Williams & Wilkins; 2001.

exercise program if the athlete remains pain free.[39] Return to regular athletic activity occurs in 12 to 14 weeks.[39]

- Management of femoral neck fractures depends on the site and extent of the stress fracture. *Compression*-side femoral neck fractures that are early and nondisplaced are managed with non–weight bearing until there is pain free and radiographic evidence of healing followed by a graduated exercise program. See interval running program, Appendix C (Fig. 22.8).[12,20]

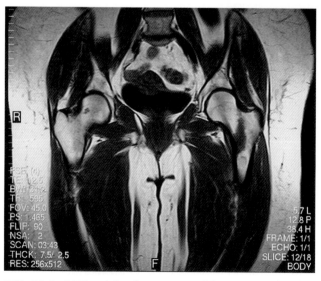

FIG. 22.8. MRI pelvis of a 50-year-old runner with a left compression-side femoral neck stress fracture. *Rockwood & Green's Fractures in Adults.* 6th ed. 2006.

Operative

- Tension-sided femoral neck stress fractures and displaced fractures are often managed with surgical internal fixation.[3,12,14,20]

Prognosis/Return to Play

Return to play when nontender on examination, radiographic evidence of healing, and with pain-free activity.[20] Healing requires 6 to 12 weeks. Pain-free interval running program (Appendix C) should be initiated once there is clinical and radiographic evidence of healing.[3,12]

Complications/Indications for Referral

Displacement, nonunion, or avascular necrosis is indication for referral. Nearly one fourth of the patients develop avascular necrosis within 5.6 years after femoral head displacement due to stress fracture.[20]

APPROACH TO THE ATHLETE WITH A SACRAL STRESS FRACTURE

Sacral stress fractures have been reported in distance runners and volleyball players and appear to be more common in female athletes.[16] They are often diagnosed in athletes who have increased training intensity or duration.

HISTORY AND PHYSICAL EXAMINATION

Vague, nonspecific low-back, buttock, or hip pain in female runners may be a sign of a sacral stress fracture. These symptoms may be confused with sacroiliac joint dysfunction, sciatica, or disc pathology.[3,16] On examination there may be tenderness on the sacrum or sacroiliac joint. Faber test and hop test may be positive on the affected side.[16]

DIAGNOSTIC TESTING

MRI is the imaging modality of choice to diagnose, grade, and make return-to-play decision.[3,16,17] CT scan can be useful to stage the *fracture line*.[16] Laboratory studies to rule out spondyloarthropathies should be considered when there is a family history.

TREATMENT

Activity modification until pain-free status is achieved. Begin interval running program once pain-free status and evidence of healing have occurred.

Prognosis/Return to Play

Healing time is 6 weeks to 8 months. Pain-free interval running program (Appendix C) should be initiated once there is clinical and radiographic evidence of healing.

Complications/Indications for Referral

It is important to diagnose sacral stress fractures because they can mimic disc disease.

APPROACH TO THE ATHLETE WITH A ACUTE SPINE STRESS FRACTURE (SPONDYLOLYSIS)

Low-back pain is a common complaint among adolescent athletes, with females appearing to be at greater risk for spine stress injuries.[16] Stress reaction of the pars interarticularis, spondylolysis, and spondylolisthesis represents a continuum of bone stress injury. These injuries are caused by hyperextension of the lumbar spine commonly performed in gymnasts and ballet dancers.

HISTORY AND PHYSICAL EXAMINATION

The most common complaint is low-back pain associated with ballet, gymnastics, diving, and soccer.[3,16,17] Pars interarticularis stress fractures may present as persistent nonradicular low-back pain worse with activity. There may be a history of menstrual irregularities and nutritional deficiencies. On examination tenderness is elicited at the affected vertebrae, most commonly L5. ROM may be limited or painful in lumbar extension.[16] Hamstring tightness was found in 80% of patients.[16] Stork test (single-legged hyperextension test) has low sensitivity and specificity in detecting spondylolysis and should not be used to exclude the diagnosis (level B).[25]

DIAGNOSTIC TESTING

Plain radiographs are the initial imaging study but will generally be positive in chronic nonunions (Scotty dog sign) and with spondylolisthesis (Figs. 22.9 and 22.10). If initial x-rays are negative and there is a high clinical suspicion, further imaging studies are warranted. Some authors recommend a SPECT bone scan followed by CT if the SPECT bone scan is positive (level A).[25,26] SPECT scans have the highest sensitivity and specificity for diagnosis of acute pars stress injury.[40]

The role of MRI in diagnosing pars stress fractures appears to be growing with advances in MRI resolution.

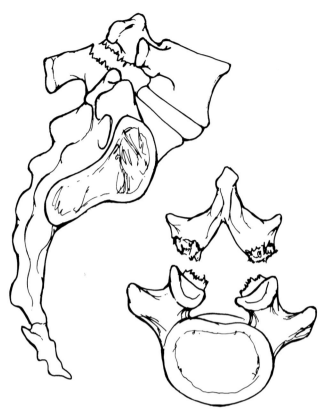

FIG. 22.9. Pars interarticularis fracture between L5 and S1 (spondylolysis) may lead to spondylolisthesis. Reprinted with permission from Oatis CA. *Kinesiology—The Mechanics and Pathomechanics of Human Movement.* Baltimore: Lippincott Williams & Wilkins; 2004.

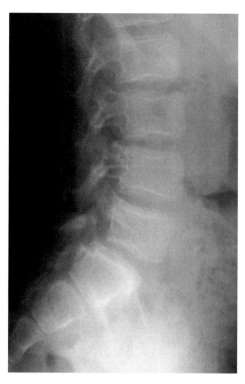

FIG. 22.10. Spondylolisthesis with anterior slippage of L5 on S1. Reprinted with permission from Fleisher GR, Ludwig S, Baskin MN. *Atlas of Pediatric Emergency Medicine.* Philadelphia: Lippincott Williams & Wilkins; 2004.

Several advantages exist, including absence of ionizing radiation and ability to image lumbar anatomy as well as disc pathology. These advantages need to be weighed against lower sensitivity and specificity compared with SPECT and CT imaging.[40]

TREATMENT

Nonoperative

Treatment involves discontinuation of all activities that cause hyperextension and impact loading of the thoracolumbar spine. Rehabilitation with emphasis on core strength, training, and hamstring flexibility should begin promptly with reevaluation in 4 to 6 weeks, especially to observe for pain-free extension. When the athlete is pain free, a gradual increase in activities may begin. If the athlete continues to be pain free, hyperextension activities may be reintroduced. The role of bracing is an area of controversy and debate, as good outcomes have been shown to occur with rigid bracing, soft bracing, and no bracing. No head-to-head trials of bracing versus nonbracing exist.

Operative

- Surgical stabilization with lumbar fusion is performed in cases of failed conservative therapy with persistent pain with sports and activities of daily living.[16] This is a very rare complication.

Prognosis/Return to Play

Return to play is allowed after progression to pain free with hyperextension activities. Healing may take as long as 6 months with conservative measures. No sports until 12 months after fusion.[16] Overall prognosis appears to be excellent in long-term studies, with incidence of back pain comparable to general population.[41]

Complications/Indications for Referral

Spondylolisthesis and cord compression may present as radicular pain, saddle numbness, and loss of bowel or bladder control, with prompt referral recommended.

17. Sofka CM. Imaging of stress fractures. *Clin Sports Med.* 2006;25:53–62.
18. Gaeta M, Minutoli F, Scribano E, et al. CT and MR imaging findings in athletes with early tibial stress injuries: comparison with bone scintigraphy findings and emphasis on cortical abnormalities. *Radiology.* 2005; 235:553–561.
19. Young AJ, McAllister DR. Evaluation and treatment of tibial stress fractures. *Clin Sports Med.* 2006;25:117–128.
20. Diehl JJ, Best TM, Kaeding, CC. Classification and return-to-play considerations for stress fractures. *Clin Sports Med.* 2006;25:17–28.
21. Fetzer GB, Wright RW. Metatarsal shaft fractures and fractures of the proximal fifth metatarsal. *Clin Sports Med.* 2006;25:139–150.
22. Johnson AW, Weiss CB, Wheeler DL. Stress fractures of the femoral shaft in athletes: more common than expected. A new clinical test. *Am J Sports Med.* 1994;22:248–256.
23. Lesho EP. Can tuning forks replace bone scans for identification of tibial stress fractures? *Mil Med.* 1997;16:802–803.
24. Arendt E, Griffiths H. The use of MR in the assessment and clinical management of stress reactions of bone in high-performance athletes. *Clin Sports Med.* 1997;16:292–306.
25. Masci L, Pike J, Malara F, et al. Use of one-legged hyperextension test and magnetic resonance imaging in the diagnosis of active spondylolysis. *Br J Sports Med.* 2006;40:940–946.
26. Gregory PL, Batt ME, Kerslake RW, et al. The value of combining photon emission computerized tomography and computerized tomography in the investigation of spondylolysis. *Eur Spine J.* 2004;13:503–509.
27. Boam S, Miser WY, Delaplain C, et al. Comparison of ultrasound examination with bone scintiscan in the diagnosis of stress fractures. *J Am Board Fam Pract.* 1996;9:414–417.
28. Munuera PV, Dominguez G, Reina M, et al. Bipartite hallucal sesamoid bones: relationship with hallux valgus and metatarsal index. *Skeletal Radiol.* 2007;36(11):1043–1050 [Epub September 2, 2007].
29. Porter D, Duncan M, Meyer, S. Fifth metatarsal Jones fracture fixation with a 4.5 mm cannulated stainless steel screw in the competitive and recreational athlete. *Am J Sports Med.* 2005;33:726–733.
30. Jones MH, Amendola AS. Navicular stress fractures. *Clin Sports Med.* 2006;25:151–158.
31. Khan K, Fuller P, Bruckner P, et al. Outcome of conservative and surgical management of navicular stress fracture in athletes. Eighty-six cases proven with computerized computerized tomography. *Am J Sports Med.* 1992;20:657–666.
32. Burne S, Mahoney C, Forster B, et al. Tarsal navicular stress injury. Long-term outcome and clinicoradiological correlation using both computed tomography and magnetic resonance imaging. *Am J Sports Med.* 2005;33:1875–1881.
33. Chisin R, Milgrom C, Giladi M, et al. Clinical significance of nonfocal scintigraphic findings in suspected tibial stress fractures. *Clin Orthop Relat Res.* 1987;220:200–205.
34. Rome K, Handoll HHG, Ashford R. Interventions for preventing and treating stress fractures and stress reactions of bone of the lower limbs in young adults. *Cochrane Database Syst Rev.* 2005;2:CD000450.
35. Beck B, Matheson GO, Bergman G, et al. Do capacitively coupled electric fields accelerate tibial stress fracture healing? A randomized controlled trial. *Am J Sports Med.* 2008;36:545–553.
36. Stewart GW, Brunet ME, Manning MR. Treatment of stress fractures in athletes with intravenous pamidronate. *Clin J Sport Med.* 2005;15(2):92–94.
37. Koester MC, Spindler KP. Pharmacologic agents in fracture healing. *Clin Sports Med.* 2006;25:63–74.
38. Varner KE, Younas SA, Litner DM, et al. Chronic anterior midtibial stress fractures in athletes treated with reamed intramedullary nailing. *Am J Sports Med.* 2005;33:1077–1084.
39. Ivkovic A, Bojanic I, Pecina M. Stress fractures of the femoral shaft in athletes: a new treatment algorithm. *Br J Sports Med.* 2006;40:518–520.
40. Campbell RS, Grainger AJ, Hide IG, et al. Juvenile spondylolysis: a comparative analysis of CT, SPECT and MRI. *Skeletal Radiol.* 2005;34(2):63–73 [Epub November 25, 2004].
41. Beutler WJ, Fredrickson BE, Murtland A, et al. The natural history of spondylolysis and spondylolisthesis: 45-year follow-up evaluation. *Spine.* 2003;28(10):1027–1035.

KEY POINTS

- Lower-extremity stress fractures are most common in running athletes, while upper-extremity stress fractures can occur in the throwing or rowing athlete

- Stress fractures are categorized as either fatigue or insufficiency stress fracture based on normal bone health versus underlying osteopenia/osteoporosis

- Early mobilization with a pneumatic brace may accelerate return to athletic activity in tibial stress fractures[34]

- Diagnostic test of choice for acute spondylolysis remains a SPECT bone scan, but MRI with STIR imaging is gaining greater use[25,26]

- There is insufficient evidence from randomized trials of preventive interventions to draw firm conclusions[34]

- There is insufficient evidence regarding the best type of shoe inserts[34]

REFERENCES

1. Snyder RA, Koester MC, Dunn WR. Epidemiology of stress fractures. *Clin Sports Med.* 2006;25:37–52.
2. Matheson GO, Clement DB, McKenzie DC, et al. Stress fractures in athletes: a study of 320 cases. *Am J Sports Med.* 1987;15:46–58.
3. Wall J, Feller JF. Imaging of stress fracture in runners. *Clin Sports Med.* 2006;25:781–802.
4. Arendt El, Agel J, Heikes C, et al. Stress injuries to bone in college athletes: a retrospective review of experience at a single institution. *Am J Sports Med.* 2003;31:959–968.
5. Iwamoto J, Takeda T. Stress fractures in athletes: review of 196 cases. *J Orthop Sci* 2003;8:273–278.
6. Pepper M, Akuthota V, McCarty EC. Pathophysiology of stress fractures. *Clin Sports Med.* 2006;25:1–16.
7. Kaeding CC, Yu JR, Wright R, et al. Management and return to play of stress fractures. *Clin J Sport Med.* 2005;15:442–447.
8. Feingold D, Hame SL. Female athlete triad and stress fractures. *Orthop Clin N Am.* 2006;37:575–583.
9. Marx RG, Saint-Phard D, Callahan LR. Stress fracture sites related to underlying bone health in athletic females. *Clin J Sport Med.* 2001;11:73–76.
10. Boden BP, Osbahr DC, Jimenez C. Low risk stress fractures. *Am J Sports Med.* 2001;29:100–111.
11. Raasch WG, Hergan DJ. Treatment of stress fractures: the fundamentals. *Clin Sports Med.* 2006;25:29–36.
12. DeFranco MJ, Recht M, Schils J, et al. Stress fractures of the femur in athletes. *Clin Sports Med.* 2006;25:89–104.
13. Zanker CL, Cooke CB. Energy balance, bone turnover, and skeletal health in physically active individuals. *Med Sci Sports Exerc.* 2004;36(8):1372–1381.
14. Bolin D, Kemper A, Brolinson PG. Current concepts in the evaluation and management of stress fractures. *Curr Sports Med Rep.* 2005;4:295–300.
15. Noonan TJ, Sakryd G, Espinoza LM, et al. Posterior rib stress fractures in professional baseball pitchers. *Am J Sports Med.* 2007;35:654–658.
16. Micheli LJ, Curtis C. Stress fractures in the spine and sacrum. *Clin Sports Med.* 2006;25:75–88.

CHAPTER

23

Athlete with Peripheral Nerve Injuries

Faren H. Williams

INTRODUCTION

Peripheral nerve injuries in athletes may serve as a diagnostic challenge for the treating clinician. They may present as acute injuries or secondary to overuse. Athletes are vulnerable due to the repetitive nature of upper- and lower-extremity movements and the superficial nature of peripheral nerves.

Peripheral nerve injuries can be underestimated in athletes due to the relative muscle hypertrophy and enhanced strength that can mask the extent of the injury. Additionally, sensory changes may not be appreciated to the same extent by athletes who are accustomed to playing with some degree of pain or discomfort. A high degree of suspicion along with an understanding of common peripheral nerve injuries in athletes will greatly enhance the proper diagnosis and treatment. Additionally, an understanding of dermatomes and peripheral nerve sensory as well as motor function is essential in differentiating peripheral nerve injuries from more central etiologies. This chapter will review the most common nerve injuries associated with different sports and address when to refer the patient for specialty electrodiagnostic consultation.

FUNCTIONAL ANATOMY

The peripheral nervous system (PNS) consists of the nerve root, the motor efferent from the anterior horn cell, the afferent sensory ganglion (usually in the neural foramina) which combines to form a spinal nerve, along with sensory and motor components. The ventral rami from these nerves coalesce to form the brachial plexus in the upper extremity and lumbosacral plexus in the lower extremity, forming trunks, divisions, and cords, which ultimately become terminal nerve branches supplying the arms or legs with motor and sensory function (Fig. 23.1).[1]

PATHOPHYSIOLOGY

Peripheral nerve injuries are most commonly classified according to Seddon's scheme.[2] The terms neuropraxia,

axonotmesis, and neurotmesis are used by electromyographers (Table 23.1).

The mildest injury, neuropraxia, has the best prognosis for recovery, with the neurotmesis having the worst prognosis, given the disruption of axons and epineurium. The latter problem may require surgical repair by a skilled peripheral nerve surgeon, with outcomes often guarded, although the surgical approximation of nerve fibers is improving.[3]

There are different degrees of axonal loss, with prognosis dependent on many factors, including the age and health of the patient, the proximity of the lesion to the muscle(s) being innervated, and the integrity of the muscle itself. In general, upper-trunk brachial plexopathies have a better prognosis than lower-trunk ones, because of the length of axonal regeneration needed for the latter.[4]

EPIDEMIOLOGY

Of 1,167 peripheral nerve injuries seen in a single orthopaedic clinic in Japan over 18 years, 5.7% were attributed to sports and 10% of them to traumatic nerve injuries.[5] Because the upper extremities are more mobile, with muscle attachments directly to the thorax, the peripheral nerves are vulnerable to injury to a greater extent than in the lower extremities. In a retrospective review of peripheral nerve injuries to athletes, 88% were to the upper extremity, with one third of the injuries being related to playing football.[6] Mechanisms for nerve injury include compression, traction, ischemia, and laceration, secondary to hyperextension of the neck or limbs, or unstable fractures or dislocations.[7]

In general, football and other contact sports such as wrestling, hockey, and basketball contribute to the majority of upper-extremity plexus injuries, while overhead throwing sports such as volleyball result in more focal nerve injury, such as the suprascapular nerve, at the sphenoglenoid notch, affecting primarily the infraspinatous muscle. Weight lifting, while a sport by itself, is also a significant part of the training program for most sports, so it can be the etiology for nerve injuries in many athletes playing different sports.[8]

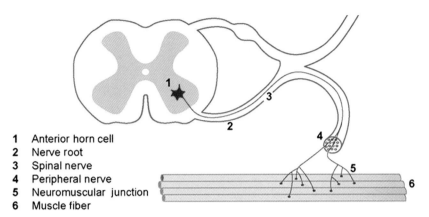

1 Anterior horn cell
2 Nerve root
3 Spinal nerve
4 Peripheral nerve
5 Neuromuscular junction
6 Muscle fiber

FIG. 23.1. Motor unit.

NARROWING THE DIFFERENTIAL DIAGNOSIS

History

The most important part of the peripheral nerve diagnosis is the patient's history of the present symptoms and the timing of any preceding trauma. Athletes may note gradually progressive weakness or atrophy after an acute injury such as a shoulder dislocation. Overuse peripheral nerve injuries may, however, present with no history of trauma but gradual-onset pain, weakness, and/or atrophy.

Athletes, especially as they age, may have underlying medical conditions such as diabetes and its associated peripheral neuropathy. Athletes with persistent numbness in the hands and feet may have a peripheral neuropathy or cervical or lumbar stenosis. Neck and upper-extremity symptoms may be alleviated by cervical traction, either manually or with weight. With lumbar stenosis, the symptoms will be exacerbated by walking or running and relieved by sitting. If there is radiation of pain into only one extremity, the athlete may have a radiculopathy from a herniated disc. Pain from this is usually worse with sitting and to a lesser extent standing; walking may relieve this type of pain.

Evidence-based Physical Examination

A thorough review of the neurologic examination is detailed below. Some common neurologic tests utilized to differenti-

ate potential peripheral nerve injury from a central etiology include the Tinel's and Phalen's tests along with the Spurlings test. The Tinel's sign involves percussion of a peripheral nerve to recreate the patients' dysthesias or paresthesias. This is most often performed at the wrist for the median nerve but can be done at the elbow for the ulnar nerve, at the tarsal tunnel for the posterior tibial nerve, and at the proximal fibula for the peroneal nerve. The sensitivity and specificity of the Tinel's sign is less than 50%, so it is not diagnostic for a nerve injury, and does not correlate well with nerve conduction studies (NCSs). Sensory testing of dermatomes and peripheral nerves, motor strength testing, and reflexes are more reliable tests.[4]

A detailed and thorough neurologic examination is warranted after a significant injury on the playing field or when the athlete presents with a suspected nerve injury. More concerning are injuries that compromise the central nervous system, which includes the spinal cord. Any athlete who has decreased motor and sensory function needs prompt evaluation, keeping in mind that a cervical injury that causes mainly symptoms in the upper extremities can be a central cord syndrome versus a cervical root or brachial plexus injury. Reflexes in a spinal cord patient acutely may be diminished due to spinal shock and become more hyperactive over time.[9]

Other common peripheral nerve injuries are cervical and to a lesser extent lumbar radiculopathies from an intervertebral disc applying pressure to a nerve root. While they may involve primarily motor function, the sensory dorsal root

TABLE 23.1 Seddon's Classification of Nerve Injuries

	Motor	Sensory	Conduction Block	Wallerian Degenerative	Perineurium Intact
Neuropraxia	Dec amp	Dec amp	Distal amp nl	No	Yes
Axonotmesis	Dec amp	Dec amp	No	Yes	Yes
Mixed (neuropraxia and axonotmesis)	Dec amp	Dec amp	Partial	Yes	Yes
Neurotmesis	No response	No response	No	Yes	No

ganglion can also be compromised in lesions that are more lateral. In these patients, the associated reflexes should be diminished compared with the contralateral side, and any sensory changes should follow a dermatomal distribution. Injuries that affect sensory may be distal to the dorsal root ganglion at the level of the brachial plexus.

The term "stingers" or "burners" is used for acute traction injuries involving the brachial plexus. Diminished reflexes and subjective sensory changes, not always objective ones, in a portion of the brachial plexus are detected on physical examination. Sensory changes may be loss of position and vibratory sensation and light touch, associated with conduction block of large myelinated fibers. Detailed examination of motor, sensory (dermatomal and peripheral nerve), and reflexes is key in helping to localize the lesion, but may be compromised in athletes who have a concomitant brain injury, which affects their ability to participate in the examination and may cause hyperreflexia. In athletes who have peripheral nerve injuries, up to 60% may have a traumatic brain injury.[10]

Diagnostic Testing

Laboratory

In the setting of an acute peripheral nerve injury, laboratory studies are rarely needed. For gradual-onset symptoms, appropriate laboratory studies may be indicated to differentiate systemic or metabolic etiology from a focal nerve injury. Complete blood count (CBC), thyroid studies, rapid plasma reagin (RPR), B_{12}, and folate are some common tests obtained. Other serology and cultures are ordered based on clinical presentation and pretest probability.

Imaging

Appropriate radiographs are indicated in cases of trauma to rule out coexisting fractures that may be associated with peripheral nerve injuries (i.e., supracondylar fractures, proximal fibula fracture, displaced or open fractures). CT may better define complex fractures and bone fragments that may be associated with traumatic peripheral nerve injuries.

MRI may play a role in visualization of potential nerve injury from both acute or overuse mechanisms. The superiority of MRI for visualization of soft tissue may be of help for visualization of mass effect along with potential visualization of the nerve itself, although a specialized MRI neurography is needed for more useful information about the nerve.

Ultrasound is growing in use for visualization of peripheral nerves due to its high resolution of superficial soft-tissue structures and its ability to visualize nerve inflammatory changes. The dynamic capabilities of ultrasound can identify conditions of nerve subluxation as can occur at the elbow with the ulna nerve. Ultrasound, however, is operator dependent, and availability is affected by access to trained individuals who understand the applications of ultrasound to peripheral nerve problems.

Other Testing

Electrodiagnostic studies can play a significant role in the diagnosis and prognosis of peripheral nerve injuries,[4] as they can assist further with prognosis. Information obtained about the integrity of the affected nerve(s) can be used to prescribe a therapeutic treatment program. Changes in amplitude occur in the motor nerve after 6 to 8 days, and the sensory nerve in 8 to 12 days; therefore, NCSs done within 1 to 2 weeks after a traumatic injury can determine whether there has been some nerve injury. Other changes with the needle electromyography (EMG) will take 3 to 4 weeks to evolve and are more suggestive of axonal loss.[11] This information about the integrity of the affected nerve(s) can be used to prescribe an appropriate therapeutic treatment program. Denervated muscle cannot be strengthened, and exercises need to focus initially on maintaining the range of motion about the involved joint.

Electrodiagnosis is quite specific in the hands of a skilled electromyographer, with specificity greater than 90%.[12] The electrodiagnostic results should complement the clinical history and physical examination. When inconsistencies are seen, one needs to question whether affected nerves were compared to similar ones on the contralateral limb, whether the athlete has a different underlying medical condition, or whether the electrodiagnostic study was thorough and technically competent.[4] One should refer patients to someone who does a complete electrodiagnostic consultation, interpreting electrodiagnostic results in the context of the patient's history, physical examination, and other pertinent studies such as imaging.[13]

Electrodiagnosis A basic understanding of this test, what it does and does not measure status post nerve injury, helps in determining when to order it. It evaluates the large myelinated (type A) peripheral nerve fibers and is useful only with injuries to these nerves, not the smaller type C pain fibers. There are two different types of electrodiagnostic testing: (1) motor and sensory NCSs and (2) needle EMG, which analyze motor units and denervation potentials seen in selected muscles after injury to the nerve innervating them.

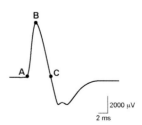

A – Distal/onset latency
A to B – CMAP amplitude
A to C – CMAP duration

FIG. 23.2. Compound motor action potential (CMAP).

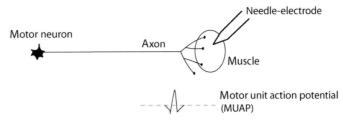

FIG. 23.3. Normal motor unit action potential (MUAP). Electrode records MUAPs from muscle fibers within the vicinity of the needle.

To perform NCSs, the peripheral nerve motor axons are stimulated electrically, causing depolarization of the muscles innervated by that nerve. By placing a recording electrode over the muscle, a compound motor action potential (CMAP) is visualized, with characteristic amplitude(s) and duration(s) for particular muscles (Fig. 23.2). Stimulation of the sensory axons results in a comparable sensory nerve action potential (SNAP). These responses are a composite of the motor or sensory fibers picked up by the recording electrodes. The motor result can be affected by neuromuscular junction problems and significant muscle atrophy or disease such as myopathies, but the sensory reflects direct nerve transmission and is usually seen before the motor response. Changes in the amplitude may suggest some axonal loss, and changes in the speed of conduction, or latency, may reflect slowing of conduction, associated with demyelination.[4]

Needle EMG is performed by inserting a needle directly into a muscle and recording motor unit action potentials (MUAPs) from the muscles in the vicinity of the needle (Fig. 23.3). Different muscles have characteristic amplitudes and durations, which indicate whether the potential is a motor unit.

Other potentials (fibs and positive waves) referred to as spontaneous activity are recorded from muscles that have sustained denervation of their nerve axons secondary to Wallerian degeneration. Normal muscle is electrically silent at rest, so this spontaneous activity at rest suggests nerve injury. Fibs and positive waves may be graded on a 1 to 4 scale depending on their prevalence with needle testing, but any axonal loss produces fibs and positive waves. Therefore, this rating does not correlate with degree of axonal loss; only the amplitude of the CMAP is proportional to the degree of axonal loss.[14]

Another EMG parameter is recruitment, or the extent to which more axons can fire in response to increasing muscle contraction. Recruitment is full and spontaneous when axonal integrity is preserved but becomes more limited as axons degenerate.[15] Decreased recruitment is often the first finding on needle EMG, suggesting axonal disruption, but should be used together with evidence for fibs and positive before commenting on whether there is evidence for acute axonal loss/denervation (Fig. 23.4). Nerves have the capacity to regenerate (1 in/month),[4] and over time the fibs and

positive waves become smaller or disappear.[16] The MUAPs may have multiple phases, suggesting that immature axons are conducting at different rates, but as axons mature, the number of phases may decrease. These findings may suggest some reinnervation (Fig. 23.5).[4]

The changes in NCSs or needle EMG are dependent on the type of injury and time from injury. These tests will help confirm a peripheral nerve injury, the one suspected or a different one(s), and are also of benefit in explaining a different etiology for the patient's pain and muscle atrophy/weakness. One limitation of early electrodiagnostic testing is the limited prognostic value, as there may not have been enough time for neurophysiologic changes to evolve. Unfortunately, a competitive athlete may not want to wait until the extent of neurologic involvement can be ascertained.

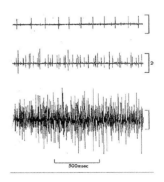

FIG. 23.4. Motor unit recruitment. Increasing force of contraction

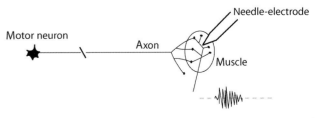

FIG. 23.5. Polyphasic motor unit reinnervation. Axonal sprouting leads to reinnervation and polyphasic MUAPs

APPROACH TO THE ATHLETE WITH STINGER/BURNER

Brachial plexus injuries are some of the more prevalent sports injuries commonly encountered in football, wrestling, hockey, basketball, baseball, and overhead throwing sports. They are transient injuries to the brachial plexus, resulting in unilateral symptoms of numbness, tingling, burning, and weakness. The primary mechanisms are forced hyperextension and lateral bending/flexion of the neck to the opposite side with downward displacement to the ipsilateral shoulder, which causes a traction-type injury to the brachial plexus. The alternative mechanism can be a forced flexion to the affected side with compression of the brachial plexus (Fig. 23.6). Younger players may be at risk because they have more mobile necks and less well-developed neck musculature.[17]

HISTORY AND PHYSICAL EXAMINATION

Stingers or burners will cause *unilateral* dysesthesias in the distribution of the brachial plexus upper trunk from the supraclavicular area radiating down the lateral or radial side of the forearm. It can resemble a C6 radiculopathy and may or may not cause motor changes. Symptoms usually resolve within seconds to minutes, and neurologic examination may be normal. There may be weakness of the shoulder abduction (deltoid), external rotation (rotator cuff muscles), and elbow flexion (biceps). If persistent subjective complaints of weakness occur, motor may need to be tested by having the person perform some aspect of the sport, that is, throwing for a quarterback.[18] Weakness on examination with stronger athletes may only be recreated on examination by stressing the area to fatigue and noting differences from side to side (i.e., resisted abduction until fatigued). Bilateral symptoms on history or examination are not consistent with a stinger and may represent a more serious central cord lesion.

DIAGNOSTIC TESTING

In the acute setting of neck pain and upper-extremity neurologic deficits, cervical radiographs may be indicated to rule out occult cervical fracture.

MRI is typically reserved for cases of single nerve root involvement, suspected cord injury, persistent symptoms, or history of recurrent stingers/burners. When a single nerve root is affected from either disc protrusion or herniation, it is more commonly C7, which may be detected with imaging studies. Occasionally the motor nerve root may be avulsed, totally or partially, causing significant motor paresis in muscles innervated by that level. The person may not experience sensory changes, as the lesion is proximal to the sensory root ganglion. Most of them are partial avulsions and recover to some extent,[4] which is good since the motor prognosis for a complete nerve root avulsion is guarded. While nerve roots are visualized on MRI scans, one needs more specialized MRI neurography to determine whether there is nerve root avulsion.[19] In general, routine MRI studies are not very specific in identifying nerve injuries and do not provide information about prognosis, given that neurophysiology changes occur over time.[20]

If symptoms of dysthesias, paresthesias, or motor weakness persist for 4 to 6 weeks, then electrodiagnostic testing may be helpful. If there are no electrodiagnostic changes after this time, then the insult to the nerve was not significant. One possibility is that dysthesias reflect intermittent pressure on any structures that have sensory input from the nervous system, joints, ligaments, muscles, etc.[21]

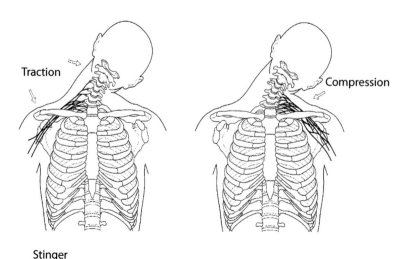

FIG. 23.6. Position of the neck.

TREATMENT

Nonoperative

- The mainstay of treatment for acute stingers/burners is nonoperative with rest from offending activities.
- Physical therapy can be initiated once symptoms have resolved and full function has returned. A focus on neck and trapezius strengthening may be helpful in preventing recurrent stingers.
- "Cowboy collars" may help prevent neck hyperextension and possible recurrent stingers.

Operative

- Operative treatment is rarely needed and is reserved for cases of nerve root avulsion, although prognosis with surgery remains guarded, as discussed earlier.

Prognosis/Return to Play

- Overall prognosis for acute stingers/burners is excellent, and return to play is based on complete resolution of symptoms.
- Most stingers/burners resolve within seconds to minutes; however, some may require weeks to months to fully heal.
- Return to play also requires that the athletes must demonstrate full range of motion and strength as well as functional stability at the shoulder to perform their required activities on examination.

Complications/Indications for Referral

Complications that can occur include brachial plexopathy or partial nerve root avulsion secondary to trauma. With these, recovery is prolonged, and there is a high incidence of recurrent stingers and burners.

Indications for referral include progressive symptoms, prolonged recovery longer than 1 to 2 weeks, or clinical picture with sensory, motor, or reflex changes. Neurodiagnostic examination in these cases is helpful to clarify the degree of axonal loss, evidence for reinnervation, and prognosis, with implications for when the athlete should return to play.

Bilateral symptoms are not consistent with a stinger and may represent a more serious central cord injury.

APPROACH TO THE ATHLETE WITH AXILLARY NERVE INJURY

Axillary nerve injuries most often present as a complication of a shoulder subluxation or dislocation in the athlete.

HISTORY AND PHYSICAL EXAMINATION

It is helpful to ask about the position of the arm following the dislocation, if the patient can recall. Abduction and external rotation may compress the axillary nerve, given the forcible extension causing the dislocation. Over time, there will be muscle atrophy of the deltoid and teres minor, causing difficulty with shoulder abduction and forward elevation. If the injury is significant, then sensory loss in the distribution of the axillary nerve and lateral brachial cutaneous nerve of the upper arm may occur.[21] The patient may experience hyperpathia, with any light touch, including clothing, against the deltoid or lateral upper arm.

DIAGNOSTIC TESTING

Electrodiagnostic testing of the axillary nerve needs to include comparison to the contralateral side to determine the normal amplitude for an individual. Loss of amplitude, which occurs in 8 to 12 days after injury, directly reflects axonal loss and provides information on the degree of axonal loss. There are no good imaging studies to evaluate this problem.

TREATMENT

Nonoperative Acute Injuries

- In the acute phase, the focus is on protecting the denervated limb to prevent further nerve injury and on reducing pain.
- Splinting is not necessary and may promote relatively more disuse atrophy and contractures.[22]
- Analgesics, muscle relaxants, and ice may be adequate initially, but heat may aggravate nerves.[23]
- As the nerve degenerates, the athlete may experience neuropathic pain. Patients may experience more intense burning pain as the nerve regenerates; they should be reassured that the increase in pain may be a good prognostic sign rather than worsening of their peripheral nerve problem.
- Strengthening of surrounding musculature, such as periscapular muscles in the upper extremities, and light aerobic exercises to maintain conditioning should be encouraged during all phases of nerve recovery and can be self-directed.

Nonoperative Chronic Injuries

- Denervated muscles (with significant axonal loss) cannot be strengthened beyond the capacity of the remaining nerve and muscle fibers to fire and contract. One needs to prescribe initially passive and active assisted range of motion exercises to adjacent joints, such as the shoulder, to prevent secondary complications like a shoulder-adhesive capsulitis. It is not possible, or helpful, to stress the muscle beyond the capacity of the nerve to fire, as there may be an increase in muscle fatigue, which will result in a temporary setback in ability to progress with strengthening. Some have termed this "overwork neuropathy."[24]

- Resistive-type exercises in water may facilitate mobilization of the joint and help strengthen the muscle, as the buoyancy of the water facilitates movement in different planes. These can be done in any swimming pool, as long as the patient can access it and understands how to perform the exercises.

- Ultrasound as a form of deep heat to the muscle bone interface may be useful in facilitating passive stretch and maintaining the range of motion of the joint or muscle along with superficial heat to relax muscle, thus preventing spasms, which may interfere with muscle contractility.[23]

- Electrical stimulation will not help denervated muscle recover any faster, may damage the motor endplate, and needs to be used almost constantly to prevent significant muscle atrophy.[24] Therefore, the usage of electrical stimulation, while common, is of limited benefit with an underlying peripheral nerve injury.

- If there is significant hyperpathia related to the nerve injury, then desensitization techniques may be helpful along with proprioceptive retraining. Both open and closed kinetic chain exercises should be done as the muscle function is improving, with dynamic exercises for strengthening and sport-specific training initiated as soon as the individual is able to perform specific maneuvers unique to that sport without recurrence or exacerbation of symptoms.

- Medications should be primarily to control inflammation and pain, with nonsteroidal or steroidal anti-inflammatories and neuropathic-type medications such as gabapentin and amitryptyline more efficacious than narcotics.[25] Muscle relaxants are helpful, especially given the sedating side effects for restful sleep, which is essential for restoration of the nerve. Medications that regulate the sleep cycle should be considered.

- Injections and manual therapy are of limited benefit for a peripheral nerve problem.

Operative

- Indications for peripheral nerve surgery are the same for all nerves, and recovery for complete reinnervation is guarded where there has been total disruption of the perineurium.

Prognosis/Return to Play

- The athletes may return to play when they have regained sufficient strength to be competitive in their sport.

- Sport-specific training should progress first in training and later in competition only after significant improvement in strength and resolution of most sensory symptoms.

- Return to play is dictated by the severity of the peripheral nerve injury and can take days to months to recover. Some chronic injuries may never fully recover, and aggressiveness of treatment is dictated by amount of disability from the injury.

- One way to objectively assess strength is to redo the motor nerve conductions and determine what improvement there has been in amplitude compared to the opposite side. The amplitude should probably be at least 50% of normal (for that person) before he or she can resume playing, although the degree of reinnervation for a pitcher probably needs to be higher.

Complications/Indications for Referral

Complications include injury of the suprascapular nerve and/or upper-trunk brachial plexopathy in addition to the axillary nerve injury, depending on the extent of nerve compression or traction. If there appears to be weakness with muscle atrophy in muscles other than the deltoid and teres minor, then the recovery period may be longer, depending on the degree of axonal loss and proximity to the lesion, as nerves regenerate approximately 1 in/month. Both may decrease sensation in the distribution of the lateral brachial cutaneous nerve of the upper arm.[26] A skilled electromyographer can assist with the prognosis for nerve recovery. If one resumes playing while the muscle(s) are still too weak, then the potential for reinjury is greater.

APPROACH TO THE ATHLETE WITH SUPRASCAPULAR NERVE INJURY

More focal injury to the shoulder in football, hockey, lacrosse, and baseball pitchers may involve the suprascapular nerve, either in the suprascapular notch, which involves both the supraspinatus and infraspinatus muscles, or in the sphenoglenoid notch in high-level volleyball players involving only the infraspinatous.

HISTORY AND PHYSICAL EXAMINATION

The mechanism of injury is probably repeated stretch of the nerve during cocking of the arm and follow-through with serving.[27,28] Players may be asymptomatic if the injury is distal to the sensory branches to the posterior capsule and acromioclavicular joint.

On examination visible atrophy may be present but can be difficult to detect in muscular athletes. Those with denervation of the infraspinatous had a 22% loss of strength of the affected arm during external rotation. Sensation is usually normal.

DIAGNOSTIC TESTING

The suprascapular nerve can be studied electrodiagnostically and compared to the contralateral side, looking for significant differences in amplitude, as slowed speed of conduction along a short segment of nerve may not be clinically significant. Needle recording is preferred to obtain the CMAPs, as recording over the surface muscles may reflect coactivation of other muscles about the shoulder girdle.[29] A careful needle EMG of both the supraspinatous and infraspinatous muscles can help localize the lesion, providing the electromyographer is studying the supraspinatous versus the upper trapezius muscle. It is important that the referring physician understands the expertise of the electromyographer, as some individuals may not perform these tests routinely.

MRI may play a role in ruling out soft-tissue mass effect as can be seen with a paralabral cyst, resulting in the suprascapula nerve injury.

FUNCTIONAL TREATMENT

Nonoperative

- Nonoperative treatment is the same as for other peripheral nerve injuries, as noted earlier in the "Approach to the Athlete with Axillary Nerve Injury" section.

Operative

- Operative treatment is as discussed earlier.

Prognosis/Return to Play

- The athletes may return to play when they have regained sufficient strength to be competitive in their sport.
- Sport-specific training should progress first in training and later in competition only after significant improvement in strength and resolution of most sensory symptoms.
- Return to play is dictated by the severity of the peripheral nerve injury and can take days to months to recover. Some chronic injuries may never fully recover, and aggressiveness of treatment is dictated by amount of disability from the injury.
- One way to objectively assess strength is to redo the motor nerve conductions and determine what improvement there has been in amplitude compared to the opposite side. The amplitude should probably be at least 50% of normal (for that person) before he or she can resume playing, although the degree of reinnervation for a pitcher probably needs to be higher.

Complications/Indications for Referral

Complications include injury of the axillary nerve and/or upper-trunk brachial plexopathy in addition to the suprascapular nerve injury, depending on the extent of nerve compression or traction. If there appears to be weakness with muscle atrophy in muscles other than the supraspinatous and infraspinatous, then the recovery period may be longer, depending on the degree of axonal loss and proximity to the lesion. A skilled electromyographer can assist with the prognosis for nerve recovery. If one resumes playing while the muscle(s) are still too weak, then the potential for reinjury may be greater.

APPROACH TO THE ATHLETE WITH SPINAL ACCESSORY, LONG THORACIC, OR MUSCULOCUTANEOUS NERVE INJURIES

KEYS TO HISTORY AND PHYSICAL EXAMINATION

The spinal accessory nerve, or cranial nerve XI, may be injured from blunt trauma, such as a hockey or lacrosse stick across the posterior neck or a traction injury from a fall. It is purely motor and can be studied electrodiagnostically. Except for some shoulder pain, the athlete may not notice any deficits, although there may be weakness in forward elevation and abduction of the shoulder and rotary winging of the scapula. Most injuries are not complete, and athletes can compensate by using other well-developed shoulder girdle muscles.

The long thoracic nerve to the serratus anterior can be injured in overhead sports such as tennis or racquetball when the arm is overhead and the neck is turned to the contralateral side. It causes significant scapular winging with forward flexion of the arms. In one study, 25% of patients had some residual nerve palsy.[30] EMG with significant fibs and positive waves in only the serratus anterior are consistent with this injury.

The musculocutaneous nerve may be injured in those who play sports with vigorous elbow motion or those involved in upper-trunk plexopathies. Localized hyperesthesia may be present along with weakness or atrophy of the biceps.[31] The electrodiagnostic study will help differentiate between neurologic involvement versus tendon rupture as the etiology for the biceps weakness.

DIAGNOSTIC TESTING

Electrodiagnostic testing of the affected nerves needs to include comparison to the contralateral side to determine the normal amplitude for an individual. Loss of amplitude, which occurs in 8 to 12 days after injury, directly reflects axonal loss and provides information on the degree of axonal loss (Fig. 23.7). There are no good imaging studies to evaluate these injuries, but MRI may be utilized to rule out mass effect, resulting in the peripheral nerve symptoms.

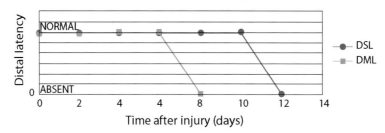

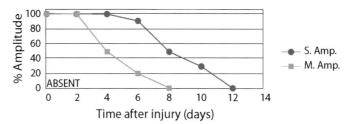

FIG. 23.7. Motor and sensory latency and amplitude changes over time.

FUNCTIONAL TREATMENT

Nonoperative

- Nonoperative treatment is the same as for other peripheral nerve injuries as noted earlier in the "Approach to the Athlete with Axillary Nerve Injury" section.

Operative

- Operative treatment is as discussed earlier.

Prognosis/Return to Play

- The athletes may return to play when they have regained sufficient strength to be competitive in their sport.
- Sport-specific training should progress first in training and later in competition only after significant improvement in strength and resolution of most sensory symptoms.
- Return to play is dictated by the severity of the peripheral nerve injury and can take days to months to recover. Some chronic injuries may never fully recover, and aggressiveness of treatment is dictated by amount of disability from the injury.
- One way to objectively assess strength is to redo the motor nerve conductions and determine what improvement there has been in amplitude compared to the opposite side. The amplitude should probably be at least 50% of

normal (for that person) before he or she can resume playing, although the degree of reinnervation for a pitcher probably needs to be higher.

Complications/Indications for Referral

Red flags include prolonged recovery that may be associated with axonal loss or progressive symptoms that do not correlate with affected nerve. A skilled electromyographer can assist with the prognosis for nerve recovery. If one resumes playing while the muscle(s) are still too weak, then the potential for reinjury may be greater.

APPROACH TO THE ATHLETE WITH MEDIAN NERVE ENTRAPMENT NEUROPATHY

Median neuropathies are the most common focal entrapment neuropathies in the upper extremities and are often used synonymously with carpal tunnel syndrome (CTS),[12] although there may be a median nerve injury at a site other than the carpal tunnel. The carpal tunnel may be compromised in football players, wrestlers, and individuals who play sports with excessive wrist motion such as cycling, tennis, and baseball. Weight lifters in particular may have findings consistent with carpal tunnel, although many of them also play different sports.[29]

HISTORY AND PHYSICAL EXAMINATION

Clinically the athlete may have numbness in the thumb, index, and long fingers and part of the ring finger (worse at night), although numbness is variable. Numbness in primarily the hand or the ring and little fingers is more commonly associated with carpal tunnel than an ulnar neuropathy due to the prevalence of carpal tunnel.[32]

Key components of the history are numbness more than pain, which is worse at night, or with prolonged activities where the wrists are flexed or experiencing vibration (driving, using vibratory tools) and involvement of the dominant hand.

The physical examination is less reliable, as sensory changes can be variable; it takes much longer for muscle atrophy to evolve, and the Tinel's and Phalen's signs are only 50% sensitive for nerve problems.[33]

DIAGNOSTIC TESTING

Focal electrodiagnostic studies of the median nerve across the carpal ligament can help to detect conduction block through the carpal tunnel and axonal loss (Fig. 23.8). Comparison studies to other upper-extremity peripheral nerves will determine how significantly the median nerve is affected. Ultrasound of the median nerve can determine the degree of inflammation and correlates with electrodiagnostic testing,[34] but it does not provide the prognostic information about the nerve integrity given by electrodiagnosis.

TREATMENT

Nonoperative

- Standard treatment for carpal tunnel includes use of wrist splints, oral or injected anti-inflammatory medication, and icing.
- A strengthening program should focus on more proximal muscles to lessen the stress on the wrist.

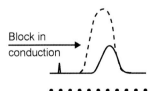

- Amplitude decreased
- Duration decreased
- Distal latency increased

Block in conduction

FIG. 23.8. Conduction block.

Operative

- For carpal tunnel with significant conduction block or axonal loss of sensory and motor responses via electrodiagnostic testing, operative treatment is the most efficacious.

Prognosis/Return to Play

- Median neuropathies are not usually associated with other injuries, so players can resume playing as soon as they are less symptomatic, or within 4 to 6 weeks following surgery.
- As usual, careful assessment of pain and strength should be done prior to the player returning to a sport that requires significant hand usage.

Complications/Indications for Referral

Indications for referrals include another underlying problem, such as a fracture, causing compression on the median nerve. Patients who are refractory to conservative treatment should have further diagnostic testing and referral to hand surgery if indicated.

Wheelchair athletes stress their upper extremities to a greater extent than most other athletes and may be more prone to focal nerve injuries such as carpal tunnel. They may also have more shoulder pathology, including rotator cuff and tendinopathy. The athlete with a lower cervical level spinal cord injury who has hyperreflexia and muscle wasting and develops a more focal cervical root impingement or nerve entrapment involving the shoulder girdle may be challenging to evaluate.[35] Referring these patients to someone who specializes in treating patients with spinal cord problems may be helpful.

APPROACH TO THE ATHLETE WITH RADIAL AND ULNAR NERVE ENTRAPMENT NEUROPATHIES

HISTORY AND PHYSICAL EXAMINATION

Fractures of the humerus commonly may involve the radial nerve at the spiral groove and can occur in arm wrestlers. Ulnar neuropathies at the elbow may be seen in pitchers who are repeatedly stressing the elbow, while compression at the wrist or in the hand is seen in performance cyclists and volleyball players.

At the level of the elbow, the radial nerve bifurcates into the motor posterior interosseous nerve (PIN), which innervates the wrist, hand, and finger extensors, and superficial radial sensory, which travels down the lateral arm and provides sensation to the lateral dorsum of the hand. With PIN lesions, the radial sensory is spared. Tennis players, who have overly developed upper-extremity muscles, may have compression of the PIN. Racquet sports with significant wrist motion may cause a superficial radial nerve injury involving only radial sensation.[7] There has been a reported radial nerve palsy related to a thrower's fracture of the humerus.[36]

Lesions of the ulnar nerve may cause weakness in specific ulnar innervated muscles, depending on the location of the injury. The dysesthesias are more variable; they may involve the ring and little fingers but can involve the entire hand and other fingers.

DIAGNOSTIC TESTING

Electrodiagnostic studies of the radial and ulnar nerves must include both motor and sensory studies to localize the lesion. There may be lesions of the peripheral nerves anywhere along the course of the nerve, which can be better localized by needle EMG. For elbow lesions, it is possible to study the ulnar nerve at 1-in intervals about the elbow to determine the exact location of a potential lesion.[32]

FUNCTIONAL TREATMENT

Nonoperative

- Nonoperative treatment is the same as for other peripheral nerve injuries, as noted earlier in the "Approach to the Athlete with Axillary Nerve Injury" section.

Operative

- Operative treatment is as discussed earlier.

Prognosis/Return to Play

- The athletes may return to play when they have regained sufficient strength to be competitive in their sport.
- Sport-specific training should progress first in training and later in competition only after significant improvement in strength and resolution of most sensory symptoms.
- Return to play is dictated by the severity of the peripheral nerve injury and can take days to months to recover. Some chronic injuries may never fully recover, and aggressiveness of treatment is dictated by the amount of disability from the injury.
- One way to objectively assess strength is to redo the motor nerve conductions and determine what improvement there has been in amplitude compared to the opposite side. The amplitude should probably be at least 50% of normal (for that person) before he or she can resume playing, although the degree of reinnervation for a pitcher probably needs to be higher.

Complications/Indications for Referral

Red flags include prolonged recovery that may be associated with axonal loss or progressive symptoms that do not correlate with affected nerve. A skilled electromyographer can assist with the prognosis for nerve recovery. If one resumes playing while the muscle(s) are still too weak, then the potential for reinjury may be greater.

APPROACH TO THE ATHLETE WITH LOWER-EXTREMITY NERVE INJURY

HISTORY AND PHYSICAL EXAMINATION

There are more musculoskeletal injuries in the lower extremities than neurologic ones, but the impairment and resulting disability from a nerve injury can be significant as it may affect one's ability to run and maneuver in physically challenging contact sports where speed and dexterity are key to success.

Injuries to the lower back in younger athletes who participate in sports requiring truncal rotation and hyperextension, such as gymnastics, usually present with posterior spinal column element injuries rather than neurologic ones. Older athletes more commonly injure the anterior elements, including the vertebral endplate and intervertebral disc, which may cause a lumbar radiculopathy, along the affected myotome. If the herniation involves the lateral recess, there may also be some sensory dermatomal changes. Repeated rotational injuries may be associated with progressive degenerative disc and facet joint disease associated with spinal stenosis, which may affect multiple nerve roots bilaterally. There may be sciatica associated with direct or indirect injury to that nerve. A routine manual muscle test may not detect the relative weakness in a high-level athlete, but careful analysis of the gait cycle and having the athlete stand on one tiptoe or heel may help detect the subtle motor changes. It is also important to isolate muscles by testing the patient in sidelying and prone positions.

Sports that may cause some compression neuropathies in the groin or lower extremities include gymnastics, which may injure the lateral femoral cutaneous nerve, or cycling, which may injure the iliofemoral cutaneous nerve or the pudendal nerve, causing numbness of the genital area or changes in miturition.

The sciatic nerve can be affected by direct trauma or traction such as in vigorous cycling. This causes significant problems with leg extension.

The peroneal nerve is vulnerable to pressure neuropathies at the lateral knee. When there is knee dislocation and ligamentous injury from blunt trauma, such as in football or martial arts, there can be peroneal nerve injury. There may be a traction injury to the peroneal nerve following an inversion ankle sprain associated with sports that involve running and jumping. It can also be compressed by knee boarding with the strap fastened too tightly around the thighs.

Dancers who wear tight ribbons and elastic in dancing shoes may have compression in the superficial peroneal nerve.[7] Runners with ankle inversion injuries may apply traction to the superficial peroneal nerve.

The tibial nerve is more commonly injured as part of a sciatic nerve injury, although the medial and lateral plantar branches in the foot may also be affected, especially in runners with tarsal tunnel syndrome.

DIAGNOSTIC TESTING

The evolution of neurophysiologic changes, detected on electrodiagnosis, is the same as in the upper extremity, except that it may take longer for needle EMG findings to appear, closer to 4 weeks, in the distal lower-extremity muscles, given the distance from the site of the pathology. As discussed earlier, changes in the motor and sensory amplitudes of the involved CMAPs and SNAPs may occur within the first week and should be compared to the contralateral limb to comment on axonal loss, but cannot provide much prognostic information until more time has lapsed.

TREATMENT

Nonoperative

• Refer to comments under upper-extremity nerve injuries, as the recommendations are similar.

Operative

• Operative possibilities are limited if there has been a severe nerve injury, although after 6 to 12 months without significant improvement in neurologic function, one may consider tendon transfers from an adjacent muscle to augment function of the denervated muscle.

Prognosis/Return to Play

• Return to play again depends on the overall condition of the athlete and extent to which the weaker muscle(s) are involved in the specific sport. For running, the athlete may need almost complete reinnervation of lower-extremity muscles to be competitive, especially of the more proximal muscles that propel the leg(s) forward and stabilize them during gait and running.

Complications/Indications for Referral

Individuals who are not showing any signs of recovery after 2 to 3 months should have more detailed electrodiagnostic studies to assist with prognosis and may benefit from looking at how the problem is affecting lower-extremity function, such as a gait analysis by someone with training to do that or a formal gait lab assessment. This information is useful in prescribing a specific physical therapy program, one designed to strengthen muscles with more optimal innervation to help compensate for any residual weakness in affected muscles.

KEY POINTS
• Peripheral nerve injuries are associated with sensory and motor changes
• Mild peripheral nerve injuries often resolve spontaneously
• Electrodiagnosis provides information about the degree of nerve injury and prognosis for recovery
• Peripheral nerve injuries in close proximity to the muscle innervated have a better prognosis for recovery
• Exercise prescriptions for patients with nerve injuries need to focus on passive range of motion and strengthening of surrounding musculature
• Disability related to peripheral nerve injuries is dependent on the type of injury and demands of the specific sport

REFERENCES

1. Leis AA, Trapani VC. *Atlas of Electromyography.* New York: Oxford University Press; 2000.
2. Seddon HJ. *Surgical Disorders of the Peripheral Nerves.* 2nd ed. New York: Churchill-Livingstone; 1975:21–23.
3. Kliot M. General principles in evaluating and treating peripheral nerve injuries in peripheral nerve injury course. American Association of Neuromuscular and Electrodiagnostic Medicine, Annual Meeting; October 2007; Phoenix, AZ.
4. Dumitru D, Amato AA, Zwarts MJ. *Electrodiagnostic Medicine.* 2nd ed. Philadelphia: Hanley and Belfus, Inc.; 2002.
5. Hirasawa Y, Sakakida K. Sports and peripheral nerve injuries. *Am J Sports Med.* 1983;11:420–426.
6. Krivickas LS, Wilbourn AJ. Sports and peripheral nerve injuries: report of 190 injuries evaluated in a single electromyography laboratory. *Muscle Nerve.* 1998;21(8):1092–1094.
7. Toth C, McNeil S, Feasby T. Peripheral nervous system injuries in sport and recreation. *Sports Med.* 2005;35(8):717–738.
8. Lodhia KR, Brahma B, McGillicuddy JE. Peripheral nerve injuries in weight training—sites, pathology, diagnosis and treatment. *Phys Sportsmed.* 2005;33(7):1–19.
9. Kirshblum S. Rehabilitation of spinal cord injury. In: DeLisa JA, Gans BM, Walsh NE, eds. *Physical Medicine and Rehabilitation: Principles and Practice.* 4th ed. Philadelphia: Lippincott Williams & Wilkins; 2005: 1715–1751.

10. Noble J, Munro CA, Prasad VS, et al. Analysis of upper and lower extremity peripheral nerve injuries in a population of patients with multiple injuries. *J Trauma.* 1998;45:116–122.

11. Williams F.H. *Supplement to Archives of Physical Medicine and Rehabilitation. Study Guide on Neuromuscular Rehabilitation and Electrodiagnosis*; March 2005.

12. Jablecki CK, Andary MT, Floeter MK, et al. Second literature review of the usefulness of nerve conduction studies and electromyography for the evaluation of patients with carpal tunnel syndrome. *Muscle Nerve.* Available at: www.interscience.wiley.com [Epub June 11, 2002]. DOI: 10.1002/mus.10215.

13. AAEM Referral Guidelines for Electrodiagnostic Consults. American Association of Neuromuscular and Electrodiagnostic Medicine (AANEM) http://www.aanem.org/practiceissues/PositionStatements/referral_guidelines_for_EDX.cfm, 1996.

14. Herbison G. EMG: waveform analysis. 33rd Annual Course in Electrodiagnostic Medicine and Clinical Neurophysiology, Jefferson Medical College; March 16, 2006; Philadelphia.

15. Dorfman LJ. Quantitative clinical electrophysiology in the evaluation of nerve injury and regeneration. *Muscle Nerve.* 1990;13:822–828.

16. Kraft GH. Fibrillation amplitude and muscle atrophy following peripheral nerve injury. *Muscle Nerve.* 1990;13:814–821.

17. Garrett WE, Speer KP, Kirkendall DT, eds. *Principles and Practice of Orthopedic Sports Medicine.* Philadelphia: Lippincott Williams & Wilkins; 2000.

18. Nissen SJ, Laskowski ER, Rizzo TD Jr. Burner syndrome: recognition and rehabilitation. *Phys Sportsmed.* 1996;24(6):57–64.

19. Chin CT. Magnetic resonance neurography in peripheral nerve injury course. American Association of Neuromuscular and Electrodiagnostic Medicine, Annual Meeting; October 2007; Phoenix, AZ.

20. Robinson L. Traumatic injury to peripheral nerves. AAEM Minimonograph #28. Rochester, MN: American Association of Electrodiagnostic Medicine; 2000.

21. American Association of Electrodiagnostic Medicine Course for Primary Care Physicians. Numbness, tingling, pain, and weakness; September 28, 1994; San Francisco, CA.

22. Visser CPJ, Coene LNJEM, Brand R. The incidence of nerve injury in anterior dislocation of the shoulder and its influence on functional recovery. *J Bone Joint Surg Br.* 1999;81(4):679–685.

23. Frontera WR, Silver JK. *Essentials of Physical Medicine and Rehabilitation.* Philadelphia: Hanley & Belfus, Inc.; 2002.

24. Kottke FJ, Lehmann JF, eds. *Krussen's Handbook of Physical Medicine and Rehabilitation.* 4th ed. Philadelphia: WB Saunders; 1990.

25. Herbison GJ, Jaweed M, Ditunno JF Jr. Exercise therapies in peripheral neuropathies. *Arch Phys Med Rehabil.* 1983;64:201–205.

26. Loeser JD, ed. *Bonica's Management of Pain.* Philadelphia: Lippincott Williams & Wilkins; 2001.

27. Cummins CA, Messer TM, Nuber GW. Current concepts review—suprascapular nerve entrapment. *J Bone Joint Surg.* 2000;82(3):415–424.

28. Ferretti A, Cerullo G, Russo G. Suprascapular neuropathy in volleyball players. *J Bone Joint Surg.* 1987;69(2):260–263.

29. Wilbourn AJ. Electrodiagnostic testing of neurologic injuries in athletes. *Clin Sports Med.* 1990;9:229–245.

30. Connor PM, Yamaguchi K, Manifold SG, et al. Split pectoralis major transfer for serratus anterior palsy. *Clin Orthop Relat Res.* 1997;341:134–142.

31. Aldridge JW, Bruno RJ, Strauch RJ. Nerve entrapment in athletes. *Clin Sports Med.* 2001;20(1):1–23.

32. American Association of Electrodiagnostic Medicine Quality Assurance Committee. Literature review of the usefulness of nerve conduction studies and electromyography in the evaluation of patients with ulnar neuropathy at the elbow. *Muscle Nerve.* 1999:22(suppl 8):S175–S205.

33. Stewart JD, Eisen A. Tinel's sign and the carpal tunnel syndrome. *Br Med J.* 1978;2:1125–1126.

34. Hobson-Webb LD, Massey JM, Juel VC, et al. The ultrasonographic wrist-to-forearm median nerve area ratio to carpal tunnel syndrome. *Clin Neurophysiol.* 2008;119(6):1353–1357.

35. DeLisa JA, Gans BM, Walsh NE, eds. *Physical Medicine and Rehabilitation: Principles and Practice.* 4th ed. Philadelphia: Lippincott Williams & Wilkins; 2005.

36. Curtin P, Taylor C, Rice J. Thrower's fracture of the humerus with radial nerve palsy: an unfamiliar softball injury. *Br J Sports Med.* 2005;39:40–43.

CHAPTER

24

Pediatric Athlete

Joseph Bernard

INTRODUCTION

Youth participation in organized sports has grown dramatically over the past couple of decades. The health care provider caring for the younger athletes should be aware of the differences in their anatomy and physiology as compared to adults.

The pediatric athlete is often still growing and many injuries are related to the changes that have or have not occurred yet during this phase of development. The specialization of sport at younger ages also places greater repetitive stress on a young athlete's body.

In evaluation of the skeletally immature pediatric athlete with bony injuries, consideration needs to be made regarding physeal (growth plate) injuries. The Salter–Harris classification, which is a radiographic classification, has been designed to further describe these fractures. Acute injuries to the growth plate are seen in an estimated 15% to 20% of injuries to the long bones and are often seen with sports participation. These are about two times more common in the upper extremity and are seen more often in boys than in girls.

FUNCTIONAL ANATOMY

The differences between adult and pediatric anatomy are crucial to the understanding of the unique types of injuries pediatric athletes sustain. Despite children's bones being weaker than those of adults, they are more plastic and absorb more energy before breaking. This means that incomplete fractures are common, that is, buckle–greenstick fractures. The periosteum is also much thicker than that in adults and is more readily elevated from the metaphysis and diaphysis of the bone and can reduce the incidence of complete periosteal rupture. The residual intact periosteum has useful functions in stabilizing the fracture and promoting healing (Fig. 24.1).[1]

The physis "growth plate" is an organized system of tissue located at the end of long bones and is primarily responsible for horizontal growth. This area of the long bones is important in the pediatric population because injury can cause growth deficiency and limb length discrepancy. The physis is

the transition zone between the metaphysis and the epiphysis. The physis is the "weakest link" in this structure. It is much more common to have an injury to the physis than to the tendons or ligaments. Salter–Harris type I fractures occur through the cartilage in the physeal zone. Salter–Harris type II fractures extend through the physis and the metaphysis. These are the most commonly seen fractures in this population. A Salter–Harris type III fracture extends through the physis to the epiphysis. Salter–Harris type IV injuries cross through the epiphysis, physis, and metaphysis. Salter–Harris type V fractures are classified as a compression-type injury to the physis and are usually not apparent on initial radiographs and can lead to growth arrest (Fig. 24.2).

Apophyses are small cartilage growth centers found at the attachment of tendons and ligaments to bones in the young athlete. The apophyses close at various rates, and common sites include the tibial tubercle (Osgood–Schlatter disease), calcaneus (Sever disease), and medial epicondyle (little league elbow). Apophyses have decreased tensile strength and are susceptible to repetitive overuse traction injury, apophysitis, as well as potential apophyseal avulsion injury (Fig. 24.3). The chronic traction injury results in microavulsions at the bone–cartilage junction. This is common during periods of rapid growth. The fusion of each apophysis occurs at differing times in development, and it is important for the sports medicine physician to be aware of this when evaluating the young athlete.

EPIDEMIOLOGY

Overuse musculoskeletal injuries should be considered in atraumatic pain in a pediatric athlete. Apophyseal injuries need to be considered in this population because of the inherent weakness of the open apophysis. Common apophyseal injuries include Osgood–Schlatter disease (patellar tendon at tibial tubercle), Sever disease (gastrocnemius–soleus complex at the calcaneus), Sinding–Larsen–Johansson syndrome (patellar tendon at the lower pole of the patella), hip flexor apophysitis (sartorius at the anterior superior iliac spine [ASIS] and rectus femoris at the anterior inferior iliac spine [AIIS]), and little league elbow (medial epicondyle of elbow).

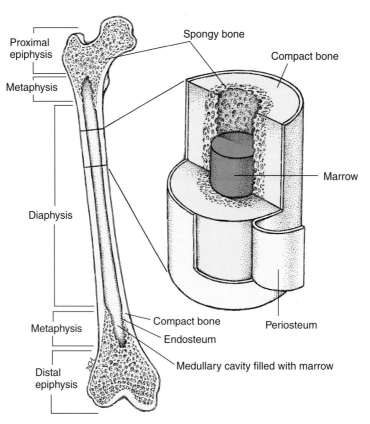

FIG. 24.1. Anatomy of pediatric long bones. Reprinted with permission from *Stedman's Medical Dictionary*. 27th ed. Baltimore: Lippincott Williams & Wilkins; 2000.

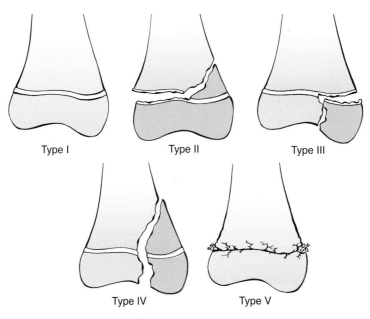

FIG. 24.2. Salter–Harris fracture classification. Reprinted with permission from Bucholz RW, Heckman JD, Court-Brown C, et al., eds. *Rockwood and Green's Fractures in Adults*. 6th ed. Philadelphia: Lippincott Williams & Wilkins; 2006.

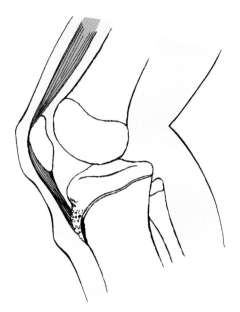

FIG. 24.3. Apophysitis with avulsion injury, Osgood–Schlatter disease. LifeART image copyright © 2008 Lippincott Williams & Wilkins. All rights reserved.

A total of 724 cases of tendinitis or apophysitis were diagnosed in 445 patients seen in the Sports Medicine Division at Boston Children's Hospital between 1980 and 1990. Of the 193 male and 253 female patients aged 8 to 19 years, boys and girls aged 16 years represented the largest groups. There were 88 injuries to the upper extremity and 636 to the lower extremity.[2]

Other common overuse injuries in the pediatric athlete include tendinosis, stress fractures, articular cartilage degeneration, and joint pain related to muscle weakness or imbalances (such as patellofemoral syndrome and multidirectional shoulder instability).

Acute injuries such as occult fractures and avulsion fractures need to be excluded. Growth plate fractures are common in the pediatric population due to incomplete closure of the physis. Mann and Rajmaira collected data on 2,650 long bone fractures, 30% of which involved the physes.[3] Neer and Horowitz evaluated 2,500 fractures to the physes (growth plate) and determined that the distal radius was the most frequently injured (44%), followed by the distal humerus (13%), and distal fibula, distal tibia, distal ulna, proximal humerus, distal femur, proximal tibia, and proximal fibula.[4]

NARROWING THE DIFFERENTIAL DIAGNOSES

History

A thorough history will guide the evaluator and help narrow the differential diagnosis. The age of the athlete is very important, as pediatric athletes present with different acute and overuse injuries than the mature athlete. The mechanism of injury will help differentiate between an overuse injury and an acute injury. This should include the sport that the athlete participates in, the position he or she plays, the level that he or she competes at, and how often he or she plays or takes time off for recovery. Asking what factors exacerbate the symptoms and what has helped to alleviate them is also important. Associated symptoms such as pain, swelling, or feeling of instability are useful.

When there is a traumatic injury in a pediatric athlete, it is important to obtain a history of when the injury occurred, the mechanism of the injury, the ability to continue to participate in the sport where the injury occurred, the area and intensity of the pain, and a history of prior fractures in that location. The age of the athlete and knowledge of when the various growth plates close are useful if a Salter–Harris fracture is suspected. Associated symptoms such as swelling, numbness, or weakness should be reviewed.

When an apophyseal injury is suspected, the immature athlete will complain of pain at or near the apophyseal site with activity. The pain will usually get better with rest. An injury or trauma preceding the development of pain would make an apophysitis less likely. The athlete may also report a recent growth spurt.

When a pediatric athlete presents with knee pain, it is important to know the age of the athlete, the history of when the pain started (acute or chronic), the location of the pain, the mechanism of injury, the sports that the athlete participates in, the level of sports participation and the amount of time for recovery between participation, the factors that make the pain better or worse, any prior history of knee pain, and what treatments have been tried. If there is not a particular event that brought on the pain, an overuse injury should be suspected. With anterior knee pain, pain associated with the patellofemoral extensor mechanism should be considered. Swelling after an acute injury may signify an internal ligamentous or meniscal derangement. Locking or catching is often seen with a meniscal tear, but the athlete may also describe some locking sensations with patellar tracking abnormalities associated with patellofemoral syndrome. If the location of the pain is near the tibial tubercle, an apophysitis may be suspected.

Evidence-based Physical Examination

When a young athlete presents with traumatic or atraumatic musculoskeletal pain, the area of pain should first be inspected for any deformities, skin changes, or swelling. The bones and joints should be palpated, assessing for deformities or tenderness. In the pediatric athlete, specific knowledge of the areas that still exhibit an open physis or apophysis should be considered. Many mild pediatric physeal and apophyseal injuries will have normal radiographs so diagnosis is based on mechanism and location of tenderness on examination.

Evaluation for range of motion of any joints in the area of pain and strength testing may help evaluate for associated muscle or tendon injuries. Strength testing can be manual or dynamic, such as single leg squat.

Ligamentous laxity would be concerning for an unstable joint due to a ligament sprain. Pediatric athletes often have hypermobile joints that may be normal. Comparison of unaffected side when dealing with an extremity can often elucidate if increased laxity is normal or pathologic.

Special tests will vary depending on the area of the body in question, but may be necessary to further rule out any specific injury. One such test is the Stork test or single-leg hyperextension test for suspected spondylolysis or spondylolisthesis.

For the pediatric knee examination, inspection of the knee is useful to evaluate for an effusion, for patellar alignment and mobility, and for ecchymosis associated with a traumatic injury. Palpation of the bony anatomy should be done to evaluate for possible fractures. If there is tenderness over the tibial tubercle or the lower patellar pole, Osgood–Schlatter disease or Sinding–Larsen–Johansson disease should be considered. Peripatellar tenderness may signify some patellofemoral pathology. Joint line tenderness would be seen if there is a meniscal tear. Special tests can also be used. A positive McMurray test is seen with meniscal pathology, a positive Lachman test is seen with a tear of the anterior cruciate ligament, and laxity or pain with varus or valgus stress would be seen with sprains of the lateral or medial collateral ligaments, respectively. A patellar compression may be seen with patellofemoral syndrome. A positive Ober test is seen with iliotibial friction syndrome.

Diagnostic Testing

Laboratory

Appropriate serologic tests are indicated largely in the setting of suspected autoimmune or infectious etiologies.

Imaging

Radiographic studies should be used judiciously due to radiation exposure. This said, many pediatric injuries warrant radiographic imaging due to risk of physeal or apophyseal injury. Bilateral views can be obtained when cortical irregularity is questioned to be pathologic or normal variant. For pediatric knee injuries, appropriate views will help determine the location of the patella in relation to the trochlear groove and the joint line space (Fig. 24.4).

Computed tomography (CT) use should be significantly reduced due to significantly greater radiation exposure with it than with plain radiographs and potential long-term risks.

Magnetic resonance imaging (MRI) is often the test of choice for soft-tissue structures but may be limited in

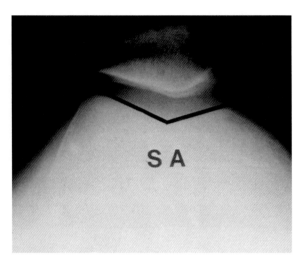

FIG. 24.4. Q-angle of knee. Reprinted with permission from Bucholz RW, Heckman JD. *Rockwood and Green's Fractures in Adults*. 5th ed. Philadelphia: Lippincott Williams & Wilkins; 2001.

young patients due to inability to remain still for prolonged periods.

Ultrasound may have an emerging role due to low cost and lack of ionizing radiation. Its use in the United States is currently limited by availability of trained technicians and physicians, as it is a highly operator-dependent modality.

Other Testing

Other testing is rarely required in the pediatric population for diagnosis and treatment of sports injuries. In the appropriate setting, electrodiagnostics may be indicated but due to patient discomfort generally not well tolerated.

APPROACH TO THE ATHLETE WITH OSGOOD–SCHLATTER

Osgood–Schlatter is a common cause of anterior knee pain in the young athlete and is most commonly found at the age of 12 to 17 years. Osgood–Schlatter is a traction apophysitis of the patella tendon at the insertion into the tibial tubercle. This is generally a benign, self-limited disorder.

HISTORY AND PHYSICAL EXAMINATION

The athlete will complain of pain at the tibial tuberosity with activity such as running and jumping. On physical examination, there will be tenderness to palpation at the tibial tubercle and usually some prominence or swelling of the tibial tubercle. Muscle imbalance with tightness in the quadriceps may be seen.

DIAGNOSTIC TESTING

Radiographs are usually not needed to make the appropriate diagnosis of Osgood–Schlatter disease. If they are obtained, they may reveal irregularity and fragmentation in the ossification at the tibial tubercle.

TREATMENT

Nonoperative

- Mainstay of treatment is conservative management with relative rest; activity modification, icing, stretching, and analgesic medications can be used.
- Knee pads for protective padding in sports at risk for landing on the tibial tubercle.

Operative

- Surgery is very rarely required and reserved for chronic severe cases that have not responded to conservative measures. Surgery involves removal of bone ossicle and debulking of the tibial tubercle.

Prognosis/Return to Play

- Osgood–Schlatter disease is usually self-limited and return to play is based on symptom relief.
- With milder pain, the athlete should be able to continue to participate as tolerated.
- More severe pain may warrant some relative rest while treating any underlying exacerbating factors.

Complications/Indications for Referral

There are rarely any long-term complications. Occasionally, the athlete will experience mild discomfort, especially with kneeling, or a persistent deformity of the tibial tubercle. Atypical or unusual symptoms or failure to respond to conservative measures 6 to 8 weeks may be indications for referral.

APPROACH TO THE ATHLETE WITH SEVER DISEASE

Sever disease is a common cause of heel pain in young athletes, usually found at the age of 5 to 12 years.[5,6] Sever disease is a traction apophysitis of the Achilles tendon at the insertion into the posterior calcaneus. This is generally a benign, self-limited disorder.

HISTORY AND PHYSICAL EXAMINATION

The athlete will report pain in the posterior aspect of the heel with running activities. Examination may reveal tenderness with medial and lateral compression of the posterior calcaneous.[5]

DIAGNOSTIC TESTING

Radiographs may be normal or reveal fragmentation at the calcaneal apophysis.

TREATMENT

Nonoperative

- Treatment consists of relative rest, activity modification, icing, stretching, and analgesic medications.
- Heel cups may provide symptomatic relief.

Operative

- Surgery is not required to treat this self-limited condition.

Prognosis/Return to Play

- Athletes can return to play as tolerated with activity.

Complications/Indications for Referral

Atypical or unusual symptoms or failure to respond to conservative measures 6 to 8 weeks may be indications for referral.

APPROACH TO THE ATHLETE WITH LITTLE LEAGUE ELBOW

Little league elbow is a traction injury to the medial epicondylar physis at the attachment site of the ulna collateral ligament secondary to repetitive valgus stress. It is a common cause of elbow pain in the young throwing athlete, particularly in baseball. Little league elbow is commonly seen between the age of 9 and 12.[5,7] More severe cases can result in significant widening or avulsion of the medial epicondylar physis with resultant compression injuries to the radial–capitellum joint.

HISTORY AND PHYSICAL EXAMINATION

When obtaining the history, hand dominance, sport and position played, and types of pitches thrown (if a baseball pitcher) should be obtained. Many athletes participate in multiple leagues simultaneously, increasing the number of throws or pitches that occur in a week. They will usually complain of pain over the medial elbow that is worse with throwing.

Physical examination will usually reveal tenderness at and around the area of the medial epicondyle. In more advanced cases, there may be some associated swelling, restricted range of motion, and a flexion contracture.

DIAGNOSTIC TESTING

Radiographs may reveal a widened or fragmented epicondylar physis in comparison to the contralateral elbow. There can be associated osteochondrosis or osteochondritis dissecans (OCD) of the capitellum or radial head as well as loose bodies in more severe cases. MRI is often unnecessary in mild cases but will show increased T2 signal along the medial epicondylar physis. MRI arthrogram is the test of choice for suspicion of loose body, osteochondrosis, or OCD.

TREATMENT

Nonoperative

- Treatment should consist of cessation of all throwing until the athlete is pain free with throwing activities. This may take 4 to 6 weeks.
- Once pain free and no tenderness on examination, a gradual return to throwing with an interval throwing program should precede return to competitive throwing.
- Rehabilitation should consist of core strengthening work and proper throwing techniques (Appendix B).

Operative

- Surgery is not indicated except in more severe cases with significant physeal widening causing functional elbow laxity.

Prognosis/Return to Play

- Once the athlete is pain free and is able to go through an interval throwing program, he or she should be able to return to his or her sport. Return to play can take up to 10 to 12 weeks.

- Prevention of these injuries is key, and pitch counts may help by limiting the number of pitches per week in these young throwing athletes.

Complications/Indications for Referral

If there is no improvement, or if radiographs show evidence of avulsion fractures or loose bodies, orthopaedic consultation may be necessary.[5,8]

APPROACH TO THE ATHLETE WITH HIP FLEXOR APOPHYSIS INJURY

HISTORY AND PHYSICAL EXAMINATION

A pediatric athlete who presents with anterior hip pain may be due to an apophyseal injury. Both the ASIS and AIIS have muscle attachment sites that could be affected. The pain is usually localized over the area of the open apophysis and there may be some associated swelling. Pain will be worsened with activities such as running and kicking and may be reproduced with active stretching of these muscles. Physical examination will reveal local bony tenderness over the ASIS or AIIS.

DIAGNOSTIC TESTING

The diagnosis is usually made clinically, but plain radiographs are necessary to evaluate for significant widening of the apophysis compared to the contralateral side.

TREATMENT

Nonoperative

Treatment usually depends on the amount of widening seen on radiographs. If no widening is seen, the athlete may be able to participate as tolerated. If symptoms were to escalate, then relative rest may be necessary. If there is widening, consistent with an avulsion injury, then initial treatment may start with protective weight bearing with crutches, with progression to full weight bearing and stretching once symptoms have resolved.[9]

Operative

Surgical treatment is rarely indicated.

Prognosis/Return to Play

- Once the athlete is pain free with ambulation and has started to improve on some of the functional causes, the athlete should be able to return to play.
- Specific hip/core strengthening and flexibility rehab is necessary to prevent the return of symptoms.

Complications/Indications for Referral

An athlete with a widened apophysis, with a displaced fragment greater than 2 cm, may require orthopaedic referral for surgical fixation.[9]

APPROACH TO THE ATHLETE WITH PATELLOFEMORAL SYNDROME

Patellofemoral syndrome is one of the most common sources of knee pain in the young athlete. This condition is reviewed in detail in Chapter 19.

APPROACH TO THE ATHLETE WITH SPONDYLOLYSIS

Spondylolysis and spondylolisthesis are common causes of low back pain in young athletes. A complete review may be found in Chapter 16.

APPROACH TO THE ATHLETE WITH A SALTER–HARRIS FRACTURE

HISTORY AND PHYSICAL EXAMINATION

A careful and thorough history should be obtained and should include the age and handedness of the athlete, a description of the injury including when the injury occurred, whether there had been any previous injury, whether prior radiographs have been taken, and a description of the treatment that has been done up until the point of the evaluation. On physical examination, the injured site should be inspected for deformities, swelling, or ecchymosis. The area should be palpated along the entire length of the bone involved, evaluating for any areas of tenderness or deformity. Range of motion of the joints relative to the area should be evaluated. Strength testing should also be done if there are no signs of an unstable fracture. With any fracture, confirmation of distal neurovascular status should be evaluated.

DIAGNOSTIC TESTING

Plain radiographs should be taken of the area of the bone that is thought to be involved. Because an open physis can often have the appearance of a fracture, comparison views of the contralateral extremity should be obtained in a skeletally immature athlete. The findings of a Salter–Harris type I fracture may be "normal" on plain radiographs, or there may be some widening or medial–lateral displacement seen. Salter–Harris type II to IV fractures can usually be seen easily when compared to the contralateral extremity. Salter–Harris type V fractures may also have "normal" appearance on plain radiographs and may only be found retrospectively after growth arrest is seen. Once a diagnosis is made, the fracture should be described in regard to its location, any separation or displacement seen, and whether any angular or rotational deformities exist. Description of the displacement may include anterior/posterior, medial/lateral, radial/ulnar, or volar/dorsal. Angulation should be described with relation of the distal fragment to the proximal fragment.

TREATMENT

Nonoperative

- Once diagnosed, a Salter–Harris fracture should be immobilized initially with splint followed by a cast once local swelling has resolved.
- Because there is rapid growth and cellular change at the physis, healing is usually rapid but can range from 4 to 12 weeks based on type and severity of the fracture.
- These should be followed with close follow-up to assure that no growth arrest occurs.

Operative

- If there is angulation, rotation, or poor alignment of the fracture site, reduction is usually necessary to achieve normal healing. This may involve closed or open reduction based on severity.

Prognosis/Return to Play

- Prior to return to participation in sports, the athlete should be pain free, there should be no tenderness to palpation at the fracture site, and he or she should have full range of motion and normal strength.
- This typically occurs in 4 to 6 weeks time, but some may require up to 12 weeks to heal. In general, pediatric fractures heal quicker than a similar fracture in a mature athlete.

Complications/Indications for Referral

Fracture management should be done in the hands of a clinician who feels comfortable following and managing pediatric fractures. Orthopaedic surgery referral is specifically warranted for complicated fractures (unstable, displaced, rotated, angulated) or one that involves a specific amount of the articular surface. This varies with the bone and joint involved. Salter–Harris type I fractures can be easily managed by a primary care physician and serial radiographs, and examinations should ensue to document healing and stability.

KEY POINTS
• The differences between adult and pediatric anatomy are crucial to the understanding of the unique types of injuries pediatric athletes sustain
• Overuse injuries are very common in pediatric population; consider apophyseal and physeal injuries when evaluating this age group
• Majority of pediatric injuries respond to conservative management
• Salter–Harris fractures involve the physis "growth plate" and need immediate attention with immobilization until pain free. Consultation depends on the degree of instability and articular surface involved

REFERENCES

1. Irwin GJ. Fractures in Children. *Imaging.* 2004;16:140–152.
2. Micheli LJ, Fehlandt AF Jr. Overuse injuries to tendons and apophyses in children and adolescents. *Clin Sports Med.* 1992;11:713–726.
3. Mann DC, Rajmaira S. Distribution of physeal and nonphyseal fractures in 2,650 long-bone fractures in children aged 0–16 years. *J Pediatr Orthop.* 1990;10(6):713–716.
4. Neer CS, Horowitz BS. Fractures of the proximal humeral epiphyseal plate. *Clin Orthop Relat Res.* 1965;41:24–31.
5. Cassas KJ, Cassettari-Wayhs A. Childhood and adolescent sports-related overuse injuries. *Am Fam Physician.* 2006;73:1014–1022.
6. Schroeder BM. American College of Foot and Ankle Surgeons: diagnosis and treatment of heel pain. *Am Fam Physician.* 2002;65:1686–1688.
7. Benjamin HJ, Briner WW Jr. Little league elbow. *Clin J Sport Med.* 2005;15:37–40.
8. Andrish JT. Osteochondritis dissecans in a young pitcher: why early recognition matters. *Phys Sport Med.* 1997;25:85–90.
9. Frank JB, Jarit GJ, Bravman JT, Rosen JE. Lower extremity injuries in the skeletally immature athlete. *J Am Acad Orthop Surg.* 2007;15(6):356–366.

Mature Athlete

Gregory Czarnecki and Jake D. Veigel

INTRODUCTION

The benefits of routine exercise can be realized throughout the spectrum of one's life. Many physiologic changes once attributed to "old age" have come into question regarding inherent physiologic change versus disuse or adaptive responses. Medical conditions including hypertension, diabetes, dyslipidemia, obesity, osteoporosis, and coronary artery disease (CAD) have been shown to be halted or slowed onset in the setting of routine exercise or addition of exercise in those previously sedentary. Advancing age traditionally leads to decreasing physical activity or incorporation of a relatively sedentary lifestyle. This is multifactorial and may include work, family, and chronic medical issues. Less than half of the U.S. adult population meets the activity recommendations of the Centers for Disease Control/American College of Sports Medicine (CDC/ACSM) and only 39% of those over 65.[1] While the "geriatric athlete" is defined as those aged 65 and up, this chapter will broaden the focus to include a much broader age range with attention to the "mature athlete" and masters-level athletes.

Masters athletes have shown that competitive exercise and "healthy aging" is possible over a broad range of ages. Masters level is defined as women and men of age 35 and up.[2] Both in organized team and in individual sports, age categories are in 5-year increments with the eldest category being those competitors aged 100 plus. The Senior Olympics, now known as the National Senior Games, includes athletes aged 50 and above. Originating in 1987 with 2,500 athletes, the National Senior Games is held every 2 years with 12,100 athletes registered in 2007.[3] Studies in previously sedentary geriatric populations with varying levels of physical function and medical comorbidities have enjoyed the benefits of renewed exercise in their daily lives. Even in masters athletes, however, there are functional declines that are observed and may be an inevitable process of aging. The ultimate question remains, how much is preventable with exercise?

PHYSIOLOGY IN THE MATURE ATHLETE

What are some of the adaptive changes associated with aging? The cardiovascular response is a 6 to 10 beats/min decline in maximum heart rate per decade. Vo$_2$max (maximal oxygen consumption) decreases 5% to 15% per decade after age 25.[4] During maximal exercise, older athletes generally demonstrate higher blood pressures and peripheral vascular resistance than their younger counterparts. The pulmonary changes of decreased lung compliance (elasticity) and decreased vital capacity may also contribute to a relative increase in perceived exertion for given workload. Loss of muscle mass, also known as sarcopenia, is a prominent feature with aging. Type 2 muscle fibers show greater relative loss. Peak muscle strength is seen around age 30 and starts to decline at age 50; in the sedentary population, there is a 15% per decade decline from age 50 to 70 and a 30% per decade decline after age 70.[5] Decreased muscle mass results in decreased lean body mass, which, in turn, leads to a lower basal metabolic rate. This decrease can contribute to central obesity and weight gain without change in caloric intake. With advancing age comes increased muscle stiffness and decreased tensile strength of tendons and ligaments. This is an important factor in the overuse injuries, and longer rehabilitation time is often needed for return to activity. Bone density declines 0.5%/year after age 40.[6] Additionally with aging, diminishing balance and coordination contributes to increased risk of falls and injury. More recently, mitochondrial dysfunction has been identified in the aging process. This dysfunction appears to stem from both electron transport chain defects and uncoupling of oxidative phosphorylation due to hydrogen leak in the inner mitochondrial membrane. These changes lead to reduced ATP generation per mitochondrion and reduced exercise efficiency with reduced ATP synthesis per O$_2$ uptake.[7] The ATP depletion at the cellular level due to the uncoupling with age is associated with apoptosis (cell death). The uncoupling is seen to a greater extent in muscles with higher percentage of type 2 fibers and may explain the preferential loss noted earlier in the text[7] (see Table 25.1).

So, with these declines, can exercise bring hope? Studies among masters athletes have shown promise. The keys to changing course include restoring fitness and maintaining a balance of cardiovascular and strength training. Some studies have shown a decrease in the rate of decline in heart rate max and Vo$_2$max with maintained levels of training. More benefit may be realized in risk reduction for the associated

TABLE 25.1	Functional Changes Associated with Aging
Cardiovascular	↑BP and PVR
	↓Vo$_2$max (5–15% per decade after age 25)
	↓HR$_{max}$ (6–10 BPM per decade)
Pulmonary	↓Elasticity
	↓Vital capacity
	↑Residual volume
Musculoskeletal	↓Muscle mass, bone mass, tensile strength of tendons/ligaments
	↓Collagen stiffness and altered collagen network structure
Neurologic	↓Balance, coordination, reaction time
	Autonomic dysfunction
	↓Thirst mechanism
Metabolic	↓BMR
	↑Cholesterol
Cellular	↓Mitochondrial function and content

BP, blood pressure; PVR, peripheral arterial resistance; HR, heart rate; BPM, beats per minute; BMR, basal metabolic rate.

comorbidities of sedentary lifestyle listed previously. Strength training in the elderly, which had often been dismissed previously, is now considered a vital component of fitness. Even the frail elderly can achieve muscle hypertrophy and increased size of muscle fibers. The benefit not only goes beyond strength itself but also contributes to maintaining balance and, in turn, fall prevention. Strength training in the frail has also demonstrated increased spontaneous activity by those previously sedentary. Bone mineral density may be improved with exercise. Activities with higher loading forces have shown greater responses to increasing bone mineral density. However, this higher impact is not always practical in the geriatric athlete. For those with osteoarthritis (OA), low-impact exercise has been shown to improve both pain and function.[6,8] Even with relatively small blood pressure reduction, risk reduction of stroke and CAD can be significant in the general population.[9] At the cellular level, reversal of mitochondrial dysfunction, uncoupling of oxidative phosphorylation, has been shown after 6 months of exercise training in elderly muscle.[7]

APPROACH TO THE MATURE ATHLETE, GENERAL CONSIDERATIONS

Vital to success of training and competition is setting and modifying goals as needed with appropriate activities for the individual. For instance, the sedentary individual who was an "athlete" years ago and is now planning to "get back into shape" or perhaps train for a marathon would need much different education than the age-matched individual who has continued to compete and whose goal is to improve his or her finish time in the same event. Overuse injuries are especially common in the mature athlete and may account for up to 70% of injuries in experienced athletes over the age of 60.[10] This may often be attributed to training errors including rapid increase in activity with inadequate recovery time, improper footwear, poor biomechanics, or training surfaces. Because of physiologic changes, recovery time for injuries is generally longer in the elder athlete. With advancing age, the thirst mechanism becomes impaired and this may put an athlete at increased risk for dehydration. Thermoregulation may also be impaired in the setting of autonomic dysfunction. In addition, certain medications, such as diuretics or β-blockers, may have side effects unsuitable for the competitive athlete. Knowledge of the athlete's medical comorbidities is imperative in counseling and physical assessment.

Prior to initiating an exercise program or significantly increasing physical activity in the mature population, one must first determine medical readiness and whether medical "clearance" is indicated. Though recommendations vary, the goal of screening is for risk stratification and identifying need for further evaluation and/or treatment prior to participation. Specific goals are to identify CAD risk factors and signs and symptoms (or current status if preexisting) of cardiovascular, pulmonary, or metabolic disease. Screening questionnaires such as American Heart Association (AHA)/ ACSM Health/Fitness Preparticipation Screening Questionnaire and the PAR-Q (Physical Activity Readiness Questionnaire) may help identify those in need of further medical screening.[11,12,13] In the absence of a positive screen, individuals are encouraged to gradually increase their level of physical activity as tolerated without need for further testing. However, this requires the participant to be current with general age-appropriate medical screenings, such as blood pressure.

NARROWING THE DIFFERENTIAL DIAGNOSES

History

Preparticipation medical screening should first assess the individual's level of previous activity and the sport or activity being planned. History and physical examination should address hearing, vision, and impairments such as glaucoma and cataracts, OA and regions affected, as well as coexisting chronic medical conditions.[12] History should include cardiac screening for chest pain, exertional dyspnea, exertional dizziness or lightheadedness, palpitations, and syncope. The presence of autonomic dysfunction increases with age and should be part of the history's screening. Medication history including supplements should be ascertained. Family history remains an important consideration, though relevance as a risk factor diminishes for many conditions in the elderly. Cardiovascular family history should question premature death (<50 years of age) or disability due to heart disease in a close relative. Additionally, consider history in family members of cardiomyopathy, long QT syndrome, Marfan syndrome, or other arrhythmias.[13]

Evidence-based Physical Examination

Examination should include assessment of blood pressure and, when indicated, orthostatic pressures, cardiac, lung, and carotid auscultation, and femoral pulses. Neurologic assessment ought to address coordination, balance, and proprioception in addition to strength and sensation. A thorough orthopaedic history and screening examination is also imperative to counsel regarding activities; see section "Approach to the Athlete with Osteoarthritis" in the following text. In essence, all organ systems are included in overall assessment in both history and physical examination, and further questioning will vary with associated comorbidities.

Diagnostic Testing

Laboratory

Preparticipation laboratory investigation again may vary by condition, but recommended screening includes hemoglobin and hematocrit, fasting blood glucose, blood urea nitrogen (BUN), creatinine, and a fasting lipid panel.

Imaging

Routine imaging studies are generally not required unless underlying medical or orthopaedic condition dictates.

Other Testing

An electrocardiogram (ECG) is recommended for masters athletes over the age of 40, and ECG and stress testing are recommended for athletes over 65.[6,13] CAD is the leading cause of sudden death during exercise in those over age 35. The ACSM recommends exercise testing for all men 45 years and older and women 55 years and older planning vigorous exercise and for those considered "high risk" planning moderate exercise (level C).[12] By age criteria alone, these age cutoffs put many of the mature athletes in the "moderate risk" category. A "high risk" individual includes those with known cardiac, peripheral vascular, or cerebrovascular disease; pulmonary disease including asthma, chronic obstructive pulmonary disease (COPD), and interstitial lung disease; and metabolic disease including diabetes, thyroid disorders, renal, or liver disease.[12] The AHA states that medically supervised exercise stress testing in men older than 40 years and women older than 55 years "may be useful," specifically

for those in competitive sports or who plan habitual vigorous training with two or more coronary risk factors.[14] Exercise testing may also be considered to assist with exercise prescription in determining maximum heart rate and heart rate reserve. Contraindications to exercise include recent myocardial infarction (MI), ischemic ECG changes, unstable angina, uncontrolled arrhythmia, third-degree heart block, and acute congestive heart failure (CHF). Relative contraindications include uncontrolled hypertension, valvular heart disease, cardiomyopathies, complex ventricular ectopy, and uncontrolled metabolic disease.[12]

APPROACH TO THE EXERCISE PRESCRIPTION FOR THE MATURE ATHLETE

Exercise prescription will vary by individual, but in general will address mode, intensity, duration, and frequency of the exercise. Mode of exercise should take into account the individual's medical conditions such as OA and patient preferences. Intensity for those previously sedentary is recommended to start low and gradually progress to individual's tolerance over weeks to months. Low- to moderate-intensity exercise itself may reduce blood pressure as well as improve other physiologic parameters described earlier in the text. Minimum duration should be in 10-minute increments with goal of 30 minutes most days of the week.[12] To promote and maintain health, as per recent updated recommendations by the ACSM, all healthy adults aged 18 to 65 years need moderate-intensity physical aerobic activity for a minimum of 30 minutes 5 days each week or vigorous-intensity aerobic activity for a minimum of 20 minutes 3 days each week (level A).[1] These minimums are in addition to activities of daily living lasting less than 10 minutes in duration. Moderate and vigorous activities can be combined to meet the minimum recommendations. In addition to aerobic activity, recommendations include incorporating strength training, flexibility, and proprioceptive/balance training. Goals and benefits of strength training are to preserve muscle mass and, in turn, the basal metabolic rate. Strength training as well as aerobic activity improves insulin action and can be a vital tool in delaying the progression from insulin resistance to type 2 diabetes (level A).[12] Additional benefits of strength training may include preservation of bone mineral density, fall prevention, and an increase in parameters of functional status in the elderly, such as walking speed and initiation of spontaneous activity.[15,16]

There are numerous tools an athlete can use to assist with determining intensity of exercise. Most common is using a percentage of the maximum heart rate or heart rate reserve as the measure of intensity. However, this will vary somewhat by individual and may not always be feasible, for example, with those on β-blockers. Maximum heart rate is estimated by 220 minus age, plus or minus 10 to 12 beats/min.

Light intensity is 50% to 63% of the maximum heart rate. Moderate intensity is 64% to 76% and vigorous 77% to 93%. Heart rate reserve is maximum heart rate minus the resting heart rate. Here, light, moderate, and vigorous intensities are 20% to 39%, 40% to 59%, and 60% to 84%, respectively.[12] The calculated numbers are added to the resting heart rate. Another method is the Borg rating of perceived exertion scale where the athlete judges the activity on a 15-point scale, as stated by his or her perceived exertion. The talk test is yet another method to grade intensity which differentiates light, moderate, and vigorous exercise by the degree of conversation that one is able to have during the activity, with vigorous exercise being unable to carry on a conversation, moderate able to, and light being able to sing, if desired. As with any athlete, adequate warm-up and cool-down is recommended with exercise to help avoid injury.

APPROACH TO THE NUTRITIONAL CONSIDERATIONS FOR THE MATURE ATHLETE

Adequate energy intake is an important reminder for the elder athlete, especially as his or her general daily intake decreases with age in part due to reduction in lean body mass. Protein intake is often suboptimal in the elderly. Long-term reduction in daily protein intake contributes to the decline in lean body mass. Current recommendations are to aim for daily protein intake of 1 to 1.25 g/kg (level C). For those 65 years of age and up, 1,500 mg/day of calcium is recommended. Vitamin D daily goals are 10 μg (400 IU) for those over 51 years and 15 μg (600 IU) for those over 70 years (level C).[17,18] With impaired thirst mechanism, elder athletes are encouraged to drink fluids at regular intervals rather than relying on sensation of thirst to guide fluid intake.

Nutritional changes with aging and in the exercising elderly can be complex. Important recommendations for the exercising elderly are as follows[17]:

- 55% to 60% of calories from carbohydrates with a focus on complex carbohydrates
- 12% to 15% of calories from protein
- 25% to 30% of calories from fat with less than 10% in saturated fat.
- No change in vitamin C recommendations
- Increase riboflavin to 1.5 mg/day
- Increase vitamin B_6 to 2.0 mg/day
- Increase vitamin B_{12} to 2.8 mg/day
- Increase folate to more than 400 μg/day
- Consume vitamin A through fruits and vegetables high in carotenoids
- Increase vitamin D to 600 IU/day
- Consider supplementation of vitamin E if at risk for coronary heart disease
- Increase calcium intake to 1,500 mg/day if there is inadequate diet, otherwise 1,200 mg is sufficient
- No change in zinc intake
- Increase iron intake to 15 mg/day in runners and vegetarians, otherwise no change

APPROACH TO THE ATHLETE WITH OSTEOARTHRITIS

It is estimated that OA affects approximately 15% of the U.S. population and the incidence increases with age.[19] Over 70% of people over the age of 70 will have x-ray evidence of OA, but symptoms may vary greatly. A key question many athletes have is, does long-term exercise increase one's risk for developing OA? Activities with heavy loading and twisting of the knee are considered risk factors for OA, but as reviewed by Griffin and Guilak, multiple studies support that moderate mechanical loading is necessary to maintain healthy articular cartilage. It is not the extended use but rather the dysfunctional use that may lead to alterations in joint homeostasis that ultimately initiates or drives the degradative process. Prolonged inactivity itself can reduce cartilage thickness and proteoglycan content.[19] Dysfunctional use, including training errors such as the overuse syndromes and biomechanical factors both inherent and external, may lead to abnormal joint forces that disrupt the balance of joint metabolism, ultimately leading to the development of OA.

HISTORY AND PHYSICAL EXAMINATION

Pain is the leading symptom with OA and varies by patient. Pain does not necessarily correlate with level of radiographic change, as many of those with radiographic "advanced arthritis" will have little to no pain. Symptoms may wax and wane and may also include joint stiffness and/or swelling. Decreased joint range of motion is characteristic and this reduction is seen in both active and passive testing. On examination, bony hypertrophy may be appreciated on inspection, and palpation may reveal crepitus. Classic findings of the hand include Heberden's and Bouchard's nodes (Fig. 25.1). Joints may be with or without effusion.

DIAGNOSTIC TESTING

Plain radiographs have been shown to follow progression of OA, rule out coexisting pathology, as well as assess for benign or malignant tumors. Whether these findings impact treatment is an area of controversy. Classic findings of knee OA include joint space narrowing, bone (subchondral) sclerosis, and bone spur formation (Fig. 25.2). Other joints may be affected as well (Fig. 25.3). Magnetic resonance imaging (MRI) may be helpful to identify early disease and exclude coexisting pathology, but adds little diagnostic value to advanced cases of OA.

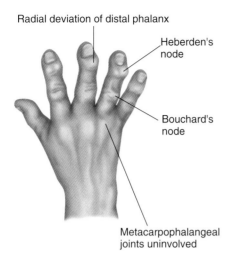

FIG. 25.1. Illustrative representation of Heberden's and Bouchard's nodes. Reprinted with permission from Bickley LS, Szilagyi P. *Bates' Guide to Physical Examination and History Taking.* 8th ed. Philadelphia: Lippincott Williams & Wilkins; 2003.

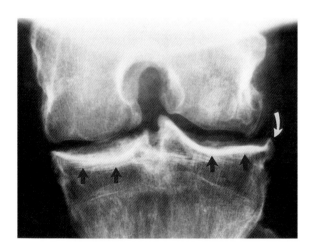

FIG. 25.2. Osteoarthritis of the knee. There is subchondral sclerosis (*straight arrows*) and a large marginal osteophyte (*curved arrow*) laterally. Reprinted with permission from Daffner RH. *Clinical Radiology: The Essentials.* 3rd ed. Philadelphia: Lippincott Williams & Wilkins; 2007.

In the presence of an effusion, alternate diagnoses should be considered such as gout or other deposition diseases. If diagnosis is unclear, diagnostic arthrocentesis may be useful in identifying inflammatory versus noninflammatory conditions and additional studies as indicated such as crystal analysis.

TREATMENT

General Measures

- Mainstays of nonpharmacologic therapy include activity modification and weight loss when indicated.
- Physical therapy to improve or maintain strength and proprioception. Joint forces must be considered and correct dysfunctional biomechanics when possible.
- There is limited evidence that bracing or neoprene sleeve can offer added benefit in pain and function than medical treatment alone in those with medial compartment OA.
- Lateral heel wedges have been shown to decrease overall nonsteroidal anti-inflammatory drug (NSAID) intake, though this reduction appears to be minor (level B).[20]

Nutritional Supplements

- The role of nutritional supplements has been fairly well studied for glucosamine with recent Cochrane review finding glucosamine to be safe as compared to placebo, but efficacy ranges from comparable to placebo to 13-point improvement in pain (scale of 0 to 100).
- The pharmaceutical brand tended to show more likelihood of favorable pain response.[21]
- The Glucosamine/Chondroitin Arthritis Intervention Trial (GAIT) is currently the largest double-blind, placebo-controlled trial comparing the efficacy and safety of glucosamine hydrochloride, chondroitin sulfate, or the two in combination that did not show statistical significance for these subgroups in pain reduction at 24 weeks. However, the combination of the two in those with moderate to severe pain at baseline did show a significantly higher response rate than placebo. The number of patients in this subgroup was relatively small and may not be powered to draw positive conclusions. Additionally, there was a 60% placebo response rate and relatively mild knee pain at baseline of the overall group, which leads to questions for the interpretation of the results.[22]
- The Osteoarthritis Research Society International (ORSI) recommends glucosamine and chondroitin as level A pharmacologic treatment of hip and knee OA with 63% strength of recommendation (95% CI).
- The American College of Rheumatology has not taken a position on the use of glucosamine and chondroitin due to the various design differences and methods among the existing studies for comparison.[23] The benefit of these supplements remains unclear in the athletic population.

Pharmacologic Treatment

- Both acetaminophen (Tylenol) and NSAIDs have been shown to be effective in reducing pain associated with OA (level A).

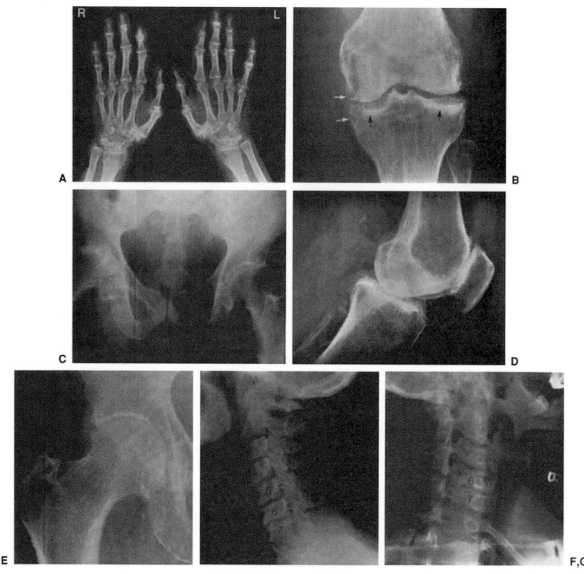

FIG. 25.3. Common findings of multiple joints with osteoarthritis.

- NSAIDS are generally superior to acetaminophen in reducing pain and improving function in moderate to severe OA.[24] Acetaminophen is generally better tolerated and side effects must be considered.
- Caution is advised with the use of an NSAID in athletes with hypertension and those on an ACE inhibitor for risk of precipitating renal failure. This also holds true for those at increased risk of dehydration.
- Intra-articular corticosteroid injections have been shown to reduce pain over weeks to months (level A) in numerous studies; however, the long-term benefits remain unclear.[25]
- Newer injection treatments include viscosupplementation, namely, with hyaluronan and hylan derivatives and

have also shown benefit in improving pain and function for those with OA of the knee.[26]
- The duration of efficacy is generally longer with these injections as compared to intra-articular corticosteroids. However, the number of injections per series and average duration of effect vary by product. While believed to add "protection" to the joint by restoring viscoelasticity and increasing concentration of hyaluronan, which is involved with counterregulation of degradative processes within the joint, there is currently no evidence to support that viscosupplementation halts or slows progression of disease.

Nonpharmacologic Treatment

- Acupuncture and massage therapy may be considered as adjunct therapies in the treatment of OA.
- Societies vary on their recommendations for level of evidence on these modalities.[22]

Surgical Treatment

- Arthroscopy, utilizing lavage and/or debridement, has long been performed in OA for persistent painful symptoms.
- Studies have shown improvement in pain and function following arthroscopic lavage alone persisting at 1-year follow-up.[27]
- Moseley et al. report in a blinded randomized trial no benefit in pain or function, comparing arthroscopic debridement or lavage with a placebo procedure in patients with OA of the knee at 2-year follow-up.[28,29]
- A Cochrane review determined level A evidence that arthroscopic debridement for undifferentiated OA provides no benefit in reducing pain and improving function.[30] Additionally, question remains to whether these data can be extrapolated to the athletic population.

Prognosis/Return to Play

- Prognosis for athletes with OA will vary by individual and severity of disease.
- For many, occasional "flares" of painful symptoms will limit activities for limited duration and return to play is individualized based on tolerance.
- With progression of disease or in "flares," activity modification is often needed and may include such factors as decreasing intensity, duration, and/or frequency of activity.
- Alternatively for some, a different mode of exercise may be the best solution.

Complications/Indications for Referral

High-impact activities and training errors can increase risk for complications including effusion and arthralgias. Effusions may limit range of motion and have an effect on competition. The presence of an undiagnosed effusion is a red flag and warrants further evaluation. Complications from injections include bleeding and infection. For corticosteroids, skin hypopigmentation, fat atrophy, and transient hyperglycemia may occur. With the viscosupplementation, there is added risk of reaction to the product and this risk increases with added exposures. Pain and stiffness may wax and wane in the course of disease, and they are the leading causes of disability with OA. Joint replacement is typically reserved for those with failed conservative measures and persistent pain or dysfunction.

APPROACH TO THE ATHLETE WITH TOTAL JOINT REPLACEMENT

Joint replacement can be an effective treatment for alleviating pain and dysfunction related to advanced OA by restoring joint mechanics, improved quality of life and increased physical activity. However, controversy remains as to what activities should or should not be performed following joint replacement. The major concerns are related to hardware failure and related complications including periprosthetic fractures.[31] Additional concern is for joint dislocation. There are no large prospective controlled studies on athletic activity following joint replacement, and recommendations remain based on expert opinion. As hardware technology has and continues to improve, joint stability following arthroplasty may lessen the risks of complications, such as loss of fixation, as compared to earlier surgical techniques and hardware. Low-impact activities are recommended (level C), but there are varied opinions for sport-specific limitations. For example, downhill skiing is generally discouraged following total knee or hip replacement, but for an experienced skier opinions vary for returning to the sport. Some would recommend allowing return with set limitations, such as type of slope or terrain or anticipated impact. There are activities deemed allowable with previous experience including cross-country skiing, speed walking, backpacking, ice skating, singles/doubles tennis, aerobics, volleyball, alpine skiing, and hiking. These are listed as intermediate recommendation by the Mayo clinic.[31] Allowable recommendations from the Mayo clinic include golf, swimming, cycling, bowling, sailing, and scuba diving after total hip and knee replacement. Contact sports and high-impact activities are not recommended by the Mayo clinic and may include such activities as basketball, racquetball, handball, running, hockey, baseball, water skiing, karate, soccer, and football (level C).[31]

KEY POINTS
• Elder athletes are growing in number, and level of competition may vary greatly. Health benefits may be numerous, but caution and appropriate screening is advised when new activities or changes in intensity are being considered
• Training errors are common in the overuse syndromes often encountered in the aging athlete. Counseling should include proper warm-up, cool-down, and allowing for recovery time following the exercise
• Training programs should include aerobic activity, strength training, flexibility, and balance training

- To promote and maintain health, achieve minimum of 30 minutes of moderate-intensity exercise minimum 5 days of the week or 20 minutes of vigorous-intensity exercise 3 days of the week with strength training at least 2 days a week

- OA is common in the aging athlete. Exercise in itself does not appear to increase the risk of developing arthritis. However, activities with heavy joint loading and twisting forces are considered risk factors. Exercise may improve pain and function in those with OA

- Low-impact activities are recommended for athletes with total joint replacement of the knee or hip. Sport-specific limitations remain unclear

REFERENCES

1. Haskell WL, Lee IM, Pate RR, et al. Physical activity and public health: updated recommendations for adults from the American College of Sports Medicine and the American Heart Association. *Circulation.* 2007;116:1081–1093.
2. http://www.world-masters-athletics.org/index.php?content=about_us/about&title=title/about_us&bild=about_us_balken.jpg
3. http://www.nsga.com/DesktopDefault.aspx?tabname=&sidebarname=History%20of%20NSGA&Params=454b04071756557a401a0c0b7b625a000000037f
4. Mazzeo RS, Cavanagh P, Evans WJ, et al. ACSM position stand: exercise and physical activity for older adults. *Med Sci Sports Exerc.* 1998;30(6):992–1008.
5. Galloway MT, Jokl P. Aging successfully: the importance of physical activity in maintaining health and function. *J Am Acad Orthop Surg.* 2000;8:37–44.
6. Powell A. Issues unique to the masters athletes. *Curr Sports Med Rep.* 2005;4:335–340.
7. Conley KE, Jubrias SA, Amara CE, et al. Mitochondrial dysfunction: impact on exercise performance and cellular aging. *Exerc Sport Sci Rev.* 2007;35(2):43–49.
8. Evans WJ. Exercise training guidelines for the elderly [Clinical sciences: Symposium: resistance training for health and disease]. *Med Sci Sports Exerc.* 1999;31(1):12–17.
9. Pescatello LS, Franklin BA, Fagard R, et al. ACSM position stand: exercise and hypertension. *Med Sci Sports Exerc.* 2004;36:533–553.
10. Chen AL, Mears SC, Hawkins RJ. Orthopaedic care of the aging athlete. *J Am Acad Orthop Surg.* 2005;13(6):407–416.
11. http://www.acsm-msse.org/pt/pt-core/template-journal/msse/media/0698c.htm. Accessed October 2008.
12. Whaley MH, Brubaker PH, Otto RM, et al. *ACSM's Guidelines for Exercise Testing and Prescription.* 7th ed. Philadelphia: Lippincott Williams & Wilkins; 2006.
13. Maron BJ, Araujo CGS, Thompson PD, et al. Recommendations for preparticipation screening and the assessment of cardiovascular disease in masters athletes: an advisory for healthcare professionals from the working groups of the World Heart Federation, the International Federation of Sports Medicine, and the American Heart Association Committee on Exercise, Cardiac Rehabilitation, and Prevention. *Circulation.* 2001;103:327–334.
14. Maron BJ, Thompson PD, Ackerman MJ, et al. Recommendations and considerations related to preparticipation screening for cardiovascular abnormalities in competitive athletes: 2007 update: a scientific statement from the American Heart Association Council on Nutrition, Physical Activity, and Metabolism. *Circulation.* 2007;115:1643–1655.
15. Hunter BR, McCarthy JP, Bamman MM. Effects of resistance training on older adults. *Sports Med.* 2004;34(5):329–348.
16. Gillespie LD, Gillespie WJ, Robertson MC, et al. Interventions for preventing falls in elderly people (review). *The Cochrane Collaboration.* Issue 3. Chichester: Wiley & Sons, Ltd; 2007.
17. Sacheck JM, Roubenoff R. Nutrition in the exercising elderly. *Clin Sports Med.* 1999;18(3):565–584.
18. Institute of Medicine, Food and Nutrition Board. *Dietary Reference Intakes for Calcium, Phosphorus, Magnesium, Vitamin D, and Fluoride.* Washington, DC: National Academies Press; 1997.
19. Griffin TM, Guilak F. The role of mechanical loading in the onset and progression of osteoarthritis. *Exerc Sport Sci Rev.* 2005;33(4):195–200.
20. Brouwer RW, Jakma TSC, Verhagen AP, et al. Braces and orthoses for treating osteoarthritis of the knee (review). *The Cochrane Collaboration.* Issue 3. Chichester: Wiley & Sons, Ltd; 2007.
21. Towheed TE, Maxwell L, Anastassiades TP, et al. Glucosamine therapy for treating osteoarthritis (review). *The Cochrane Collaboration.* Issue 3. Chichester: Wiley & Sons, Ltd; 2007
22. Clegg DO, Reda DJ, Harris CL, et al. Glucosamine, chondroitin sulfate, and the two in combination for painful knee osteoarthritis. *N Engl J Med.* 2006;354(8):795–808.
23. Recommendations for the medical management of osteoarthritis of the hip and knee: 2000 update. American College of Rheumatology Subcommittee on Osteoarthritis Guidelines. *Arthritis Rheum.* 2000;43(9):1905–1915.
24. Towheed TE, Maxwell L, Judd MG, et al. Acetaminophen for osteoarthritis (review). *The Cochrane Collaboration.* Issue 3. Chichester: Wiley & Sons, Ltd; 2007.
25. Bellamy N, Campbell J, Robinson V, et al. Intraarticular corticosteroid for treatment of osteoarthritis of the knee (review). *The Cochrane Collaboration.* Issue 3. Chichester: Wiley & Sons, Ltd; 2007.
26. Bellamy N, Campbell J, Robinson V, et al. Viscosupplementation for the treatment of osteoarthritis of the knee (review). *The Cochrane Collaboration.* Issue 3. Chichester: Wiley & Sons, Ltd; 2007.
27. Edelson R, Burks RT, Bloebaum RD. Short-term effects of knee washout for osteoarthritis. *Am J Sports Med.* 1995;23(3):345–349.
28. Moseley JB, Wray NP, Kuykendall D, et al. Arthroscopic treatment of osteoarthritis of the knee: a prospective, randomized, placebo-controlled trial results of a pilot study. *Am J Sports Med.* 1996;24(1): 28–34.
29. Moseley JB, O'Malley K, Petersen NJ, et al. A controlled trial of arthroscopic surgery for osteoarthritis of the knee. *N Engl J Med.* 2002;347(2):81–88.
30. Laupattarakasem W, Laopaiboon M, Laupattarakasem P, et al. Arthroscopic debridement for knee osteoarthritis. *Cochrane Database Syst Rev.* 2008;(1):CD005118. DOI: 10.1002/14651858.CD005118.pub2.
31. Nicholls MA, Selby JB, Hartford JM. Athletic activity after total joint replacement. *Orthopedics.* 2002;25(11):1283–1287.

26 Athletes Using Performance Enhancers

Lee A. Mancini

INTRODUCTION

In 1987 a poll of Olympic-level power athletes offered the following scenario: the athletes were offered a banned substance with two guarantees—you would not get caught and you would win the gold medal. Out of 198 athletes, 195 said yes and only 3 said no. Another question posed in that 1987 poll was, would you take a banned substance if it would let you win every competition you entered for the next 5 years, but would kill you in the sixth year? Over half of these athletes responded yes, that is, they would take the substance.[1] It is estimated that between one to three million athletes in the United States have used steroids. Nearly 60% of all high school students play on formal sports teams.[2] There is enormous pressure on athletes to gain any sort of competitive advantage. This chapter will review the most common types of performance enhancers used by athletes and help the medical provider approach this challenging issue in an organized fashion with their patients.

PATHOPHYSIOLOGY/PHARMACOLOGY

Erythropoietin

Erythropoietin is an alternative to blood doping. It is a hormone naturally produced in the kidney. The recombinant form is used to artificially increase hematocrit mass and to increase oxygen-carrying capacity of blood. It has been proven to increase hematocrit, Vo_2max, and time to exhaustion. Side effects of erythropoietin are an increased risk of cerebral vascular accident, myocardial infarction, and pulmonary embolism. Erythropoietin is banned by the International Olympic Committee (IOC), the International Cycling Union, and the International Ski Federation. The governing bodies have adopted an upper limit of hemoglobin as a rule for competition.[3]

Blood Doping

Blood doping is an autologous transfusion of blood into an athlete. Blood doping artificially increases the hematocrit mass and increases oxygen-carrying capacity of blood. It has been shown to increase hematocrit, Vo_2max, and time to exhaustion in athletes. Side effects of blood doping are an increased risk of cerebral vascular accident, myocardial infarction, pulmonary embolism, and blood pathogens such as HIV, hepatitis B, and hepatitis C. Blood doping is banned by the IOC, the International Cycling Union, and the International Ski Federation. Governing bodies have adopted an upper limit of hemoglobin as a rule for competition.[3]

Anabolic–Androgenic Steroids (AAS)

The goal of synthetic steroids is to maximize anabolic effects while minimizing androgenic effects. Synthetic steroids have alkylation of the 17-α position on sterol D ring and carboxylation of the 17-β hydroxyl group on the sterol D ring. Stacking is taking multiple steroids at the same time. Pyramiding is increasing the doses to peak toward the middle of a cycle.

Synthetic steroids have been proven to increase fat-free mass. Most studies have shown increases in lean body mass (LBM) of an average of 2 to 5 kg in a 10-week period.[4] Steroids have been proven to increase strength.[2] The effects of steroids are dose related, with higher doses leading to greater gains.

Steroids have been shown to have a wide array of side effects that range from nuisances to life threatening. The side effects of steroids affect every organ system in the body.

Cardiovascular Effects

Steroid use by athletes causes a significant decrease in high-density lipoprotein (HDL) cholesterol and an increase in low-density lipoprotein (LDL) and very low density lipoprotein (VLDL) cholesterol. Athletes taking steroids have a greater risk of myocardial ischemia and infarction, hypertension, and cerebral vascular accident.[5] Chronic steroid use can cause left ventricular hypertrophy and left ventricular wall thickness.[2,6] All cardiovascular effects reversed when examined 3 months after cessation of steroids.[1]

Psychologic Effects

Steroid use has been shown to increase the risk of aggressive behavior. There have been reports of steroids causing mood disturbances.[4]

Toxicologic Effects

There have been documented cases of steroid users contracting hepatitis B, hepatitis C, and HIV.[7] There have also been documented cases of fungal and bacterial abscesses from injection of steroids.[8] As with any injectable substances, athletes are at risk if they are sharing needles.

Musculoskeletal Effects

There is an increased risk of tendon ruptures in athletes using steroids. There is evidence of premature closure of growth plates in younger athletes using steroids.

Dermatologic Effects

Steroid use has been shown to cause alopecia, striae distensae (stretch marks), and acne.

Male Reproductive Effects

Male athlete steroid use decreases testes size, sperm count, and sperm quality and can cause gynecomastia.

Female Reproductive Effects

Female athlete steroid use causes voice deepening, sterilization, enlargement of clitoris, menstrual irregularities, hirsutism, male pattern baldness, and breast atrophy. Sterilization is irreversible in women after discontinuing steroids.

Hepatic Effects

Steroid use elevates liver enzymes, can create peliosis hepatis (blood-filled cysts in the liver) and cholestatic jaundice, and can cause hepatocellular carcinoma (Table 26.1).[4,8]

Legal Issues

Steroids are banned by the IOC, the National Collegiate Athletic Association (NCAA), the National Football League (NFL), the National Basketball Association (NBA), and Major League Baseball (MLB). A positive test has a testosterone-to-epitestosterone ratio greater than 6:1 for both men and women. The normal ratio in healthy male is 1.3:1, and only one male in 1,000 has a ratio of 4:1.

Possession of steroids carries both a 1-year prison sentence and minimum $1,000 fine. Selling or the intent to sell steroids carries a 5-year prison sentence and $250,000 fine.[2]

Prohormones

Prohormones are the androgenic testosterone precursors. Examples of prohormones are androstenedione and dehydroepiandrosterone (DHEA). The proposed mechanism is that prohormones would increase serum testosterone.

Performance Effects

There are no proven performance effects of androstenedione. DHEA has been shown to decrease body fat in some studies and no effect in others. DHEA has shown no increase in testosterone levels.[9]

TABLE 26.1 **Adverse Effects of Steroid Use**

CNS	Derm	Musculoskeletal	Liver	Men	Women	Cardiac	Immune
Increased aggression	Oily hair and skin	Premature closure of growth plates	Increased LFTs	Gynecomastia	Hirsutism	Increased total cholesterol, LDL, VLDL, and triglycerides	Increased risk of HIV
Mood swings	Alopecia	Increased risk of tendon ruptures	Peliosis hepatis (blood-filled liver cysts)	Increased risk of prostate cancer	Voice deepening	Increased risk of stroke	Increased risk of hepatitis B
Increased sexual aggression	Striae distensae (stretch marks)			Decreased testicle size	Clitoral hypertrophy	Decreased HDL	Increased risk of hepatitis C
Increased major mood disorders	Acne on the face and back			Decreased sperm count	Decrease in breast size and amenorrhea	Increased risk of myocardial infarction	
	Increased sebaceous cysts			Decreased fertility	Male pattern baldness	Hypertension	

LFTs, liver function tests; LDL, low-density lipoprotein; VLDL, very low density lipoprotein; HDL, high-density lipoprotein.

Side Effects

Androstenedione has been shown to increase estrone and estradiol levels in male athletes. It has been shown to decrease HDL cholesterol. There have been case reports of hair loss, hirsutism, and virilization in women.

DHEA

DHEA has been shown to increase estrone and estradiol levels in male athletes. It has been shown to decrease HDL. It has been shown to cause gynecomastia. There have been case reports of hair loss, hirsutism, and virilization in women.[2] There is an increased risk of breast, uterine, and prostate cancers.

Legal Issues

Prohormones like DHEA and androstenedione are banned by the IOC, the NFL, MLB, and the NCAA. Prohormones were banned by the government on February 1, 2005, but this banned list does not include DHEA.[2]

Human Growth Hormone (hGH)

hGH is an endogenous hormone secreted in anterior pituitary gland. Patients deficient in hGH are short in stature. Patients with an overabundance of hGH have gigantism. There is a high association with steroid use as well. hGH stimulates the release of somatomedins like the insulin-like growth factor. Also, hGH stimulates renal and hepatic gluconeogenesis and lipolysis. There is no evidence that supplementation with hGH leads to an increase in performance. There has been evidence that it decreases fat mass.[10] Side effects of hGH supplementation are water retention, increased insulin resistance, and an increased risk of carpal tunnel syndrome. Athletes who supplement with hGH also have an increased risk of contracting Creutzfeldt–Jakob disease if hGH is obtained in the black market.[10] In younger athletes who have not reached skeletal maturity, there is an increased risk of developing slipped capital femoral epiphysis, an increased risk of premature closure of growth plates, and an increased risk of developing hypertension. hGH is banned by the IOC, the NFL, the MLB, and the NCAA. Olympic athletes are not officially tested for hGH. Testing in professional sports in the United States lacks an accurate method.

Ephedra

Ephedra has been around for over 5,000 years, dating back to the ancient Chinese. It is also known as guarana or ma huang. Ephedra is a stimulant that mimics the effect of norepinephrine and epinephrine. It increases resting metabolism rate and calorie expenditure and causes appetite suppression. A proven effect of ephedra is that it promotes fat loss of 1.0 kg/month greater than placebo. With ephedra

use it is a dose-related effect, with doses in various studies ranging from 25 to 120 mg daily. Ephedra was been shown to cause a number of cardiovascular side effects such as hypertension, cardiac arrhythmias, and heart palpitations. Ephedra has also been shown to cause headaches, hyperthermia, and anxiety. All reported side effects stopped within 48 hours of the person discontinuing the drug. The FDA has reported 800 adverse incidents, and in greater than 90% of those cases, the recommended dose was exceeded. In 2003, it accounted for less than 1.0% of all supplement sales, yet accounted for 64% of all adverse supplement reactions. There have even been several case reports of fatal arrhythmias and myocardial infarctions. Ephedra has been banned by the IOC, the NFL, MLB, and the NCAA. In March 2004, the government banned the sale of ephedra, but the ban was overturned in April 2005 by a U.S. District Court judge.[2]

Caffeine

Caffeine is the number one used drug in the world with 82% to 92% of adults using caffeine daily. It is a methylated xanthine alkaloid derivative, and its structure is similar to adenosine. Caffeine binds to adenosine cell membrane receptors; stimulates the central nervous system (CNS); increases release of epinephrine, heart rate, metabolic rate, respiratory center output, and fat oxidation; and decreases fatigue and perceptions of pain. There is evidence that caffeine increases endurance performance by increasing time to exhaustion. It has also been shown to improve concentration. With caffeine there is a dose-related effect, with doses in studies ranging from 2 to 9 mg/kg daily. Side effects of caffeine include hypertension, cardiac arrhythmias, heart palpitations, facial flushing, and anxiety. Tolerance to caffeine appears after *only* 4 to 5 days of taking the supplement. It *only* takes 3 days of use to develop dependency on caffeine. The withdrawal symptoms from stopping caffeine may last 12 hours to 7 days. Caffeine withdrawal causes mood shifts, headaches, tremors, and fatigue. In 2005, caffeine was removed from banned list by the IOC. It is allowed in MLB, the NFL, the NHL, and the NBA. The NCAA also allows caffeine but only below a certain level tested for in the urine.

Creatine

Creatine was first described by the French chemist Chevreul, and its name is derived from the Greek word flesh. Creatine is made of three amino acids: arginine, glycine, and methionine. Creatine is involved in the chemical process where creatine phosphate + ADP $\Rightarrow$ ATP + creatine using the enzyme creatine kinase. In intense exercise, ATP is used in the first 0 to 10 seconds. Creatine phosphate is the next energy source that is used in the next 5 to 15 seconds.[11] Creatine also serves to buffer muscle pH, which delays muscle fatigue. A meta-analysis showed that creatine supplementation led to an increase in strength of 1.09% per week. Creatine also increases LBM by 0.36% per week. Creatine supplementation improved strength in 1RM bench press by an average of 15 lb over 6 weeks versus placebo. It improved strength in 1RM squat by an average of 25 lb over 6 weeks versus placebo.[12] Creatine has been proven to improve performance in *repeated* high-intensity sprints lasting 30 seconds to 3 minutes. However, creatine has *not* been shown to improve performance in long-distance endurance events and has even been shown to decrease performance.

Side effects of creatine supplementation include gastrointestinal distress, diarrhea, and flatulence. There have been case reports of muscle cramping, but no studies confirming this. Studies have shown no effect on kidney function.[13] However, recently there have been two reported cases of compromised renal function, but renal function returned to normal after discontinuing creatine.[11] Creatine is not banned by the IOC, the NFL, MLB, and the NCAA. The American College of Sports Medicine advocates against creatine use in any athlete under the age of 18.[11]

β-Hydroxy-β-methylbutyrate (HMB)

HMB is a metabolite of the branched chain amino acid leucine. The goal of HMB supplementation is to prevent exercise-induced muscle damage. The mechanism of action is unknown at present. Supplementation with HMB has been shown to have no effect on 1RM performance on bench press and leg press. There are some studies showing that supplement with HMB leads to significant increases in fat-free mass and decreases in body fat percentage. However, other studies showed no significant changes in body composition. There are no studies showing any negative side effects from HMB supplementation. Some positive side effects in studies showed lowered total cholesterol, lowered LDL cholesterol, and lowered blood pressure from HMB use. HMB is not banned by the IOC, the NFL, MLB, the NCAA, or any other sport-governing body.

EPIDEMIOLOGY

Steroids

A survey of more than 1,600 Canadian students in grade 6 and above showed that 2.8% used steroids. Of the students who had used steroids, 29% injected steroids and 29% of those injecting admitted to sharing needles. Also 54% of the steroid users felt that steroids were bad, but had used them anyway. Another survey of high school football players in Indiana found that 6% used steroids. The mean age for first use was 14, and 15% of steroid users started before the age of 10.[1] The overall rates of steroid use in high school athletes is 4% to 12% in male athletes and 1% to 2% in female athletes. From an NCAA survey in 2001, it was reported that 1.4% of all college athletes had used steroids within the past year.[2] High-risk behaviors are associated with steroid use, such as suicidal behavior, needle sharing, increased sexual activity, smoking, weapon possession, and multiple drug use. Most

athletes use steroid doses 5 to 20 times the doses that have been studied.[4]

hGH

A study of 432 10th graders in the Midwest showed 5% had taken hGH.[1] An NCAA study showed 3.5% of all college athletes had taken hGH in the past 12 months.[2]

Creatine

Creatine is the most widely used supplement. Different studies have reported creatine use between 25% and 78% in NCAA college athletes. Fourteen percent of high school students have used creatine. Seventy-five percent of users admitted to either not knowing how much creatine they were taking or were taking more than the recommended dose.[2] One study showed that 5.6% of middle school and high school athletes had used creatine.[11]

Caffeine

Caffeine is the most widely used drug in the world, with 82% to 92% of adults using it daily.

Ephedra

An NCAA survey in 2001 reported 3.9% of college athletes had taken ephedra in the past 12 months. A study in 2004 of NCAA Division I male ice hockey teams found that 38% used ephedra and 46% used pseudoephedrine.

NARROWING THE DIFFERENTIAL DIAGNOSIS

History

There are many important questions that need to be asked if an athlete presents to your office after taking a specific supplement. Ask the athlete what supplement has he or she been taking? It is important to have him or her bring in the exact bottle or container. If the athlete does not have bottle or container, then have him or her bring in the ingredient list or the website or store name from which the supplement was purchased. This enables the physician to see the specific active ingredients and determine which class of supplement it is. Specific questions to be asked about the particular supplement are, for how long have you been using the supplement? How often have you been using this supplement? Having you been using it daily, weekly, or monthly? What dose have you been using? What is the recommended use or recommended dose? It is important to compare the athlete's dose and regimen to the recommended label use. Have you noticed any effects from taking the supplement? Any performance changes? Any physique changes? Have you experienced any side effects? Have you noticed any changes in mood?

Evidence-based Physical Examination

Dermatologic Examination

For the dermatologic examination, the physician should examine the athlete for acne on the upper back. Examine for increased oiliness of the skin. Evaluate for striae distensae (stretch marks). Have male athletes remove their shirts to evaluate for gynecomastia. Evaluate for hirsutism and alopecia. Evaluate thighs, buttocks, and shoulders for injection sites or abscesses. In male athletes evaluate for atrophy of testes. Eighty percent of steroid users exhibit at least one of these physical signs.[7]

Cardiovascular Examination

Auscultate the athlete's heart for cardiac murmurs.

Abdominal Examination

Evaluate the athlete for hepatomegaly.

Diagnostic Testing

Laboratory

For the athlete taking a performance enhancer, a basic metabolic profile, a complete blood count, a fasting lipid panel, liver function studies, a testosterone level, an estrogen/estradiol level, and a thyroid function test should be obtained.

Imaging

An echocardiogram should be ordered if the athlete has been taking steroids or if there is a new cardiac murmur appreciated on the physical examination.

Other Testing

An EKG, blood pressure, and heart rate should be obtained on any athlete taking a performance enhancer.

APPROACH TO THE ATHLETE USING PERFORMANCE ENHANCERS

HISTORY AND PHYSICAL EXAMINATION

Important questions for the athlete taking performance enhancers include the following:

- What supplement or supplements have you been taking?
- How long have you been taking this supplement or supplements?

If the athlete is using steroids, the physician needs to ask:

- How did the athlete obtain the steroids?
- Was the athlete injecting the AAS?
- Was the athlete sharing needles?
- From where did the athlete get the needles?
- How is the athlete disposing of the needles?
- What doses of steroids has the athlete been taking?
- Is the athlete cycling or stacking other steroids, masking agents, or supplements with this?
- Are these doses more or less than prior cycles?
- Has the athlete noticed any changes in his or her body?
- Has the athlete lost or gained any weight?
- Is the athlete having any chest pain?
- Is the athlete having any difficulty breathing?
- Has the athlete noticed any loss of hair?
- Has the athlete noticed any new hair growth in other parts of the body?

The physical examination should include but not be limited to a thorough cardiovascular examination. It is important on the cardiovascular examination to listen for any cardiac murmurs, to document heart rate, and to measure blood pressure. Tachycardia or arrhythmia may indicate stimulant use. The dermatologic examination should examine for signs of steroid use including acne on the upper back, increased oiliness of the skin, striae distensae (stretch marks), gynecomastia (male athletes), hirsutism, and alopecia. Evaluate thighs, buttocks, and shoulders for injection sites or abscesses. Abdominal examination should evaluate for presence of hepatomegaly. In male athletes evaluate for atrophy of testes. Eighty percent of steroid users exhibit at least one of these physical signs.[7]

DIAGNOSTIC TESTING

If the athlete has admitted to having taken steroids, his or her blood pressure and heart rate should be taken. A fasting lipid panel including LDL, total cholesterol, HDL, VLDL, and triglycerides should be ordered. Testosterone, estrogen (estrone or estradiol), a basic metabolic panel, and liver function studies should also be ordered. An EKG and an echocardiogram should be obtained. If the athlete has been injecting steroids or sharing needles, then a hepatitis panel should be ordered, and the athlete should be consented for an HIV test.

If the athlete has admitted to taking caffeine, ephedra, or another stimulant, then he or she should have a basic metabolic panel and a thyroid function test. Heart rate and blood pressure should be measured.

If the athlete has admitted to blood doping, then a complete blood count should be ordered. If the athlete has been injecting or sharing needles, then a hepatitis panel should be ordered, and the athlete should be consented for an HIV test.

TREATMENT

General Measures

For the athlete who presents to your office and is interested in starting to take a specific supplement, he or she should be asked questions that every athlete needs to have addressed about the supplement.

- Is this supplement legal?
  - Athlete needs to check with his or her sports-governing organization's banned substance list.
  - NCAA—http://www1.ncaa.org/membership/ ed_outreach/health-safety/drug_testing/ banned_drug_classes.pdf.
  - World Anti-Doping Agency—http://www.theathlete.org/ wada.htm.
  - Athlete must be informed of the position statement that any athlete who takes a supplement does so at his or her own risk of committing a doping violation.
  - Athlete must be informed that cross-contamination in production facilities does occur between different classes of supplements and may result in a positive test.[14]
- Is this supplement safe?
  - Athlete must be informed of any proven negative side effects.
  - Athlete must be informed of any health-related issues that taking the supplement might cause.
- Is this supplement effective?
  - Athlete must be informed of any proven benefits of taking the supplement.
  - Athlete must make sure that the proven benefits are applicable to his or her sport as well.
- Advise that the athlete must first adhere to the training and nutrition pyramid protocol before starting any supplement that has met the above criteria of being legal, safe, and effective.
  - Athlete must be following a proper, healthy nutrition program.
  - Athlete must be following a proper training program.
  - Athlete must bring in the actual product or product ingredient list for the physician to review prior to the athlete starting supplementation.
- Education of athletes as individuals or as a member of a team, known as thoughtful discouragement.[11]
  - Education interventions have been shown to be effective.
    - Athletes more knowledgeable about the dangers of steroids
    - Athletes less likely to believe unsubstantiated supplement claims
    - Athletes more knowledgeable about supplements in general[2]

Pharmacologic Treatment

None indicated.

Prognosis/Return to Play

- Good for supplements such as HMB, creatine, caffeine, and other over-the-counter substances.
- Good for athletes having taken AAS and having had cardiac, dermatologic, or hepatic function changes—these are all reversible once the athlete discontinues the supplements.
- Poor for skeletally immature athletes having taken AAS and now have had premature closure of the growth plates—this is irreversible.
- Poor for female athletes having taken AAS and now are suffering from sterilization—this is irreversible.
- If athlete has tested positive for a banned substance, he or she must serve the required suspension.
- If athlete has taken an illegal substance, then the athlete is subject to the fines and penalties of the legal system.
- If an athlete has taken an approved substance without any significant medical side effects, then the athlete can return to play without any restrictions.
- If an athlete has taken a performance-enhancing substance and has had negative health side effects, then the athlete should be held out until he or she can be medically cleared for those side effects.

Complications/Indications for Referral

- Athletes who discontinue taking AAS should be closely monitored for increasing signs of depression, suicidal ideation, and erratic behavior.
- Athletes who have taken AAS and have cardiac changes on EKG or echocardiogram should be referred to a cardiologist.
- Athletes who have shared needles and tested positive for hepatitis C or HIV should be referred to an infectious disease specialist.

KEY POINTS
• Performance enhancers are commonly used by athletes to obtain a competitive edge
• Have athletes answer the questions, is it legal, is it safe, and is it effective, about any supplement they are interested in taking
• AAS have proven serious health risks
• Educating athletes about all performance-enhancing drugs has been shown to be effective in decreasing the number of new steroid or illegal supplement users

REFERENCES

1. Tokish JM, Kocher MS, Hawkins RJ. Ergogenic aids: a review of basic science, performance, side effects, and status in sports. *Am J Sports Med.* 2004;32:1543–1553.
2. Calfee R, Fadale P. Popular ergogenic drugs and supplements in young athletes. *Pediatrics.* 2006;117:e577–e589.
3. Robinson N, Giraud S, Saudan C, et al. Erythropoietin and blood doping. *Br J Sports Med.* 2006;40:30–34.
4. Hartgens F, Kuipers H. Effects of androgenic–anabolic steroids in athletes. *Sports Med.* 2004;34(8):513–554.
5. Payne JR, Kotwinski PJ, Montgomery HE. Cardiac effects of anabolic steroids. *Heart.* 2004;90:473–475.
6. Urhausen A, Albers T, Kindermann W. Are the cardiac effects of anabolic steroid abuse in strength athletes reversible? *Heart.* 2004;90: 496–501.
7. Evans NA. Current concepts in anabolic–androgenic steroids. *Am J Sports Med.* 2004;32:534–542.
8. Maravelias C, Dona A, Stefanidou M, et al. Adverse effects of anabolic steroids in athletes. *Toxicol Lett.* 2005;158(3):167–175.
9. Ciocca M. Medication and supplement use by athletes. *Clin Sports Med.* 2005;24(3):719–738.
10. Saugy M, Robinson N, Saudan C, et al. Human growth hormone doping in sport. *Br J Sports Med.* 2006;40(S1):i35–i39.
11. Laos C, Metzl JD. Performance-enhancing drug use in young athletes. *Adolesc Med Clin.* 2006;17:719–731.
12. Nissen SL, Seifert JG, Burke E. Effect of dietary supplements on lean mass and strength gains with resistance exercise: a meta-analysis. *J Appl Physiol.* 1999;94(2):651–659.
13. Crowe MJ, O'Connor DM, Lukins JE. The effects of β-hydroxy-β-methylbutryrate (HMB) and HMB/creatine supplementation on indices of health in highly trained athletes. *Int J Sport Nutr Exerc Metab.* 2003;13(2):184–198.
14. Delbeke FT, Van Eenoo P, Van Thuyne W, et al. Prohormones and sport. *J Steroid Biochem Mol Biol.* 2002;83(1–5):245–251.

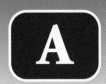

APPENDIX

A

Injection Techniques

Kelton Burbank

INTRODUCTION

Injection therapies are common office-based procedures utilized for the short-term reduction of pain and inflammation. They can be employed for diagnostic and therapeutic benefits. Injections that induce even a transient reduction or relief of a patient's symptoms can help identify the pathologic structures or site involved. Additionally, an aspiration of fluid can assess for cell counts, cultures, and fluid analysis.

Common therapeutic indications for injection include treatment of osteoarthritis, bursitis, synovitis, tendonitis, and tenosynovitis. Their use continues despite the lack of consistent level 1 evidence of their efficacy. Complicating assessing the efficacy of injection therapy is the challenge of accurate needle placement and the potential benefit of image guidance (fluoroscopic or ultrasound). A sound understanding of anatomy and appropriate landmarks is essential for appropriate efficacy and reduction of risk or discomfort to the patient.

MATERIALS

Appropriate preparation and materials is essential to the success of injection therapy. For joint or soft-tissue injections, a combination of corticosteroid and anesthetic is the author's preferred method, as the combined volume will distribute more evenly and in a less concentrated fashion. Some will inject anesthetic first, then corticosteroid. The preferred medications of the author are listed in the following text. There is no evidence of one corticosteroid being superior, but it is felt that medium- to long-acting preparations enhance efficacy and decrease systemic absorption. The injectable corticosteroid preparations are manufactured such that a milliliter of one product is efficaciously equivalent to another. Lidocaine or bupivacaine are the preferred anesthetics that can be utilized alone or in combination based on provider's preference. Bupivacaine allows for longer anesthesia (6 to 8 hours) versus lidocaine (2 to 4 hours) but has a slower onset and time to full anesthesia. The author prefers to use lidocaine if rapid anesthesia is required

in the case of an aspiration, while for most soft-tissue or joint injections bupivacaine provides excellent anesthesia.

- Corticosteroids
  - Triamcinolone, dexamethasone, and methylprednisolone (medium- to long-acting corticosteroids)
- Local anesthetics
  - Lidocaine and/or bupivacaine
- Betadine or antiseptic
- Alcohol wipe
- 22- or 25-gauge × 1.5-in needle for injection
- 18-gauge needle for aspiration of medication
- 5- or 10-cc syringe

METHODS

Sterile technique should be utilized to minimize the risk of infection. We typically use betadine to paint the field, and then we use a sterile glove in one hand to palpate the landmarks underneath the betadine preparation. The hand holding the needle/syringe does not need to be sterile. This allows for maximum efficiency in finding the site and preventing infection at the site. Injection site can be marked prior to application of betadine with a pen cap or syringe cap. This will be visible even after betadine application.

Typically, a 25-gauge needle is used, as this seems to cause less discomfort. However, a larger needle can be used, if the patient is particularly muscular, to avoid deflection of the tip. A 22-gauge needle is usually sufficient in these cases. Needle length is also important to ensure the material is deposited in the area of interest, such as the joint, rather than in the subcutaneous tissues surrounding it. For aspirations an 18-gauge needle is preferred but generally requires administering a small subcutaneous anesthesia with lidocaine.

We use a separate needle to draw up the solution, typically an 18-gauge needle, as this hastens the process. The top of the bottle of the steroid and the local anesthetic should be wiped with an alcohol pad prior to insertion of the needle when drawing the medicine into the syringe. This also ensures sterility of the solution.

RISKS AND COMPLICATIONS

Potential local complications include infection, tendon rupture, skin depigmentation, tissue atrophy, and nerve injury. Because of the potential for tendon rupture, intratendinous injections of weight-bearing tendons (Achilles and patella tendons) with corticosteroids are a contraindication and should be avoided. Potential systemic complications include facial flushing, allergic reaction, and hyperglycemia. Most patients will experience a postinjection pain flare ranging from 24 to 72 hours; for a small percentage this can be significant. Thus, the relative risk/benefit of each injection should be assessed prior to undertaking any procedure.

AFTER CARE/RETURN TO PLAY

Injection site should be kept clean and relatively dry. Ice and over-the-counter (OTC) analgesic can be utilized for expected short-term postinjection pain flare. Most recommend avoidance of heavy or impact-loading activities to the affected site for 5 to 7 days to prevent rapid disbursement away from the injection site. Injections in or around non–weight-bearing tendons subjected to excessive strain may benefit from 1 to 2 weeks' relative rest to avoid potential tendon rupture risk.

SHOULDER INJECTIONS

The three most common types of injections in the shoulder are subacromial injection, acromioclavicular (AC) joint injection, and glenohumeral joint injection.

Subacromial Injection

Approaching the patient from behind can lead to less anxiety on the part of the patient. Identify the posterior lateral edge of the acromion. Palpate the anterior aspect of the acromion to help judge the angle of the acromion. The bursa sits in the anterior half of the subacromial space, so the needle will need to be placed under the acromion and advanced anteriorly. Take care to avoid injecting either above the acromion (too superiorly) or into the rotator cuff muscles (too inferiorly). The fluid should flow easily. Do not force the injection, as this is more likely to lead to poor placement of the solution. A 1.5-in 25- or 22-gauge needle can be used. Typically, 2 cc of corticosteroid along with 6 to 8 cc of local anesthetic is injected (Fig. A.1).

Acromioclavicular Joint Injection

This injection can be difficult as the space is quite narrow and slanted. Plain films can be helpful as the AC joint is often angled in the sagital plane. Palpate the clavicle as it traverses

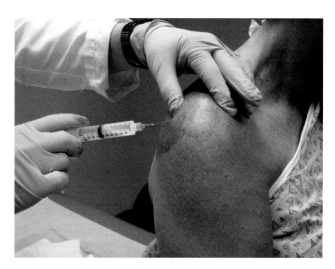

FIG. A.1. Subacromial injection.

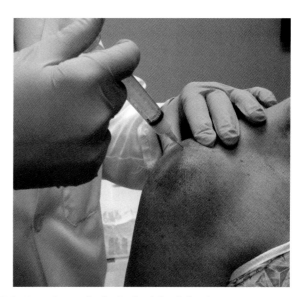

FIG. A.2. Acromioclavicular joint injection.

to meet the acromion. Palpate the acromion. Often, one can feel the ridge at the AC joint. A 25-gauge needle is used to enter the joint from a superior approach with a slight 20-degree lateral angulation from the sagital plane. It is important to make sure the needle enters the joint for maximal effect. Typically, a total of 2 cc is injected with equal parts of corticosteroid and anesthetic (Fig. A.2).

Glenohumeral Joint Injection

Several studies have questioned the ability to reach the glenohumeral joint without x-ray guidance. For this reason, it is the author's opinion that these injections should be performed with x-ray or ultrasound guidance.

KNEE INJECTION

There are two approaches to the knee. One is from a superior lateral approach, where the needle is guided under the patella with the patient supine. Another approach is into the anterior lateral aspect of the knee with the patient seated and the knee bent to 90 degrees. The superior lateral approach is generally more accurate and well tolerated by the patient. It is also the approach for aspiration of the knee joint.

Superior Lateral Approach

With the patient supine and the knee relaxed in near-full extension (the patella should move freely), the edges of the patella are palpated. The superior and lateral edge is most important. The needle is placed underneath the superior–lateral edge of the patella. Care should be taken to start posteriorly enough so that the needle does not graze the patella, but anteriorly enough that it does not hit the trochlea. Both of these mistakes may cause injury to the articular cartilage. Once the needle has penetrated the lateral retinaculum, the needle tip is intra-articular and medication can be injected. A 1.5-in 25- or 22-gauge needle can be used. Typically, 2 cc of corticosteroid along with 6 to 8 cc of local anesthetic is injected (Fig. A.3).

ELBOW INJECTIONS

The tendinous insertions on the medial and lateral epicondyles are a frequent source of pain and a frequent site of injection. The joint itself is not routinely injected in the office.

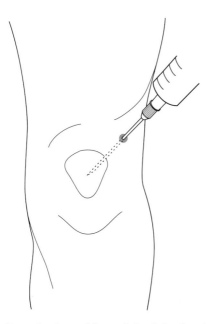

FIG. A.3. Superior lateral knee joint injection/aspiration approach.

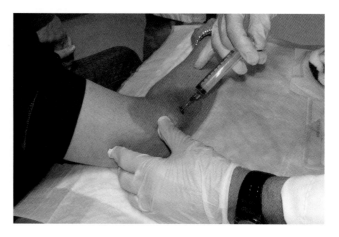

FIG. A.4. Lateral epicondyle injection.

Lateral Epicondyle

The lateral epicondyle is easily palpated. Typically, the patient's pain is located just distal to the epicondyle itself. Injection should be superficial and into the area of maximal tenderness. Care must be taken to avoid the radial–capitellar joint, which sits deep in this area. A very superficial injection risks depigmentation of the skin and some fat atrophy. Typically, a total of 2 cc is injected with equal parts of corticosteroid and anesthetic, utilizing a 22- or 25-gauge 1- or 1.5-in needle (Fig. A.4).

Medial Epicondyle

The medial epicondyle is also very superficial. Directly underneath this structure lies the ulnar nerve, which must be avoided. Typically, the pain is located distal and anterior to the epicondyle. This is the direction in which the needle should be angled, toward the large flexor–pronator mass and not toward the nerve. Typically, a total of 2 cc is injected with equal parts of corticosteroid and anesthetic, utilizing a 22- or 25-gauge 1- or 1.5-in needle.

HIP INJECTIONS

The hip joint itself is deep and not easily accessible. It should only be injected under x-ray or ultrasound guidance due to the neurovascular bundle that must be avoided.

Greater Trochanteric Bursa Injection

The trochanteric bursa, however, is a frequent source of discomfort and is easy to palpate and inject safely. The borders of the greater trochanter on the lateral aspect of the proximal femur are palpated. The area of maximal tenderness is then defined. The area is typically near the anterior/superior edge of the greater trochanter. With the patient lying on his or her side with the painful hip facing upward, the needle is

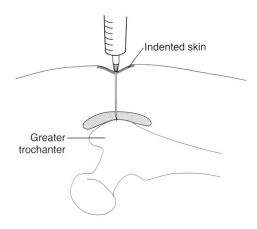

FIG. A.5. Greater trochanteric bursa injection.

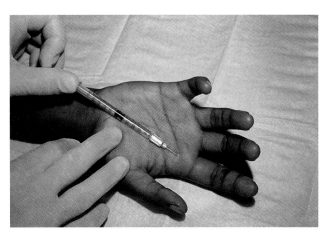

FIG. A.6. Trigger finger injection. Needle should be angled at 45 degrees to allow injection into tendon sheath. Reprinted with permission from Strickland JW, Graham TJ. *Master Techniques in Orthopaedic Surgery: The Hand.* 2nd ed. Philadelphia: Lippincott Williams & Wilkins; 2005.

injected at a 90-degree angle in the coronal plane. Advance the needle till the greater trochanter is felt and then withdraw 1 to 2 mm prior to injection. A 1.5-in 25- or 22-gauge needle can be used. Typically, 2 cc of corticosteroid along with 6 to 8 cc of local anesthetic is injected (Fig. A.5).

HAND/WRIST INJECTIONS

Two common areas around the hand and wrist are the A1 pulley in trigger fingers and the first dorsal compartment in de Quervain syndrome.

Trigger Finger Injection

Trigger fingers occur on the volar surface of the palm at the proximal end of the A1 pulley. This is also the metacarpal–phalangeal (MCP) joint. It is easy to see on the dorsal surface, but on the volar surface it lies much more proximally than one would intuit. It is at the level of the distal palmar crease. To alleviate the symptoms of a trigger finger, the injection is best placed at the entry to the A1 pulley. The MCP joint is palpated on the volar surface of the hand. Asking the patient to gently flex and extend the fingers can help localize the area. The injection needs to be placed in the midline of the tunnel entrance to avoid injury to the digital nerves. It also needs to be placed between the tendon and the tendon sheath. After the midline, proximal edge of the tunnel is palpated, and the needle is directed from proximal to distal at about a 45-degree angle. One can usually feel the needle pierce the tissue anterior to the joint. Often, the tendon is hit lightly. If this occurs, withdraw the needle slightly. Ask the patient to flex and extend the digit. If the needle is too deep and in the tendon, it will move as the patient moves the digit. Otherwise, it will remain still. The injection should flow easily. Typically, 1 to 2 cc is injected with a 50:50 mixture ratio of corticosteroid to local anesthetic with a 25-gauge needle (Fig. A.6).

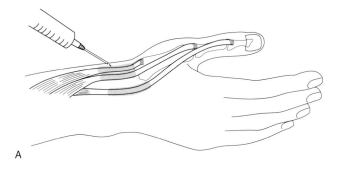

A

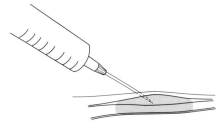

B

FIG. A.7. de Quervain tenosynovitis injection. Angle needle at 45 degrees and withdraw slightly once tendon is felt; injection should flow smoothly.

de Quervain Tenosynovitis Injection

This area can usually be reached with a needle angled at about 45 degrees from proximal to distal. The goal of the injection is to deposit the medicine in the tendon sheath, but not in the tendon or in the superficial radial nerve which lies nearby. Typically, 1 to 2 cc is injected with a 50:50 mixture ratio of corticosteroid steroid to local anesthetic with a 25-gauge needle (Fig. A.7).

B

Interval Throwing Program

Benjamin M.J. Thompson

INTRODUCTION

Interval throwing programs (ITPs) are utilized by athletes in a variety of sports to help train, condition, and rehabilitate the throwing athlete's arm after injury.[1] The program should always be initiated under the careful watch of a team physician and the training staff in case of injury. Wilk and Arrigo have suggested a four-stage rehabilitation program for the injured throwing shoulder, of which the ITP falls into the fourth phase.[2] In phase 1, management is focused on the reduction of pain and inflammation. As the rehabbing throwing athlete progresses into phase 2, a strengthening program is gradually introduced. Advanced strengthening occurs in phase 3, prior to beginning competitive throwing in phase 4. There are a variety of different interval programs that have been created, and often these are specifically tailored for a particular sport.[1,3–6] Regardless of the differences in each individual program, there is generally a separation into short and long toss components: the objective of the short toss component being simulation of game time situations, while the long toss component serves to work on endurance and strengthening via low-intensity and long-duration exercises.[1]

DESCRIPTION OF PROGRAM

It must be made clear from the beginning that there is no set timetable for completion of the program, as this puts unnecessary stress on the participant to move on to the next step when pain may be present. Each level of the program is therefore designed to be accomplished *two to three times without pain three times per week* with a day off in between each session prior to progression to the start of the next step. On the off day the athlete may work on flexibility exercises.[2] If the athlete develops pain, especially in the joint, then he or she must stop the program immediately and return to the previous step once pain free. After the completion of the indicated daily program, a high-repetition, low-weight exercise program should be utilized to increase resistance to fatigue and injury. It is imperative that the throwing athlete should not attempt to move quickly to the next step by over- or underthrowing. By following the prescribed number of throws rather than the indicated times, better and more predictable results may be obtained with the ITP.[4]

CRITERIA FOR PROGRESSION

Light jogging prior to stretching is essential prior to beginning the ITP to increase flexibility.[2] Stretching should begin with a focus on the legs, then moving to incorporate the trunk and upper extremities. Warm-up throws are begun at whatever distance is comfortable and pain free. For example, if the athlete is throwing pain free at 60 ft, progression is made to 90 ft in keeping with the specifics of the individual throwing program. There is no set correct starting distance. Once the athlete is able to throw from each distance without pain, normal pitching or fielding mechanics may begin off from flat ground at 60 ft 6 in.[2] Throwing from flat ground is beneficial because it will produce a shorter stride as well as less shoulder external rotation at foot contact compared to normal full-effort pitching.[1,4] Other benefits of flat-ground throwing include more elbow varus torque during arm cocking and a more upright trunk at ball release.[1,4] Overall the combined benefits of flat-ground throwing help to reduce reinjury by producing less shoulder and elbow compressive forces during deceleration.[1,2,4]

PHASE 1

The first phase of the ITP as outlined by Wilk and Arrigo[7] is listed in the following text. Throughout the entirety of the ITP, it is crucial that there be a strong focus on proper throwing mechanics so as not to put unnecessary stresses on the recovering arm. The *crow-hop method* is well known as the best way to simulate the act of throwing. In this method throwing is preceded by a hop and a skip. This method helps to avoid the type of reinjury that can occur by throwing flat-footed. Flat-footed throwing places increases stresses on the thrower's arm and encourages improper body mechanics.[2] Once phase 1 is completed, position players are able to return to play while pitchers progress to phase 2: Throwing off the Mound (Table B.1).

TABLE B.1 **Interval Throwing Program Phase 1**[8,9]

45′ Phase	60′ Phase	90′ Phase
Step 1: A. Warm-up throwing B. 45′ (25 throws) C. Rest 5–10 min D. Warm-up throwing E. 45′ (25 throws)	**Step 3:** A. Warm-up throwing B. 60′ (25 throws) C. Rest 5–10 min D. Warm-up throwing E. 60′ (25 throws)	**Step 5:** A. Warm-up throwing B. 90′ (25 throws) C. Rest 5–10 min D. Warm-up throwing E. 90′ (25 throws)
Step 2: A. Warm-up throwing B. 45′ (25 throws) C. Rest 5–10 min D. Warm-up throwing E. 45′ (25 throws) F. Rest 5–10 min G. Warm-up throwing H. 45′ (25 throws)	**Step 4:** A. Warm-up throwing B. 60′ (25 throws) C. Rest 5–10 min D. Warm-up throwing E. 60′ (25 throws) F. Rest 5–10 min G. Warm-up throwing H. 60′ (25 throws)	**Step 6:** A. Warm-up throwing B. 90′ (25 throws) C. Rest 5–10 min D. Warm-up throwing E. 90′ (25 throws) F. Rest 5–10 min G. Warm-up throwing H. 90′ (25 throws)

120′ Phase	150′ Phase	180′ Phase
Step 7: A. Warm-up throwing B. 120′ (25 throws) C. Rest 5–10 min D. Warm-up throwing E. 120′ (25 throws)	**Step 9:** A. Warm-up throwing B. 150′ (25 throws) C. Rest 5–10 min D. Warm-up throwing E. 150′ (25 throws)	**Step 11:** A. Warm-up throwing B. 180′ (25 throws) C. Rest 5–10 min D. Warm-up throwing E. 180′ (25 throws)
Step 8: A. Warm-up throwing B. 120′ (25 throws) C. Rest 5–10 min D. Warm-up throwing E. 120′ (25 throws) F. Rest 5–10 min G. Warm-up throwing H. 120′ (25 throws)	**Step 10:** A. Warm-up throwing B. 150′ (25 throws) C. Rest 5–10 min D. Warm-up throwing E. 150′ (25 throws) F. Rest 5–10 min G. Warm-up throwing H. 150′ (25 throws)	**Step 12:** A. Warm-up throwing B. 180′ (25 throws) C. Rest 5–10 min D. Warm-up throwing E. 180′ (25 throws) F. Rest 5–10 min G. Warm-up throwing H. 180′ (25 throws)

Step 13:
A. Warm-up throwing
B. 180′ (25 throws)
C. Rest 5–10 min
D. Warm-up throwing
E. 180′ (25 throws)
F. Rest 5–10 min
G. Warm-up throwing
H. 180′ (20 throws)
I. Rest 5–10 min
J. Warm-up throwing
K. 15 throws progressing from 120 to > 90′

Step 14: Return to respective position or progress to step 14 below

Flat-ground Throwing for Baseball Pitchers
Step 14:
A. Warm-up throwing
B. Throw 60′ (10–15 throws)
C. Throw 90′ (10 throws)
D. Throw 120′ (10 throws)
E. Throw 60′ (flat ground) using pitching mechanics (20–30 throws)

All throws should be on an arc with a crow hop

Warm-up throws consist of 10–20 throws at ~30′

TABLE B.1 *(Cont.)*

120′ Phase	150′ Phase	180′ Phase
Step 15: A. Warm-up throwing B. Throw 60′ (10–15 throws) C. Throw 90′ (10 throws) D. Throw 120′ (10 throws) E. Throw 60′ (flat ground) using pitching mechanics (20–30 throws) F. Throw 60–90′ (10–15 throws) G. Throw 60′ (flat ground) using pitching mechanics (20 throws) **Progress to phase 2—Throwing Off the Mound**		**Throwing program should be performed every other day, 3 times/wk unless otherwise specified by your physician or rehabilitation specialist** **Perform each step 2–3 times before progressing to next step**

45 ft = 13.7 m
60 ft = 18.3 m
90 ft = 27.4 m
120 ft = 36.6 m
150 ft = 45.7 m
180 ft = 54.8 m

TABLE B.2   **Interval Throwing Program: Phase 2–Throwing Off the Mound[9,10]**

Stage 1: Fastballs Only[a]	Stage 2: Fastballs Only	Stage 3
Step 1: A. Interval throwing[b] B. 15 throws off mound 50%[c]	Step 9: A. 60 throws off mound 75% B. 15 throws in batting practice	Step 12: A. 30 throws off mound 75% warm-up B. 15 throws off mound, 50% breaking balls C. 45–60 throws in batting practice (fastball only)
Step 2: A. Interval throwing B. 30 throws off mound 50%	Step 10: A. 50–60 throws off mound 75% B. 30 throws in batting practice	
Step 3: A. Interval throwing B. 45 throws off mound 50%	Step 11: A. 45–50 throws off mound 75% B. 45 throws in batting practice	Step 13: A. 30 throws off mound 75% B. 30 breaking balls 75% C. 30 throws in batting practice
Step 4: A. Interval throwing B. 60 throws off mound 50%		
Step 5: A. Interval throwing B. 70 throws off mound 50%		Step 14: A. 30 throws off mound 75% B. 60–90 throws in batting practice (25% breaking balls)
Step 6: A. 45 throws off mound 50% B. 30 throws off mound 75%		Step 15: A. Simulated game: progressing by 15 throws per workout B. Begin with 18–20 pitches per inning for 7 innings with 8-min rest between innings. Pitchers should return to their preinjury repertoire[3]
Step 7: A. 30 throws off mound 50% B. 45 throws off mound 75%		
Step 8: A. 10 throws off mound 50% B. 60 throws off mound 75%		

[a]All steps/phases done in the presence of a pitching coach or sport biomechanist to stress proper throwing mechanics.
[b]Use interval throwing 120 ft (36.6 m) phase as warm-up.
[c]Percentage effort.

PHASE 2: THROWING OFF THE MOUND

Once the throwing athlete has progressed to phase 2, he or she is ready to throw off of the mound. As with phase 1, there is a gentle, pain-free achievement model that must be followed to avoid reinjury. In general, pitchers will begin at 50% capacity, advancing as tolerated to full throwing capacity. Half-effort pitching produces 85% ball and joint speed and 77% kinetics correlating with a more upright throwing posture and reduction of arm rotation serving to minimize stresses on the shoulder and elbow.[4]

The emphasis of phase 2 is to avoid reinjury to athlete's shoulder and elbow as he or she progresses through his or her repertoire of pitches using normal pitching mechanics. Initially only fastballs are used, as they provide the lowest amount of stress on the thrower's arm. Once the pitcher is able to throw at his or her normal full fastball capacity, the more strenuous breaking pitches are phased in to gradually increase the tolerance of the shoulder joint to the stresses of throwing.[2] While the majority of the literature stresses the use of the ITP for the pitcher, position players may use a modified schedule, which simulates gamelike situations once phase 2 is achieved, once again limiting initial efforts to half to prevent reinjury (Table B.2).

LITTLE LEAGUE INTERVAL THROWING PROGRAM

In recent years there has been an emphasis on the development of ITPs for younger athletes. As there has been an explosion in the single-sport athlete at a younger and younger age, there has been a new rash of injuries that the sports medicine doctor as well as the athletic trainer must contend with. The majority of these injuries have been shown to involve the upper extremity.[6,7,11–13] Table B.3 outlines a modified version of the ITP for the Little League–level players. Given the large age range of Little League players, the distances and number of throws should be decreased for the younger player, and supervision by an experienced physical therapist or pitching coach is recommended. Some general guidelines for a Little League ITP developed by Axe et al. are as follows[1]:

1. If sore when throwing, take the day off and drop down one level the following day.
2. If sore after throwing and it does not improve after warm-up, take that day off and drop down one level the following day.
3. If not sore while throwing, but sore the following day and the soreness disappears after warm-up, continue with the program at that level.
4. Do not advance more than two levels per week.
5. Shoulder strengthening exercises follow throwing program.

TABLE B.3 Little League Interval Throwing Program[9,14]

30′ Phase	45′ Phase
Step 1:	Step 3:
A. Warm-up throwing	A. Warm-up throwing
B. 30′ (25 throws)	B. 45′ (25 throws)
C. Rest 15 min	C. Rest 15 min
D. Warm-up throwing	D. Warm-up throwing
E. 30′ (25 throws)	E. 45′ (25 throws)
Step 2:	Step 4:
A. Warm-up throwing	A. Warm-up throwing
B. 30′ (25 throws)	B. 45′ (25 throws)
C. Rest 10 min	C. Rest 10 min
D. Warm-up throwing	D. Warm-up throwing
E. 30′ (25 throws)	E. 45′ (25 throws)
F. Rest 10 min	F. Rest 10 min
G. Warm-up throwing	G. Warm-up throwing
H. 30′ (25 throws)	H. 45′ (25 throws)

60′ Phase	90′ Phase
Step 5:	Step 7:
A. Warm-up throwing	A. Warm-up throwing
B. 60′ (25 throws)	B. 90′ (25 throws)
C. Rest 15 min	C. Rest 15 min
D. Warm-up throwing	D. Warm-up throwing
E. 60′ (25 throws)	E. 90′ (25 throws)
Step 6:	Step 8:
A. Warm-up throwing	A. Warm-up throwing
B. 60′ (25 throws)	B. 90′ (20 throws)
C. Rest 10 min	C. Rest 10 min
D. Warm-up throwing	D. Warm-up throwing
E. 60′ (25 throws)	E. 60′ (20 throws)
F. Rest 10 min	F. Rest 10 min
G. Warm-up throwing	G. Warm-up throwing
H. 60′ (25 throws)	H. 45′ (20 throws)
	I. Rest 10 min
	J. Warm-up throwing
	K. 45′ (15 throws)

30 ft = 9.1 m
45 ft = 13.7 m
60 ft = 18.3 m
90 ft = 27.4 m

REFERENCES

1. Axe MJ, Snyder-Mackler L, Konin JG, et al. Development of a distance-based interval throwing program for Little League-aged athletes. *Am J Sports Med.* 1996;24(5):594–602.
2. Kolt GS, Snyder-Mackler L. Regional sport and exercise injury management. In: Kolt GS, Snyder-Mackler L, eds. *Physical Therapies in Sport and Exercise: Principles and Practice.* St Louis, MO: Churchill Livingstone Inc; 2003:306–308.
3. Axe MJ, Windley T, Snyder-Mackler L. Data-based interval throwing programs for collegiate softball players. *J Athl Train.* 2002;37(2): 194–203.
4. Axe MJ, Konin JG. Distance based criteria interval throwing program. *J Sport Rehab.* 1992;1: 4.

5. Wilk KE, Arrigo CA. Interval sports programs for the shoulder. In: Andrews JR, Wilk KE, eds. *The Athlete's Shoulder.* New York, NY: Churchill Livingstone; 1994:669–671.

6. Medich G. Interval throwing program for baseball players. *Sports Med Update.* 1987;2:1.

7. American Academy of Pediatrics Committee on Sports Medicine. Risk of injury from baseball and softball in children 5 to 14 years of age. *Pediatrics.* 1994;93:690–692.

8. Andrews JR. Interval throwing program: phase I. http://www.andrewsortho.com/education/IntervalThrowingProgramPhaseI.pdf

9. Reinold MM., Wilk K, Reed J, et al. Interval sport programs: guidelines for baseball, tennis and golf. *J Orthop Sports Phys Therap.* 2002;32(6): 293–298.

10. Andrews JR. Interval throwing program: phase II: throwing off the mound. http://www.andrewsortho.com/education/IntervalThrowingProgramPhase2.pdf

11. Gugenheim JJ Jr, Stanley RF, Woods GW, et al. Little league survey: the Houston study. *Am J Sports Med.* 1976;4:189–200.

12. Pappas AM. Elbow problems associated with baseball during childhood and adolescence. *Clin Orthop.* 1982;164:30–41.

13. Micheli LJ. Overuse injuries in children's sports: the growth factor. *Orthop Clin North Am.* 1983;14:337–360.

14. Andrews JR. Little League interval throwing program. http://www.andrewsortho.com/education/LittleLeagueIntervalThrowingProgram.pdf

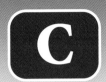

Interval Running Program

J. Herbert Stevenson, MD

he goal of the interval running program is to progress from each successive stage when activity is pain free. The athlete must be *pain free with activity, after activity, and the next day.* If pain recurs, then the athlete must rest for 1 to 2 days and drop to the exercise level at which there is *no pain with activity or the next day.* If athlete is pain free with activity as well as the next day for 3 consecutive days, then he or she may progress to next stage. One may use bike/pool running or elliptical to complete a cardio session after the interval session, depending upon stage of progression (i.e., if running 15 minutes, then can use bike/pool run or elliptical to complete a cardio session). This is a general example, and one may consider modification based on severity of injury and with consult of the supervising medical provider (Table C.1).

STAGES

1. Bicycle 30 to 45 minutes or pool running.
2. Elliptical trainer, start 15 minutes and work up to 30 to 45 minutes. May substitute walking if elliptical trainer not available, with time as mentioned earlier with starting at 5 to 10 minutes.
3. Speed walking. Start 10 to 15 minutes and work up to 30 to 45 minutes.
4. Start with light running (50% max, i.e., jogging). Begin with half mile and increase by half mile every other day. Once you are light running 2 miles, increase running intensity from 50% to 75%, then 100%, while maintaining pain-free status. Some will employ a walk–run on a track with running straight section and walking the corners.
5. Progress to sport-specific drills. If pain free after 3 days, then resume full activity.

TABLE C.1   **Interval Running Program Example**

Week	Monday	Tuesday	Wednesday	Thursday	Friday	Saturday	Sunday
1	Bike/pool running	Bike/pool running	Bike/pool running	Bike/pool running	Bike/pool running	Bike/pool running	Rest
2	Elliptical 10–15 min	Elliptical 15–20 min	Elliptical 20–25 min	Elliptical 25–30 min	Elliptical 30–35 min	Elliptical 30–45 min	Rest
3	Speed walk 10–15 min	Speed walk 15–20 min	Speed walk 20–25 min	Speed walk 25–30 min	Speed walk 30–35 min	Speed walk 30–45 min	Rest
4	Run $\frac{1}{2}$ mile	Cross-train	Run $\frac{1}{2}$ mile	Cross-train	Run 1 mile	Rest	Run 1 mile
5	Cross-train	Run 1$\frac{1}{2}$ miles	Cross-train	Run 1$\frac{1}{2}$ miles	Cross-train	Run 2 miles	Rest
6	Run 2 miles	Cross-train	Run 3 miles	Cross-train	Run 3 miles	Rest	Return to sport-specific drills